IMMUNOBIOLOGY OF CANCER AND AIDS
ETIOLOGY, DIAGNOSIS, AND MANAGEMENT

IMMUNOBIOLOGY OF CANCER AND AIDS
ETIOLOGY, DIAGNOSIS, AND MANAGEMENT

**Selected Papers Presented at the First International
Symposium on Immunobiology of Cancer and Allied Immune
Dysfunctions Held in Copenhagen, Denmark**

Editors

HERBERT E. NIEBURGS

Professor of Pathology
University of Massachusetts
Medical School
at Berkshire Medical Center
Pittsfield, Massachusetts

J. GEORGE BEKESI

Professor of Neoplastic Diseases
Department of Neoplastic Diseases
Mount Sinai School of Medicine and Hospital
New York, New York

These papers are also being published as the journal *Cancer
Detection and Prevention*, Supplement 1, 1987; Herbert E.
Nieburgs, Editor; J. George Bekesi, Guest Editor.

ALAN R. LISS, INC. • NEW YORK

Library of Congress Cataloging-in-Publication Data

International Symposium on Immunobiology of Cancer and
 Allied Immune Dysfunction (1st : 1985 : Copenhagen,
 Denmark)
 Immunobiology of cancer and AIDS.

 Has also been published as Cancer detection and
prevention, supplement 1, 1987.
 Includes bibliographies and index.
 1. Cancer—Immunological aspects—Congresses.
2. AIDS (Disease)—Congresses. I. Nieburgs, Herbert E.
II. Bekesi, J. George. III. Title. [DNLM: 1. Acquired
Immunodeficiency Syndrome—immunology—congresses.
2. Neoplasms—immunology—congresses. W3 IN918SD 1st
1985i / QZ 200 I61235 1985i]

RC268.3.I5 1985   616.99'4079   87-17060
ISBN 0-8451-4236-4

Contents

Contributors . . . . **xiii**

Introduction
H.E. Nieburgs and J.G. Bekesi . . . . **xxi**

BIOLOGY AND ETIOLOGY OF IMMUNE DYSFUNCTION

Nutrition and Immunological Responses
Adrianne E. Rogers and Paul M. Newberne **1**

Protein Deficiency Reduces Natural Antitumor Immunity
Ralf Ruffmann, Erich Schlick, Tamara Tartaris, Wladyslaw Budzynski,
and Michael A. Chirigos **15**

Immunotoxicology: Environmental Contamination by Polybrominated Biphenyls and Immune Dysfunction Among Residents of the State of Michigan
J. George Bekesi, Julia P. Roboz, Alf Fischbein, and Patricia Mason **29**

Immunocompetence in Pregnancy: Production of Interleukin-2 by Peripheral Blood Lymphocytes
G.J. Hauser, A. Lidor, V. Zakuth, H. Rosenberg, T. Bino, M.P. David, and Z. Spirer . **39**

Influence of Factor Substitution on the B-Cell Response in Hemophiliacs
J. Kekow, H. Plendl, and W.L. Gross **43**

Impaired Natural Killer Cytotoxicity During Recrudescence of Recurrent Herpes Simplex Virus Type 1 Infection
Yuh-Chi Kuo, Ching-Yuang Lin, Sai-Foo Cheng, Ching-Chi Lin, and Wu-Tse Liu . . . **51**

Stress-Related Modulation of Immunity: A Review of Human Studies
Jan E.W. Palmblad **57**

IMMUNOBIOLOGY OF CANCER

Antibody-Induced Modulation of H-2K^b Antigens on Mouse Tumor Cells In Vitro
Jan Stagsted and Lennart Olsson **65**

Cell Surface Glycoprotein Differences Between a Highly Malignant Murine Tumor Line and a Plastic-Adherent, Less Malignant Variant
Elke Lang, Peter Altevogt, and Volker Schirrmacher **73**

The Tumor Promoter 12-0-Tetradecanoylphorbol-13-Acetate (TPA) Accelerates Expression of Differentiation Markers in Cultures of Rat Palatal Epithelial Cells
Dorthe Arenholt and Erik Dabelsteen **81**

Escape of Hybridomas From Cellular Defense Mechanisms: An In Vitro Study Using Autologous and Allogeneic Lymphocytes
K.S. Zänker, G. Blümel, J. Lange, and J.R. Siewert **91**

Relevance of Aging Research for Cancer
P. Ebbesen   97

Phenotypic and Functional Analyses of Tumour-Infiltrating Leu 7 + Natural Killer-Like Cells in Non-Hodgkin Lymphomas
Diponkar Banerjee   103

Novel Tumor-Specific Antigen(s) Response Observed in a Syngeneic Lymphoma-Bearing Host
Lionel A. Manson   111

High Incidence of Stomach Cancer in Relatives of Patients With Malignant Lymphoproliferative Disorders
A. Genčík, M. Buser, B. Temminck, J.P. Obrecht, W. Weber, and Hj. Müller   121

Lectin Binding Pattern of Hodgkin Disease-Derived Cell Lines in Comparison to Other Human Cell Lines
Marin Schwonzen, Gerhard Uhlenbruck, Michael Schaadt, Detlev Funken,
Heinz Burrichter, and Volker Diehl   127

Production of Interleukin-2 and Expression of Tac Antigen in Hodgkin Disease
Narendra N. Joshi, Rabindranath Mukhopadhyay, Suresh H. Advani, and
Sudha G. Gangal   137

Correlative Studies on Antigenicity of Pancreatic Cancer and Blood Group Types
Eiji Uchida, Margaret A. Tempero, David A. Burnett, Zenon Steplewski, and
Parviz M. Pour   145

ORGAN TRANSPLANTATION

Neoplastic Consequences of Transplantation and Chemotherapy
Israel Penn   149

Malignant Lymphoproliferative Disorders of Viral Origin in Transplant Patients Undergoing Immunosuppressive Therapy
J.L. Touraine and J. Traeger   159

Difficulty in Establishing Diagnosis From Lung Biopsies and Bronchial Washing Analysis in Children With Leukemia Following Bone Marrow Transplantation
Thomas Miale, Nat Mody, Barrett Dick, Parashar Nanavati, Lilly Mathew,
R. Frederick Boedy, Michael Steinberg, Diane Davis, Subhash Chaudhary, and
L. Gilbert Thatcher   165

BIOMARKERS

Flow Cytofluorometric Analysis of Choriogonadotropin-Like Material on the Surface of Human and Mouse Malignant Cells
Radmila B. Raikow, Hernan F. Acevedo, Alexander Krichevsky, Mary Jo Buffo, and
Patricia Fogarty   173

A Subset of Normal Human B Lymphocytes Expresses an Antigen Cross-Reactive With gp52 of Murine Mammary Tumor Virus
Anne Tax and Lionel A. Manson   183

Monoclonal Antibody to HSV$_2$ Protein as an Immunodiagnostic Marker in Cervical Cancer
Silvano Costa, Antonia D'Errico, Walter F. Grigioni, Camillo Orlandi,
Cinthya C. Smith, Antonio M. Mancini, and Laure Aurelian   189

Human-Human Hybridomas Generated With Lymphocytes From Patients With Colorectal Cancer
Per Borup-Christensen, Karin Erb, Jens Christian Jensenius, Sven-Erik Svehag, and
Bjarne Nielsen **207**

Immunologic Markers for Epstein-Barr Virus in the Control of Nasopharyngeal Carcinoma and Burkitt Lymphoma
Paul H. Levine **217**

Common Acute Lymphoblastic Leukemia Antigen: Partial Characterization by In Vivo Labeling and Isolation of Its Messenger RNA
Susanne Heinsohn and Hartmut Kabisch **225**

Comparison of CEA Polyclonal Antibodies, CEA Monoclonal Antibodies, Tissue Polypeptide Antigen in the Sera of Supposedly Healthy Individuals
Eric P. Pluygers, Marc P. Beauduin, and Paul E. Baldewyns **231**

IMMUNODIAGNOSIS

Screening of Hybridoma Supernatants Raised Against Membrane Fractions From Breast Cancer Using an Immunodot Assay
Ralf Heinsohn, Christiane R. Seitz, Ariel C. Hollinshead, William Hyun, and
Alois Poschmann **235**

Strategies for the Development of Monoclonal Antibodies for In Vivo Imaging: Their Use in the Imaging of Ovarian Carcinoma
Joy Burchell, Joyce Taylor-Papadimitriou, and Andrew B. Griffiths **241**

Imaging of Primary and Metastatic Colorectal Carcinoma With Monoclonal Antibody 791T/36 and the Therapeutic Potential of Antibody-Drug Conjugates
M.V. Pimm, N.C. Armitage, K. Ballantyne, R.W. Baldwin, A.C. Perkins,
L.G. Durrant, M.C. Garnett, and J.D. Hardcastle **249**

Monoclonal Islet Antibody Hisl-19 as a Tool in the Diagnosis of Neuroendocrine Carcinomas of the Skin
Peter Buxbaum, Gabriele Horvat, Christian Gamper, and Klaus Krisch **263**

Monoclonal Antibodies Detecting Plasminogen Activators on the Membrane of Leukemic Lymphoid Cells of T-Cell Origin
Klaus G. Stünkel, Eckhard Thiel, Hans G. Opitz, H.D. Schlumberger, Uta Opitz,
Daniel Catovsky, and Volker Klimetzek **269**

IMMUNOTHERAPY

Passive, Adoptive, and Active Immunotherapy: A Review of Clinical Trials in Cancer
Georges Mathé **279**

Metastasis Models for Human Tumors in Athymic Mice: Useful Models for Drug Development
Donald L. Fine, Robert Shoemaker, Adi Gazdar, Joseph G. Mayo, Oystein Fodstad,
Michael R. Boyd, Betty J. Abbott, and Patricia A. Donovan **291**

Effect of Red Ginseng on Natural Killer Cell Activity in Mice With Lung Adenoma Induced by Urethan and Benzo(a)pyrene
Yeon S. Yun, Hae S. Moon, Yeong R. Oh, Sung K. Jo, Young J. Kim, and
Taik K. Yun **301**

DNA Methylating Activity in Murine Lymphoma Cells Treated With Xenogenizing Chemicals
P. Puccetti, M. Allegrucci, C. Borri Voltattorni, L. Romani, P. Dominici, and M.C. Fioretti 311

Cell Regulatory and Immunorestorative Activity of Picibanil (OK432)
Michael A. Chirigos, Tohru Saito, James E. Talmadge, Wladyslaw Budzynski, and Eilene Gruys 317

Imunovir in the Treatment of Immunodepression of Diverse Etiology
B.B. O'Neill and A.J. Glasky 329

Clinical Efficacy of Lentinan on Patients With Stomach Cancer: End Point Results of a Four-Year Follow-Up Survey
T. Taguchi 333

Serological Evaluation of Melanoma Patients in a Phase I/II Trial of Vaccinia Melanoma Oncolysate (VMO) Immunotherapy
Marc K. Wallack, Jerry A. Bash, Katherine R. McNally, and Eleuthere Leftheriotis . . 351

BM 41.440: A New Antineoplastic, Antimetastatic, and Immune-Stimulating Drug
Dieter B.J. Herrmann, Uwe Bicker, and Wulf Pahlke 361

Transfer Factor For Adjuvant Immunotherapy in Cervical Cancer
G. Wagner, W. Knapp, E. Gitsch, and S. Selander 373

Immunosuppressive Effects of Isoprinosine in Man: A Comparison to Chlorambucil Effects in Multiple Sclerosis
Alain Pompidou, Gérald Rancurel, Marie-C. Delsaux, Claude Meunier, Louise Telvi, Véronique Cour, and André Buge 377

BIOLOGICAL RESPONSE MODIFIERS

Immune Response by Biological Response Modifiers
Michael A. Chirigos, Erich Schlick, and Wladyslaw Budzynski 385

Modulation of Antitumor Immune Responses
E. Mihich 399

Correction of Secondary T-Cell Immunodeficiencies With Biological Substances and Drugs
John W. Hadden 409

Antitumor and Metastasis-Inhibitory Activities of Lentinan as an Immunomodulator: An Overview
Goro Chihara, Junji Hamuro, Yukiko Y. Maeda, Tsuyoshi Shiio, Tetsuya Suga, Nobuo Takasuka, and Takuma Sasaki 423

Do Tuftsin and Bestatin Constitute a Biopharmacological Immunoregulatory System?
G. Mathé 445

Immunological Effects of Isoprinosine as a Pulse Immunotherapy in Melanoma and ARC Patients
Alain Pompidou, Claude Soubrane, Véronique Cour, Louise Telvi, Claude Meunier, and Claude Jacquillat 457

Modulation of NK Activity in Regional Lymph Nodes by Preoperative Immunotherapy With OK-432 in Patients With Cancer of the Oral Cavity
K. Vinzenz, M. Matejka, G. Watzek, H. Porteder, N. Neuhold, and M. Micksche . . 463

Effects of Immunization Against Human Choriogonadotropin on the Growth of
Transplanted Lewis Lung Carcinoma and Spontaneous Mammary Adenocarcinoma
in Mice
Hernan F. Acevedo, Radmila B. Raikow, John E. Powell, and Vernon C. Stevens . . .   477

LAS (LYMPHADENOPATHY SYNDROME), ARC (AIDS RELATED COMPLEX), AND AIDS

A. BIOLOGY, ETIOLOGY, AND RISK FACTORS

AIDS in Subsaharan Africa
R.J. Biggar   487

Genetic Comparison of LAV-Related Isolates
Samuel Magasiny, Bruno Spire, Francoise Rey, Francoise Barre-Sinoussi, and
Jean-Claude Chermann   493

Simian Models for AIDS
M.D. Daniel, R.C. Desrosiers, N.L. Letvin, N.W. King, D.K. Schmidt, P. Sehgal, and
R.D. Hunt   501

Extrathecal and Intrathecal IgG Response to the AIDS Virus LAV/HTLV-III in
Experimental Infection of Chimpanzees
Jaap Goudsmit, Clarence J. Gibbs Jr., David M.A. Asher, and D. Carleton Gajdusek   509

Human Lymphocyte Subpopulations: Analysis by Multiparameter Flow Cytometry and
Monoclonal Antibodies
Noel L. Warner   515

AIDS and Lymphadenopathy Syndrome (LAS) Patients Display Similar Abnormal In
Vitro Proliferation and Differentiation of T-Colony Forming Cells (T-CFC)
Yanto Lunardi Iskandar, Vassilis Georgoulias, Willy Rozenbaum, Daniel Vittecoq,
Patrice Meyer, Marc Gentilini, and Claude Jasmin   525

Immune Status of Drug Abusers
D. Fuchs, A. Hausen, G. Reibnegger, D. Schönitzer, B. Unterweger, H.G. Blecha,
P. Hengster, H. Rössler, T. Schulz, E.R. Werner, M.P. Dierich, H. Hinterhuber,
K. Schauenstein, K. Traill, and H. Wachter   535

B-Cell Reactivity in Homosexuals With Persistent Generalized Lymphadenopathy (PGL)
J. Kekow, P. Kern, H. Schmitz, and W.L. Gross   543

Imbalance of the Epstein-Barr Virus-Host Relationship in AIDS-Related Complex
Patients
Giuseppe Ragona and Maria Caterina Sirianni   549

Distribution of P24 HTLV3 Major Core Protein in Lymph Nodes of LAS Patients
Carlo D. Baroni and Francesco Pezzella   553

B. NEOPLASTIC RELEVANCE

Lymphomas Associated With the Acquired Immune Deficiency Syndrome (AIDS): A
Study of 35 Cases
Harry L. Ioachim, Marvin C. Cooper, and Gerard C. Hellman   557

Exposure to Hair Dyes and Polychlorinated Dibenzo-p-Dioxins in AIDS Patients With
Kaposi Sarcoma: An Epidemiological Investigation
Lennart Hardell, Andrew Moss, Dennis Osmond, and Paul Volberding   567

Lymphocyte Subsets, Natural Killer Cytotoxicity, and Perioperative Blood Transfusion for Elective Colorectal Cancer Surgery
Paul Ian Tartter and Giorgio Martinelli 571

C. DIAGNOSIS AND MANAGEMENT

Immunohistochemical Studies of Lymph Nodes From LAS and AIDS Patients
H. Müller, S. Falk, and H.J. Stutte 577

Activated T Cells in Addition to LAV/HTLV-III Infection: A Necessary Precondition for Development of AIDS
D. Fuchs, A. Hausen, E. Hoefler, D. Schönitzer, E.R. Werner, M.P. Dierich,
P. Hengster, G. Reibnegger, T. Schulz, and H. Wachter 583

Modified Nucleosides in Patients With Acquired Immune Deficiency Syndrome (AIDS) and Individuals at High Risk of AIDS: Correlations With Lymphadenomegaly and Immunological Parameters
Alf Fischbein, J. George Bekesi, Stephen Solomon, Ernest Borek, and
Opendra K. Sharma 589

Isoprinosine (Inosine Pranobex BAN, INPX) in the Treatment of AIDS and Other Acquired Immunodeficiencies of Clinical Importance
Alvin J. Glasky and Judy F. Gordon 597

Normalization of Immunoregulatory T-Helper T-Suppressor Sublineages and Cell-Mediated Immunity by Isoprinosine In Vitro in the Early Stages of AIDS
Peter Tsang and J. George Bekesi 611

Immunological Studies in Acquired Immunodeficiency Syndrome: Effect of TCGF and Indomethacine on the In Vitro Lymphocyte Response
Bo Hofmann, Lars Fugger, Lars P. Ryder, Johannes Gaub, Niels Ødum, Per Platz,
Jan Gerstoft, and Arne Svejgaard 619

Subject Index and List of References Cited 627

IN APPRECIATION

Special contributions in support of the Immunobiology of Cancer and Allied Immune Dysfunctions have been made by the following:

Ajimomoto Company, Inc.

Becton Dickinson Inc.

Cetus Inc.

Coulter Immunology Inc.

Cyanamid

Danish Cancer Society

F. Hoffman La Roche, Inc.

Institut Merieux

Newport Pharmaceuticals International

Scandinavian Airlines

Contributors

Betty J. Abbott [291] Developmental Therapeutics Program, National Cancer Institute/Frederick Cancer Research Facility, Frederick, Maryland

Hernan F. Acevedo [173,477] Department of Laboratory Medicine, Allegheny-Singer Research Institute, Allegheny General Hospital, Pittsburgh, Pennsylvania

Suresh H. Advani [137] Department of Medicine Hospital, Parel, Bombay, India

M. Allegrucci [311] Institute of Pharmacology, University of Perugia, Perugia, Italy

Peter Altevogt [73] Institut für Immunologie und Genetik, Deutsches Krebsforschungszentrum, Heidelberg, Federal Republic of Germany

Dorthe Arenholt [81] Department of Oral Pathology, Royal Dental College, Aarhus, Copenhagen, Denmark

N.C. Armitage [249] Department of Surgery, Queen's Medical Centre, Nottingham, England

David M.A. Asher [509] Laboratory of Central Nervous System Studies, NINCDS, National Institutes of Health, Bethesda, Maryland

Laure Aurelian [189] Division of Biophysics, The Johns Hopkins Medical Institutions, Baltimore, Maryland

Paul E. Baldewyns [231] Cancer Detection Unit and Radioimmunology Laboratory, Oncology and Nuclear Medicine Department, Jolimont Hospital, La Louvière, Belgium

R.W. Baldwin [249] Cancer Research Campaign Laboratories, University of Nottingham, England

K. Ballantyne [249] Department of Surgery, Queen's Medical Centre, Nottingham, England

Diponkar Banerjee [103] Department of Pathology, St. Joseph's Health Centre and the University of Westen Ontario, London, Canada

Carlo D. Baroni [553] Section of Immunopathology, Department of Biopathology, University of Rome "La Sapienza," Rome, Italy

Francoise Barre-Sinoussi [493] Viral Oncology Unit, Institut Pasteur, Paris, France

Jerry A. Bash [351] Department of Surgery, Mount Sinai Medical Center, Miami Beach, Florida

Marc P. Beauduin [231] Cancer Detection Unit and Radioimmunology Laboratory, Oncology and Nuclear Medicine Department, Jolimont Hospital, La Louvière, Belgium

J. George Bekesi [29,589, 611] Department of Neoplastic Diseases, The Mount Sinai School of Medicine of the City University of New York, New York, New York

Uwe Bicker [361] Doehringer Mannheim GmbH, Department of Immunopharmacology and Cancer Research, Mannheim, Federal Republic of Germany

R.J. Biggar [487] Environmental Epidemiology Branch, National Cancer Institute, Bethesda, Maryland

T. Bino [39] The Israel Institute for Biological Research, Ness-Ziona, Israel

H.G. Blecha [535] Clinic of Psychiatry, Institute for AIDS Research, University of Innsbruck, Innsbruck, Austria

G. Blümel [91] Institute for Experimental Surgery, Technical University Munich, Munich, Federal Republic of Germany

R. Frederick Boedy [165] Department of Pediatrics, Southern Illinois University School of Medicine, Springfield, Illinois

Ernest Borek [589] Department of Molecular Biology, AMC Cancer Research Center, Denver, Colorado

Per Borup-Christensen [207] Biomedical Laboratory, Institute of Surgery, University of Odense, Odense, Denmark

Michael R. Boyd [291] Developmental Therapeutics Program, Bethesda, Maryland

Wladyslaw Budzynski [15,317,385] Biological Therapeutics Branch, Division of Cancer Treatment, National Cancer Institute, NIH, Frederick Cancer Research Facility, Frederick, Maryland

The number in brackets is the opening page number of the contributor's article.

Mary Jo Buffo [173] Department of Laboratory Medicine, Allegheny-Singer Research Institute, Allegheny General Hospital, Pittsburgh, Pennsylvania

André Buge [377] Service de Neurologie, Hôpital Pitié-Salpêtrière, Paris, France

M. Buser [121] University Computer Center and Institute for Informatics, Basel, Switzerland

Joy Burchell [241] Imperial Cancer Research Fund, London, England

David A. Burnett [145] Department of Internal Medicine, University of Nebraska Medical Center, Omaha, Nebraska

Heinz Burrichter [127] Medizinische Klinik 1 der Universität zu Köln, Köln, Federal Republic of Germany

Peter Buxbaum [263] Department of Pathology, University of Vienna, Medical School, Vienna, Austria

Daniel Catovsky [269] Royal Postgraduate Medical School, Hammersmith Hospital, London, England

Subhash Chaudhary [165] Department of Pediatrics, Southern Illinois University School of Medicine, Springfield, Illinois

Sai-Foo Cheng [51] Department of Dermatology, Veterans General Hospital, Taipei, Taiwan, Republic of China

Jean-Claude Chermann [493] Viral Oncology Unit, Institut Pasteur, Paris, France

Goro Chihara [423] National Cancer Center Research Institute, Tokyo, Japan

Michael A. Chirigos [15,317,385] Biological Therapeutics Branch, Division of Cancer Treatment, National Cancer Institute, NIH, Frederick Cancer Research Facility, Frederick, Maryland

Marvin C. Cooper [557] Department of Medicine, Lenox Hill Hospital, New York, New York

Silvano Costa [189] Department of Obstetrics and Gynecology, University of Bologna Medical School, Bologna, Italy

Véronique Cour [377,457] Laboratoire d'Anatomie-Pathologique, Hôpital Saint-Vincent de Paul, Paris, France

Erik Dabelsteen [81] Department of Oral Diagnosis, Royal Dental College, Copenhagen, Denmark

M.D. Daniel [501] New England Regional Primate Research Center, Harvard Medical School, Southborough, Massachusetts

M.P. David [39] Department of Obstetrics and Gynecology "B", Tel-Aviv Medical Center and The Leon Alcalay Chair in Pediatric Immunology, Tel-Aviv University, Tel-Aviv, Israel

Diane Davis [165] Department of Pediatrics, Southern Illinois University School of Medicine, Springfield, Illinois

Marie-C. Delsaux [377] Laboratoire d'Anatomie-Pathologique, Hôpital Saint-Vincent de Paul, Paris, France

Antonia D'Errico [189] Department of Pathology, University of Bologna Medical School, Bologna, Italy

R.C. Desrosiers [501] New England Regional Primate Research Center, Harvard Medical School, Southborough, Massachusetts

Barrett Dick [165] Department of Pathology, Southern Illinois University School of Medicine, Springfield, Illinois

Volker Diehl [127] Medizinische Klinik 1 der Universität zu Köln, Köln, Federal Republic of Germany

M.P. Dierich [535,583] Institute of Hygiene, Ludwig Boltzmann Institute for AIDS Research, University of Innsbruck, Innsbruck, Austria

P. Dominici [311] Institute of Biochemistry, University of Perugia, Perugia, Italy

Patricia A. Donovan [291] Program Resources, Inc., National Cancer Institute/Frederick Cancer Research Facility (NCI-FCRF), Frederick, Maryland

L.G. Durrant [249] Cancer Research Campaign Laboratories, University of Nottingham, Queen's Medical Centre, Nottingham, England

P. Ebbesen [97] The Institute of Cancer Research, The Danish Cancer Society, Radiumstationen, Aarhus, Denmark

Karin Erb [207] Institute of Pathology, University of Odense, Odense, Denmark

S. Falk [577] Zentrum der Pathologie, J.W. Goethe Universität, Frankfurt, Federal Republic of Germany

Donald L. Fine [291] Program Resources, Inc., National Cancer Institute/Frederick Cancer Research Facility (NCI-FCRF), Frederick, Maryland

M.C. Fioretti [311] Institute of Pharmacology, University of Perugia, Perugia, Italy

Alf Fischbein [29,589] Environmental Sciences Laboratory, The Mount Sinai School of Medicine of the City University of New York, New York, New York

Oystein Fodstad [291] Norsk Hydros Institute for Cancer Research, Oslo, Norway

Patricia Fogarty [173] Department of Laboratory Medicine, Allegheny-Singer Research Institute, Allegheny General Hospital, Pittsburgh, Pennsylvania

D. Fuchs [535,583] Institute of Medical Chemistry and Biochemistry, Ludwig Boltzmann Institute for AIDS Research, University of Innsbruck, Innsbruck, Austria

Lars Fugger [619] Tissue Typing Laboratory of the Department of Clinical Immunology, University Hospital (Rigohospitalet), Copenhagen, Denmark

Detlev Funken [127] Medizinische Klinik 1 der Universität zu Köln, Köln, Federal Republic of Germany

D. Carleton Gajdusek [509] Laboratory of Central Nervous System Studies, NINCDS, National Institutes of Health, Bethesda, Maryland

Christian Gamper [263] Department of Pathology, University of Vienna, Medical School, Vienna, Austria

Sudha G. Gangal [137] Immunology Division, Cancer Research Institute, Parel, Bombay, India

M.C. Garnett [249] Cancer Research Campaign Laboratories, University of Nottingham, Queen's Medical Centre, Nottingham, England

Johannes Gaub [619] University Clinic for Infectious Diseases, University Hospital (Rigohospitalet), Copenhagen, Denmark

Adi Gazdar [291] NCI-Naval Medical Oncology Branch, Bethesda, Maryland

A. Genčík [121] Laboratory of Human Genetics, Department of Medicine, Cantonal Hospital, Basel, Switzerland

Marc Gentilini [525] Département de Santé Publique et de Médecine Tropicale, Hôpital Pitié Salpêtrière, Paris, France

Vassilis Georgoulias [525] Unité d'Oncogénèse Appliquée, Hôpital Paul Brousse, Villejuif, France

Jan Gerstoft [619] State Serum Institute, Department of Rubella, Copenhagen, Denmark

Clarence J. Gibbs, Jr. [509] Laboratory of Central Nervous System Studies, NINCDS, National Institutes of Health, Bethesda, Maryland

E. Gitsch [373] 1st Department of Obstetrics and Gynecology, University of Vienna, Vienna, Austria

A.J. Glasky [329,597] Newport Pharmaceuticals Int. Inc., Newport Beach, California

Judy F. Gordon [597] Newport Institute for Medical Research, Newport Beach, California

Jaap Goudsmit [509] Virology Department, Academic Medical Center of the University of Amsterdam, Amsterdam, The Netherlands

Andrew B. Griffiths [241] Imperial Cancer Research Fund, London, England

Walter F. Grigioni [189] Department of Pathology, University of Bologna Medical School, Bologna, Italy

W.L. Gross [43,543] Department of Internal Medicine, Christian Albrecht University, Kiel, Federal Republic of Germany

Eilene Gruys [317] Immunopharmacology Section, Division of Cancer Treatment, National Cancer Institute, NIH, Frederick Cancer Research Facility, Frederick, Maryland

John W. Hadden [409] Program of Immunopharmacology, University of South Florida Medical College, Tampa, Florida

Junji Hamuro [423] Ajinomoto Central Laboratory, Yokohama, Japan

J.D. Hardcastle [249] Department of Surgery, Queen's Medical Center, Nottingham, England

Lennart Hardell [567] School of Public Health, University of California, Berkeley, California

A. Hausen [535,583] Institute of Medical Chemistry and Biochemistry, Ludwig Boltzmann Institute for AIDS Research, University of Innsbruck, Innsbruck, Austria

G.J. Hauser [39] Pediatric Immunology Unit, Tel-Aviv Medical Center and The Leon Alcalay Chair in Pediatric Immunology, Tel-Aviv University, Tel-Aviv, Israel

Ralf Heinsohn [235] Universitätskrankenhaus Eppendorf Kinderklinik, Abteilung für Klinische Immunopathologie, Hamburg, Federal Republic of Germany

Susanne Heinsohn [225] Kinderklinik, Abteilung für Hämatologie und Onkologie, Universitätskrankenhaus Eppendorf, Hamburg, Federal Republic of Germany

Gerard C. Hellman [557] Department of Medicine, Lenox Hill Hospital, New York, New York

P. Hengster [535,583] Institute of Hygiene, Ludwig Boltzmann Institute for AIDS Research, University of Innsbruck, Innsbruck, Austria

Dieter B.J. Herrmann [361] Boehringer Mannheim GmbH, Department of Immunopharmacology and Cancer Research, Mannheim, Federal Republic of Germany

H. Hinterhuber [535] Clinic of Psychiatry, Ludwig Boltzmann Institute for AIDS Research, University of Innsbruck, Innsbruck, Austria

E. Hoefler [583] Institute for Blood Transfusion and for Immunology, and Ludwig Institute for AIDS Research, University of Innsbruck, Innsbruck, Austria

Bo Hofmann [619] Tissue Typing Laboratory of the Department of Clinical Immunology, University Hospital (Righospitalet), Copenhagen, Denmark

Ariel C. Hollinshead [235] Department of Medicine, The George Washington University Medical Center, Washington, DC

Gabriele Horvat [263] Department of Pathology, University of Vienna, Medical School, Vienna, Austria

R.D. Hunt [501] New England Regional Primate Research Center, Harvard Medical School, Southborough, Massachusetts

William Hyun [235] Department of Medicine, The George Washington University Medical Center, Washington, DC

Harry L. Ioachim [557] Department of Pathology, Lenox Hill Hospital, New York, New York

Yanto Lunardi Iskandar [525] Unité d'Oncogénèse Appliquée, Hôpital Paul Brousse, Villejuif, France

Claude Jacquillat [457] Hôpital Pitié-Salpêtrière, Paris, France

Claude Jasmin [525] Unité d'Oncogénèse Appliquée, Hôpital Paul Brousse, Villejuif, France

Jens Christian Jensenius [207] Institute of Medical Microbiology, University of Odense, Odense, Denmark

Sung K. Jo [301] Laboratory of Immunology, Korea Cancer Center Hospital, Korea Advanced Energy Research Institute, Seoul, Korea

Narendra N. Joshi [137] Immunology Division, Cancer Research Institute, Parel, Bombay, India

Hartmut Kabisch [225] Kinderklinik, Abteilung für Hämatologie und Onkologie, Universitätskrankenhaus Eppendorf, Hamburg, Federal Republic of Germany

J. Kekow [43,543] Department of Internal Medicine, Christian Albrecht University, Kiel, Federal Republic of Germany

P. Kern [543] Clinical Department, Bernhard-Nocht-Institut, Hamburg, Federal Republic of Germany

Young J. Kim [301] Laboratory of Cancer Pathology, Korea Cancer Center Hospital, Korea Advanced Energy Research Institute, Seoul, Korea

N.W. King [501] New England Regional Primate Research Center, Harvard Medical School, Southborough, Massachusetts

Volker Klimetzek [269] Bayer AG, Wuppertal, Federal Republic of Germany

W. Knapp [373] Institute of Immunology, University of Vienna, Vienna, Austria

Alexander Krichevsky [173] Department of Medicine, College of Physicians and Surgeons, Columbia University, New York, New York

Klaus Krisch [263] Department of Pathology, University of Vienna, Medical School, Vienna, Austria

Yuh-Chi Kuo [51] Graduate Institute of Microbiology and Immunology, National Yang-Ming Medical College, Veterans General Hospital, Taipei, Taiwan, Republic of China

Elke Lang [73] Institut für Immunologie und Genetik, Deutsches Krebsforschungszentrum, Heidelberg, Federal Republic of Germany

J. Lange [91] Surgical Clinic, Technical University Munich, Munich, Federal Republic of Germany

Eleuthere Leftheriotis [351] Institut Merieux, Lyon, France

N.L. Letvin [501] New England Regional Primate Research Center, Harvard Medical School, Southborough, Massachusetts

Paul H. Levine [217] Environmental Epidemiology Branch, National Cancer Institute, National Institutes of Health, Bethesda, Maryland

A. Lidor [39] Department of Obstetrics and Gynecology "B", Tel-Aviv Medical Center and the Leon Alcalay Chair in Pediatric Immunology, Tel-Aviv University, Tel-Aviv, Israel

Ching-Chi Lin [51] Department of Internal Medicine, Mackay Memorial Hospital, Taipei, Taiwan, Republic of China

Ching-Yuang Lin [51] Department of Medical Research, Veterans General Hospital, Taipei, Taiwan, Republic of China

Wu-Tse Liu [51] Graduate Institute of Microbiology and Immunology, National Yang-Ming Medical College, Veterans General Hospital, Taipei, Taiwan, Republic of China

Yukiko Y. Maeda [423] The Tokyo Metropolitan Institute of Medical Sciences, Tokyo, Japan

Samuel Magasiny [493] Viral Oncology Unit, Institut Pasteur, Paris, France

Antonio M. Mancini [189] Department of Pathology, University of Bologna Medical School, Bologna, Italy

Lionel A. Manson [111,183] The Wistar Institute of Anatomy and Biology, Philadelphia, Pennsylvania

Giorgio Martinelli [571] Department of Surgery, The Mount Sinai Medical Center, New York, New York

Patricia Mason [29] Department of Neoplastic Diseases, The Mount Sinai School of Medicine of the City University of New York, New York, New York

M. Matejka [463] Division of Oral Surgery, Dental School, Vienna University, Vienna, Austria

Georges Mathé [279,445] Service des Maladies Sanguines et Tumorales and ICIG, Hôpital Paul-Brousse, Villejuif, France

Lilly Mathew [165] Department of Pediatrics, Southern Illinois University School of Medicine, Springfield, Illinois

Joseph G. Mayo [291] Developmental Therapeutics Program, National Cancer Institute/Frederick Cancer Research Facility (NCI-FCRF), Frederick, Maryland

Katherine R. McNally [351] Department of Surgery, Mount Sinai Medical Center, Miami Beach, Florida

Claude Meunier [377,457] Laboratoire d'Anatomie-Pathologique, Hôpital Saint-Vincent de Paul, Paris, France

Patrice Meyer [525] Institut de Cancérologie et d'Immunogénétique, Hôpital Paul Brosse, Villejuif, France

Thomas Miale [165] Department of Pediatrics, Southern Illinois University School of Medicine, Springfield, Illinois

M. Micksche [463] Institute of Applied and Experimental Oncology, Vienna University, Vienna, Austria

E. Mihich [399] Grace Cancer Drug Center, Roswell Park Memorial Institute, New York State Department of Health, Buffalo, New York

Nat Mody [165] Department of Pathology, Southern Illinois University School of Medicine, Springfield, Illinois

Hae S. Moon [301] Laboratory of Immunology, Korea Cancer Center Hospital, Korea Advanced Energy Research Institute, Seoul, Korea

Andrew Moss [567] Department of Epidemiology and International Health, University of California, San Francisco General Hospital, San Francisco, California

Rabindranath Mukhopadhyay [137] Immunolog Division, Cancer Research Institute, Parel, Bombay, India

H. Müller [577] Zentrum der Pathologie, J.W. Goethe Universität, Frankfurt, Federal Republic of Germany

Hj. Müller [121] Laboratory of Human Genetics, Department of Medicine, Cantonal Hospital, Basel, Switzerland

Parashar Nanavati [165] Department of Radiation Therapy, Southern Illinois University School of Medicine, Springfield, Illinois

N. Neuhold [463] Department of Pathology, Medical School, Vienna University, Vienna, Austria

Paul M. Newberne [1] Department of Pathology, Boston University School of Medicine, and Mallory Institute of Pathology, Boston City Hospital, Boston, Massachusetts

Bjarne Nielsen [207] Institute of Pathology, University of Odense, Odense, Denmark

J.P. Obrecht [121] Department of Research of the University Clinics and Division of Oncology, Department of Medicine, Cantonal Hospital, Basel, Switzerland

Niels Ødum [619] Tissue Typing Laboratory of the Department of Clinical Immunology, University Hospital, (Rigohospitalet), Copenhagen, Denmark

Yeong R. Oh [301] Laboratory of Cancer Pathology, Korea Cancer Center Hospital, Korea Advanced Research Institute, Seoul, Korea

Lennart Olsson [65] Cancer Biology Laboratory, State University Hospital (Righospitalet), Copenhagen, Denmark

B.B. O'Neill [329] Newport Pharmaceuticals Int. Inc., Newport Beach, California

Hans G. Opitz [269] Bayer AG, Wuppertal, Federal Republic of Germany

Uta Opitz [269] Bayer AG, Wuppertal, Federal Republic of Germany

Camillo Orlandi [189] Department of Obstetrics and Gynecology, University of Bologna Medical Center, Bologna, Italy

Dennis Osmond [567] Department of Epidemiology and International Health, University of California, San Francisco General Hospital, San Francisco, California

Wulf Pahlke [361] Boehringer Mannheim GmbH, Department of Immuno-pharmacology and Cancer Research, Mannheim, Federal Republic of Germany

Jan E.W. Palmblad [57] Department of Medicine III, The Karolinska Institute, Stockholm, Sweden

Israel Penn [149] Department of Surgery, University of Cincinnati Medical Center, Cincinnati Veterans Administration Medical Center, Cincinnati, Ohio

A.C. Perkins [249] Department of Medical Physics, Queen's Medical Centre, Nottingham, England

Francesco Pezzella [553] Section of Immunopathology, Department of Biopathology, University of Rome "La Sapienza," Rome, Italy

M.V. Pimm [249] Cancer Research Campaign Laboratories, University of Nottingham, Queen's Medical Centre, Nottingham, England

Per Platz [619] Tissue Typing Laboratory of the Department of Clinical Immunology, University Hospital (Rigohospitalet), Copenhagen, Denmark

H. Plendl [43] Department of Human Genetics, Christian Albrecht University, Kiel, Federal Republic of Germany

Eric P. Pluygers [231] Cancer Detection Unit and Radioimmunology Laboratory, Oncology and Nuclear Medicine Department, Jolimont Hospital, La Louvière, Belgium

Alain Pompidou [377,457] Laboratoire d'Anatomie-Pathologique, Hôpital Saint-Vincent de Paul, Paris, France

H. Porteder [463] Clinic for Maxillo-Facial Surgery, Vienna University, Vienna, Austria

Alois Poschmann [235] Universitätskrankenhaus Eppendorf Kinderklinik, Abteilung für Klinische Immunopathologie, Hamburg, Federal Republic of Germany

Parviz M. Pour [145] The Eppley Institute for Research in Cancer and Allied Diseases, University of Nebraska Medical Center, Omaha, Nebraska

John E. Powell [477] Department of Obstetrics and Gynecology, The Ohio State University, Columbus, Ohio

P. Puccetti [311] Institute of Pharmacology, University of Perugia, Perugia, Italy

Giuseppe Ragona [549] Department of Experimental Medicine, University of Rome, "La Sapienza," Rome, Italy

Radmila B. Raikow [173,447] Department of Laboratory Medicine, Allegheny-Singer Research Institute, Allegheny General Hospital, Pittsburgh, Pennsylvania

Gérald Rancurel [377] Service de Neurologie, Hôpital Pitié-Salpêtrière, Paris, France

G. Reibnegger [535,583] Institute of Medical Chemistry and Biochemistry, Ludwig Boltzmann Institute for AIDS Research, University of Innsbruck, Innsbruck, Austria

Francoise Rey [493] Viral Oncology Unit, Institut Pasteur, Paris, France

Julia R. Roboz [29] Department of Neoplastic Diseases, The Mount Sinai School of Medicine of the City University of New York, New York, New York

Adrianne E. Rogers [1] Department of Pathology, Boston University School of Medicine, and Mallory Institute of Pathology, Boston City Hospital, Boston, Massachusetts

L. Romani [311] Institute of Pharmacology, University of Perugia, Perugia, Italy

H. Rosenberg [39] The Israel Institute for Biological Research, Ness-Ziona, Israel

H. Rössler [535] Clinic of Psychiatry, Ludwig Boltzmann Institute for AIDS Research, University of Innsbruck, Innsbruck, Austria

Willy Rozenbaum [525] Département de Santé Publique et de Médecine Tropicale, Hôpital Pitié-Salpêtrière, Paris, France

Ralf Ruffmann [15] Division of Cancer Treatment, National Cancer Institute, NIH, Frederick Cancer Research Facility, Frederick, MD; presently at: Recordati Chemical and Pharmaceutical Industries, Milano, Italy

Lars P. Ryder [619] Tissue Typing Laboratory of the Department of Clinical Immunology, University Hospital (Rigohospitalet), Copenhagen, Denmark

Tohru Saito [317] Immunopharmacology Section, Division of Cancer Treatment, National Cancer Institute, NIH, Frederick Cancer Research Facility, Frederick, Maryland

Takuma Sasaki [423] National Cancer Center Research Institute, Tokyo, Japan

Michael Schaadt [127] Medizinische Klinik 1 der Universität zu Köln, Köln, Federal Republic of Germany

K. Schauenstein [535] Institute of Experimental Pathology, Ludwig Boltzmann Institute for AIDS Research, University of Innsbruck, Innsbruck, Austria

Volker Schirrmacher [73] Institut für Immunologie und Genetik, Deutsches Krebsforschungszentrum, Heidelberg, Federal Republic of Germany

Erich Schlick [15,385] Division of Cancer Treatment, National Cancer Institute, NIH, Frederick Cancer Research Facility, Frederick, Maryland

H.D. Schlumberger [269] Bayer AG, Wuppertal, Federal Republic of Germany

D.K. Schmidt [501] New England Regional Primate Research Center, Harvard Medical School, Southborough, Massachusetts

H. Schmitz [543] Department of Virology, Bernhard-Nocht-Institut, Hamburg, Federal Republic of Germany

D. Schönitzer [535,583] Institute for Blood Transfusion and Immunology, Ludwig Boltzmann Institute for AIDS Research, University of Innsbruck, Innsbruck, Austria

T. Schulz [535,583] Institute of Hygiene, Ludwig Boltzmann Institute for AIDS Research, University of Innsbruck, Innsbruck, Austria

Marin Schwonzen [127] Medizinische Klinik 1 der Universität zu Köln, Köln, Federal Republic of Germany

P. Sehgal [501] New England Regional Primate Research Center, Harvard Medical School, Southborough, Massachusetts

Christiane R. Seitz [235] Universitätskrankenhaus Eppendorf Kinderklinik, Abteilung für Klinische Immunopathologie, Hamburg, Federal Republic of Germany

S. Selander [373] 2nd Department of Obstetrics and Gynecology, University of Vienna, Vienna, Austria

Opendra K. Sharma [589] Department of Molecular Biology, AMC Cancer Research Center, Denver, Colorado

Tsuyoshi Shiio [423] Ajinomoto Central Laboratory, Yokohama, Japan

Robert Shoemaker [291] Developmental Therapeutics Program, National Cancer Institute/Frederick Cancer Research Facility (NCI-FCRF), Frederick, Maryland

J.R. Siewert [91] Surgical Clinic, Technical University Munich, Munich, Federal Republic of Germany

Maria Caterina Sirianni [549] Department of Allergology and Clinical Immunology, University of Rome, "La Sapienza," Rome, Italy

Cinthya C. Smith [189] Divisions of Biophysics and Comparative Medicine, The Johns Hopkins Medical Institutions, Baltimore, Maryland

Stephen Solomon [589] Department of Neoplastic Diseases, Mount Sinai School of Medicine, The City University of New York, New York, New York

Claude Soubrane [457] Hôpital Pitié-Salpêtrière, Paris, France

Bruno Spire [493] Division de Radiobiologie et de Radioprotection, Centre de Recherches du Service de Santé des Armées, Clamart, France

Z. Spirer [39] Pediatric Immunology Unit, Tel-Aviv Medical Center and The Leon Alcalay Chair in Pediatric Immunology, Tel-Aviv University, Tel-Aviv, Israel

Jan Stagsted [65] Cancer Biology Laboratory, State University Hospital (Righospitalet), Copenhagen, Denmark

Michael Steinberg [165] Department of Pediatrics, Southern Illinois University School of Medicine, Springfield, Illinois

Zenon Steplewski [145] The Wistar Institute of Anatomy and Biology, Philadelphia, Pennsylvania

Vernon C. Stevens [477] Department of Obstetrics and Gynecology, The Ohio State University, Columbus, Ohio

Klaus G. Stünkel [269] Bayer AG, Wuppertal, Federal Republic of Germany

H.J. Stutte [577] Zentrum der Pathologie, J.W. Goethe Universität, Frankfurt, Federal Republic of Germany

Tetsuya Suga [423] National Cancer Center Research Institute, Tokyo, Japan

Sven-Erik Svehag [207] Institute of Medical Microbiology, University of Odense, Odense, Denmark

Arne Svejgaard [619] Tissue Typing Laboratory of the Department of Clinical Immunology, University Hospital (Rigohospitalet), Copenhagen, Denmark

T. Taguchi [333] Department of Oncologic of Oncologic Surgery, Research Institute for Microbiol Diseases, Osaka University, Osaka, Japan

Nobuo Takasuka [423] National Cancer Center Research Institute, Tokyo, Japan

James E. Talmadge [317] Program Resources, Inc., National Cancer Institute, NIH, Frederick Cancer Institute, NIH, Frederick Cancer Research Facility, Frederick, Maryland

Tamara Tartaris [15] Division of Cancer Treatment, National Cancer Institute, NIH, Frederick Cancer Research Facility, Frederick, Maryland

Paul Ian Tartter [571] Department of Surgery, The Mount Sinai Medical Center, New York, New York

Anne Tax [183] Wistar Institute of Anatomy and Biology, Philadelphia, Pennsylvania

Joyce Taylor-Papadimitriou [241] Imperial Cancer Research Fund, London, England

Louise Telvi [377,457] Laboratoire d'Anatomie-Pathologique, Hôpital Saint-Vincent de Paul, Paris, France

B. Temminck [121] Laboratory of Human Genetics, Department of Medicine, Cantonal Hospital, Basel, Switzerland

Margaret A. Tempero [145] Department of Internal Medicine, University of Nebraska Medical Center, Omaha, Nebraska

L. Gilbert Thatcher [165] Department of Pediatrics, Southern Illinois University School of Medicine, Springfield, Illinois

Eckhard Thiel [269] Hematology, GSF, Munich, Federal Republic of Germany

J.L. Touraine [159] Transplant Unit and INSERM U80, Hôpital Edouard Herriot, Lyon, France

J. Traeger [159] Transplant Unit and INSERM U80, Hôpital Edouard Herriot, Lyon, France

K. Traill [535] Institute of Experimental Pathology, Ludwig Boltzmann Institute for AIDS Research, University of Innsbruck, Innsbruck, Austria

Peter Tsang [611] Department of Neoplasic Diseases, Mount Sinai School of Medicine and Hospital, New York, New York

Eiji Uchida [145] The Eppley Institute for Research in Cancer and Allied Diseases, University of Nebraska Medical Center, Omaha, Nebraska

Gerhard Uhlenbruck [127] Medizinische Klinik 1 der Universität zu Köln, Köln, Federal Republic of Germany

B. Unterweger [535] Clinic of Psychiatry, Ludwig Boltzmann Institute for AIDS Research, University of Innsbruck, Innsbruck, Austria

K. Vinzenz [463] Clinic for Maxillo-Facial Surgery, Vienna University, Vienna, Austria

Daniel Vittecoq [525] Départment de Maladies Infectieuses, Hôpital Saint-Louis, Service du Pr. Modai, France

Paul Volberding [567] Department of Medical Oncology, University of California, San Francisco General Hospital, San Francisco, California

C. Borri Voltattorni [311] Institute of Biochemistry, University of Perugia, Perugia, Italy

H. Wachter [535,583] Institute of Medical Chemistry and Biochemistry, Ludwig Boltzmann Institute for AIDS Research, University of Innsbruck, Innsbruck, Austria

G. Wagner [373] 1st Department of Obstetrics and Gynecology, University of Vienna, Vienna, Austria

Marc K. Wallack [351] Department of Surgery, Mount Sinai Medical Center, Miami Beach, Florida

Noel L. Warner [515] Becton Dickinson Monoclonal Center, Inc., Mountain View, California

G. Watzek [463] Division of Oral Surgery, Dental School, Vienna University, Vienna, Austria

W. Weber [121] Laboratory of Human Genetics, Department of Medicine, Cantonal Hospital, Basel, Switzerland

E.R. Werner [535,583] Institute of Medical Chemistry and Biochemistry, Ludwig Boltzmann Institute for AIDS Research, University of Innsbruck, Innsbruck, Austria

Taik K. Yun [301] Laboratory of Cancer Pathology, Korea Cancer Center Hospital, Korea Advanced Energy Research Institute, Seoul, Korea

Yeon S. Yun [301] Laboratory of Immunology, Korea Cancer Center Hospital, Korea Advanced Energy Research Institute, Seoul, Korea

V. Zakuth [39] Pediatric Immunology Unit, Tel-Aviv Medical Center and The Leon Alcalay Chair in Pediatric Immunology, Tel-Aviv University, Tel-Aviv, Israel

K.S. Zänker [91] Institute for Experimental Surgery, Technical University Munich, Munich, Federal Republic of Germany

INTRODUCTION

HERBERT E. NIEBURGS, MD
J. GEORGE BEKESI, PhD

University of Massachusetts, Medical School at Berkshire Medical Center, Pittsfield, Massachusetts
Department of Neoplastic Diseases, Mount Sinai School of Medicine and Hospital, New York, New York

This compendium presents an update of information on virally and nonvirally induced immune deficiencies. The new developments in basic and clinical immunology have occurred as a result of the explosive increase in the number of patients with HIV infection. Exposure to environmental and occupational hazards, nutrition, sexually transmitted diseases, intravenous drug abusers, and blood transfusions may lead to immune dysfunctions with enhancement of tumor development.

The mounting number of cases of death from AIDS, the incidence of neoplastic complications, and decreased immunocompetence from use of drugs for cancer treatment and organ transplantation have precipitated global efforts for improved management of immune-suppressed patients.

This book provides information in the form of original research reports and comprehensive overview articles. The text, arranged in eight chapters, deals with biology and etiology of immune dysfunctions, immunobiology of experimental and clinical oncology, organ transplantation, biomarkers, immunodiagnosis, and immunotherapy. Emphasis is focused on the multifactorial etiology of immune deficiencies and assessment of risk for immune dysfunctions. The use of monoclonal antibodies for immunodiagnosis and therapy of cancer patients and choice of biological response modifiers is extensively described.

A large chapter is devoted to LAS, ARC, and AIDS. It includes reports of studies on the biology of acquired immune deficiency, neoplastic complications, risk assessment, diagnosis, and the clinical control of HIV-infected patients.

It is hoped that the large number of selected articles serves as an overview of recent advances, offers insights into the biology of immune dysfunctions, and provides useful theoretical and clinical information that may permit the improved management of immune-compromised patients.

Acknowledgment is due to the contributing authors, to many colleagues who reviewed the submitted papers, to the assistant editor Suzanne A. Kay, to the production editor Ms. Mary Walsh, and to all those who were involved in the preparation of this volume.

Cancer Detection and Prevention Supplement 1:1–14 (1987)

Nutrition and Immunological Responses

Adrianne E. Rogers, MD
Paul M. Newberne, DVM, PhD

*Department of Pathology, Boston University School of Medicine, Boston, MA
and Mallory Institute of Pathology, Boston City Hospital*

ABSTRACT   Interactions between severe malnutrition and immunity have been described in clinical and experimental studies. Effects of marginal malnutrition or deficiency of single nutrients are less well-defined and should be investigated. Studies indicate that T cell function, in particular, is sensitive to many nutritional deficits or abnormalities and may compromise clinical immunological responses.

Key words: alcohol, calories, lipid, lipotropes, protein, T cells, vitamin A, vitamin B_6

INTRODUCTION

In 1980, in a comprehensive review of nutritional effects on immune function, Gross and Newberne [1] summarized data that supported the following conclusions. 1) There is extensive evidence from studies of patients with protein calorie malnutrition (PCM) and from laboratory animal models that nutritional status plays a role in immunocompetence. 2) Both quality and quantity of protein ingested determine the extent of immunological impairment in PCM. 3) Cell-mediated immunity (CMI) is affected more markedly than humoral immunity in PCM; phagocytic activity of leukocytes is diminished; serum content of components of complement is decreased. 4) Vitamin deficiencies contribute to the immunological abnormalities found in PCM; isolated vitamin deficiencies also may induce clinically significant depression of immunologic function. Deficiencies of vitamins A and B6, folate, thiamine, and riboflavin occur frequently in children with PCM. All are required for normal immunological responses in laboratory animals. Isolated deficiencies of vitamin A or folate depress responses to tests of CMI in humans; deficiency of vitamin A is associated with increased susceptibility to infection, but the major mechanism for that effect is failure of epithelial barrier functions rather than of immunological responses. 5) Minerals probably influence immunocompetence. There is evidence that iron deficiency increases susceptibility to infection and depresses cellular and humoral immunity, but the results of clinical and experimental studies are highly variable. In laboratory animals, severe zinc deficiency has marked effects on lymphoid tissue and on function of T lymphocytes in particular. 6) Humoral immunity and CMI are depressed by high intakes of fat, particularly the polyunsaturated acids, in laboratory animals. 7) Clinical and experimental studies show persistent immunological defects following intrauterine PCM.

Address reprint requests to Dr. Adrianne E. Rogers, Department of Pathology, Boston University School of Medicine, Boston, MA 02118.

Experimental studies have shown defective CMI and response to bacterial infection after intrauterine deficiency of vitamin B6 or lipotropes. 8) Obesity is associated with increased susceptibility to infection, but specific changes in immune function have not been reported.

Since that review, many studies of immune function and nutritional status in hospitalized and other patients have been published, and experimental studies have expanded the information available on effects of several nutrients on immunological responses.

CLINICAL STUDIES

Close interactions of nutrition and susceptibility to infectious disease are evident in the spectrum of childhood diarrheas, the first or second cause of childhood death worldwide [2]. Increased susceptibility of malnourished children to microbial and parasitic gastrointestinal infection probably is the result of several factors including diminished immune responses and failure of barrier and phagocytic systems. Since diarrheas occur also in measles, and other systemic infections, as well as after exposure to toxins, the roles of malnutrition and immunological responses undoubtedly vary. In turn, diarrhea intereferes with food ingestion, absorption, and utilization, increases nutrient loss in gi secretions, and is accompanied by fever and hormonal alterations that accelerate tissue breakdown and increase nutrient need.

Immune mechanisms that may be important in intestinal infection include antigen processing by macrophages and lamina propria lymphocytes, formation of IgA anbtibodies, and interactions between lymphocytes and possibly between cells of the immune system and the epithelium, but the general mechanisms and role of intestinal immunity are not known [2,3]. Recovery from diarrhea occurs with elimination of the reponsible agent and regeneration of damaged epithelium. Early provision of adequate food reduces recurrence rates of diarrhea, probably by increasing rate of epithelial repair as well as by enhancing immune mechanisms [2].

Malnutrition and childhood diarrheas occur in settings in which exposure to infectious [1], parasitic [4], and toxic agents can be expected and in which antenatal as well as postnatal, malnutrition may be common. If fetal and neonatal development of the immune system is abnormal, it may be incapable of responding normally even with a subsequent complete nutrient supply. The cellular subsets of the immune system directly and indirectly regulate each other's activity and may respond differently to nutrient supply, infection, or toxins [5].

Cunningham-Rundles [6] cited reports of reduced BCG immunization response, response to DNCB, and in vitro lymphocyte activation by mitogen in malnourished Colombian infants and diminished indices of CMI in malnourished hospitalized patients. The nutritional deficits reviewed were generally more damaging to cellular than to humoral immunity. Methods to evelute the immune system were reviewed.

In a review on the mucosal immune system, Allardyce and Bienenstock [7] make the following points. 1) Malnutrition is the major cause of immunodeficiency in the world. Deficiencies of Zn and vitamin A in addition to PCM probably are of major importance. 2) Investigation should be focused on mucosal immune responses, since mucosal infections are common and lethal in malnourished populations. 3) Resistance to intestinal and other mucosal surface infections correlates more strongly with specific IgA antibodies in the local secretions than in the blood. 4) IgA has a regulatory as well as a defense role. 5) Exclusion of infections agents, food antigens, and chemical toxins is dependent, at least in part, on SIgA at the mucosal surface. 6) Uptake, transport, and breakdown of agents that cross the epithelium depend on IgA.

The specialized epithelial (M) cells over the lymphoid areas of the gut (GALT) are the primary sites for antigen uptake, which is diminished by the presence of Ab or An-Ab complexes and mucous. IgE responses, mucosal mast cells, and lymphocytes expressing NK activity all contribute to mucosal immunity. Mucous (goblet) cell hyperplasia and secretion are probably induced by sensitized T cells, immune complexes, and IgE-mediated inflammation.

In PCM, atrophy of GALT and depletion of intraepithelial lymphocytes, mucosal T cells, and sIgA-bearing B cells have been reported [7,8].

Interactions of malnutrition and immunity appear to be important in the etiology of sepsis in postoperative or other severely ill patients from generally healthy and well nourished populations as well as from chronically malnourished populations. Nutrient requirements can be altered by physiological, environmental, and dietary factors; by drug and alcohol intake, smoking, and physical activity; and by disease or treatment of disease. Evidence of malnutrition may appear during illness and hospitalization in a patient not malnourished on admission. Patients who sustain significant trauma or burns, have surgery, or are septic are particularly at risk for developing malnutrition.

Caloric requirements can be increased 10–20% in the hypermetabolic states associated with surgery and trauma and by as much as 50% by infection or severe burns. Electrolytes and protein are lost in fistula drainage, diarrhea, ascites formation, and burns. Cancer patients may have increases in their resting metabolic rates of 20–42%, a change that represents a major increase in nutrient demand [9]. Cancer treatment can induce severe malnutrition [10]. Inflammatory bowel disease presents recurring nutritional problems, often of severe degree.

Definitions of malnutrition vary and may include as criteria dietary intake of some percent of the RDA, reduced growth or recent weight loss, biochemical measurements in blood, serum, or urine that fall outside the normal, and abnormalities on clinical examination [11]. History of dietary intake should include alcohol; chronic illness, drug intake, and recent surgery all should be documented. Physical examination in many studies has included measurement of midarm muscle circumference and triceps skinfold thickness. Laboratory studies generally include hematology and serum proteins (albumin, transferrin, or retinol-binding protein).

Evaluation of protein status is generally made using albumin, which has a half-life of 14 days. Transferrin, which has a half-life of 8 days and proteins with shorter half-lives, such retinol-binding protein, have been used but might not give a significant advantage.

Nutritional assessment methods were studied by Evans et al [12] in evaluation of effectivenes of TPN. A group of patients with small-cell carcinoma of the lung were given 30 days of intensive TPN at initiation of chemotherapy. At the outset, 91% of the patients were defined as nutritionally depleted by any one of the following criteria: weight loss $\geqslant 5\%$, albumin < 3.4 g%, TIBC < 270 μg%, creatinine-height index (CHI) $< 90\%$, urine urea N > 2 g/liter, midarm muscle circumference (MAMC) < 21 cm (women) or < 23 cm (men). They were, however, in a high-performance status category and essentially symptomless. Immunocompetence was not measured. TPN resulted only in expansion of ECF volume and intracellular water. Toxicity of chemotherapy and patient survival were not altered, and the authors concluded that TPN was not useful in this minimally malnourished group.

Functional assessment of nutritional status has been proposed as more significant than biochemical or chemical assessment [13]. When an essential nutrient becomes limiting, homeostatic mechanisms often maintain blood levels at the expense of body stores and reduce turnover or excretion or alter metabolic pathways to spare the limiting nutrient. Response to physiological supplements of a nutrient can be used to indicate preexisting deficiency if the response stabilizes with nutrient sufficiency rather than continuing to increase with excess nutrient supply. Solomons and Allen [13] gave a comprehensive listing and discussion of functional indices of nutritional status, including immunological assessment.

Preoperative nutritional status and postoperative morbidity and mortality have been known to be correlated for many years [10]. The earliest publication generally cited [14] was one in which major weight loss (20% or more of body weight) before surgery for chronic peptic ulcer disease was associated with significantly worse prognosis than no weight loss. Many subsequent studies have documented PCM and other deficiencies in hospitalized surgical and medical patients and shown a negative effect of poor nutritional status on prognosis. The portion of the effect that is due to immunological impairment is not clear, but many investigators have concluded that it is significant.

Burritt and Anderson [15] reviewed the evidence for PCM in hospitalized patients and discussed the value of several clinical laboratory tests in its detection and in monitoring response to nutritional therapy. Serum albumin is decreased in patients with infection or cancer, and a decreased value on admission predicts a longer hospital stay because of complications, including infection. Reduced retinol-binding protein also predicts complications and may be more useful than albumin in monitoring nutritional therapy. However, albumin is a widely used and a good indicator of both malnutrition and immune competence [16,17].

Evaluation of nutritional replenishment can include recovery of antibody synthesis and delayed cutaneous hypersensitivity (DCH). The value of lymphocyte counts in indicating malnutrition is controversial, but values of $1,200$–$2,000/mm^3$ have been associated with mild and < 800 with severe deficiency [9].

In retrospective and prospective studies in surgical patients, Lewis and Klein [18] reported a correlation between low serum albumin (< 2.7 g/100 ml), lymphocytopenia ($< 1,000/mm^3$), and postoperative sepsis.

Evaluation of nutritional replenishment in reducing operative morbidity and mortality in several recent studies showed that 1–2 weeks of therapy, with evidence of a response in transferrin levels, improved prognosis in patients with moderate to severe malnutrition. Reversal of anergic skin tests was reported in hemodialysis patients given 3 months of nutritional supplementation [9].

Mullen [19] proposed calculation of a nutritional index to assess prognosis in surgical patients using four nutritional variables, serum albumin and transferrin, response to recall skin test antigens, and triceps skinfold thickness, and demonstrated its usefulness.

McIrvine and Mannick [20] introduced a discussion of lymphocyte function in critically ill surgical patients by stating that improved intensive care of critically ill patients increases their short-term survival, but death from sepsis then occurs in the weeks to months following, despite antibiotic treatment, because of failure of host defenses against infection. Organisms responsible for lethal sepsis in hospitalized patients represent a broad spectrum from organisms thought to be eliminated solely by humoral antibodies to organisms eliminated by cellular immunity, the latter being the larger group. The authors concluded that nutritional repletion is a reasonably safe method to use in attempting to restore immune and other host defenses, but the evidence for its effectiveness is not strong.

Endocrine responses and anesthetic or other drug treatment are major complicating factors in assessing interactions between severe illness or trauma, immunity, and nutrition. The adrenal cortical hormones, several antibiotics, antiinflammatory drugs, and cancer chemotherapeutic agents are immunosuppressive; epinephrine increases wbc; cimetidine and other H-2 receptor blockers diminish suppressor T-cell function [20].

Host defenses comprise elements that interact in complex and, in many cases, unknown ways. The many cell types required for defense have varying nutrient requirements for maintenance of cell division, differentiation, and synthesis of specific protein or other components needed for their immunologic, phagocytic, destructive, and other activities. Many tests for the number and competence of the white cell components of host defenses are used clinically and in experimental studies (see Table 2 in ref. 20). Their significance for predicting response to infection and their correlations with each other are variable. An important consideration is that repeated testing in vivo with antigen may itself elicit a response. This arises in assessing effects of nutritional therapy on DCH. Measurement of killer cell activity of lymphocytes may give better correlations with major changes in nutritional status and can be performed repeatedly [20].

In assessing nutritional effects on in vitro measures of CMI, spurious results can be obtained. In PCM, reduced lymphocyte transformation indices can be the result of lower serum trace elements, particularly Zn, reduced number rather than reactivity of circulating T cells, or increased ratio of suppressor to helper T cells [3,21]. Immune suppressor cells and suppressive serum factors have been reported in patients and laboratory animals following burn and other trauma; their nature, function, interactions, and response to nutritional support are not known [20].

In clinical and experimental studies, indications are that secondary antibody responses are increased or unchanged by surgical or other trauma but that primary responses are depressed, probably because of reduced antigen recognition systems. The intimate and extensive interactions between B and T cells make attempts at isolation of nutritional influences somewhat artificial and largely impossible.

Diminished activity of NK cells was observed in patients with alcoholic cirrhosis and evidence of malnutrition. Lysis of two different NK cell target cell lines by peripheral blood mononuclear cells (PBMC) was significantly reduced in cirrhotics compared to normal controls or to alcoholic patients without evidence of cirrhosis or malnutrition. Within the cirrhotic group, NK-cell activity was significantly inversely related to severity of malnutrition. The authors concluded that PCM, and not alcohol, was responsible for the immunological defects in alcoholic patients (Table I) [22].

Patients with alcoholic hepatitis were evaluated for nutritional and immunological status. Indices of nutritional deficiency and immunological deficits increased as severitiy of liver disease increased. Some evidence of malnutrition was found in all patients with alcoholic liver disease [23].

Severe head injury leads to increased catabolism and elevated caloric needs. Early parenteral nutrition was compared to standard delayed enteral nutrition in head-injured patients and was found to prevent early deaths. Mortality within 18 days of admission was 44% in the enteral nutrition group and zero in the TPN group (P < 0.0001). Of the eight patients who died, six were septic; death was ascribed primarily to sepsis in two of them [24]. Nitogen and caloric intake and balance were significantly greater in the TPN group, and they had a much smaller decline in serum transferrin than the delayed-feeding group. Total lymphocyte counts were not significantly different in the two groups, but DCH increased more rapidly in TPN patients (Table II).

In adult Crohn's disease patients, a 2 month period of full nutritional supplementation of about 500 kcal/day supported increased serum albumin and prealbumin and T lymphocytes in

TABLE I. Immunological and Nutritional Status in Alcoholic Cirrhotic Patients [22]

Group	No.	Malnutrition* (%) Moderate	Severe	Skin test anergy (%)	T cells† per mm^3	Stimulation Index PHA	PWM	Ig (mg%)† A	G	M
Cirrhosis	59	67	33	39	605 ± 63	132	83	763	2,094	277
Control	37	0	0	—	159 ± 46	203	120	194	1,251	172

*Criteria: arm circumference < 80% normal, serum albumin < 3.3 g%, transferrin < 240 mg/ml.
†The differences are significant ($P < 0.05$).

TABLE II. Nutritional and Immunological Indices in Head-Injured Patients [24]

Index	Feeding regimen EARLY TPN (day) 1	10	16	STANDARD ENTERAL (day) 1	10	16	P value
N balance	−14	−12	−10	−16	−22	−14	0.002
(%) Change transferrin	−4	+3	−18	−17	−32	−34	0.06
Albumin	−16	−24	−26	−17	−33	−41	0.75
Day	1	7	14	1	7	14	
Positive skin test (%)	19	41	42	12	14	27	0.04

peripheral blood. (Values before supplementation were in the low-normal range.) Monocyte phagocytosis and adherence and Ig production also were completely or partially corrected by nutritional supplementation [3].

Ambulatory male outpatients at a VA Center were placed into two age groups (45–65 and >65 years) and classified by nine markers of malnutrition (Table III). Patients with evidence of infection, autoimmune disease, or major medical illness were excluded. Lymphocyte responses were decreased and serum IgA increased in patients with three or more markers of malnutrition not including immunological markers (lymphocyte count, DCH). Chemotactic responses of neutrophils and serum IgG or IgM content were not different from controls [25].

High-risk patients undergoing vascular surgery were evaluated for nutritional status and immunocompetence before surgery and for wound healing and infection postoperatively (Table IV). Reduced serum albumin and transferrin were significantly associated with septic and other complications of wound healing. Reduced DCH appeared also to be associated, although the incidences of wound complications in anergic patients (71%) and reactive patients (44%) were not significantly different [26].

In 215 surgical patients, a group from which cancer patients were excluded, admission nutritional status and postoperative course were evaluated (Table V). In the 12% judged to be malnourished, complications of surgery were significantly increased (45% vs 23%). Of the nutritional markers used, serum albumin had the greatest predictive value; proteins with shorter half-lives were of the same or less value. Recent weight loss and reduced weight index (percent

TABLE III. Incidence of Markers of Malnutrition in a Male Outpatient Population [25]

Marker	Incidence (%) at age	
	45–65 Years	65+ Years
Albumin <3.5 g%	44	34
Alcoholism	35	16
Triceps skinfold <70%	28	32
MAMC <90%	25	28
Lymphocytes <1,200/mm^3	14	18
Anergic DCH	10	14
<90% Ideal weight	10	16
Cachexis	7	8
Hgb <10 g%	6	8
Three or more markers	29*	38*

*These patients had a significant decrease in lymphocytes responding to mixed lymphocyte culture, PHA; increase in response to PWM; increased serum IgA.

TABLE IV. Nutritional and Immunological Indices in Relation to Wound Healing in 75 High-Risk Vascular Surgery Patients [26]

INDEX	Abnormal (%)
Albumin <3 g%	21*
Transferrin <150 mg%	32*
Lymphocytes <1,000/mm^3	23
Zn <80 mg%	9
DCH	22
PMN phagocytosis	38

*Significantly associated with septic or other complication of wound healing. Anthropometric indices showed no association.

TABLE V. Admission Nutritional Status of 215 Surgical Patients [27]

Marker	(%)
Weight index <0.8	14
Arm muscle circumference*	6
Weight Loss >5%	16
Albumin <3.3 g%, 3.8 g%†	16
At least two markers abnormal	12

*<18–23 cm depending on age, sex.
†Women, men respectively; predictive value was not increased by consideration of three additional proteins: transferrin <210 mg%; prealbumin <21 mg%, 23.5 mg%, retinol-binding protein <3.5 mg%.

of ideal weight) also had predictive value, but anthropometric measurements were not helpful [27]. About one-third of the patients tested for DCH showed some degree of anergy, but the results did not correlate with nutritional assessment.

Nutritional assessment was made of 277 new pediatric tumor patients using dietary history and physical, anthropometric, biochemical, hematological, and immunological examination. There was no evidence of significant malnutrition in any patient. In patients with solid tumors, body weight index and iron intake by history correlated with lymphocyte reactivity to mitogens; in patients with benign tumor, vitamin A intake by history correlated with lymphocyte responses. The authors concluded that nutritional status and immunological reactivity are normal on presentation in pediatric and tumor patients and that subsequent abnormalities are iatrogenic [28].

Growth, intestinal function and morphology, and nutritional status were evaluated in nine children given 3 years of maintenance therapy for acute lymphoblastic leukemia studied within days after the last dose of drug. Growth was retarded in all patients. Morphometry of jejunal biopsies showed elongation of villi and crypts and increased crypt mitoses in all patients. Intestinal disaccharidases were decreased in three; intraepithelial lymphocytes and IgA-containing cells were reduced in all; IgM-containing cells were normal. Serum immunoglobulins were reduced in four patients. D-xylose absorption was reduced in one patient, but serum nutrient content was normal except for reduced Fe and Cu in one patient each. The authors concluded that intestinal absorptive function and nutritional status were essentially normal, but that musocal immunity had been depressed by the therapy administered [29].

Chandra et al [30] evaluated DCH and nutritional status in a group of 51 adult medical and surgical patients with inflammatory bowel disease, short bowel syndrome, anorexia nervosa, or chronic idiopathic malabsorption. Lean body mass and serum albumin and DCH using ten recall antigens were used. Anergy was present in 80% of cases whose albumin was less than 2.25 g%; response was normal in almost all patients whose albumin was 3 g% or higher. Among responders, the diameter of induration correlated with lean body mass.

Malnutrition in human populations varies in the significant components with place, time, age, sex, and culture and is often complicated by infectious diseases or other severe medical or surgical illness. Studies of malnutrition in laboratory animals can be made much more specific but may miss significant interactions that contribute to the results in humans, such as the close link between protein quality and quantity, calorie and trace mineral quantity in human diets. Correlation of serum Zn and albumin has been demonstrated in many studies, and correlation of both with lymphocyte counts has been reported [31].

Proceedings of a workshop on single-nutrient effects on immune function were summarized and single-nutrient deficiencies reviewed in detail [32,33]. Patients at increased risk for single-nutrient deficiency include people with chronic disease, particularly if therapy includes hemodialysis or parenteral nutrition, the elderly, pregnant women, growth-retarded or premature children, the obese, those with chronic or recurrent infection, and food faddists. In humans, the best evidence for an effect on immunological responses has been provided for folate, iron, and zinc [32].

EXPERIMENTAL STUDIES

There are several recent studies of effects of caloric, protein, or zinc depletion on immune responses in laboratory animals. Immunological effects of immediate postnatal under- and overfeeding were studied in mice distributed into litters of four, nine, or 20 pups immediately after birth. [34]. At weaning, the mice showed the expected differences in body and organ weight, but weights of the lymphoid organs relative to body weight were the same in all groups, and mitogen responses of thymus and spleen cells were normal. Serum albumin and A- and B-globulins were decreased in the underfed mice; IgG was normal. Overfeeding had no effect. Primary and secondary antibody responses to immunization were normal in all mice, although the number of responding cells per spleen paralleled milk intake.

When the underfed mice were repleted for 4 weeks, their serum proteins became normal. If the underfeeding was continued after weaning, however, at 75% of ad libitum intake, thymus and spleen atrophied; all three serum globulin fractions, antibody response, and cutaneous response to DNFB were significantly reduced. The results showed, therefore, a rather minor effect of underfeeding during a critical period in immunological maturation in the mouse (the first 4 weeks of age) but increasing deficiency with prolonged underfeeding [34].

Listeria monocytogenes infection and peritoneal macrophage activity were studied in mice starved for 48 hr and in fed controls. Starved mice had markedly increased resistance to bacterial sepsis compared to fed controls, and their macrophages inhibited proliferation of *Listeria* and a tumor cell line in vitro to a significantly greater extent than macrophages from fed mice. However, macrophage activity against *Toxoplasma gondii* was reduced by starvation [35].

Five weeks of protein deprivation in rats previously immunized with KLH led to cutaneous anergy in 60% of the rats. Mortality from an IP injection of virulent bacteria was similar in control and malnourished reactive rats but was significantly greater in the malnourished anergic rats [36].

Protein or specific amino acid deprivation probably accounted for results of a study reporting increased antibody response to foreign antigen by mice fed lactalbumin compared to mice fed other protein sources (casein, wheat, or soy) [37]. The response in lactalbumin-fed mice was similar to the responses in mice fed a natural ingredient diet, whereas responses in the other three groups were depressed. Wheat and soy proteins are not complete, but casein should have given results comparable to the natural ingredient and lactalbumin diets; failure to do so may have been the result of the high level of corn oil (18%) in the purified diet.

Immune responses in animals deficient in single amino acids have been reviewed [38]. In mice, single deficiencies of several amino acids reduced NK-cell activity, production of blocking antibody by T-helper cells, and resistance to *Salmonella typhimurium* infection despite normal phagocytic and bactericidal and nearly normal antibody responses to infection.

A deficiency in rats closely related to protein deficiency is deficiency of lipotropic agents, since one of the two major lipotropes is methionine, an amino acid often limiting in poor-quality proteins. The others, choline, vitamin B12, and folate, are needed for normal methylation pathways in all animals. The immune response, which requries rapid proliferation of sensitized cells, is affected by a deficiency of folic acid and other methyl group sources (Table VI). Alterations in CMI have been reported in patients with megaloblastic anemia resulting from folate deficiency and in both humoral and CMI in folate-deficient animals [39].

Impaired humoral [40–42] and cell-mediated [43] immune responses have been reported in folate-deficient rats. They were more susceptible to infection with *Trypanosoma lewisi* [44] and had increased blood parasite counts and longer duration of infection.

Weaning Sprague-Dawley rats fed a folate-deficient diet for 3 months had decreased numbers of T cells in the spleen and peripheral blood, decreased cytotoxic activity of splenic

TABLE VI. Lipotrope Deficiency and the Immune System in Rats [43,46–48]

Dietary deficiency	Age	Immune system
Folate	1–3 months	Decreased T cells in spleen, blood Decreased cell-mediated cytotoxicity Decreased DCH (PHA)
B12	1–3 months	Normal response to Salmonella
B12	Gestation to 3 months	Increased mortality from Salmonella
Choline and methionine	Gestation to 3 months	Increased mortality from Salmonella Decreased size of thymus, spleen, nodes Decreased mitogen responses of splenic lymphocytes Decreased serum antibody responses Decreased DCH

lymphocytes, and depressed cutaneous response to intradermal PHA. If deficient diet was fed for 12 months, however, there were no longer significant differences between the experimental and control groups [43, 45, 46]. Folate requirements, like other nutrient requirements, decrease with decreasing growth rate as animals age.

Rats littered to dams fed diets marginally deficient in methionine and choline during gestation were switched to complete diet at birth or maintained on the deficient diet. Three months later they were infected with *S. typhimurium*. Deficient rats had a high mortality rate compared to the normal controls, and diet supplementation after weaning did not reduce the mortality [46]. The thymus, spleen, and lymph nodes of deficient rats showed marked hypoplasia; response to T-cell and B-cell mitogens was depressed in spleen or thymus cells [47,48].

Vitamin A deficiency is associated with decreased resistance to infection; recent studies have examined its effects on CMI. Vitamin A deficiency in rats does not affect serum complement levels [49], has moderate effects on antibody production [40,50], and diminishes local immune responses [51]. In a well controlled animal model, mitogen-induced transformation of splenic lymphocytes was depressed in the early stages of vitamin A deficiency [52], but the depression was not paralleled by alterations in the dose-response curve or stimulation kinetics [53] and could be reversed by 3 days of repletion with retinyl acetate. As deficiency progressed, the number and mitogen responses of splenic lymphocytes decreased, but response of cells isolated from lymph nodes increased [54].

In an experimental model for studying ocular infections with herpes simplex virus (HSV) type 1 in vitamin A-deficient (A$^-$) and pair-fed control (A$^+$) rats, the severity and course of the disease were evaluated by clinical examination, slit lamp biomicroscopy, and histopathology [55]. Rats were infected in the early stages of deficiency, prior to or at the beginning of the weight plateau. The onset of herpetic keratitis was more rapid, and the clinical disease more severe, in A$^-$ rats than in A$^+$ controls. The inflammatory response in the cornea and uveal tract of A$^-$ rats was significantly greater than in A$^+$ animals. Even mild vitamin A deficiency increased the severity of corneal HSV infection resulting in a high incidence of epithelial ulceration and necrosis.

In additional studies, local and regional immune functions were examined in vitamin A-deficient rats infected with HSV [56]. Specific or non-specific immune responses were studied. Cell-mediated responses and natural killer activity were monitored during the course of infection. Prior to infection, the concanavalin A (con A)-induced response of splenic lymphocytes from A$^-$ rats was significantly reduced. Three days after application of HSV to the corneas, the splenocyte response was decreased in both A$^-$ and A$^+$ animals, and it remained low for 10 days. The cervical lymph node (CLN) response to con A was depressed in both groups but was higher in the A$^-$ group than in the A$^+$ group. In vitro responses to inactivated

HSV appeared on day 7 in the spleen and day 10 in the CLN, were higher in A^- animals than in A^+ pair-fed controls, and were related to severity of the disease. Splenic NK cytotoxic responses were initially higher in A^+ than in A^- animals and decreased in both groups after infection; cervical lymph node NK responses were not affected by diet or HSV infection.

It appears that vitamin A deficiency has a significant effect on response to HSV infection and on indices of immunocompetence. The effects vary among the segments of the system, as do effects of infection. It is important to note that immune functions were altered before clinical signs of the deficiency were detected. High doses of vitamin A and some of its metabolites or analogues potentiate immunity in animal models and have been reported to enhance or suppress human lymphocyte activity in vitro. In a study of separated T and B cells, retinoic acid enhanced the T-cell response to mitogen but suppressed B-cell response [57].

In animals, vitamin B6 deficiency has consistent and severe effects on the immune system. Effects include atrophy of lymphoid organs, lymphocytopenia, reduced Ab responses, and reduction in many indices of CMI [5,32].

Using the immunologically responsive mouse Moloney sarcoma virus (MSV)-induced tumor model, Ha et al [58] examined the effect of dietary vitamin B6 content on immunity. Tumors induced at the site of virus injection regress after 14 days because of an immunological response, primarily of cytotoxic T lymphocytes but involving also cytotoxic antibodies, macrophages, and NK cells. Following regression, animals are immune to challenge by transplanted tumor. The model can, therefore, be used to test both primary and secondary immune responses to tumor.

Female mice were fed a fully nutritious diet to which was added the recommended amount of vitamin B6 (1 mg/kg) or lower amounts (0.5, 0.1, or 0 mg/kg). (The basal diet contained an additional 0.1 mg/kg of B6 in the casein.) After 4 weeks, at which time mice fed the two lower levels of B6 were demonstrably deficient, MSV was injected. Tumors appeared, grew at the same rate, and achieved peak size at the same time in all groups. Rate of regression was directly correlated with dietary B6 content, and tumors recurred only in mice given no added B6 in the diet. Secondary tumor takes was not influenced by dietary B6 content.

The role of zinc in clinically important immunological responses is being investigated intensively, and results have been reviewed recently [3,59]. Genetically determined immuno-deficiency syndromes in cattle and humans are alleviated by increasing intake on Zn above the levels generally required. Thymic atrophy in Zn-deficient people and animals and failure of thymus development in animals made Zn-deficient in utero are evidence that Zn is required for normal function of serum thymic factor [60]. Zn deficiency in patients given TPN was associated with defective CMI, which was corrected by Zn supplementation. In dialysis patients, lowered neutrophil Zn content was associated with reduced motility, but lymphocyte Zn content and function were normal. Uremia-related immunosuppression in patients has been reported to be reversed by supplementation with Zn [3].

There are experimental data showing defective T-cell function in vivo and in vitro and defective primary antibody response and interferon production in Zn deficiency. Pregnant rhesus monkeys fed a diet low, but not severely deficient, in Zn manifested clinical and biochemical signs of Zn deficiency in the third trimester and showed small decreases in response of lymphocytes to mitogens. No abnormality of immunologulin, complement, or percent E-rosette-positive cells was detected [61].

Studies of effects of amount and type of dietary fat on CMI were reviewed [62,63]. Polyunsaturated oils have been studied in animal models of autoimmune diseases and tissue transplantation. In studies largely uncontrolled for nutritional effects of increased lipid supply, linoleic acid or oenothera oil (7.5% γ-linolenic acid) decreased development of allergic encephalomyelitis following injection of myelin basic protein and decreased lymphokine production by lymphocytes compared to results in essential fatty acid (EFA)-deficient mice or adequately nourished guinea pigs. Skin transplant survival increased in some studies in mice fed or injected with polyunsaturated fatty acids (PUFA); however, other investigators could not demonstrate an effect or found oleic acid (monounsaturated) to be as effective as PUFA in suppressing transplant rejections.

Direct effects of fatty acids on in vitro measures of CMI were summarized [62]. Addition of certain fatty acids to cultures in concentrations similar to concentrations in serum decreased a number of indices of response. The effect of type of fatty acid was controversial, probably because of the use of serum containing lipoproteins and unknown quantities of fatty acids and albumin. Sera from hyperlipoproteinemic patients inhibited lymphocyte responses to mitogens and contained an LDL that had in vivo suppressing activity in mice; it was postulated to act by binding to receptors on lymphocytes and blocking their activation. In serum-free medium, PUFA and oleate stimulated lymphocyte responses at low concentrations but were inhibitory at higher levels. The reviewer concluded that there might be a graded in vitro response of lymphocytes to certain fatty acids, and a possible role of prostaglandins was discussed.

The effects of dietary fat on lymphocyte function may be the result of highly specific changes in lymphocyte membrane composition and function. In rats fed purified diets containing different ratios of n-2 and n-3 fatty acids, subpopulations of lymphocytes accumulated different relative amounts of fatty acids in their phospholipids [63]. Early in lymphocyte activation, long-chain fatty acids are transferred from intracellular sites to membrane phospholipids. There is rapid turnover of fatty acyl species mediated by an acyl transferase with a high affinity for PUFA that is activated when the ligand (mitogen or antigen) is bound. Increased unsaturation of the membrane phospholipids appears crucial to the events of activation. Prostaglandin (PG) synthesis by macrophages, and perhaps by T and B cells, and production and control of the amount of fatty acid precursors for PG appear to be key events.

Rats fed diets containing 10% fat with increasing ratios of 18:3n-3 to 18:2n-6 fatty acids were studied. Splenocytes and peripheral blood lymphocytes isolated from second-generation rats fed the higher 18:3n-3 diets had depressed PG synthesis. The depression was attributed to competition of 18:3n-3 and its metabolites with 18:2n-6 and its metabolites for key enzymes. Peritoneal macrophages showed the same effect on PG synthesis but still had normal phagocytic capacity. Similar competitive effects are thought to explain decreased leukocyte product generation and reactivity of leukocytes from humans fed the 18:3n-3 fatty acids [64].

The conclusions of both reviews [62,63] can be summarized as follows: 1) Effects of lipids on immune function probably exist and may be important in immunoregulation. Overall, diets high in PUFA depress lymphocyte mitogen response. Results comparing different types and amounts of fat are, however, highly variable. 2) Important effects should be demonstrable using physiological concentrations and appropriate fatty acid binding proteins. 3) Study of lipid effects on immune reactivity in vivo and in vitro should be improved by careful consideration of diet design, changes in LDL and other serum lipoproteins, in vitro alterations of plasma membrane composition, and responses of prostaglandins and other mediators. Measurement of the entire eicosanoid profile should be made. 4) Widely differing results can be explained in part by the detailed studies of Locniskar et al [65] that showed that the effect of dietary fat on lymphocyte mitogen response is governed by the duration of feeding and the tissue of origin of the lymphocytes.

The question of the effect of lipid on immunological responses is important in design of both general diet recommendations and recommendations for nutritional therapy for surgical and other critically ill patients. Recently, two types of oral and parenteral solutions were tested in comparable groups of septic and nonseptic patients. In one solution, energy was provided by a mixture of fat and carbohydrate and in the other carbohydrate only; total daily protein and energy supply were essentially the same with the two solutions. Lymphocyte total and subset counts, DCH response and serum immunoglobulins were the same in both groups at the end of therapy, and there was no evidence of a deleterious effect of the lipid administered [66].

Lipids and lipotropes are, of course, closely related metabolically and can be used experimentally to investigate further immunological interactions. One area of possible interest is in macrophage function and phospholipids in cell membranes. Macrophage recognition of abnormal cells is apparently governed in part by the phospholipid content of the cell membrane, a content that changes with lipid supply and with choline suppply [67].

REFERENCES

1. Gross RL Newberne PM. Role of nutrition in immunologic function. Physiol Rev 1980; 60:188–302.
2. Rohde JE. Selective primary health care: Strategies for control of disease in the developing world. XV. Acute diarrhea. Rev Infect Dis 1984; 6:840–54.
3. Dowd PS Heatley RV. The influence of undernutrition on immunity. Clin Sci 1984; 66:241–8.
4. Chandra RK. Parasitic infection, nutrition, and immune response. Fed Proc 1984; 43:251–5.
5. Brandon DL. Interactions of diet and immunity Adv Exp Med V 1984; 177:65–90.
6. Cunningham-Rundles S. Effects of nutritional status on immunological function. Am J Clin Nutr 1982; 35:1202–10.
7. Allardyce RA, Bienenstock J. The mucosal immune system in health and disease, with an emphasis on parasitic infection. Bull WHO 1984; 62:7–25.
8. Chandra RK. Mucosal immune responses in malnutrition. Ann NY Acad Sci 1983; 409:345–52.
9. Orr JW Jr, Shingleton HM. Importance of nutritional assessment and support in surgical and cancer patients. J Reprod Med 1984; 29:635–50.
10. Diehl JT, Steiger E,, Hooley R. The role of intravenous hyperalimentation in intestinal disease. Surg Clin North Am 1983; 63:11–26.
11. Sauberlich HE. Implications of nutritional status on human biochemistry, physiology and health. Clin Biochem 1984; 17:132–42.
12. Evans WK, Makuch R, Clamon GH, et al. Limited impact of total parenteral nutrition on nutritional status during treatment for small cell lung cancer. Cancer Res 1985; 45:3347–53.
13. Solomons NW, Allen LH. The functional assessment of nutritional status: Principles, practice and potential. Nutr Rev 1983; 41:33–50.
14. Studley HO. Percentage of weight loss. A basic indicator of surgical risk in patients with chronic peptic ulcer. J Am Med Assoc 1936; 106:458–60.
15. Burritt MF, Anderson CF. Laboratory assessment of nutritional status. Hum Pathol 1984; 15:130–3.
16. Bistrian BR, Blackburn GL, Hallowell R. Protein status of general surgical patients. J Am Med Assoc 1974; 230:858–60.
17. Bistrian BR, Blackburn GL, Scrimshaw NS. Cellular immunization in semistarved states in hospitalized adults. Am J Clin Nutr 1975; 28:1148–55.
18. Lewis RT, Klein H. Risk factors in post-operative sepsis. J Surg Res 1979; 26:365–71.
19. Mullen JL. Consequences of malnutrition in the surgical patient. Surg Clin North Am 1981; 61:465.
20. McIrvine AJ, Mannick JA. Lymphocyte function in the critically ill surgical patient. Surg Clin North Am 1983; 63:245–61.
21. Wirth JJ, Fraker PJ, Kierszenbaum F. Changes in the levels of marker expression by mononuclear phagocytes in zinc-deficient mice. J Nutr 1984; 114:1826–33.
22. Charpentier B, Franco D, Paci L, et al. Deficient natural killer cell activity in alcoholic cirrhosis. Clin Exp Immunol 1984; 58:107–15.
23. Mendenhall CL, Anderson S, Weesner RE. Protein-calorie malnutrition associated with alcoholic hepatitis. Am J Med 1984; 76:211–22.
24. Rapp RP, Young B, Twyman D. The favorable effect of early parenteral feeding on survival in head-injured patients. J Neurosurg 1983; 58:906–12.
25. Linn BS, Jensen J. Malnutrition and immunocompetence in older and younger outpatients. Southern Med J 1984; 77:1098–102.
26. Casey J, Flinn WR, Yao JST. Correlation of immune and nutritional status with would complications in patients undergoing vascular operations. Surgery 1983; 93:822–7.
27. Warnold I, Lundholm K. Clinical significance of preoperative nutritional status in 215 noncancer patients. Ann Surg 1983; 199:299–305.
28. Ramirez I, van Eys J, Carr D. Immunologic evaluation in the nutritional assessment of children with cancer. Am J Clin Nutr 1985; 41:1314–21.
29. Perkkio M, Rajantie J, Savilahti E, Siimes MA. Jejunal mucosa after leukemia treatment in children. Acta Pediatr. Scand 1984; 73:680–4.

30. Chandra RK, Baker M, Kumar V. Body composition, albumin levels, and delayed cutaneous cell-mediated immunity. Nutr Res 1985; 5:679–84.
31. Gellert SA, Woldseth R. Trace element analysis as part of the nutritional assessment of geriatric patients. Nutr Res 1985; Suppl I:217–23.
32. Beisel WR., Edelman R, Nauss K, Suskind RM. Single nutrient effects on immune functions. J Am Med Assoc 1981; 245:53–8.
33. Beisel WR. Single nutrients and immunity. The American J Clin Nutr 1982; 35:417–68.
34. Wade S, Lemonnier D, Bleiberg F, Delorme J. Early nutritional experiments: Effects on the humoral and cellular immune responses in mice J Nutr 1983; 113:1131–9.
35. Wing EJ. Effect of acute nutritional deprivation on host defenses against *Listeria monocytogenes*—Macrophage function. Adv Exp Med Biol 1983; 162:245–50.
36. Ing AFM, Meakins JL, McLean APH, Christou NV. Determinants of susceptibility to sepsis and mortality: Malnutrition vs anergy J Surg Res 1982; 32: 249–55.
37. Bounos G, Letourneau L, Kongshaun PAL. Influence of dietary protein type on the immune system of mice. J Nutr 1983; 113:1415–21.
38. Hill CH. Interaction of dietary amino acids with the immune response. Fed Proc 1982; 41:2818–20.
39. Newberne PM, Rogers AE. Labile methyl groups and the promotion of cancer. Ann Rev Nutr 1986; 6:407–32.
40. Ludovici PP, Axelrod AE. Circulating antibodies in vitamin deficiency states, pteroylglutamic acid, niacin-tryptophan, vitamins B_{12}, A and D deficiencies. Proc Soc Exp Biol Med 1951; 77:526.
41. Kumar M, Axelrod AE. Cellular antibody synthesis in thiamin, riboflavin, biotin and folic acid-deficient rats. Proc Soc Exp. Biol Med 1978; 157:421.
42. Pruzansksy J, Axelrod AE. Antibody production to diptheria toxoid in vitamin deficiency status. Proc Soc Exp Biol Med 1955; 89:323.
43. Williams EAJ, Gross RL, and Newberne PM. Effects of folate deficiency on the cell-mediated immune response in rats. NRI 1975; 12:137.
44. Aboko-Cole GF, Lee CM. Interaction of nutrition and infection: Effect of folic acid deficiency on resistance to *Trypanosoma Lewisi* and *Trypanosoma Rhodesiense*. Int J Biochem 1974; 5:693.
45. Gross RL, Newberne PM. Malnutrition, the thymolymphatic system and immunocompetence. In Friedman H, Escobar MR, Reichard SM, eds. The reticuloendothelial system in health and disease: Immunologic and pathologic aspects. New York: Plenum Publishing Corp., 1976, 179–87.
46. Nauss KM, Newberne PM. Effects of dietary folate, vitamin B_{12} and methionine/choline deficiency on immune function. In Phillips M, Baetz A, eds: Diet and resistance to disease. New York: Plenum, 1981; 63–91.
47. Newberne PM, Gerhardt BM. Pre- and postnatal malnutrition and responses to infection. NRI 1973; 7:407.
48. Newberne PM, Wilson RB. Prenatal malnutrition and postnatal responses to infection. NRI 1972; 5:151.
49. Madjid B, Sirisinha S, Lamb AJ. The effect of vitamin A and protein deficiency on complement levels in rats. Proc Soc Exp Biol Med 1978; 158:92–5.
50. Krishnan S, Bhuyan UN, Talwar GP, Ramalingaswami V. Effect of vitamin A and protein-calorie undernutrition on immune responses. Immunology 1974; 27:383–93.
51. Sirishinha S, Sarip MD, Moongkarndi P, Ongsakul M, Lamb AJ. Impaired local immune response in vitamin A-deficient rats. Clin Exp Immunol 1980; 40: 127–35.
52. Nauss KM, Mark DA, Suskind RM. The effect of vitamin A deficiency on the in vitro cellular immune response of rats. J Nutr 1979;109:1815–23.
53. Mark DA, Nauss KM, Baliga BS, Suskind RM. Depressed transformation response by splenic lymphocytes from vitamin A-deficient rats. Nutr Res 1981; 1:489–97.
54. Nauss KM, Phua C-C, Ambrogi L, Newberne PM. Immunological changes during progressive stages of vitamin A deficiency in the rat. J Nutr 1985; 115:909–18.
55. Nauss KM, Anderson CA, Conner MW, Newberne PM. Ocular infection with herpes simplex virus (HSV-1) in vitamin A-deficient and control rats. J Nutr 1985; 115:1300–15.
56. Nauss KM, Newberne PM. Local and regional immune function of vitamin A-deficient rats with ocular herpes simplex virus (HSV) infections. J Nutr 1985; 115:1316–24.
57. Oalone RH, Payan DG. Potentiation of mitogen-induced human T-lymphocyte activation by retinoic acid. Cancer Res 1985; 45:4128–31.
58. Ha C, Kerkvliet I, Miller LT. The effect of vitamin B-6 deficiency on host susceptibility to Moloney sarcoma virus-induced tumor growth in mice. J Nutr 1984; 114:938–45.

59. Watson RR, Mohs ME. Determination of requirements for nutrients with critical roles in lymphocyte functions: Zinc and vitamin A. Nutr Res 1984; 4:951–5.

60. Dardenne M, Pleau JM, Nabarra B, LeFrancier P, Derrien, Choay J, Bach JF. Contribution of zinc and other metals to the biological activity of the serum thymic factor. Proc Natl Acad Sci USA 1982; 79:5370–3.

61. Golub MS, Gershwin ME, Hurley LS, Baly DL, Hendrick AG. Studies of marginal zinc deprivation in rhesus monkeys. I. Influence on pregnant dams. Am J Clin Nutr 1984; 39:265–80.

62. Gurr MI. The role of lipids in the regulation of the immune system. Prog Lipid Res 1983; 22:257–87.

63. Johnston PV. Dietary fat, eicosanoids, and immunity. Adv Lipid Res 1985; 21:103–41.

64. Lee TH, Hoover RL, Williams JD, Sperling RI. Effect of dietary enrichment with eicosapentaenoic and docosahexaenoic acids on in vitro neutrophil and monocyte leukotriene generation and neutrophil function. N. Engl J Med 1985; 312:1217–24.

65. Locniskar M, Nauss KM, Newberne PM. The effect of quality and quantity of dietary fat on the immune system. J Nutr 1983; 113:951–61.

66. Mullin TJ, Kirkpatrick JR. Substrate composition and sepsis, effects on immunity. Arch Surg 1983; 118:176–80.

67. Fidler IJ. Macrophages and metastasis-A biological approach to cancer therapy: Presidential address. Cancer Res 1985; 45:4714–26.

Cancer Detection and Prevention Supplement 1:15–27 (1987)

Protein Deficiency Reduces Natural Antitumor Immunity

Ralf Ruffmann
Erich Schlick
Tamara Tartaris
Wladyslaw Budzynski
Michael A. Chirigos

Biological Therapeutics Branch (R.R., T.T., W.B., M.A.C.) and Laboratory of Molecular Immunoregulation (E.S.), Biological Response Modifiers Program, Divison of Cancer Treatment, National Cancer Institute, NIH, Frederick Cancer Research Facility, Frederick, MD

ABSTRACT Clinical data have shown that neoplastic diseases and/or related therapies frequently result in protein depletion of tumor-bearing patients. Depressions of acquired and specific immunity caused by protein depletion are well known. In an experimental model protein depletion was induced by lack of nutritional protein in otherwise isocaloric conditions in BALB/c and C57BL/6 mice over various time periods (max. 35 days). The results show that natural immune effector cells, natural killer cells, and monocyte/macrophages also during treatment with biological response modifiers (BRM) are depressed in their cytotoxic potentials in vitro and in vivo. Substantial and critical reductions of bone marrow cellularity (bone marrow nucleated cells) were also observed. In contrast, preliminary results show that if, following protein depletion, mice were treated parenterally with amino acids (Neo-aminomel, Boehringer-Ma. Co., FRG) complete restoration of immune parameters takes place. Adequate protein status is shown to be a crucial factor for natural immunity and therapy with BRM.

Key words: protein deficiency, natural immunity, macrophages, biological response modifiers, MVE-2

INTRODUCTION

In recent years, research on biological response modifiers (BRM) has been intense. BRM by definition are agents that modify the relationship between tumor and host by modifying the host's biological response to tumor cells [1]. This definition indicates that a variety of possible biologic alterations might be considered. However, most efforts have been devoted to either increasing host defense mechanisms against tumors or improving the host's ability to tolerate damage caused by conventional tumor reductive therapies.

Erich Schlick is now at the Department of Oncology, BASF Pharma-KNOLL Ag, Postfach 210805, D-67 Lu, FRG.

Dr. Ruffmann is now at Recordati Chemical and Pharmaceutical Industries S.p.A. Via Civitali 1, 1-20148 Milano, Italy. Address reprint requests there.

The efforts to increase host defense mechanisms have focused on cytotoxic T lymphocytes and cytotoxic natural immune effector cells, that is, natural killer (NK) cells, and monocyte/macrophages (Mϕ) [2,3]. A considerable number of biologic agents or chemically defined substances have been identified as being stimulatory for these host defense compartments [1]. At the same time, however, it has also become evident that therapy with BRMs may be quite unpredictable in its effects depending on such conditions as kind of drug and dose [4–7], route of administration [7–9], frequency of treatments [8–11], additional tumor reductive therapies [12,13], and tumor burden [14–18]; recently we and others were able to show that precise timing in combined treatment modalities of cyclophosphamide and the synthetic BRM maleic anhydride divinyl ether (MVE-2) is another factor of outstanding importance [9,12,13]. Maintaining an appropriate interval between the end of chemotherapy and onset of biologic modification improved effector cell numbers and cytotoxic activity recruitments and increased the tumor reductive effect of chemotherapy significantly. Any interval that was smaller than the ideal resulted in significantly reduced effects; any larger interval favored tumor recruitment and regrowth [9,13].

The present investigations examine how protein deficiency would affect natural immune effector cell activities and MVE-2 treatment. There is abundant evidence that malignant diseases of different sites and stages result in severe depletions of body protein [19–21]. This condition could become important, since BRMs are projected for therapy of cancer-bearing patients especially in an advanced stage of disease. Furthermore, there is substantial evidence from a survey [22] that reduced body protein supplies cause strong decreases of T lymphocyte-mediated immunity and humoral immunity. Regarding natural immune effector cells and particularly BRM treatments, so far only incomplete and limited information is available.

MATERIALS AND METHODS
Animals

BALB/c and C57BL/6 male mice, 6–10 weeks old, weighing 25 g, were used for experiments. The animals were supplied by the Animal Production Section, Division of Cancer Treatment, National Cancer Institute (Frederick, MD).

Feeds and Weight Control of Animals

Mice were kept ad libitum on normal feed (18% protein, energy value 4.02 kcal/g, diet No. 170593) or on a protein-deficient feed (<1% protein, energy value 3.97 kcal/g, diet No. 170597). Both feeds were purchased from TEKLAD (Madison, WI). The feeds were weighed and allotted in equal amounts to the comparison groups, and consumption of both feeds was monitored closely to make sure that both feeds were eaten in equal amounts. All animals were given water ad libitum. Animals were weighed three times per week on an Ohaus Brainway Electronic Balance (Ohaus Florham Park, NJ) to monitor weight behavior.

Drugs

MVE-2 was kindly supplied by Dr. R. Corrano (Adria Laboratories, Columbus, OH). MVE-2 was diluted for in vivo use with phosphate-buffered saline (PBS; Grand Island Biological Company, Grand Island, NY) and the pH adjusted to 7.0 with 0.1 N Na OH.

Tumor Cells

The tissue culture line of YAC-1, a Moloney virus-induced lymphoma of A/Sn origin, was used as the target for NK cells. MBL-2, a Moloney virus-induced lymphoblastic leukemia cell line (C57BL/6), was used as the target for Mϕ. Both cell lines were maintained in tissue culture with RPMI 1604 with 4 mM L-glutamine (GIBCO), 100 μg/ml of gentamycin (Microbiological Associates, Bethesda, MD), and 10% fetal bovine serum (Associated Biomedic Systems, Buffalo, NY). MBL-2 was also carried in vivo by weekly intraperitoneal passage of tumor cell-containing ascites fluid.

Assay of Macrophage-Mediated Cytotoxicity

The assay for measuring the ability of agents to induce Mϕ-mediated cytotoxicity has been previously described [23]. Briefly, for in vivo activation, all groups were sacrificed on day 0, and peritoneal exudate cells were harvested by lavaging the abdominal cavity of the mice with 8 ml of RPMI 1640 and washing the cells in fresh tissue culture medium. Mϕ (4 $\times$ 10^5) were seeded onto 11.3-mm wells of Costar 48-well plates, centrifuged at 200 g, and incubated at 37°C in 5% CO_2 in air for 2 hr. The monolayers were washed three times with PBS to eliminate nonadherent cells. The remaining adherent monolayers ($>95\%$ Mϕ as judged by esterase and Wright's staining) were then overlaid with 1 $\times$ 10^5 viable MBL-2 cells resuspended in medium containing 10 ng/ml of LPS (*Salmonella typhimurium*; Difco Laboratories, Detroit, MI). The ratio of Mϕ to tumor target cells was 4:1 at the beginning of each experiment. All cultures were incubated at 37°C in 5% CO_2 in air for 48 hr and/or 72 hr, and the number of viable MBL-2 cells as determined by trypan blue dye exclusion was counted in a hemocytometer; mean counts and standard errors (SE) were calculated. Triplicate cultures were maintained for each group.

The percentage of growth inhibition of MBL-2 cells induced by Mϕ was calculated by the following formula: % inhibition = 1 − (mean of MBL-2 cells incubated with drug-treated Mϕ/mean of MBL-2 cells incubated with nontreated Mϕ) $\times$ 100.

Assay for Splenic Natural Killer (NK) Cell Activity

A conventional ^{51}Cr-release assay was employed as previously described [24]. In brief, 1 $\times$ 10^4 radiolabeled YAC-1 cells (100 μCi of ^{51}CR [New England Nuclear; specific activity 250–800 mCi mg^{-1}] per 1.0 $\times$ 10^7 YAC-1 cells at 37°C for 45 min) in 0.1 ml volume were added to graded numbers of splenic effector cells in round-bottomed 96-well microtiter plates. Triplicate cultures were maintained at 37°C in 5% CO_2 for 4 hr. At the end of the incubation period the plates were centrifuged for 10 min at 800 g, and the supernatants were harvested using a Titertek automatic harvesting system and measured in a γ-counter. The percentage of cytotoxicity was calculated from the formula: % cytotoxicity = (experimental CPM − SR CPM/TR CPM − SR CPM) $\times$100. SR is the spontaneous release as determined by incubation of 1.0 $\times$ 10^4 tumor cells in 0.2 cc of RPMI 1640 in round-bottomed 96-well microtiter plates for 4 hr at 37°C in 5% CO_2, and TR is the total release of radioactivity as determined by adding 0.1 ml of SDS 0.5% to 0.1 ml of 1 $\times$ 10^4 radiolabeled YAC-1 cells.

Bone Marrow Cells (BMC)

Single cell suspensions from femoral bone marrow were prepared as described previously [25]. The total number of viable nucleated cells per femur was counted for each individual mouse in a hemocytometer.

Serum Protein Determinations

Serum was obtained from whole nonheparinized blood. Quantatitive colorimetric determinations were performed for albumin by Sigma procedure No. 630 [26] and total protein by Bio Rad protein assay [27]. Semiquantitative determination of prealbumin was performed by reading levels of prealbumin off a gradient slab gel electrophoresis (5–20% polyacrylamide). The complete procedure is described elsewhere [28].

Statistical Analysis

The Student's t test was used for statistical analysis.

RESULTS
Weight Development Caused by Protein-Deficient Feed (Fig. 1)

Mice on protein-deficient (PD mice) progressively lost weight throughout an observation period of 41 days, with the strongest reduction in weight between days 0 and 8 (17% of weight loss) and days 8 and 17 (additional 16% of weight loss) (Fig. 1). Until day 41, the weight loss was up to 46% of the original weight. Mice on a normal 18% protein feed (ND mice) maintained or increased slightly their initial weight during the same period. PD mice started to develop diarrhea and polyuria around days 5–7. Their fur became ruffled, and mice repeatedly became subject to partial alopecia.

Prealbumin, Albumin, and Total Protein Serum Concentration Changes Caused by the Protein-Free Feed

To assess whether protein-deficient feed indeed led to a lack of protein in thus fed animals, prealbumin, albumin, and total serum concentration changes were determined (Table I; Fig. 2). Because of nutritional lack of protein, the typical prealbumin band disappeared completely and albumin underwent a 22% reduction. The amount of total protein in the serum was reduced by 23%. These findings reflect typical clinical patterns of protein depletion [29–

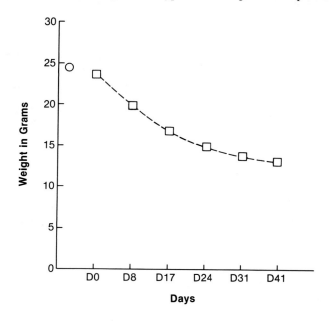

Fig. 1. BALB/c mice were kept on a normal diet (18% protein, energy value 4.02 kcal/g) (○) or a protein-deficient diet (<1% protein, energy value 3.97 kcal/g) (□). Mice were weighed at the days indicated. Results are the mean values of a typical experiment (15 mice for each time point). SD was less than 15% of the mean. The experiment was repeated twice with similar results.

TABLE I. Serum Concentrations of Albumin and Total Protein in Mice on a Normal or Protein-Deficient Diet

Feed of mice*	Albumin (g/dL)†	Total protein (g/dL)†
Normal	3.11 ± 0.25‡	4.26 ± 0.74
Protein-deficient	2.43 ± 0.21§	3.26 ± 0.86

*BALB/c mice were kept on normal (18% protein) or protein-deficient (<1% protein) isocaloric diets for 5 days prior to sacrifice.
†Albumin and total protein were determined in serum from whole blood after tail vein bleeding 5 days after start of diets.
‡Each value represents the mean and SEM of three separate experiments (five mice for each value).
§P < 0.05 compared to normal control.

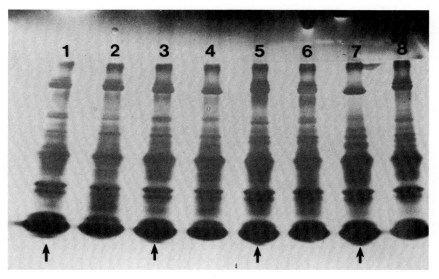

Fig. 2.   Gradient slab gel electrophoresis of serum proteins. BALB/c mice were kept on normal (18% protein) diets (uneven numbers) and on protein-deficient (<1% protein) isocaloric diets (even numbers) for 5 days prior to sacrifice. Electrophoresis was performed with serum from whole blood after tail vein bleeding (N = 5 mice). Arrows indicate the prealbumin band. Total loss of this band occurs in protein-deficient mice (even numbers). Results of a typical experiment are shown. Similar results were found in two additional experiments.

33]. The determinations were performed 5 days after the onset of the diet, showing that even a short depletion period was sufficient to induce characteristic symptoms of lack of protein.

Spleen Natural Killer Cell Cytotoxic Activity (Spontaneous and After Stimulation by MVE-2) During Nutritional Protein Depletion

Spontaneous NK activity was compared in the PD and ND for 35 days (Fig. 3). Spontaneous NK activity was not significantly altered in the PD mice. Administration of MVE-2 (25 mg/kg) at intermittent periods resulted in an augmentation of NK activities in both PD mice and ND mice. ND mice consistently achieved cytotoxic activities of about 30%, whereas PD mice at best reached 18% in the beginning of the diet and then progressively lost activity down to 8%.

Bone Marrow Nucleated Cell Counts (BMC)

Mice on a protein-deficient diet showed a marked progressive decrease in the number of bone marrow nucleated cells (Fig. 4). Whereas mice on ND regularly had counts of 10×10^6 cells/femur, PD mice after 5 days of diet only had 8.6×10^6 of cells (13% reduction), which progressively decreased to 6.9×10^6 of cells/femur (30% reduction). In all cases administration of MVE-2 resulted in an increase of BMC 3 days after injection. In the ND mice, injection of MVE-2 consistently led to a substantial increase of BMC. In contrast, although MVE-2 treatment led to a reconstitution of BMC in the PD mice, a return to normal levels was never achieved.

Macrophage Cytotoxicities In Vitro and In Vivo During Nutritional Protein Depletion

When evaluated in vitro in a 48 hr or 72 hr assay, Mϕ cytotoxicities were distinctly enhanced by MVE-2 but were not altered because of protein-depleted feedings (Fig. 5). On a per-cell basis, Mϕ cells displayed equivalent amounts of antitumor resistance. Peritoneal Mϕ

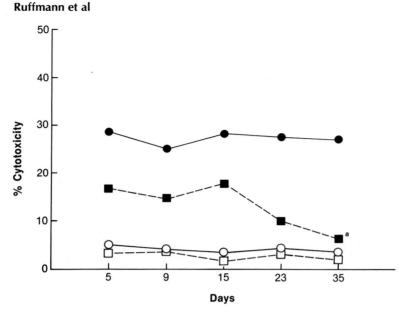

Fig. 3.   Spleen natural killer cell cytotoxicity (E/T 100:1, E/T of 50:1 and 25:1 showed similar results) of BALB/c mice on normal (18% protein) diets (○), normal diets plus intraperitoneal injection of 25 mg/kg MVE-2 (●), protein-deficient (<1% protein) isocaloric diets (□), and protein-deficient diets plus intraperitoneal injection of 25 mg/kg MVE-2 (■). Mice were sacrificed at the indicated days after start of diets. MVE-2 was injected each time 3 days prior to sacrifice. Results shown here are the mean of a typical experiment (SD less than 5%, N = 5 mice). Additional experiments were performed yielding similar results. [a]P < 0.05 compared to ○.

cell numbers of individual animals, however, as assessed after peritoneal lavage were profoundly decreased because of nutritional protein depletion (data not shown).

As the in vivo antitumor resistance of a given effector cell population is determined by the percentage of cytotoxicity (in vitro) multiplied by the number of the total effector cell population (in vivo), losses of Mφ cell numbers might have a detrimental effect for the in vivo Mφ-mediated tumor resistance.

To investigate this possibility, C57BL/6 mice were fed normally or given a protein-depleted diet for 7 days. On day 8 all animals received 100 mg/kg cyclophosphamide (Cy) intraperitoneally, which eliminates concurring NK and T-cell activities while leaving mono-cyte/Mφ reactivity [12,13,34,35] largely intact. On day 9 all animals were injected intraperi-toneally with 2×10^6 MBL-2 tumor cells per mouse, which grow as an ascites tumor. Six hours later activation of peritoneal Mφ was induced by injection of 25 mg/kg MVE-2 intraperitoneally. Subsequently, depending on the amount of in vivo Mφ cytotoxicity, tumor cell lysis and reduction of tumor burden would take place. On day 11, all animals were sacrificed, and, after standardized individual peritoneal lavage, tumor cells were recovered from mice. Tumor cells were counted and thus tumor burden (reductions of tumor burden and in vivo Mφ cytotoxicity) assessed. In addition, in vivo macrophage cell numbers per mouse and in vitro Mφ cytotoxicity were determined.

Confirming earlier data, Mφ cytotoxicity in vitro was enhanced by MVE-2 but was not influenced by any changes of the feed. Mφ cell numbers, however, were found to be strongly decreased in protein-depleted animals. They amounted to only 30% of numbers found in normally fed animals. MVE-2 enhanced cell numbers irrespective of the type of feed but was never able to change the basic pattern set by the type of feed. The in vivo ability of Mφ to lyse and eliminate tumor cells was significantly increased by MVE-2 in animals on normal feed.

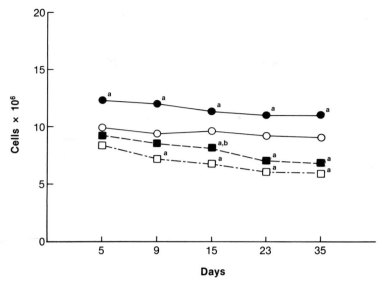

Fig. 4. Counts of nucleated bone marrow cells (BMC/femur) of BALB/c mice on normal (18% proteins) diets (○), normal diets plus intraperitoneal injection of 25 mg/kg MVE-2 (●), protein-deficient (< 1% protein) isocaloric diets (□), and protein-deficient diets plus intraperitoneal injection of 25 mg/kg MVE-2 (■). Mice were sacrificed at the indicated days after start of diets. MVE-2 was injected each time 3 days prior to sacrifice. Results shown here are the mean of a typical experiment (SD less than 15%, N = 5 mice). Additional experiments had similar results. [a]P < 0.05 compared to ○; [b]p < 0.05 compared to □.

Tumor burden in these animals was decreased by some 80%. In mice that underwent protein depletion overall slower tumor development took place in vivo. Although this would mean a lower tumor burden, the effectiveness of MVE-2 was much lower (around 20%) and did not result in significant decreases of tumor load.

DISCUSSION

In recent years immunotherapy directed against neoplastic disease has largely focused on natural immune effector cells as opposed to the more conventional host defense mechanism such as T cell-mediated immune responses [1]. In fact, in contrast to the latter, which are not spontaneously present in normal, nonstimulated individuals and develop only after a latent period of approximately 2 weeks upon sensitization, natural immune effector cells also exert spontaneous activity in normal individuals even when they have never been exposed to tumor cells. The natural immune system is quite heterogeneous, including Mφ, NK cells, granulocytes, further cytotoxic effector cells, and natural antibodies [2].

NK cells and Mφ have received growing attention. Mφ have a major role in the phagocytosis and disposal of effete cells, cellular debris, and serum proteins. Evidently Mφ have a considerable ability to differentiate between old and young, damaged and healthy, and normal and neoplastic cells [36]. In addition, Mφ play major parts in the host's response to injury (inflammation), infections, and parasitic diseases and as mediators of immune regulations [36,37].

Mφ have been proposed to be crucial elements of immune surveillance. Studies of Norbury and Kripke [38] dealing with skin carcinogenesis in mice induced by ultraviolet radiation demonstrated that treating mice with pyran copolymer, which is a strong Mφ activator, prolonged the latent period of tumor development. In contrast, administration of Mφ suppressants, such as carrageenan or silica, shortened the latent period of tumor development.

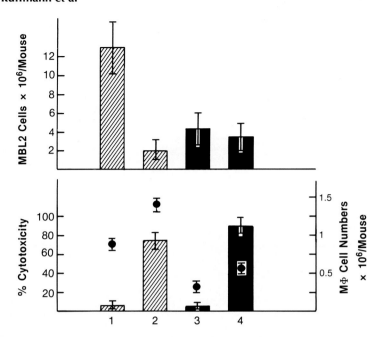

Fig. 5. Peritoneal macrophage cytotoxicity in vitro and in vivo: C57BL/6 mice were kept on a normal diet (18% protein, hatched bars) or on an isocaloric protein deficient diet (<1% protein, closed bars) beginning on day 0. On day 7 all groups were treated with cyclophosphamide (100 mg/kg) and on day 8 received 2×10^6 MBL-2 tumor cells per mouse intraperitoneally. Six hours later groups 2 and 4 had additional IP treatment with MVE-2 (25 mg/kg) for in vivo enhancement of macrophage cell numbers and cytotoxicities. On day 11 all animals were sacrificed and underwent peritoneal lavage. After peritoneal cell counts were determined, the mean tumor volume per mouse (**top**) and the mean macrophage cell number per mouse (**●, bottom**) were calculated. Cytotoxicity (bar graphs, **bottom**) was determined for 4×10^5 macrophages/well in vitro (E/T 4:1). Results of a typical experiment (N = 5 mice per group) are shown. Similar results in additional experiments.

Furthermore, abundant evidence has accumulated showing that in vivo activation [39,40] or adoptive transfer of Mϕ [41,42] are highly effective in tumor therapy even against established tumors [36,37].

The phenomenon of natural killing was discovered 13 years ago. During studies regarding the cytotoxic activity of lymphocytes obtained from tumor-bearing patients or animals on autologous or allogeneic tumor target cells, effector cells derived from normal nontumor-bearing controls also expressed considerable activity against these targets [43]. This activity was found to be linked to lymphocytes, termed NK cells, with spontaneous lytic activity against various targets [2]. The profound and widespread research during following years accumulated an impressive amount of evidence as to the vital role that NK cells have for in vivo resistance against disease, particularly against neoplastic disease [2,44,45].

Typical examples that emphasize the impact of NK cells on host defense are the enhancement of tumor growth in the presence of low NK activity as in beige mice [46–48] or after selective inhibition of NK activity by antiasialo GMI antibody [45,49], whereas adoptive transfer of NK-enriched cell populations has resulted in diminished local tumor growth and reduced metastatic spread [45,49].

Both monocyte/Mϕ and NK cells are bone marrow derived [13,50–53]. This is why the in vivo efficiency of both compartments is appreciably linked to the bone marrow's ability to proliferate and provide these cells. Considerations regarding the in vivo role of Mϕ and NK compartments should also include this aspect.

The BRM MVE-2 has been shown to be a potent in vitro and in vivo activator for Mϕ and NK cytotoxic activities [54]. Treatments of tumor-bearing animals with MVE-2 have frequently resulted in significant increases of median survival time and overall survival. It is essential, however, to emphasize that success or failure may largely depend on whether recommendations for treatments with BRM such as MVE-2 as far as they have been identified are duly respected or not. Since BRM mostly have indirect action on tumor cells as opposed to traditional cytotoxic drugs, directives for BRM treatments (dose, optimum time point, route, frequency, mode of integration into schedules, and so forth) are harder to define [5,6,8,12,13]. In fact, besides identifying new BRM, "setting up the rules for BRMs" in general and also for particular substances has become a large field of research [5,6,8,12,13,16,39,40,55–59]. In this respect, protein depletion caused by neoplastic disease has to be examined for its effects on natural immune effector cells, bone marrow cells, and BRM treatments related to these cells.

In fact, an impressive amount of information has accumulated showing that protein-calorie malnutrition occurs with high frequency in tumor-bearing patients [19–21], which is documented by reduction in body weight, anthropometric measurements, serum albumin, transferrin concentrations, and the creatinine height index [33]. The causes of malnutrition in cancer patients are manifold and comprise anorexia, local consequences of tumor growth, tumor-related therapies such as chemotherapy and radiotherapy [21,60], psychological factors, and interference of the tumor with the host metabolism. Contrary to most normal cells, tumor cells obtain nearly all their energy from metabolism of glucose to lactate rather than from metabolism to carbon dioxide and water, which is the energy source for the majority of normal cells. The ensuing conversion of amino acids to glucose to meet the tumor's energy demands depletes muscle tissue of amino acids and reduces the body's protein supplies in general [21].

This chain of events exemplifies how body protein becomes subject to biochemical cannabalism [21]. Evaluations of body protein consistently reveal serious reductions in serum levels of albumin, prealbumin, transferrin, and retinol-binding protein in states of cancer and protein deficiency [19,20,30,31,32,61–63]. Unfortunately, malabsorption of proteins is a major negative consequence of protein deficiency [20], thus accelerating the deterioration of body protein supplies. At the same time, sparing of vital body functions during malnutrition is heavily dependent on an adequate maintenance of body protein. This is why parameters like serum albumin concentration as markers for clinically significant malnutrition have outstanding importance independent of weight loss [64,65].

There is no way to correlate in a general way tumor stage or extent with the degree of protein calorie malnutrition. For gastrointestinal tumors malnutrition, as judged roughly by weight loss, occurred in some 65% of all cases when first diagnosed [66], whereas metastatic bone disease of various primaries in children presented overt malnutrition in 37% of the cases [20]. Even small primary lesions not involving the gastrointestinal tract such as certain carcinomas of the lung are frequently accompanied by clinical signs of protein-calorie malnutrition that often appear to exceed that which might be reasonably expected on the ground of the extent to the neoplastic disease [66]. In any event, weight loss and reduced body protein, while not being characteristic symptoms of early cancer but rather of growing and advanced neoplasms, are by no means restricted to terminal states of tumor disease and cachexia.

The negative effects of protein depletion on specific and acquired immunities such as T cell- and B cell-mediated host defense reactions have been amply studied and documented. These data are summarized [22,67]. Since natural immune effector cells have moved into the center of interest regarding immunotherapy, it has become essential to investigate the effects of lacking body protein on these cells and how their ability to respond to BRM therapy would be affected.

Our findings show that shortage of nutritional protein results in distinct depressions of bone marrow cellularity (BMC) (Fig. 4). It is true that administration of MVE-2, which normally results in effective increases of BMC [13] even under these conditions, augments the numbers of bone marrow nucleated cells. However, it is also true that the effected increases never reach the levels of normally fed mice on MVE-2 treatment and even fail to return to the levels of nonstimulated mice on normal feed.

In agreement with these findings, we also observed decreases of spleen cell numbers in the respective treatment groups (data not shown). These findings could already account for a reduced in vivo NK activity. In addition, NK activity, when evaluated on a per cell basis (Fig. 3), also showed decreases when the animals had undergone protein depletion in vivo. The differences for spontaneous NK activity were not significant; however, after MVE-2 treatment cells derived from normally fed mice responded readily with substantial augmentation of NK cytotoxicity, whereas the response in protein-depleted mice was considerably weaker. In the latter, MVE-2 was able to achieve some boosting of NK cytotoxicity but significantly failed to reach the levels attained in normally fed animals after MVE-2 boosting.

In vitro Mϕ cytotoxicity was also enhanced by MVE-2 but did not change because of lack of protein. In vivo cell numbers, however, were strongly reduced after protein depletion (Fig. 5). Mice on normal feed showed impressive in vivo Mϕ activity and equally strong tumor reductions. Mice on protein-free feed had slower developments of tumor burden. This fact has been well known and frequently described [63,68,69]. Food restrictions generally slow down the developments of transplanted tumors but have no positive effect on median survival time or overall survival. In fact, there are indications that in these conditions the nitrogen balance of the host is negative, wherease the tumor's is positive [70]. Apart form these considerations, the data as presented in Figure 5 indicate that administration of MVE-2 to protein-depleted animals does result in some in vivo Mϕ activation and tumor reduction, but the differences in tumor cell counts between MVE-2-treated and nontreated groups are only about 20% and never turned out to be significant. In normally fed animals injections of MVE-2 maintained the injected tumor volume at its initial size, whereas in protein-depleted mice even in a situation of reduced tumor growth rate MVE-2 treatment did not succeed in doing so.

In conclusion, protein depletion has negative consequences for natural immune effector cells and BMC. Most importantly, biological activities triggered by MVE-2 are severely compromised. Additional investigations have shown that not only spleen NK cytotoxic activity but also peritoneal and blood NK activities are equally depressed during protein depletion and that natural immune responses after treatment with the BRM polyriboinosinic-polycytidylic acid poly-L-lysine stabilized with carboxylmethyl cellulose (Poly ICLC) show depressions similar to those that occur after MVE-2 treatments (Ruffman and Tartaris, unpublished observations). Seemingly, there is a difference between NK and Mϕ cytotoxicity in vitro, one being affected and the other not by protein depletion. It has to be noted, however, that the NK-cytotoxicity assay was performed with total lymphocyte populations and not with purified populations of large granular lymphocytes (LGL). Current investigations on how protein depletion affects LGL numbers, percentages, and activities are being performed.

Preliminary results indicate that parenteral (intraperitoneal) administration of a mixture of amino acids (Neo-aminomel) to previously protein-depleted mice is able to revert the negative effects on natural immune effector cells discussed above [71]. This information is still limited, and further investigations are needed to determine more precisely conditions of Neo-aminomel treatments. Nevertheless, the present conclusion is that diagnosis of protein depletion and subsequent protein restoration have to be included as directives for BRM treatments in neoplastic disease.

Recently a prospective study into the nutritional status of 114 patients with untreated primary squamous cell carcinomas of the head and neck was undertaken to assess its possible prognostic value for survival [72]. Nutritional status turned out to be of significant importance as a prognostic factor. The investigators concluded that the effects of insufficient nutrition were at least in part caused by secondary immunologic dysfunctions. These findings emphasize the role of tumor-related nutritional imbalances in the success or failure of BRM treatments.

ACKNOWLEDGMENTS

R.R. is the recipient of a grant from Deutsche Forschungsgemeinschaft, Bonn, FRG.

REFERENCES

1. Mihich E, Fefer A, eds. Biological responses modifiers: Subcommittee report, Natl Cancer Inst Monogr 1983; 63.
2. Herberman RB. Natural killer cells and other effector cells. In Herberman RB, Friedman H, eds: The reticuloendothelial system. New York: Plenum, 1983; 5:279–313.
3. Chirigos MA, Mitchell M, Mastrangelo MJ, Krim, M. Mediation of cellular immunity in cancer by immune modifiers, New York: Raven, 1981: 1–269.
4. Reizenstein P, Mathé G. Immunomodulating agents. In: Fenichel RL, Chirigos M A, eds: Immune modulation agents and their mechanisms. New York: Marcel Dekker, 1984: 347–63.
5. Herberman RB. Biological response modifiers for the therapy of cancer. Ann Allergy 1985: 54:376–81.
6. Aoki T, Lentinan. In Fenichel FL, Chirigos MA, eds: Immune modulation agents and their mechanisms. New York: Marcel Dekker, 1984: 63–79.
7. Cummins CS. Corynebacterium parvum and its fractions. In Fenichel FL, Chirigos MA, eds: Immune modulation agents and their mechanisms. New York: Marcel Dekker, 1984.
8. Megel H, Gibson JP. Tilosone and related analogs. In Fenichel FL, Chirigos MA, eds: Immune modulation agents and their mechanisms. New York: Marcel Dekker, 1984: 97–120.
9. Ruffman R, Schlick E, Welker RD, Chirigos MA. Cytoreductive chemotherapy followed by MVE-2: Impact of interval between treatment modalities and therapeutic results against MBL2 tumor. AACR Proc 1984; 25:1284 (abstract).
10. Saito T, Ruffmann R, Welker RD, Herberman RB, Chirigos MA. Development of hyporesponsiveness of natural killer cells to augmentation of activity after multiple treatments with biological response modifiers. Cancer Immunol Immunother 1985; 19:130–5.
11. Saito T, Welker RD, Fukui H, Herberman RB, Chirigos MA. Development of hyporesponsiveness to augmentation of natural killer cell activity after multiple doses of maleic anhydride divinyl ether: Association with decreased numbers of large granular lymphocytes. Cell Immunol 1985; 90:577–89.
12. Berd D, Maguire HC Jr, Mastrangelo MJ. Immunopotentiation by cyclophosphamide and other cytotoxic agents. In Fenichel RL, Chirigos MA, eds: Immune modulation agents and their mechanisms. New York: Marcel Dekker, 1984: 39–63.
13. Schlick E, Ruffmann R, Chirigos MA, Welker RD, Herberman RB. In vivo modulation of myelopoiesis and immune functions by MVE-2 in tumor-free and MBL-2 tumor-bearing mice treated with cyclophosphamide. Cancer Res 1985; 45:1108–14.
14. Mathé G, Kenis Y. La chimiothé rapie des cancers. Expansion Scientifique Francaise 1975; 3: 222–6.
15. Herberman RB ed. Natural cell-mediated immunity against tumors. New York: Academic Press, 1980.
16. Carrano RA, Iuliucci D, Luce JK, Page JA, Imondi AR. MVE-2 development of an immunoadjuvant for cancer treatment In Fenichel RL, Chirigos MA, eds: Immune modulation agents and their mechanisms. New York: Marcel Dekker, 1984: 243–61.
17. Tsang KY, Fudenberg HH, Hoehler FK, Hadden JW. Immunostimulating compounds isoprinosine and NPT 15396. In Fenichel RL, Chirigos MA, Immune modulation agents and their mechanisms, New York: Marcel Dekker, 1984: 79–97.
18. Takasugi M, Ramseyer A, Takasugi J. Decline of natural nonselective cell-mediated cytotoxicity in patients with tumor progression. Cancer Res 1977; 37:413–8.
19. Harvey RB, Bothe, A Jr, Blackburn GL. Nutritional assessment and patient outcome during oncological therapy. Cancer 1979; 43:2065–9.
20. Van Eys J. Malnutrition in children with cancer: Incidence and consequence. Cancer 1979; 43: 2030–5.
21. DeWys WD. Nutritional care of the cancer patient. JAMA 1980; 244:374.
22. Chandra RK. Nutrition, immunity and infection (mechanisms of interactions). New York: Plenum 1977.
23. Ruffmann R, Welker RD, Saito T, Chirigos MA, Varesio L. In vivo activation of macrophages but not natural killer cells by picolinic acid (PLA). J Immunopharmacol 1984; 6:291–304.

24. Herberman RB, Nunn ME, Lavrin DH. Natural cytotoxic reactivity of mouse lymphoid cells against syngeneic and allogeneic tumors. I. Distribution, reactivity and specificity. Int J Cancer 1975; 16:216–28.
25. Schlick E, Friedberg KD. Bone marrow cells of mice under the influence of low lead diseases. Arch Toxicol 1982; 49:227–36.
26. Anon. Sigma Tech Bull No. 630 (9–80). St. Louis, MO: Sigma Chemical Co., revised, 1983 .
27. Anon. Bio Rad protein assay instruction manual. Richmond, CA: Bio Rad Laboratories, 1981.
28. Anderson L, Anderson NG. High resolution two-dimensional electrophoresis of human plasma proteins. Proc Natl Acad Sci USA 1977; 74:5421–5.
29. Daly JM, Dudrick SJ, Copeland EM III. Effects of protein depletion and repletion in cell mediated immunity in experimental animals. Ann Surg 1978; 188:791–804.
30. Bistrian BR, Blackburn GL, Hallowell E, Heddle R. Protein status of general surgical patients. JAMA 1974; 230:858.
31. Bistrian BR, Blackburn GL, Vitale J, Cochran D, Naylor J. Prevalence of malnutrition in general medical patients. JAMA 1976; 235:1567.
32. Ingenbleek Y, Visscher M, De Nayer R. Measurement of prealbumin as index of protein-calorie malnutrition. Lancet 1972; 2:106–8.
33. Blackburn GL, Schlamm HT. Nutritional assessment and treatment of hospital malnutrition. In van Eys J, Seelig MS, Nichols BL, eds: Nutrition and cancer. New York: SP Medical and Scientific Books, 1979: 1–54.
34. Kempf RA, Mitchell MS. Effects of chemotherapeutic agents on the immune response. I. Cancer Invest 1984; 2:459–66.
35. Turk JL, Parker D. The effect of cyclophosphamide on the immune response. J Immunopharmacol 1979; 1:127–37.
36. Fidler IJ, Poste G. Macropohage-mediated destruction of malignant tumor cells and new strategies for the therapy of metastatic disease. Springer Semin Immunopathol 1982; 5:161–74.
37. Fidler IJ. Macrophages in host defense against cancer metastasis. Cancer Bull 1984; 36:226–30.
38. Nobury KC, Kripke ML, Ultraviolet-induced carcinogenesis in mice treated with silica, trypan blue or pyran copolymer. J Reticuloendothel Soc 1979; 26:827–35.
39. Sone S, Fidler IJ. In situ activation of tumoricidal properties in rat alveolar macrophages and rejection of experimental lung metastases by intravenous injection of *Nocardia rubra* cell wall skeleton. Cancer Immunol Immunother 1982; 12:203–9.
40. Hisano G, Fidler IJ. Systemic activation of macrophages by liposome-entrapped muramyl tripeptide in mice pretreated with the chemotherapeutic agent adriamycin. Cancer Immunol Immunother 1982; 14:61–6.
41. Fidler IJ. Inhibition of pulmonary metastasis by intravenous injection of specifically activated macrophages. Cancer Res 1974; 34:1074–8.
42. Liotta LA, Gattozzi C, Kleinerman J. Reduction in tumor cell entry into vessels by BCG-activated macrophages, Br J Cancer 1977; 36:639–41.
43. Rosenberg EB, Herberman RB, Levine PH, Halterman RH, McCoy JL, Wunderlich JR., Lymphocyte cytotoxicity reactions to leukemia-associated antigens in identical twins. Int J Cancer 1972; 2:648–58.
44. Herberman RB. NK cells and other natural effector cells. New York: Academic Press, 1982.
45. Herberman RB. Multiple functions of natural killer cells, including immunoregulation as well as resistance to tumor growth. Concepts Immunopathol 1985; 1:96–132.
46. Roder J, Duwe A. The beige mutation in the mouse selectively impairs natural killer cell function. Nature 1979; 278:451–3.
47. Talmadge TE, Meyers KM, Prieur DJ, Starkey JR., Role of NK cells in tumor growth and metastasis in beige mice. Nature 1980; 284:622–4.
48. Kärre K, Klein GO, Kiessling R, Klein G, Roder JC. Low natural in vivo resistance to syngeneic leukaemias in natural killer-deficient mice. Nature 1980; 284:624–6.
49. Barlozzari T, Reynolds CW, Herberman RB. In vivo role of natural killer cells: Involvement of large granular lymphocytes in the clearance of tumor cells in anti-asialo GM_1-treated rats. J Immunol 1983; 131:1024–7.
50. Miller SC. Production and renewal of murine natural killer cells in the spleen and bone marrow. J Immunol 1982; 129:2282–6.
51. Haller O, Wigzell H. Suppression of natural killer activity with radioactive strontium: Effector cells are bone marrow dependent. J Immunol 1977; 118:1503–12.

52. Haller OA, Gidlund M, Kurnick JT, Wigzell H. In vivo generation of mouse natural killer cells: Role of the spleen and thymus. Scand J Immunol 1978; 8:207–15.

53. Trenton JJ, Kiessling R, Wigzell H, et al. Bone marrow transplantation immunobiology. In Baum SJ, Ledney GD, eds: Experimental hematology today. New York: Springer-Verlag, 1977: 181.

54. Talmadge JE, Maluish AE, Collins M, et al. Immunomodulation and antitumor effects of MVE-2 in mice. J Biol Response Modif 1984; 3:634–52.

55. Herberman, RB In Rationale of biological response modifers in cancer treatment. 6th Hakone Symposium, 1985. Unpublished.

56. Mowshowitz SL, Chin-Bow ST, Smith GD. Inteferon and cis-DDP: Combination chemotherapy for P388 leukemia in CDFl mice. J Interferon Res 1982; 2:587–91.

57. Purnell DM, Bartlett GL, Kreider JW, Biro TG. *Corynebacterium parvum* and cyclophosphamide as combination treatment for a murine mammary adenocarcinoma. Cancer Res 1977; 37:1137–40.

58. Scott MT. Analysis of the principles underlying chemo-immunotherapy of mouse tumours. Cancer Immunol Immunother 1979; 6:107–19.

59. North RJ. Cyclophosphamide-facilitated adoptive immunotherapy of an established tumor depends on elimination of tumor-induced suppressor T cells. J Exp Med 1982; 55:1063–74.

60. Donaldson SS, Lenon RA. Alterations of nutritional status: Impact of chemotherapy and radiation therapy. Cancer 1979; 43:2036–52.

61. Van eys J. Nutrition and neoplasia. Nutr Rev 1982; 40: 353–9.

62. Fabris C, Piccoli A, Meani A, et al. Study of retinol-binding protein in pancreatic cancer. J Cancer Res Clin Oncol 1984; 108:227–9.

63. Copeland EM III, Rodman CA, Dudrick SJ. Nutritional concepts of neoplastic disease, In Van Eys J, Seelig MS, Nicholas BL, eds: Nutrition and cancer. New York: SP Medical and Scientific Books, 1979: 133–56.

64. Bistrian BR, Blackburn GL, Scrimshaw NS, Flatt JP. Cellular immunity in semistarved states in hospitalized adults. Am J Clin Nutr 1975; 28:1148–55.

65. Bistrian BR, Sherman M, Blackburn GL, Marshall R, Shaw C. Cellular immunity in adult marasmus. Arch Intern Med 1977; 137:1408–11.

66. Shils ME. Nutritonal problems associated with gastrointestinal and genitourinary cancer. Cancer Res 1977; 37:2366–72.

67. Shizgal HM. Nutrition and immune function. Surg Annu 1981; 13:15–29.

68. Brennan MF. Uncomplicated starvation versus cancer cachexia. Cancer Res 1977; 37:2359–64.

69. Copeland EM III, Daly JM, Dudrick SJ. Nutrition as an adjunct to cancer treatment in the adult. Cancer Res 1977; 37:2451–6.

70. Buzby GP, Mullen JL, Stein P, Miller EE, Hobbs CL, Rosato EF. Host-tumor interaction and nutrient supply. Cancer 1980; 45:2940–8.

71. Ruffmann R, Tartaris T, Schlick E, et al. Auswirkungen des Protein-mangels auf die natuerliche Immunitaet. In Striebel JP, Henningsen B, Kluther R, eds: Klinische Ernaehrung Im Gespraech. Munich: Zuckschwerdt Verlag 1985: 102–11.

72. Brookes GB. Nutritional status—A prognosic indicator in head and neck cancer. Otolaryngol Head Neck Surg 1985; 93:69–74.

Immunotoxicology: Environmental Contamination by Polybrominated Biphenyls and Immune Dysfunction Among Residents of the State of Michigan

J. George Bekesi
Julia P. Roboz
Alf Fischbein
Patricia Mason

Department of Neoplastic Diseases (J.G.B., P.M., J.P.R.) and Environmental Sciences Laboratory (A.F.), The Mount Sinai School of Medicine of the City University of New York, New York, NY

ABSTRACT   In 1973, inadvertent contamination occurred in a special farm feed supplement for lactating cows. Polybrominated biphenyls (PBBs) were used in place of magnesium oxide resulting in serious harm to farm animals, including cattle, chickens, geese, ducks. Farm families, accustomed to eating their own products, were most heavily exposed. To study the impact of PBBs, 336 adult Michigan farm residents, 117 general consumers for comparison, 75 dairy farm residents in Wisconsin, who had not eaten PBB-contamined food, were examined, as were 79 healthy subjects in New York City. Abnormalities in the Michigan groups included hypergammaglobulinemia, exaggerated hypersensitive response to streptococci, significant decrease in absolute numbers and percentage of T and B-lymphocytes, and increased number of lymphocytes with no detectable surface markers ("null cells"). Significant reduction of in vitro immune function was noted in 20–25% of the Michigan farm residents who had eaten food containing PBB. The decreased immune function detected among the PBB-exposed farm residents tended to affect families as a unit and was independent of exposed individuals' age or sex, pointing against the possibility of genetic predisposition.

Key words: T and B-cell functions, phenotypes, immunoglobulins, clinical symptoms

INTRODUCTION

It is presently recognized that certain chemicals can adversely affect the immune system. The relatively new field of immunotoxicology is therefore gaining wide interest. The objective of this article is to review briefly recent studies on the immunotoxicology of polybrominated biphenyls (PBB).

In 1973, a mixture of polybrominated biphenyls (PBB), a fire retardant chemical, was inadvertently used instead of magnesium oxide in the commercial preparation of a special feed supplement for lactating cows in the state of Michigan [1,2]. The mixture of brominated

Address reprint requests to Dr. J. George Bekesi, Mount Sinai School of Medicine, 10 East 102nd Street, New York, NY 10029.

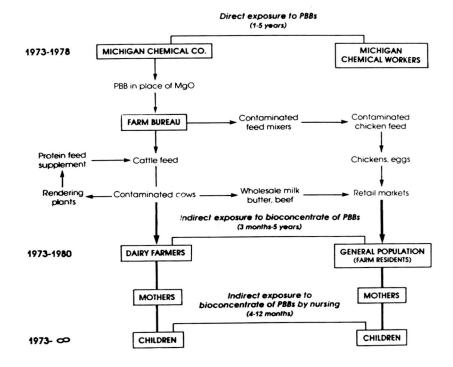

Fig. 1.   Course of polybrominated biphenyl (PBB) contamination in Michigan.

biphenyls consisted of 2 penta-, 4 hexa-, and 2 octabromobiphenyl isomers, a combination developed for use as the flame retardant Firemaster FF-1 [3].

Adverse effects of PBB on dairy cattle, including anorexia and decrease in milk production a few weeks after ingestion of the contaminated feed, were first reported in 1974 [4]. In addition, some animals developed hematomas, abscesses, abnormal hoof growth, alopecia, and thickening of the skin. Others developed cachexia and died within 6 months. Consequently, more than 500 of Michigan's dairy and poultry farms were quarantined in 1973 and 1974. More than 30,000 cattle and 1.5 million chickens died, and 5 million eggs had to be destroyed. Unfortunately, dairy products containing PBB were widely consumed in the state until 1978. PBB was subsequently found in the serum and/or adipose tissues of dairy farm residents and workers who manufactured the fire retardant and who may have been occupationally exposed to the chemical as well as most Michigan residents [5–9]. Figure 1 shows the course of contamination in the state of Michigan.

PBB, which has a chemical structure similar to that of polychlorinated biphenyls (PCB), is fat soluble and is stored in the thymus, liver, brain, and adipose tissues for long periods of time [10]. Following PBB exposure in animals, effects such as intrahepatic bile duct hyperplasia, skin and preneoplastic changes, and enzyme induction have been reported (Table I). PBB has been shown to promote tumors and together with several (purified) cogeners has inhibited the metabolic cooperation between 6-thioquanine sensitive and resistant Chinese hamster V79 cells in a manner similar to known tumor promoters (phorbol ester) [11,12].

METHODS OF STUDY

Investigation of the consequences of PBB exposure in humans was undertaken in 1976–1977 and again in 1981–1983. Those studied included 332 adult dairy farmers from Michigan, 156 individuals from the general population of that state, and 29 chemical workers who were

TABLE I. Experimental Evidence for the Toxicity of Polybrominated Biphenyls

Species	Route of entry to the body	Exposure or dose levels	Toxic signs, target organs, and processes
Heifers and bulls	Oral	Suspected feed ad libitum	Prostration, liver, testicles spermatozoa, hyperkeratosis
Dairy cattle	Oral	50 ppm PBB in diet	Nil effect
Dairy cattle	Oral	5,000 ppm PBB in diet	Liver, kidney, skin
Dairy cattle	Oral	10 mg PBB/day (0.71 ppm in diet)	Nil by 1975
Cow	Oral	1.13 gm PBB	Intrahepatic bile duct hyperplasia; liver + gall-bladder
Chickens	Oral	45, 125, and 625 ppm PBB in diet	Hatchability depressed; egg production declined; egg production ceased; liver, spleen, thyroid, heart, male hormone
Rats	Oral	Up to 500 ppm PBB in diet	Liver weight and size increase
Rats (timed-pregnant)	Oral	50 ppm PBB	Fatal gastrointestinal hemorrhage; decreased fetal weight
Rats	Oral	100 ppm PBB in diet	No reproductive interference, birth defects, or cytogenic aberrations
Rats	Oral	300 ppm PBB in diet	Liver enzyme induction
Rats	Oral	0–500 ppm PBB in diet	Microsomal enzyme induction + increased liver weight
Mice	Oral	50 ppm PBB and 100 ppm in diet	Decreasing fetal weight with dosage; weak tetra-togen; fat storage
Mice (pregnant)	Oral	0, 100, and 200 PBB in diet	Dead or resorbed fetuses; fetal weight down
Mice (pregnant)	Oral	0, 50, and 100 ppm PBB in diet	Mortality of offspring increased
Rabbits (albino)	Dermal	2 and 0–5.0 g BP-6 per kg body weight	Skin irritation
Rabbits	Dermal	5 g BP-6 per kg body weight	Liver enlargement of 1 gm/kg and higher

Based on the study of Kay [10].

TABLE II. Analysis of Immunological Parameters for Husbands and Wives in PBB-Exposed Michigan Dairy Farmers

Immune parameter	Means ± SD (N)		Absolute mean difference (SD)	N	t	Spearman correlation coefficient (RHO)
	Husband	Wife				
Surface markers						
T Cells (%)	59.17 ± 10.94 (101)	60.93 ± 10.83 (102)	1.80 (11.88)	101	1.52	0.298†
Null cells (%)	22.14 ± 13.17 (98)	20.59 ± 11.74 (100)	1.56 (13.57)	97	1.13	0.337†
Lymphocyte functions						
T cell by PHA (cpm × 1,000)	77.83 ± 23.06 (100)	73.30 ± 17.96 (100)	4.30 (24.33)	98	1.75	0.303†
B cells by PWM (cpm × 1,000)	72.84 ± 24.92 (92)	73.91 ± 24.77 (99)	0.241 (29.63)	89	0.077	0.282†
Immunoglobulins						
IgG (mg/dl)	1,637.24 ± 491.89 (100)	1,616.55 ± 510.58 (102)	27.34 (564.76)	100	0.484	0.324†
IgA (mg/dl)	323.24 ± 140.30 (100)	280.98 ± 133.61 (102)	41.09 (197.11)	100	2.085*	0.053
IgM (mg/dl)	121.09 ± 69.64 (100)	147.40 ± 84.97 (101)	27.80 (102.62)	99	2.695*	0.150

*P < 0.05.
†P < 0.01.

TABLE III. Prevalence of Multiple Symptoms Among PBB-Exposed Michigan Farm Residents With Immune Dysfunctions

Symptoms	% with symptoms	
	Abnormal immunology group	Normal immunology group
Headaches	28.0*	14.1
Dizziness	16.0*	6.5
Paresthesias	24.0*	11.1
Loss of balance/clumsiness	16.0*	2.5
Fatigue	38.5*	16.6
Nervousness	28.0*	6.5
Sleepiness	24.0*	3.5
Sleeplessness	24.0*	7.5
Loss of memory	24.0*	13.6
Joint pain	32.0*	12.6
Swelling in joints	20.0*	3.5
Slower healing of cuts	18.0*	4.5
Frequent colds	19.2*	6.5

*Difference between normal immunology group and abnormal immunology group is statistically significant, $P < 0.001$.

involved in the manufacturing of PBB. One hundred fifty dairy farm residents from Wisconsin served as the control group.

An attempt was made to study whether a toxic PBB syndrome profile existed in the exposed Michigan population. The prevalence of multiple clinical symptoms was examined among the Michigan farm residents with multiple immune dysfunctions.

The immunobiological abnormalities and clinical symptoms were also examined with respect to distribution within family units. This was to investigate whether the observed effects might be genetically determined rather than related to the potential exposure. Cluster analysis of clinical data and various immunological parameters (T, B and lymphocytes without surface markers. T and B lymphocyte function [PHA, ConA, and PWM], and levels of immunoglobulins [IgG, IgA, and IgM]) were performed for husbands and wives in the 101 family units (Table II).

RESULTS
Clinical Manifestations

A high prevalence of clinical symptoms was found among the adult Michigan subjects (Table III). Four major categories of symptoms were recognized in particular: neurological, musculoskeletal, dermatological, and gastrointestinal. Neurological symptoms were the most prominent and included fatigue, decreased capacity for physical and intellectual work, increased sleeping time, memory impairment, headaches, dizziness, and irritability. Musculoskeletal symptoms consisted of arthritis-like abnormalities including swelling of joints with deformities in some cases, joint pain, and various degrees of movement limitation in knees, ankles, fingers, and hands. The prevalence of symptoms among dairy product consumers was similar to that among dairy farmers [13–15]. Significant differences, however, were found in the prevalence of most symptoms between the Michigan dairy farmers and the Wisconsin control group.

Immunological Findings

Significant deviations from normal in both percentage and absolute number of T lymphocytes were observed in subgroups of PBB-exposed Michigan dairy farm residents and chemical workers [5–7]. Thirty-four percent of the farm residents and 59% of the chemical workers manifested reduced T-cell and increased null cell values. The percentages and absolute numbers of T and B lymphocytes and lymphocytes without detectable surface markers (null cells) measured in the Michigan general population group were, in most cases, within the normal range. Direct occupational (chemical workers) and indirect (Michigan farm residents and consumers) exposure to PBB also resulted in various degrees of abnormalities in cell-mediated immunity. Marked decreases were observed in lymphocyte responses to T and B cell-specific mitogens as well as in the proliferative T lymphocyte responses in the MLC reaction. Five subgroups emerged with levels of immune dysfunctions ranging from no or one abnormal function (subgroup 1) to the most serious multiple immune dysfunctions (subgroup 5) (Table IV).

Subgroup 2, consisting of 52 individuals with significantly reduced lymphocyte function of both T and B cells, showed a high prevalence of neurological and musculoskeletal symptoms. Subgroup 3 had numerical (T and null cells) and functional (T and B cells) defects in addition to multiple clinical symptoms. Increased levels of IgG and IgA (with prominent monospecific peak) were reflected in subgroup 4; C_3 levels in this group were elevated, while C_4 values were reduced. This aberration in serological profile was not accompanied by numerical or functional alterations in lymphocytes. The abnormalities found in this group were accompanied by significantly heightened in vivo response to recall antigens such as mumps, varidase, and multiple neurological and musculoskeletal symptoms. Subgroup 5 included 25 Michigan dairy farm residents with such serious dysfunctions as polyclonal hypergammaglobulinemia, reduced T-cell population and dysfunction, and an increased number of null cells (Table V).

The plasma levels of PBB in the subgroups ranged between 0.6 and 70 ppb; in 25% of the subjects an increase in PBB levels was noted between 1976 and 1978. There was no apparent relationship between serum PBB levels and the prevalance of clinical symptoms and/or immunobiological findings. However, the PBB content of white blood cells, particularly in the apolipoprotein B fraction of the affected individuals, appeared to correlate with the most severe immune dysfunction(s) [9, 16–18].

The Persistence of Immune Dysfunction in Michigan Dairy Farm Residents Exposed to Polybrominated Biphenyls

The original Michigan farm residents and the controls were examined on two separate occasions in 1976 and again in 1981. This enabled us to study the persistence of immunological abnormalities. Seventeen of the 40 Michigan farmers examined at these times showed devia-

TABLE IV. Breakdown of Michigan Dairy Farm Residents (N = 331) According to Abnormal Values on Immune Parameters

Subgroup	Michigan farm residents
1. No or only one abnormal immune parameter	199
2. Low lymphocyte stimulation induced by PHA, Con A, PWM with normal surface markers (T, B, and null cells)	52
3. Low lymphocyte stimulation induced by PHA, Con A, PWM, with abnormal surface markers (T and null cells)	30
4. Increased levels of IgG, IgA, C_3, LOW C_4, with normal surface markers (T, B, and null cells) and lymphocyte function (PHA, Con A, and PWM)	25
5. Increased levels of IgG, C_3, with abnormal surface markers (T and null cells) and lymphocyte function (PHA, Con A)	25

TABLE V. Mean and Standard Deviation Values* of Immunological Parameters in Subgroup 5

Subjects	IgG (mg/dl)	IgA (mg/dl)	C_3	T cells (%)	Null cells (%)	PHA (cpm $\times$ 10^{-3})	Con A (cpm $\times$ 10^{-3})
Control	924 ± 264	174 ± 80	76.9 ± 21	69.1 ± 4.6	11.4 ± 1.2	99 ± 18	94.0 ± 19
PBB-exposed dairy farm residents							
With normal serology, number, and lymphocytes	1,223 ± 266	202 ± 68	101 ± 32	69.8 ± 6.1	10.1 ± 8	97.6 ± 22	91.2 ± 17
	(510–1,700)	(54–261)	(33–120)				
With abnormal serology, number, and lymphocytes	2,519 ± 632†	451 ± 172†	1,512 ± 27	48.0 ± 7.9	36.5 ± 9.3	50.7 ± 7.2	54.9 ± 7.8
Lymphocyte functions	1,829–4,085	382–666	129–234	36–60	21–49	10–68	30–62

*Ranges are given in parentheses.
†Difference between control and the study group is statistically significant p < .001.

tions from the normal range in both percentage and absolute number of T lymphocytes. Also, significant group differences were found between PBB-exposed subjects and control populations with respect to percentage and total number of T lymphocytes. On both occasions, the Michigan farmers fell within the normal range with regard to B lymphocytes.

A second important feature of lymphocytes among the PBB-exposed farmers was a marked prevalence of lymphocytes without detectable surface markers (null cells). The functional integrity of PBL was assessed by lymphoblastogenesis to mitogens (phytohemagglutinin [PHA] for T cells and pokeweed mitogen [PWM] for B cells). Differences between control group and PBB-exposed subjects were significant for both parameters in 1976 and 1981. Fifteen of the 39 Michigan farmers exhibited persistently lower PHA values. The persistence of this effect was further reflected in the high correlations between the two surveys for both T-cell ($r = 0.87$, $P = 0.01$) and B-cell functions ($r = 0.85$, $P = 0.01$). In a large number of cases a decreased response to the T-cell mitogen was accompanied by a corresponding decrease in the number of T lymphocytes [6,7].

While no significant abnormalities were found in the number of B lymphocytes among PBB-exposed individuals, a functional anomaly reflected by a decreased response to the B-cell mitogen was observed. This could represent either a defect in the B cells per se and/or some alteration in the ratio between helper T-cell and suppressor T-cell subpopulations.

Family Clustering of Immune Dysfunction and Clinical Symptoms

Strong family clustering was noted for abnormalities in the immunological, neurological, and musculoskeletal systems for husbands and wives. Moreover, there were significant correlations between multiple symptoms and immune dysfunctions for both sexes, independent of age and serum or fat levels of PBB [7,9,19,20]. Intrafamily clustering was similarly observed for serum and adipose PBB levels of quarantine and nonquarantined families. This suggested the importance of a common dietary source rather than genetic factors for the observed multiple clinical symptoms and immune dysfunctions in Michigan dairy farm populations exposed to PBB.

DISCUSSION

Based on longitudinal studies of PBB-exposed Michigan farmers, the presence of a toxic syndrome related to this chemical has been established. This investigation identified, for the first time, the presence of a "human toxic PBB syndrome" characterized by effects on the neurological and musculoskeletal organ systems in a large segment of the Michigan residents. The low numbers and impaired function of T lymphocytes observed some 8 years after the onset of PBB exposure in this group of Michigan dairy farm residents suggest persistence of a PBB-induced immune deficiency.

The persistence of symptoms and immunological manifestations is of interest and warrants follow-up investigations. It is also known that PBB is transmitted to nursing infants via breast milk. The long-term health effects of the described PBB exposure in both adults and children have not yet been assessed, and this matter requires future epidemiological surveillance. The long latency between exposure to potential carcinogens and its clinical effects should be recognized in this regard.

ACKNOWLEDGMENTS

This work was supported by NIEHS grant NO1-ES-9-0004 and in part by the T.J. Martell Memorial Foundation for Leukemia and Cancer Research.

The authors gratefully acknowledge the technical assistance of Mrs. Sophie Kurdziel, the editorial help of Mrs. Susan Zanjani, and the secretarial assistance of Ms. Diane Andujar.

REFERENCES

1. Carter LT. Michigan's PBB incident: Chemical mix-up leads to disaster. Science 1976; 192:240–3.
2. Dunckel AE. An updating on the polybrominated biphenal disaster in Michigan. J Am Vet Med Assoc 1975; 167:838–41.
3. Sundstrom G, Hutzinger O, Safe S. Environmental chemistry of flame retardants. II. Identification of 2, 2′, 4, 4′, 5, 5′-hexabromobiphenyl as the major constituent of flame retardant Firemaster BP-6. Chemosphere 1976; 5:11–4.
4. Jackson TF, Halbert FL. A toxic syndrome associated with the feeding of polybrominated biphenals-contaminated concentrate to dairy cattle. J Am Vet Med Assoc 1974; 165:437–9.
5. Bekesi JG, Holland JF, Anderson HA, et al. Lymphocyte function of Michigan dairy farmers exposed to polybrominated biphenyls. Science 1978; 199:1207–9.
6. Bekesi JG, Roboz JP, Solomon J, Fischbein A, Roboz J, Selikoff IJ. Persistent immune dysfunction in Michigan dairy farm residents exposed to polybrominated biphenyls. In Hadden JW, Chedid L, Ducor P, Spreafiro S, Willoughby D, eds: Advances in immunopharmacology, New York: Pergamon Press, 1983: 33–9.
7. Bekesi JG, Roboz JP, Solomon S, Fischbein AS, Selikoff IJ. Altered immune function in Michigan residents exposed to polybrominated biphenyls. In Gibson GG, Hubbard R, Parke DV, eds. Immunotoxicology. New York: Academic Press, 1983: 181–91.
8. Kreiss K, Roberts C, Humphrey HEB. Serial polybrominated biphenyl levels, polychlorinated biphenyl levels and clinical chemistries in the polybrominated biphenyl cohort of Michigan (USA). Arch Environ Health 1982; 37:141–7.
9. Roboz J, Suzuki RK, Bekesi JG, Holland JF, Rosenman K, Selikoff IJ. Mass spectral identification and quantification of polybrominated biphenyls in blood compartments of exposed Michigan chemical workers. J Environ Pathol Toxicol Oncol 1979; 3:363–78.
10. Kay K. Polybrominated biphenyls (PBB) environmental contamination in Michigan. Environ Res 1977; 13:74–93.
11. Trosko JE, Dawson B, Chang CC. PBB inhibits metabolic cooperation in Chinese hamster cells in vitro: Its potential as a tumor promoter. Environ Health Perspect 1981; 37:179–82.
12. Tsushimoto G, Trosko JE, Change CC, Aust SD. Inhibition of metabolic cooperation in Chinese hamster V79 cells in culture by various polybrominated biphenyl (PBB) congeners. Carcinogenesis 1982; 3:181–6.
13. Anderson HAR, Lilis R, Selikoff IJ, Rosenman KD, Valciukas JA, Freedman S. Unanticipated prevalence of symptoms among dairy farmers in Michigan and Wisconsin. Environ Health Perspect 1978; 23:217–26.
14. Lilis R, Anderson HA, Valciukas JA, Freedman S, Selikoff IJ. Comparison of findings among residents on Michigan dairy farms and consumers of produce purchased from these farms. Environ Health Perspect 1978; 23:105–9.
15. Humphrey HEB, Hayner NS. Polybrominated biphenyls: an agricultural incident and its consequences. An epidemiological investigation of human exposure. Lansing, MI: Michigan Department of Health, 1974.
16. Roboz J, Greaves J, Holland JF, Bekesi JG. Determination of polybrominated biphenyls in serum by negative chemical ionization mass spectrometry. Anal Chem 1982; 54:1104–8.
17. Greaves J, Bekesi JG, Roboz J. Halogen anion formation by polybrominated compounds in negative chemical ionization mass spectrometry. Biomed Mass Spectrom 1982; 9:406–10.
18. Wolff MS, Anderson HA, Selikoff IJ. Human tissue burdens of halogenated aromatic chemicals in Michigan. JAMA 1982; 247:2112–6.
19. Wolff MS, Haymes N, Anderson HA, Selikoff IJ. Family clustering of PBB and DDE values among Michigan dairy farmers. Environ Health Perspect 1978; 23:315–9.
20. Wolff MS, Anderson HA, Camper E, et al. Analysis of adipose tissue and serum from PBB (polybrominated biphenal) exposed workers. J Environ Pathol Toxicol Oncol 1979; 2:1397–411.

Cancer Detection and Prevention Supplement 1:39–42 (1987)

Immunocompetence in Pregnancy:
Production of Interleukin-2 by Peripheral Blood Lymphocytes

G.J. Hauser, MD
A. Lidor, MD
V. Zakuth, MSc
H. Rosenberg, PhD

T. Bino, PhD
M.P. David, MD
Z. Spirer, MD

Pediatric Immunology Unit (G.J.H., V.Z., Z.S.) and Department of Obstetrics and Gynecology "B" (A.L., M.P.D.), Tel-Aviv Medical Center and The Leon Alcalay Chair in Pediatric Immunology, Tel-Aviv University, Tel-Aviv; the Israel Institute for Biological Research, Ness-Ziona, Israel (H.R., T.B.)

ABSTRACT   Pregnancy is a natural allograft and the mechanisms for its non-rejection are obscure. Depression of maternal cellular immunity was suggested as a possible explanation. Interleukin-2(IL-2) is a lymphokine release from OKT4+ lymphocyte. This factor has a crucial role in the proliferation and differentiation of T cell subsets, and controls functions associated with immune rejection mechanisms. We therefore examined the ability of lymphocytes from women in the 3 trimesters of pregnancy to produce IL-2 in culture. Mononuclear cells were cultured with PHA for 48 h. The IL-2-containing supernatant was added to and supported the proliferation of an IL-2 dependent T cell line. Proliferation of this line indicated the IL-2 content of the added supernatant. Using this assay, IL-2 production in all 3 trimesters of pregnancy was adequate and comparable to that of lymphocytes from non-pregnant women. These results suggest that the proposed defect in cellular immunity during pregnancy is not mediated by an inability of the lymphocytes to produce IL-2.

Key words: tolerance, immunity, lymphocytes

INTRODUCTION

After many years of research in reproductive immunology, the mechanisms leading to nonrejection of the fetal allograft are still obscure [1]. Depression of maternal cellular immunity during pregnancy has been sought to explain the survival of this allotransplantation. Such depression may be induced by an intrinsic block of the maternal immune system or by humoral suppressing agents originating in either the fetus [2] or the mother [3].

Interleukin-2 (IL-2) is a lymphokine released by T lymphocytes after stimulation with mitogen or antigen. It has a crucial role in the proliferation and differentiation of the various T cell subsets. Through this involvement, IL-2 controls many cellular and humoral immune functions, including graft rejection [4].

Address reprint requests to Vera Zakuth, Pediatric Immunology Lab, P.O. Box 51, Tel-Aviv, Israel.

We examined the ability of lymphocytes from pregnant women to produce IL-2 in culture to assess immunocompetence in pregnancy.

MATERIALS AND METHODS
Patients

Thirty-one pregnant healthy women who came for a routine check-up were asked to participate in the study and signed informed consent forms. None had a history of recurrent abortions or sterility. Twelve were in the first trimester of pregnancy, ten in the second trimester, and nine in the third trimester. Ten healthy nonpregnant women, volunteers of the hospital staff, served as controls. The age range of the patient groups was 17–40 years (means 24.8, 30.7 and 29.4 years for the first, second, and third trimester groups, respectively). The age range in the control group was 23–37 years (mean 28.1 years).

Separation of Mononuclear Cells

Mononuclear cells were obtained from the heparinized peripheral venous blood by Ficoll-Paque gradient centrifugation, as previously described [5].

Interleukin-2 Production

Mononuclear cells from pregnant women and controls (10^6 cells/ml) were cultured for 48 hr with PHA-M (Wellcome) at a dose of 1 μg/ml. The supernatants were then harvested and added to IL-2-dependent long-term cultured mouse T cells (CTLL-2), placed in 96-well flat-bottomed microtiter plates (5×10^3 cells/well). The cultures were pulsed the last 4 hr with ^{3}H-thymidine (1 μCi/well), harvested after 24 hr, and counted in a liquid scintillation counter.

RESULTS

The mean age of the three pregnancy groups did not differ significantly from that of the control group. The amount of IL-2 secreted by the cultured lymphocytes into the supernatant is indicated by the proliferation of the IL-2-dependent mouse T cells to which the supernatant was added.

The supernatant obtained from lymphocyte cultures from pregnant women and controls (diluted 1:2 and 1:4) contained comparable titers of IL-2, indicating normal IL-2 production by the lymphocytes during pregnancy (Fig. 1.).

DISCUSSION

Attempts to elucidate the exact mechanisms through which survival of the fetal allograft is maintained have been so far unsuccessful. Current theories suggest that depression of the maternal cellular immune response may be responsible for this nonrejection [6]. The delayed rejection of skin allografts reported during pregnancy [7] as well as the depressed response to intradermal tuberculin [8] support these theories. In vitro studies have shown impairment of cellular immunity during pregnancy. The percentage of T and B lymphocytes was found to be normal [9], but lymphocyte proliferation after mitogenic stimulation and in the mixed leukocyte cultures was found to be depressed [10,11], and the proportions of suppressor and helper cells were abnormal [3]. The true clinical significance of these findings has, however, been questioned [1].

IL-2 is a lymphokine released by sensitized lymphocytes. It controls the differentiation and proliferation of T lymphocytes [4], affects natural killer cell activity [12], and influences the production of other lymphokines such as γ-interferon [13]. Because of its vast range of action, IL-2 has gained recognition as an important factor in the regulation and control of the normal immune response.

We have shown that cultured lymphocytes obtained from pregnant women are capable of producing sufficient IL-2 in culture. The lymphocytes in our study were cultured in the absence of maternal serum, so one cannot rule out the possibility of an in vivo depression of

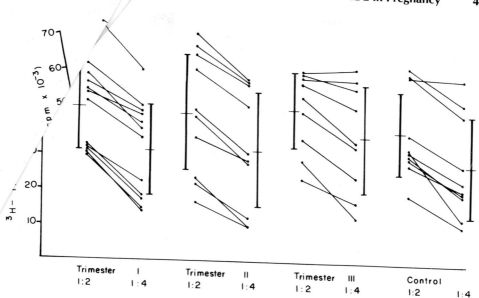

Fig. 1. Interleukin-2 production by cultured lymphocytes from pregnant women and controls, expressed by the proliferation of an IL-2–dependent mouse T cell line to which the IL-2 containing supernatant was added in two dilutions (1:2 and 1:4).

IL-2 production during pregnancy by a blocking factor present in maternal serum. Indeed, Nicholas et al [14] have shown that human pregnancy serum inhibits IL-2 production by lymphocytes from nonpregnant donors. Since it has been reported that normal human serum also has an inhibitory effect on IL-2 production, the true significance of the findings of Nicholas et al is yet to be proved [15]. Nevertheless, evidence of humoral immunosuppressive agents present in maternal serum are constantly emerging. These factors may originate from maternal suppressor cells [12], fetal suppressor cells [2], decidual cells [16], or perhaps steroid hormones [17].

The relevance of these in vitro findings to the clinical setting is yet to be determined. Hopefully they will be of some help in the future management of women with unexplained recurrent abortions in whom an immune-related pathogenesis has already been implicated [18].

REFERENCES

1. Sargent IL, Redman CWG. Maternal cell mediated immunity to the fetus in human pregnancy. J Reprod Immunol 1985; 7:95–104.
2. Froelich CJ, Goodwin JS, Bankhurst AD, Williams RC. Pregnancy, a temporal fetal graft of suppressor cells in autoimmune disease. Am J Med 1980; 69:329–31.
3. Hirahara F, Gorai I, Tanaka K, et al. Cellular immunity in pregnancy: Subpopulations of T lymphocytes bearing Fc receptors for IgG and IgM in pregnant women. Clin Exp Immunol 1980; 41:353–7.
4. Watson J, Mochizuki D. Interleukin-2: A class of T cell growth factors. Immunol Rev 1980; 51:257–78.
5. Boyum A. Isolation of mononuclear cells and granulocytes from human blood. Scand J Clin Lab Invest 1968; 21 [Suppl 97]:77–89.
6. Mukherjee AB, Laki K, Agrawal AR. Possible mechanism of success of an allotransplantation in nature: Mammalian pregnancy. Med Hypoth 1980; 6:1043–55.
7. Andersen RH, Monroe CW. Experimental study of the behaviour of adult human skin homografts during pregnancy. Am J Obstet Gynecol 1962;84: 1096–9.

8. Finn G, Hill CA, StGoven GJ, et al. Immunological responses in pregnancy and survival of fetal homograft. Br Med J 1972; 3:150–2.
9. Birkeland SA, Kristoffersen K. T and B lymphocytes during normal pregnancy: longitudinal study. Scand J Immunol 1979; 10:415–9.
10. Tomoda Y, Fuma M, Muva T, et al. Cell mediated immunity in pregnant women. Gynecol Invest 1976; 7:280–4.
11. Kasakura S. A factor in maternal plasma during pregnancy that suppresses the reactivity of mixed leukocyte cultures. J Immunol 1971; 107:1296–301.
12. Domzig W, Stadler BM, Herberman RB. Interleukin-2 dependence of human natural killer (NK) cell activity. J Immunol 1983; 130:1970–3.
13. Reem GH, Yeh NH. Interleukin-2 regulates expression of its receptor and synthesis of gamma interferon by human T lymphocytes. Science 1984; 225:429–30.
14. Nicholas NS, Panayi GS, Nouri ME. Human pregnancy serum inhibits Interleukin-2 production. Clin Exp Immunol 1984; 58:587–95.
15. Rodrick ML, Saporoschetz I, Wood JJ, et al. Inhibition of human interleukin-2 (IL-2) production and action by human serum. Lymphokine Res 1984; 3:269 (Abstr).
16. Golander A, Zakuth V, Shechter Y, Spirer Z. Suppression of lymphocyte reactivity in vitro by a soluble factor secreted by explants of human decidua. Eur J Immunol 1981; 11:849–51.
17. Lawrence R, Church JA, Richards W, Borzy M. Immunological mechanisms in the maintenance of pregnancy. Ann Allergy 1980; 44:166–72.
18. Rocklin RE, Kitzmuller JC, Carpenter CB, et al. Maternal-fetal relation. Absence of an immunologic blocking factor from the serum of women with chronic abortions. N Engl J Med 1976; 295:1209–11.

Cancer Detection and Prevention Supplement 1:43–49 (1987)

Influence of Factor Substitution on the B-Cell Response in Hemophiliacs

J. Kekow, MD
H. Plendl, MD
W.L. Gross, MD

Departments of Internal Medicine (J.K., W.L.G.) and Human Genetics (H.P.), Christian Albrecht University, Kiel, Federal Republic of Germany

ABSTRACT Studies in hemophiliacs receiving factor concentrates demonstrated T-cell defects in vitro. Recently, B-cell dysfunctions were described in AIDS and pre-AIDS and in some hemophiliacs. To investigate the B-cell function in hemophiliacs in relation to factor substitution, we examined five patients with mild (substitution < 20,000 U/year) and seven with severe (> 100,000 U/year) hemophilia A and compared the data with normal control individuals. The B-cell proliferative response (^{3}H-thymidine uptake) to *Staphylococcus aureus* Cowan I and the differentiation response (Ig secretion into culture supernatants) to T-cell-dependent or -independent polyclonal B-cell activators (PBAs) were studied in vitro. In contrast to T-cell dysfunctions, which correlate with the amount of clotting factor concentrates, the B-cell proliferative response was not affected. Stimulation with PBAs however failed to increase elevated spontaneous IgG levels and showed a diminished increase in IgM levels in severe, but not in mild, hemophilia. Our data give evidence of a T-cell-independent B-cell dysfunction in asymptomatic hemophiliacs that correlates with factor substitution.

Key words: B-cell function, HTLV III/LAV, AIDS, hemophilia

INTRODUCTION

Patients with hemophilia receiving factor concentrates are reported to show opportunistic infections and malignancies (eg, Kaposi sarcoma) with an incidence of about 0.8% [1]. In a high percentage of cases, HTLV III/LAV antibodies have been detected in hemophiliacs, suggesting contact with this retrovirus considered to be the most likely cause of the acquired immunodeficiency syndrome (AIDS) [2]. As in the case of AIDS, the examination of immunologic abnormalities in otherwise healthy hemophiliacs revealed T-cell abnormalities and evidence of abnormal B-cell function, as reported recently by Brieva et al [3] and Seki et al [4].

To evaluate the nature of abnormal B-cell activation, we applied a previously reported model of human B-cell activation to hemophiliacs receiving different amounts of factor

Address reprint requests to Dr. W.L. Gross, I. Medizinische Klinik, Klinikum der CAU, Schittenhelmstrasse 12, D-23 Kiel, Federal Republic of Germany.

concentrates. This model works in a T-cell-independent polyclonal manner [5,6] and uses membrane preparations of gram-negative bacteria. With mice, Mosier et al [7] recently demonstrated that T-cell-independent polyclonal B-cell activators (PBAs) are a useful tool for elaborating B-cell function after infection with a retrovirus. Although the B-cell proliferative response was normal in all the patients we investigated, the B-cell differentiation response showed an abnormal pattern, which correlated with the annual consumption of factor VIII concentrates.

MATERIALS AND METHODS
Patients

Twelve asymptomatic patients with hemophilia A were investigated. Seven severely affected hemophiliacs were being treated prophylactically with factor concentrates. The moderately affected cases received concentrates on demand. Table I contains detailed clinical aspects and the preliminary laboratory evaluation. A control group consisted of healthy heterosexual men paired by age.

Cell Preparation and Culture Conditions

Mononuclear cells (MNC) were separated by Ficoll-hypaque gradient centrifugation [8] and cultivated in microtiter plates (2×10^5 MNC in 200 μl per well) at 37°C in a 5% CO_2-95% air humidified atmosphere. For stimulation, *Staphylococcus aureus* Cowan I (SAC) (Calbiochem, Frankfurt/Main Federal Republic of Germany), pokeweed mitogen (PWM) (Difco, Detroit, MI), concanavalin A (Con A) (Difco), or a membrane preparation of A-*Streptococcus* (AScM) was added [for details, see 8]. For T-cell-independent B-cell differentiation, *Klebsiella* and *Salmonella* membrane preparations (Klebs M, Salm) were employed [for detailed methods, see 6]. All cultures were carried out in triplicate.

Lymphocyte Proliferation Assay

DNA synthesis was determined by measuring ^{3}H-thymidine incorporation. The culture periods (SAC 3 days, PWM 5 days) were terminated after a 4 hr pulse with 0.5 μCi/well. The trichloroacetic acid-insoluble ^{3}H-thymidine in the cells was collected on Millipore filters and radioactivity counted in a liquid scintillation counter.

Lymphocyte Differentiation Assay

Secreted immunoglobulins (IgM and IgG) in culture supernatants were assessed by ELISA [9]. After a 6 day culture period, appropriate dilutions of culture supernatants were transferred into microtiter plates, precoated with anti-IgM or anti-IgG, and incubated overnight. Following extensive washing, anti-IgM or anti-IgG peroxidase conjugates were added. Two hours later, the plates were washed and orthophenylendiamindihydrochloride was added as substrate. Then extinction was measured at 492 nm.

Statistics

The results of the different groups were compared, and the significance was analyzed with Wilcoxon's rank sum test. Correlation coefficients were calculated according to Spearman. Data are expressed as arithmetic means $\pm$ SEM when appropriate.

RESULTS

Table II shows details of the proliferation studies. MNC were stimulated with PWM or SAC, and, for comparison, with Con A and AScM. Similar to PWM, a T-cell-dependent B-cell mitogen, SAC, a T-cell-independent B-cell mitogen [10], induced significant ^{3}H-thymidine uptake (stimulation index > 3 [11]) in all groups of hemophiliacs investigated. In addition, Con A and AScM induced substantial blastogenesis. The statistical analysis (P $\leqslant$ 0.01) did not demonstrate any differences between the hemophiliacs and the control group.

TABLE I. Main Clinical Characteristics and Laboratory Data of the Hemophiliacs

Group	Age ($\overline{X}$)	Clinical features	Serum immuno-globulins (mg/dl)*	No delayed cut. hypersensitivity[†]	Ratio OKT4/OKT8[‡] (range)	HTLV III antibodies[§]
Moderate hemophilia A	45 (range 36–58)	Factor VIII substitution <20,000 U/year	IgA 222 ± 20 IgG 1,425 ± 97 IgM 149 ± 34	1/5	1.6 (1.0–2.3)	0/5
Severe hemophilia A	25 (range 16–42)	Factor VIII substitution >100,000 U/year PGL (2/7)	IgA 297 ± 46 IgG 3,024 ± 423 IgM 175 ± 15	5/7	0.8 (0.4–1.5)	5/7

*Normal values: IgA 90–450, IgG 800–1,800, IgM 69–280 mg/dl. Results are expressed as means ± SEM.
[†]Response to three different antigens, namely Mumps, *Candida*, SK-SD.
[‡]Detected by indirect immunofluorescence and monoclonal antibodies (Ortho, Heidelberg); values of the control group: $\overline{X}$ = 2.0 (1.6–2.4).
[§]HTLV III antibodies were kindly investigated by Dr. Vettermann, Robert-Koch-Institut (West Berlin) using ELISA [12].

TABLE II. Proliferative and Differentiation Responses of Mononuclear Cells From Hemophiliacs*

Stimulant	Dose	Control group (n = 6)	Moderate hemophilia (n = 5)	Severe hemophilia (n = 7)
Proliferative response (cpm)				
None (day 3)		568 ± 98	287 ± 90	275 ± 84
SAC	1:5000 v/v	2,898 ± 221	2,495 ± 645	2,037 ± 261
ConA	20.0 μg/ml	20,067 ± 8,192	11,579 ± 2,022	9,129 ± 1,585
None (day 5)		1,764 ± 289	1,258 ± 116	955 ± 183
PWM	1.5 μl/ml	9,373 ± 2,043	12,131 ± 2,957	12,601 ± 1,861
AScM	100.0 μg/ml	13,794 ± 3,728	19,183 ± 1,996	10,906 ± 3,404
Differentiation response (IgG; ng/ml)				
None		126 ± 49	408 ± 78	762 ± 220
PWM	1.5 μl/ml	969 ± 243	1,095 ± 346	926 ± 211
Klebs M	100.0 μl/ml	1,032 ± 192	2,026 ± 578	587 ± 143
Salm	100.0 μl/ml	1,193 ± 173	1,928 ± 722	677 ± 129
Differentiation response (IgM; ng/ml)				
None		199 ± 46	127 ± 24	136 ± 47
PWM	1.5 μl/ml	1,113 ± 190	1,172 ± 358	445 ± 117
Klebs M	100.0 μl/ml	4,182 ± 491	1,952 ± 505	458 ± 96
Salm	100.0 μl/ml	5,140 ± 898	1,205 ± 368	408 ± 87

*Results are expressed as means ± SEM

The Ig levels of the supernatants were calculated by ELISA. The spontaneous IgG levels were remarkably high, especially in the hemophiliacs who were treated prophylactically. In this group, stimulation with PWM, and especially Klebs M and Salm, two T-cell-independent polyclonal B-cell activators [5,6] failed to increase the spontaneous IgG levels. In contrast, in the moderate forms of hemophilia, the initial IgG levels increased by a factor of 2.5–5 after stimulation with PWM, Klebs M, or Salm. No characteristic increase in the IgM isotype could be observed in unstimulated cultures from the hemophiliacs. When PWM was used, the hemophiliacs receiving continuous factor VIII substitution responded weakly in comparison with the other hemophiliacs and the control group. The same results were obtained using Klebs M or Salm for stimulation. The moderately affected hemophiliacs showed a decreased IgM production compared with the control group after the application of Klebs M or Salm for stimulation. Nevertheless, these responses ranged from nine to 15 times above the spontaneous level (for detailed results, see Table II). A positive correlation between Klebs M/Salm-induced IgG/IgM production in the hemophiliacs and their annual consumption of clotting factor was found (Klebs M $P < 0.01/P < 0.01$, Salm $P < 0.1/P < 0.01$).

DISCUSSION

This study demonstrates a B-cell dysfunction in hemophiliacs that correlates with the annual consumption of factor VIII concentrates. Although none of our hemophiliacs could be diagnosed as having AIDS or an AIDS-related complex [for definition, see 13], a number of these patients had persistent generalized lymph node enlargement. The severely affected hemophiliacs showed immunologic abnormalities similar to those seen in AIDS: no delayed type cutaneous hypersensitivity responses to recall antigens, an inverse ratio of T4/T8-positive cells, and elevated serum IgG levels. HTLV III antibodies could not be detected in moderate hemophilia, whereas five of seven patients with severe hemophilia were positive for HTLV III. The in vitro study of two different steps in the B-cell maturation process, the proliferative and the differentiation responses, revealed normal B-cell proliferation but an impaired differentiation response to T-cell-independent PBAs in all patients. Characteristic of the severely affected hemophiliacs were the elevated spontaneous IgG levels in the culture supernatants with no further elevation after stimulation with several PBAs. However, in concordance with the normal serum IgM values, no increased IgM secretion into the culture supernatants was found. Furthermore, stimulation with all PBAs used so far resulted in merely a threefold increase in IgM. In the moderately affected hemophiliacs, the IgG levels in culture supernatants ranged between the normal controls and severe hemophilia when no stimulant was added. However, their MNCs did respond to PWM, Klebs M, or Salm.

T-cell-independent B-cell dysfunctions in AIDS were first reported by Lane et al in 1983 [14]. These now occupy a substantial portion of the reviews on the wide spectrum of immunologic abnormalities in AIDS [15]. Both the proliferative and the differentiation responses are affected, and these findings are thought to be a result of polyclonal B-cell activation in vivo by the numerous infective agents (eg, Epstein-Barr virus, etc) commonly seen in AIDS. Recently, we found these abnormal B-cell functions in homosexuals before symptoms of ARC/AIDS were apparent [16]. The detection of the HTLV III retrovirus in B-cell fractions or B-cell lines [17–19] suggests the possibility of a direct interference with these lymphocytes and therefore another source of B-cell dysfunction.

Previous studies undertaken in hemophiliacs focused on phenotypical and functional aspects of the T-cell system. Many investigators reported phenotypical abnormalities correlating with the amount of clotting factor concentrates [20–22]. Only a few investigators have dealt with the humoral immune response in hemophiliacs, especially those patients who are more likely to develop AIDS because they have HTLV III antibodies. Allogenetic coculture experiments using B cells from hemophiliacs and T cells from normal controls in a PWM-driven system showed results similar to those reported by Lane et al in 1983 [14]., indicating a separate B-cell dysfunction [3]. With respect to T-cell abnormalities that influence the humoral response, Köller et al in 1985 [23] and Seki et al in 1984 [4] presented data showing increased numbers of in vivo activated T-suppressor cells in hemophiliacs. Other functional studies concerning proliferative capacities of lymphocytes from these patients gave evidence of some abnormalities, mainly in T lymphocytes [21]. We were able to confirm the data for a normal proliferative response to PWM [24] and extend these findings to stimulation with the B-cell mitogen SAC. The assessment of the B-cell differentiation response to true (ie, T-cell-independent) polyclonal B-cell activators produced results similar to those with PWM-driven allogenetic coculture experiments. However, our experiments indicate that the B cell appears to be refractory to B-cell activators, which bypass the network of B-cell-triggering T cells necessary for PWM-induced B-cell activation. An influence of large amounts of T8-positive cells on the Klebs M-induced differentiation response could be excluded, since former experiments have demonstrated that this PBA-response is absolutely independent of T-suppressor cell influences [25].

The underlying event(s) of the apparent immunologic abnormalities in hemophiliacs is subject to speculation. The first studies comparing immune dysfunction and the detection of HTLV III antibodies failed to find a correlation [22]. It has been stressed that the presence of antibodies to HTLV III can indicate immunization, infection, or an asymptomatic carrier state [2]. The lymphocyte dysfunction in our patients clearly correlates with the substitution doses of factor VIII concentrates needed per annum and could also be related to our HTLV III antibody results. This suggests that the abnormalities were caused primarily by the retrovirus. The two HTLV III-negative patients would then have to be interpreted as having a severe immune defect rendering them incapable of producing specific antibodies. This explanation, however, does not fit the healthy clinical appearance of our patients. The hypothesis that B cells can be activated by recurrent viral infections (eg, Epstein-Barr virus, cytomegalovirus, herpes simplex virus) may be considered for homosexuals. Hemophiliacs, however, do not show evidence of higher rates of these infections as compared with normal controls [3]. Thus in hemophiliacs a follow-up is necessary to elucidate the significance of the partial B-cell dysfunction, which is distinct from AIDS but obviously a reaction to the active/inactive HTLV III virus and/or a variety of allogenetic factors contained in the factor concentrates [26,27]. For abnormalities in the T-cell system, Ludlam et al [28] were recently able to demonstrate that an inverse T4/T8 ratio is also seen in hemophiliacs before HTLV III antibodies are present. From this point of view, the occurence of immunologic abnormalities in hemophiliacs, indicating an activated immune system, could support the hypothesis that infection with AIDS virus can be considered an opportunistic infection in an immunomodulated host [29].

ACKNOWLEDGMENTS

This work was supported by the BMFT "Forschungsförderung AIDS."

REFERENCES

 1. Jones P. Acquired immunodeficiency syndrome, hepatitis, and haemophilia. Br Med J 1983; 287:1737–8.
 2. Kitchen LW, Barin F, Sullivan JL, Mc Lane MF, Brettler DB, Levine PH, Essex M. Aetiology of AIDS–Antibodies to human T-cell leucaemia virus (type III) in haemophiliacs. Nature 1984; 312:367–9.
 3. Brieva JA, Sequi J, Zabay JM, Pardo A, Campos A, Luz de la Sen M, Bootello A. Abnormal B cell function in haemophiliacs and their relationship with factor concentrates administration. Clin Exp Immunol 1985; 59:491–8.
 4. Seki H, Taga K, Nagaoki T, Barot-Ciorbaru R, Miyawaki T, Taniguchi N. Some evidence for the in vivo functional activation of suppressor T cells in asymptomatic patients with hemophilia A receiving factor VIII concentrates. Clin Immunol Immunopathol 1985; 34:27–38.
 5. Chen WY, Fudenberg HH. Polyclonal activation of human peripheral blood B-lympocytes. III. Cellular interaction and immunoregulation of immunoglobulin-secreting cells induced by formalde-hyd-fixed Salmonella paratyphy B. Clin Immunol Immunopathol 1982; 22:279–90.
 6. Gross WL, Rucks A. Klebsiella pneumoniae stimulate highly purified human blood B cells to mature into plaque forming cells without prior proliferation. Clin Exp Immunol 1983; 52:372–80.
 7. Mosier DE, Yetter RA, Morse HC. Retroviral induction of acute lymphoproliferative disease and profound immunosuppression in adult C57/ B1/6 mice. J Exp Med 1985; 161:766–84.
 8. Gross WL. Lymphozytenantwort auf humanpathogene Streptokokkenantigenpräparationen. Stutt-gart; Thieme, 1982.
 9. Voller A, Bartlett A, Bidwell D. Enzyme immunoassay with special reference to ELISA techniques. J Clin Pathol 1978; 31:507–20.
10. Schuurman RKB, Gelfand EW, Dosch HM. Polyclonal activation of human lymphocytes in vitro. I. Characterisation of the lymphocyte response to a T-cell-independent B cell mitogen. J Immunol 1980; 125:820–6.
11. Ling NR, Kay JE. Lymphocyte stimulation. New York: Elsevier, North Holland, 1975; 179.
12. Sarngadharan MG, Popovic M, Bruch L, Schüpbach J, Gallo RC. Antibodies reactive with human T-lymphotrophic retroviruses (HTLV-III) in the serum of patients with AIDS. Science 1984; 224:506–8.
13. Quinn TC. Early symptoms and signs of AIDS and the AIDS-related complex. In Ebbesen P, Biggar RJ, Melbye M, eds: AIDS. Copenhagen: Munksgaard, 1984; 69–83.
14. Lane HC, Masur H, Edgar LC, Whalen G, Rook AH, Fauci AS. Abnormalities of B-cell activation and immunoregulation in patients with the acquired immunodeficiency syndrome. N Engl J Med 1983; 309:453–8.
15. Seligmann M, Chess L, Fahey JL, Fauci AS, Lachmann PJ, L'Age-Stehr J, Ngu J, Pinching AJ, Rosen FS, Spira TJ, Wybran J. AIDS—An immunologic reevaluation. N Engl J Med 1984; 311:1286–97.
16. Kekow J, Kern P, Dietrich M, Gross WL. T- und B-Zellreaktionen bei AIDS und AIDS-Risikogrup-pen. Immun Infekt 1985; 13:26–8.
17. Longo DL, Gelmann EP, Cossman J, Young RA, Gallo RC, O'Brian SJ, Matis LA. Isolation of HTLV-transformed B-lymphocyte clone from a patient with HTLV-associated adult T-cell leucae-mia. Nature 1984; 310:505–6.
18. Montagnier L, Gruest J, Charmaret S, Dauguet C, Acler C, Guétard D, Nugeyre MT, Barré-Sinoussi F, Chermann JC, Brunet JB, Klatzmann D, Gluckman JC. Adaptation of lymphadenopathy associated virus (LAV) to replication in EBV-transformed B lymphoblastoid cell lines. Science 1984; 225:63–6.

19. Volsky DJ, Sinangil F, Sonnabend J, Casareale D. Isolation of HTLV-III and EBV-positive B lymphoblastoid cell lines from peripheral blood lymphocytes of AIDS patients. Ann Intern Med (in press).

20. Lechner K, Niessner H, Bettelheim P, Deutsch E, Fasching I, Fuhrmann M, Hinterberger W, Korninger C, Neumann E, Liszka K, Knapp W, Mayr WR, Stingl G, Zeitlhuber U. T-cell alterations in haemophiliacs treated with commercial clotting factor concentrates. Thrombos Hemostas 1983; 50:553–6.

21. Lederman MM, Ratnoff OD, Scillan JJ, Jones PK, Schacter B. Impaired cell-mediated immunity in patients with classic haemophilia. N Engl J Med 1983; 308:79–83.

22. Tsoukas C, Gervais F, Shuster J, Gold P, O'Shaughnessy M, Robert-Guroff M. Association of HTLV-III antibodies and cellular immune status of haemophiliacs. N Engl J Med 1984; 311:1514–5.

23. Köller U, Majdic O, Liszka K, Stockinger H, Pabinger-Pasching I, Lechner K, Knapp W. Lymphocytes of haemophilia patients treated with clotting factor concentrates display activation—linked cell-surface antigens. Clin Exp Immunol 1985; 59:613–21.

24. Schneider H, Sutor AH, Thaiss H, Künzer W. Alterations of T-cell subsets in hemophiliacs during treatment. Blut 1984; 49:225–6.

25. Kekow J, Sieg J, van de Venn D, Gross WL. Regulation of B-cell activity in man induced by T cell-dependent and "true" polyclonal B-cell activators. I. Role of suppressor cells. Paper presented at the 14th Leukozytenkulturen Konferenz, Hamburg, März, 1984.

26. Kienast K, Trobisch H. Vergleichende proteinchemische Untersuchungen von Faktor VIII-Konzentraten. Arzneim-Forsch Drug Res 1984; 34:895–900.

27. Tilsner V, Reuter H. Neberwirkungen der Faktor VIII -Substitution bei Patienten mit Hämophilie A. Münch Med Wochenschr 1982; 124:553–7.

28. Ludlam CA, Steel CM, Cheinsong-Popov R, et al. Human T-lymphotrophic virus type III (HTLV-III) infection in seronegative haemophiliacs after transfusion of factor VIII. Lancet 1985; ii:233–6.

29. Levy JA, Ziegler JL. Acquired immune deficiency syndrome (AIDS) is an opportunistic infection and Kaposi's sarcoma results from secondary immune stimulation. Lancet 1983; ii:78–81.

Cancer Detection and Prevention Supplement 1:51–55 (1987)

Impaired Natural Killer Cytotoxicity During Recrudescence of Recurrent Herpes Simplex Virus Type 1 Infection

Yuh-Chi Kuo, MA
Ching-Yuang Lin, MD, PhD
Sai-Foo Cheng, MD
Ching-Chi Lin, MD
Wu-Tse Liu, PhD

Graduate Institute of Microbiology and Immunology, National Yang-Ming Medical College (Y.-C.K., W.-T.L.), Department of Medical Research (C.-Y.L.) and Department of Dermatology (S.-F.C.), Veterans General Hospital, and Department of Internal Medicine, Mackay Memorial Hospital (C.-C.L.), Taipei, Taiwan, Republic of China

ABSTRACT We investigated natural killer (NK) cytotoxicity in patients with recurrent herpes infection by using K562 cells infected with Herpes simplex virus type 1 (HSV-1) as target. The NK cytotoxicity was lower than during convalescence and in controls during recrudescence (0 to 3 days postonset of clinical symptoms; $P < 0.001$). In the convalescent phase (4 to 14 days postonset of symptoms) the NK cytotoxicity was significantly higher than in controls ($P < 0.05$). These results suggest that low NK cytotoxicity is related to the recurrence of herpes.

Key words: K562 cells, mononuclear cells, recrudescence

INTRODUCTION

Approximately one-half of individuals infected by herpes simplex virus (HSV) develop recurrent lesions that occur as a consequence of the reactiviation of the latent virus. Human defense against viral infection is related to the development of cell-mediated immunity, specific cellular cytotoxicity, and/or combined humoral and cellular immunity. However, one of the most important antiviral actions in the human defense system is natural killer (NK) cytotoxicity [1].

NK cells have been found in virtually all mammalian species tested, including nude mice, which lack mature T lymphocytes [2–7]. The NK cells are a particular subpopulation of lymphocytes that possess cytotoxic activity against a wide variety of targets, including transformed and virus-infected cells [8,9]. In man, as well as in mice, evidence is accumulating that NK cells may play an important role in antiviral defense, tumor immunity, and immune

Address reprint requests to Dr. Ching-Yuang Lin, Pediatric Research Laboratory, Department of Medical Research, Veterans General Hospital, Shih-Pai, Taipei, Taiwan 112, ROC.

surveillance [10–13] and may also be involved in the regulation of growth and differentiation of normal cells [8,14,15].

In an attempt to investigate the role of NK cells in patients with HSV infection, we used K562 cell infection with HSV-1 as a target cell and compared the NK cytotoxicity between recrudescence (0 to 3 days postonset of lesion) and convalescence (4 to 14 days postonset).

MATERIALS AND METHODS
Patient Population

Sixteen patients were included with a history of recurrent oral herpes (defined as at least four eruptions per year) seen from April to the end of September 1985. Their ages ranged from 10 to 40 years; there were six males and ten females. Diagnosis was made clinically and by cytologic findings of positive immunofluorescent staining with anti-HSV-1 antibody (M.A. Bioproducts, Maryland, U.S.A.). All patients were seropositive.

Twenty-three healthy, seropositive normal, age and sex-matched persons with no history of recurrent genital or facial herpetic lesions were used as controls.

Methods

All blood samples were taken during recrudescence (0 to 3 days postonset of clinical symptoms) and convalescence (4 to 14 days postonset of clinical symptoms). The NK cytotoxicity assay was performed as described previously [16]. Briefly mononuclear cells (MNC) at 2×10^6 cells/ml were suspended in RPMI 1640 plus 10% fetal calf serum (FCS) as target cells, and 1×10^6 cells of K562 were infected with 0.2 ml HSV-1 (KOS strain) at a multiplicity of 0.1 PFU/cell. After 18 hours of infection, the K562 cells infected with HSV-1 (K562-HSV-1) were labeled with ^{51}Cr (New England Nuclear Research Products, Boston, U.S.A.; 150 μCi for 1×10^6 cells) for 2 hours in a 37°C water bath, washed three times, and resuspended in RPMI 1640 plus 10% FCS at 1×10^5/ml as target cells. The infecting HSV-1 had been expressed on the surface of K562 cells, which was proved by immunofluorescent method. Effector (100 μl) cells were added to the round-bottomed microtiter plate wells, with dilutions for effector cells to target cells at ratios of 50:1 and 25:1. They were incubated for 4 hours at 37°C in a 5% CO$_2$ incubator. At the end of incubation the plates were centrifuged at 150g for 10 minutes, and 100 μl samples of the supernatant were harvested for counting in a gamma counter. Spontaneous release of ^{51}Cr from labeled K562 HSV-1 target cells was measured in RPMI 1640 plus 10% FCS with no added effector cells. Maximal lysis of the labeled K562 HSV-1 target cells was measured in 2% Triton X-100 (Sigma, St. Louis, MO). NK cytoxicity against K562 HSV-1 was calculated as

$$\% \text{ lysis} = \frac{\text{cpm (experimental lysis)} - \text{cpm (spontaneous release)}}{\text{cpm (maximal release)} - \text{cpm (spontaneous release)}} \times 100.$$

The differences between groups were assessed by the Student's t test or approximate t test.

RESULTS

To study the role that NK cells play in the defense against HSV infection, K562 cells were infected with HSV-1 and used as target cells. The direct immunofluoresence method was used to identify whether the HSV-1 infected K562 cells and expressed its antigen on the cell surface after 18 hours of infection. Then NK cell activities were assayed when E:T ratios were 50:1 and 25:1 during recrudescence and convalescence. As shown in Figure 1 and Table I the NK cytotoxicity distribution of 15 patients at recrudescence and convalescence were observed. The NK cell activity was lower during recrudescence than in the convalescent phase, with a

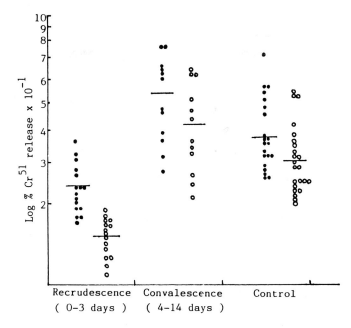

Fig. 1. NK cytotoxicity in normal control and in HSV-1 facial herpes patients during recrudescence and convalescence. ●, E:T ratio at 50:1; ○, E:T ratio at 25:1.

TABLE I. Comparison of the NK Cytotoxicity Between Recrudescence and Convalescence of Recurrent HSV-1 Facial Patients

NK cytotoxicity	Recrudescence (N = 16)	Convalescence (N = 12)	Controls (N = 23)
E:T = 25:1	11.88 ± 4.17*	41.75 ± 15.32*,§	31.65 ± 10.61§
E:T = 50:1	23.56 ± 6.45†	53.92 ± 17.46*,‡	38.22 ± 12.39‡

*,†Approximate t test is used (against same symbol, P < 0.001).
‡Student's t test is used (against same symbol, 0.005 < P < 0.01).
§Student's t test is used (against same symbol, 0.02 < P < 0.05).

significant decrease when E:T ratios were either 50:1 or 25:1. In the convalescent phase, the NK cytotoxicity was significantly higher than in controls (P < 0.001).

DISCUSSION

In this study, NK cytotoxicity was measured during the recrudescent and convalescent stages. During the recrudescent stage, the lesions in these patients were serious and the virus was highly active. Patients harboring herpes simplex are known to have neutralizing antibodies to this virus in their sera and saliva, but the antibodies do not protect against recurrent infections [17,18]. At the same time, cellular immunity plays an important role in the inhibition of virus activity [19,20]. Nevertheless, it is known that NK cells have the ability to inhibit tumor growth and viral infection. We therefore investigated NK cytotoxicity during the recrudescent and convalescent phases to understand the mechanism of frequent recurrences of infection with herpes simplex.

Because antigens of herpes simplex virus are related to cell-mediated immunity, the K562 cells were infected with HSV-1 and used as target cells [21]. Mononuclear cells were isolated from patients during the recrudescent and convalescent phases. Based on the results of the NK cytotoxicity assay, we concluded that NK cytotoxicity during recrudescence was lower than in the convalescent state and in normal controls. Possibly in recrudescence the T helper cell (T_h) had not been activated and did not proliferate. Corresponding lymphokines secreted by (T_h), for example, interleukin-2 (IL-2) were at low concentrations. Furthermore γ-interferon induced by IL-2 was also not increased. NK cell activity is related to IL-2 and γ-interferon [22–24]. The NK cytotoxicity in recrudesence was not enhanced by IL-2 and interferon and was therefore decreased. In contrast to recrudescence, in the convalescent state the NK cytotoxicity was higher than in normal controls. It may be suggested that 4 to 14 days after recrudescence the cellular immunity and humoral immunity were at the higest level, and the NK cytotoxicity was also elevated by increased IL-2 and γ-interferon. After 14 days, the NK cytotoxicity gradually decreased and was restored to the normal range. It is suggested that in clinical therapy enhancement of NK cytotoxicity may prevent and possibly cure the frequent recurrence of HSV infection.

Further studies of the immunobiological basis of these cellular immune responses and their roles may help to define the host factors that contribute to recurrent disease, in opposition to prolonged latency, and further elucidate the relationship between host immune functions and the control of latent viral infections.

ACKNOWLEDGMENTS

We thank the staff of the Laboratory of Clinical Virology, Veterans General Hospital, who helped us to identify the virus.

REFERENCES

1. Herberman RB, Djeu JY, Kay HD, et al. Natural killer cells: Characteristics and regulation of activity. Immunol Rev 1979; 44:43–70.
2. Kiessling R, Petrany G, Klein G, Wigzell H. Non-T-cell resistance against a mouse moloney lymphoma. Int J Cancer 1976; 17:275–81.
3. Warner NL, Woodruff MF, Burton RC. Inhibition of the growth of lymphoid tumors on syngeneic, athymic (nude) mice. Int J Cancer 1977; 20:146.
4. Minato N, Bloom Br, Jones C, Holland J, Reid LM. Mechanism of rejection of virus persistently infected tumor cells by athymic nude mice. J Exp Med 1979; 149:1117–33.
5. Zawatzky R, Hilfenhaus J, Kirchner H. Resistance of nude mice to herpes simplex virus and correlation with in vitro production of interferon. Cell Immunol 1979; 47:424–8.
6. Armerding D, Rossiter H. Induction of natural killer cells by HSV-2 in resistant and sensitive inbred mouse strains. Immunobiol 1981; 158:369.
7. Lopez C. Resistance to herpes simplex type 1. Curr Top Microbiol Immunol 1981; 92:15–24.
8. Kiessling R, Wigezell H. Surveillance of primitive cells by natural killer cells. Curr Top Microbiol Immunol 1981; 92:107–23.
9. Welsh RM. Natural cell-mediated immunity during viral infections. Curr Top Microbiol Immunol 1981; 92:83–106.
10. Nair PNM, Ferandes G, Onoe K, Day K, Good RA. Inhibition of effector cell functions in natural killer cell activity and antibody-dependent cell-mediated cytotoxicity in mice by normal and cancer sera. Int J Cancer 1981; 25:667–77.
11. Moore M, Vose BM. Extravascular natural cytotoxicity in man: anti-K562 activity if lymph node and tumor-infiltrating lymphocytes. Int J Cancer 1981; 27:265–72.
12. Ziegler HW, Kay NE, Kay NE, Zarling JM. Deficiency of natural killer cell activity in patients with chronic lymphocytic leukemia. Int J Cancer 1981; 27:321–7.
13. Ching C, Lopez C. Natural killing of herpes simplex virus type 1-infected target cells: Normal human responses and influence of antiviral antibody. Infect Immun 1977; 26:49–56.
14. Cudkowicz G, Hochman PS. Do natural cells engage in regulated reactions against self to insure homeostasis? Immunol Rev 1979; 44:13–41.
15. Nair PNM, Schwartz SA. Suppression of natural killer activity and antibody-dependent cellular cytotoxicity by cultured human lymphocytes. J Immunol 1981; 126:2221–9.
16. Boeyum A. Isolation of mononuclear cells and granuclocytes from human blood. Scand J Clin Lab Invest 1968; 21:77–80.

17. Gentifanto YM, Little JM, Kaufman HE. The relationship between virus chemotherapy, secretory antibody formation and recurrent herpetic disease. Ann NY Acad Sci 1970; 173:649–55.

18. Douglas RG, Couch RB. A prospective study of chronic herpes simplex virus infection and recurrent herpes labialis in humans. J Immunol 1970; 104:289–95.

19. Lopez C, Oreilly RJ. Cell-mediated immune responses in recurrent herpesvirus infection. J Immunol 1977; 118:895–902.

20. Russell AS. Cell-mediated immunity to herpes simplex virus in man. J Infect Dis 1974; 129:142–6.

21. Eberle R, Russell RG, Rouse BT. Cell-mediated immunity to herpes simplex virus: Recognition of type-specific and type-common surface antigens by cytotoxic T cell populations. Infect Immun 1981; 34:795–803.

22. Handa K, Suzuki R, Matsui H, Shmizu Y, Kumagai K. Natural killer (NK) cells as a responder to interleukin 2 (IL2). I. Proliferative response and establishement of cloned cells. J Immunol 1983; 130:981–7.

23. Handa K, Suzuki R, Matsui H, Shimizu Y, Kumagai K. Natural killer (NK) cells as a responder to interleukin 2 (IL 2) II. IL 2-induced interferon production. J Immunol 1983; 130:988–92.

24. Gidlund M. Orn A, Wigzell H, Senik A, Gresser I. Enhanced NK cell activity in mice injected with interferon and interferon inducers. Science 1978; 273:759–61.

Cancer Detection and Prevention Supplement 1:57–64 (1987)

Stress-Related Modulation of Immunity:
A Review of Human Studies

Jan E.W. Palmblad, MD, PhD

Section of Hematology, Department of Medicine III, The Karolinska Institute, Stockholm, Sweden

ABSTRACT   The assumption that life changes and stressful events can alter host defense is based mainly on studies of changes in a variety of immune and inflammatory reactions. Whether those changes also confer an increased susceptibility to infectious agents and neoplasms, or modify the course of such diseases, is still less well substantiated. Nonetheless, psychological and neural modulation of immunity has recently been possible to approach from a mechanistic viewpoint. For instance, generation of a variety of lipid mediators from arachidonic acid may be under control of dietary and endocrine factors that can be affected by stress. Since these lipids, eg, lipoxygenase products, are potent regulators of leukocyte functional responses, their significance as one of several mechanisms is discussed. The role of various neuropeptides in leukocyte function has only recently been discovered. Since the release of, eg, substance P, enkephalins, and endorphins, which all have modulating effects on leukocyte functional responses, is under neural control and can occur in the vicinity of immunocompetent cells, they might constitute one of several links between the mind and the immune system.

Key words: fatty acids, neuropeptides, steroids

INTRODUCTION

The thesis that mind can modulate immunity rests on animal as well as human studies. A growing body of evidence suggests that stress, distress, grief, and depression can confer immunosuppression and, sometimes, immunostimulation. Since it also has been shown that one's ability to cope with stress-elicited events and life changes is an important feature in the expression of SAID (stress-associated immunodeficiency), studies of humans will be given priority in this paper. Reviews of animal studies are available elsewhere [1–4].

Most studies on SAID have followed a selected group of individuals for a period of time, either during a rather intensive experience lasting for a few days to 1-2 weeks or lasting for several months. In the following paper, these two categories will be referred to as short-term and long-term studies. The rationale for this division is that it is probable (although not shown) that different mechanisms are operating.

Short-term exposure to stressors have involved various academic examinations, sleep deprivations, space flights, etc. Also, effects of hypnosis can for temporal reasons be grouped

Address reprint requests to Dr. J. Palmblad, Med. Klin. 3, Södersjukhuset, S-100 64 Stockholm, Sweden.

here, although no stressor in the classical sence is involved. Long-term exposure comprises events such as bereavement, unemployment, depression or, less dramatically but very appropriately, everyday events. It is in these studies that the significance of coping with life events has been most evidently an influence on immune responsiveness. This review will start by giving a few examples of relevant situations, categorized as outlined above, and then proceed to possible mechanisms involved.

SHORT-TERM STUDIES

In the majority of these studies, a selected group of individuals is followed prior to and following what is considered as a stressor. Academic examination was accompanied by depressed NK-cell cytotoxicity [5], impaired lymphocyte plaque-forming and mitogen responsiveness [6], reduced salivary IgA excretion [7], and increased serum IgA concentrations but without changes in salivary IgA [5]. Sleep deprivation for 48–72 hr was followed by reduced lymphocyte stimulability and neutrophil phagocytosis and gradually enhanced interferon production (Fig. 1) [8,9]. After space shuttle missions, lymphocytes exhibited reduced blastogenic transformation [10], whereas immunoglobulin concentrations were not affected [11].

Noteworthy is that the most reduced responses, regardless of which immunological variable was examined, were found in individuals who reported difficulties in coping adequately with the stressor or life events [5]. The psychological assessments concerned not only the stress perceived from the actual stressor but also recent or preceding year life changes, degree of feeling of loneliness, and behavior patterns. These or similar divisions of subjects in to categories with regard to psychological vulnerability or stability have proved to be an important part of studies of psychoimmunology.

As discussed in more detail below efforts have been made to research the mechanisms for recorded changes. Changes in corticosteroid and catecholamine as well as growth hormone and prolactin concentrations or output have been the main targets. Hitherto, results are at best described as conflicting.

Another feature assessed in some studies is immunological reactivity following termination of the stressor exposure. In the few experiments concerned with this period, an enhanced responsiveness of human neutrophils and of interferon production [8] has been observed and, in animals, of antibody [12] and interferon [13] generation. More research is needed to

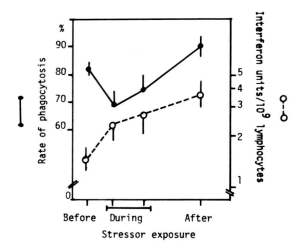

Fig. 1.   Phagocytosis of human neutrophils and interferon generation in lymphocytes during a stressful 72 hr vigil. Adapted from Palmblad et al [8], with permission.

substantiate the hypothesis that timing of the interaction between stressor exposure and assessments of immune functions is of significance [14].

There are also some studies of the effect of hypnosis on skin hypersensitivity. These studies deal with situations in which no stress of the classical Selye-Levi concept [15] is involved and in which no systemic or general endocrine changes are expected [16]. Black and colleagues [17,18] and Smith and McDaniel [19] conducted series of experiments in which they showed that suggestion under hypnosis and a paradigm similar to behavioral conditioning reduced edema and erytema in response to intradermally administered tuberculin extracts. That was found both for immediate and delayed skin reactions. In contrast, cell accumulation was not influenced. The mechanisms for that discrepancy is not known, but it suggests that part of the inflammatory reaction, particularly the vasoactive component, is inhibited by hypnosis. These intriguing studies point to a possible role for, eg, neural and neuropeptide modulation of inflammation, a concept that is reviewed further below. Support for the hypothesis that vascular permeability can be modified by stress comes also from a study of electric foot shock treatment on rats in which reduced vascular permeability was found [20]. In the same study, adherence of neutrophils was reduced, and decreased accumulation of neutrophils in experimental inflammatory lesions was also observed.

LONG-TERM STUDIES

Studies that concerns mainly what happens months after a major or repeated minor life changes are reviewed here. The pioneering work was done by Bartrop et al [21], who found that, 6 weeks after the death of a spouse, T lymphocytes of the bereaved spouse exhibited decreased proliferation, whereas B and T-cell numbers and antibody and various hormone concentrations were similar compared to controls and other time points for the bereaved. Similar findings were also reported by Schleifer et al [22]. They also noted that the effects were significant 1–2 months after bereavement but returned towards normality after 4–14 months (Fig. 2).

Apart from bereavement, which certainly ranges high on life-change scales, loss of job also constitutes a major change. In a recent study, Arnetz et al [23] found that unemployed

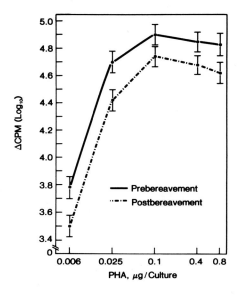

Fig. 2. PHA-induced lymphocyte stimulation before and 1–2 months after bereavement. Reprinted from Schleifer et al [22], with permission

persons showed reduced lymphocyte stimulability several months after loss of job. An interesting aspect was also introduced by offering psychological support to a subgroup in order to see whether that could reduce immunosuppression. However, no difference was noted from those who did not receive such support (Fig. 3).

Locke et al [24] approached the problem in a different way. In assessing NK-cell activity and relating that to reported life-change stress of healthy undergraduate students, they did not find any significant relationship when the results of the whole group were considered. However, when the results were divided according to whether the subjects had few psychologic symptoms despite larger amount of stress ("good copers"), or the opposite, a significantly lower NK-cell activity was found for the "poor copers." Once more, this study emphazises the need for evaluation of the individual's actual response to stress particulary important when the effects of rather weak stimuli are assessed.

DOES STRESS AFFECT HOST DEFENSE AGAINST INFECTIONS?

Although it can be regarded as an established hypothesis that stress will modulate a number of immune and inflammatory variables, it is less well documented that stress also will affect morbidity (or mortality) in diseases in which those host defense mechanisms are significant elements. Only a few studies have addressed this question. In fact, none of the above-mentioned studies has assessed illness in relation to recorded changes in immunity.

One of the first to do so [25] reported that more hemolytic streptococcal infections occurred in families among whom an acute or chronic family stress situation was evident. Kasl et al [26] have contributed one of the most interesting studies in this respect. Cadets at West Point were followed prospectively for development of infectious mononucleosis with symptoms or only a seroconversion. Those cadets with high motivation and poor academic performance had significantly more clinically evident mononucleosis than those who performed well. Thus clinical expression of an infectious disease might be related to life stress.

Pizzo et al [27] followed patients with neutropenia secondary to cytostatic treatment. Because of the neutropenia, patients were at risk for acquiring infections so they were given prophylactic antibiotics. The efficacy of this treatment was assessed by comparing infection incidence to a placebo-treated control group identical in all other respects. An important feature of the study was that compliance to drug therapy was assessed and related to rate of infections.

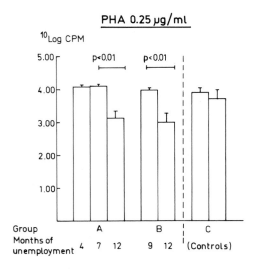

Fig. 3. PHA-induced lymphocyte stimulation in unemployed women who received no (A) or some (B) psychosocial support. Reprinted from Arnetz et al [23] with permission.

It was found that only 32% of the placebo-treated patients showing excellent compliance became infected, compared to 100% of those with poor compliance. There is no clear indication of what constitutes the mechanisms for this difference between two groups receiving an inactive drug. We can only speculate that poor compliance reflects personality and psychological traits that are of significance also for host defense.

CORTICOSTEROIDS

Secretion of corticosteroids has long been considered to be a major mechanism of stress-induced modulation of immunity and inflammation [1,2,5–8,12,13,15,21,22]. Doubtless, steroid levels in body fluids can be elevated during a stressor exposure. However, during the past years, a large number of studies have made us aware that this hypothesis requires reconsideration. In fact, it can be questioned whether corticosteroids are important as mediator of stress-associated immune dysfunction. The basis for this statement is that so many studies in humans reported rather uniform changes of inflammatory or immune reactions in response to stressors, whereas steroid hormone levels were affected in a nonuniform manner [5–9,14,21,22]. It is true that the absence of a direct relation between these particular immune and endocrine systems might be described partly to technical factors, eg, that cortisol samples were obtained too seldom or that urinary output might reflect the total turnover of cortisol better than serum concentration assessments. Also, the steroid-induced generation of the phospholipase inhibitor lipmodulin or macrocortin [28], which has been suggested to be one molecular mechanism for the antiinflammatory action of corticosteroids, requires considerable time to be expressed. Steroids may also modulate receptor density/affinity, eg, to catecholamins, so that immunocompetent and inflammatory cells react differently [29]. Although factors and circumstances of this kind clearly can obscure a role for steroids, Stein [30] demonstrated recently that stress-induced immunosuppression can occur in adrenalectomized animals and is as severe as in sham-operated animals, emphasising that SAID can occur in absence of corticosteroids in certain situations.

LIPIDS AS MEDIATORS

The emergence of a role for fatty acids as mediators of a great variety of inflammatory and immune functions has offered unique possibility to explore how stress-reduced immuno-modulation may occur. The background for this idea is very simple: We are what we eat.

In times of life changes, such as bereavement and divorce, changes in eating habits are frequently evident. Not only will grief modify appetite (we are prone either to loose appetite or, maybe less often, to overeat), but loneliness will also affect food preferences and cooking habits. For example, a widower, who rarely prepared meals when his wife was alive, might envisage practical difficulties in the kitchen, conceivably resulting in a monotonous menu. Thus energy and nutrient intake can be changed considerably and may remain so for extend periods before a new life-style can be adopted. In addition, alcohol and tranquilizer intake can be expected to increase, possibly having effects of their own on the immune systems.

A decreased energy intake clearly affects the immune system, as demonstrated from studies of starving individuals in developing countries. Less dramatic but to a similar end is the often inconspicuous undernutrition among hospitalized and elderly persons in industrialized countries. Such malnutrition-associated immune dysfunction (MAIDS) confers an increased risk of acquiring infectious diseases [reviewed in 31].

Several mechanisms might be operative in MAIDS. Apart from effects of protein, vitamin, and trace metal deficiencies, it has been documented that intake of lipids also affects immunity. In particular, intake of fatty acids is now believed to be of considerable consequences for inflammatory responses. The main interest has been given linoleic and linolenic acids since they, particularly the former, are essential fatty acids for humans and are parent compounds of arachidonic acid and eicosapentaenoic acids. Deficiency as well as increased intake of the parent compounds or their metabolites influence generation of a spectrum of other metabolites derived by their cyclooxygenation and lipoxygenation. These latter metabolites include substances such as prostaglandins, thromboxanes, and leukotrienes. Leukotriene B_4 (LTB$_4$), generated from arachidonic acid, is one of the most potent endogenously formed inducers of adherence, chemotaxis, and enzyme release for neutrophil, eosinophil, and basophil granulocytes [32]. It will also modify functional responses of various classes of lymphocytes and NK cells [33]. Lipoxins are a recently described group of compounds that also affect these cells [34].

The generation of these substances are under dietary control. Although it appears rather difficult for a previously well nourished adult to exclude, eg, linoleic acid from the diet to such a degree that deficiency arises, other manipulations can result in lack of metabolites of linoleic acid. First, reduced intake of proteins was recently shown to reduce the expression of enzymes that converts linoleic acid to arachidonic acid [35], the parent substance for most prostaglandins and leukotrienes. That resulted in hampered synthesis of, eg, LTB$_4$ within 3 weeks. It has been suggested that an increased susceptibility to infection in protein-energy undernutrition might indeed be mediated by such impaired enzyme synthesis [31]. This suggestion is supported by findings from studies of essential fatty acid deficiency (EFAD). EFAD [reviewed in 31] may also occur rapidly. It is associated with impaired leukocyte function and leukotriene generation and increased susceptibility to infectious diseases. Moreover, EFAD has been associated with reduced autoimmune disease manifestation, reduced delayed cutaneous hypersensitivity, and fever responses. Second, the relative proportion of linoleic vs linolenic acid metabolites in the diet is of significance in leukocyte function and fatty acid-mediator production. Recently it was reported that a rather modest addition of eicosapentaenoic acid and docosahexaenoic acid to a standard diet was associated with markedly reduced adhesion capacity of neutrophils to endothelial cells and LTB$_4$ generation [36]. A similar addition of eicosapentaenoic acid ameliorated manifestations of rheumatoid arthritis [37]. It has also been found that extra linoleic acid modifies rheumatoid symptoms and immunity [38] and neutrophil functional responses. (Palmblad et al, unpublished observations).

One recent and probably pertinent finding is that leukotriene C_4 is a potent activator of ACTH release from the pituitary gland [39]. Once more, if fatty acid content of the diet is changed, it might be expected also to influence such a messenger system. Taken together, changes in intake of lipids and protein of an order that might be expected to occur in a rather every day manner have been shown to influence inflammatory and immune systems in a definite way and confer increased susceptibility to infectious agents and modify the course of autoimmune diseases. Although no studies of stress-induced immunosuppression have assessed the occurrence and possible effects of dietary habit changes, this clearly is one important variable to be taken into account, particularly in situations in which long-term effects are expected, such as bereavement and divorce.

NEUROANATOMY OF LYMPHOID TISSUE

K. Bulloch [40] has pioneered knowledge in this area. Her work has shown that there exists a direct and significant innervation of lymphoid tissues. This might represent a basis for explanation of how immune functional responses can be directly modulated by the autonomic nervous system. The suggestions for a role of neurotransmitters, such as catecholamines, substance P, enkephalins, and endorphins, in this context have met with considerable interest. Despite rather intriguing findings of immunosuppressive effects of these substances, conflicting results have not yet permitted a clear-cut understanding [reviewed in 2,3,41]. Nonetheless, since the autonomic nervous system and neurotransmitters regulate blood flow, vascular permeability, and the functions of immune and inflammatory cells, it is conceivable that they are significant mechanisms in rapidly occurring responses, as discussed above for short-term studies.

FUTURE RESEARCH

Despite ample evidence that mind influences immunity (and vice versa) [42], research has not come any closer to the critical issue of whether any of the recorded in vitro responses are of significance for health. If so, that might have implications also for health care, ie, whether psychosocial support can influence disease incidence or course.

Such issues can be approached. The study of Pizzo et al [27] on infections in neutropenic patients (where neutropenia and infections are easily predictable) provides an intriguing model. Following other patient populations at risk for acquiring infections might also lead to answers.

ACKNOWLEDGMENTS

This study was supported by a grant from the Swedish Medical Research Council (19P-7095). The author wishes to thank Mrs. S. Riddez for the preparation of the manuscript.

REFERENCES

1. Ader R, ed. Psychoneuroimmunology. New York: Raven Press; 1981.
2. Guillemin R, Cohn M, Melnechuk T, eds. Neural modulation of immunity. New York: Raven Press; 1985.
3. Tecoma ES, Huey LY. Psychic distress and the immune response. Life Sci 1985; 36:1799–1812.
4. Rodgers MP, Dubey D, Reich P. The influence of the psyche and the brain on immunity and disease susceptibility. Psychosom Med 1979; 41:147–64.
5. Kiecolt-Glaser JK, Garner W, Speicher C, Penn GM, Holliday J, Glaser R. Psychosocial modifiers of immunocompetence in medical students. Psychosom Med 1984; 46:7–14.
6. Dorian B, Garfinkel P, Brown G, Shore A, Gladman D, Keystone E. Aberrations in lymphocyte subpopulations and function during psychological stress. Clin Exp Immunol 1982; 50:132–8.
7. Jemmott JB, Borysenko M, Chapman R, Borysenko JZ, McClelland DC, Meyer D, Benson H. Academic stress, power motivation and increase in secretory rate of salivary secretory immunoglobulin A. Lancet 1983; i :1400–2.
8. Palmblad J, Cantell K, Strander H, Fröberg J, Karlsson CG, Levi L, Granström M, Unger P. Stressor exposure and immunological response in man; interferon producing capacity and phagocytosis. J Psychosom Med 1976; 20:193–9.
9. Palmblad J, Petrini B, Wasserman J, Akerstedt T. Lymphocyte and granulocyte reactions during sleep deprivation. J Psychosom Med 1979; 41:273–8.
10. Taylor GR, Dardano JP. Human cellular immune responsiveness. Aviation Space Environ Med 1983; 54:S55–8.
11. Voss EW. Prolonged weightlessness and humoral immunity. Science 1984; 225:214–5.
12. Salomon GF. Stress and antibody response in rats. Int Arch Allerg Appl Immunol 1969; 35:97–104.
13. Salomon GF, Merigan TC, Levine S. Variations in adrenal cortical hormones within physiological ranges, stress and interferon production in mice. Proc Soc Exp Biol Med 1967; 126:74–9.
14. Palmblad J. Stress and immunologic competence–Studies in man. In Ader R, ed: Psychoneuroimmunology. New York: Academic Press 1981; 229–57.
15. Levi L. Stress and distress in response to psychosocial stimuli. Acta Med Scand 1972; Suppl 528.
16. Bovbjerg D, Ader R, Cohen N. Behaviorally conditioned suppression of a graft-versus-host response. Proc Natl Acad Sci USA 1982; 79:583–5.
17. Black S. Inhibition of immediate-type hypersensitivity response by direct suggestion under hypnosis. Br Med J 1963; 1:925–9.
18. Black S, Humphrey JH, Niven JSF. Inhibition of Mantoux reaction by direct suggestion under hypnosis. Br Med J 1963; 1:1649–52.
19. Smith RG, McDaniel SM. Psychologically mediated effect on the delayed hypersensitivity reaction to tuberculin in humans. Psychosom Med 1983; 45:65–9.
20. Harmsen AG, Turney TH. Inhibition of in vivo neutrophil accumulation by stress. Inflammation 1985; 9:9–20.
21. Bartrop RW, Luckhurst E, Lazarus L, Kiloh LG, Penny R. Depressed lymphocyte function after bereavement. Lancet 1977; i:834–6.
22. Schleifer SJ, Keller SE, Camerino M, Thornton JC, Stein M. Suppression of lymphocyte stimulation following bereavement. JAMA 1983; 250:374–7.
23. Arnetz DB, Wasserman J, Petrini B, Brenner SO, Levi L, Eneroth P, Salovaara H, Hjelm R, Salovaara L, Theorell T, Hall E, Pettersson IL. Immune function in unemployed women. Psychosom Med, (in press).

24. Locke SE, Krans L, Leserman, Jurst MW, Heisel JS, Williams RM. Life change stress, psychiatric symptoms and natural killer cell activity. Psychosom Med 1984; 46:441–53.

25. Meyer RJ, Haggerty RJ. Streptococcal infections in families: Factors altering individual susceptibility. J Pediatr 1962; 29:539–49.

26. Kasl SV, Evans AS, Niederman JC. Psychosocial risk factors in the development of infections mononucleosis. Psychosom Med 1979; 41:445–66.

27. Pizzo PA, Robichaud KJ, Edwards BK, Schumaker C, Kramer BS, Johnson A. Oral antibiotic prophylaxis in patients with cancer. J Pediatr 1983; 102:125–33.

28. Flower RJ. Macrocortin and the antiphospholipase proteins. In Weissmann G, ed: Advances in inflammation research. New York: Raven Press, 1984; Vol 8, 1–34.

29. Davies AO, Lefkowitz RJ. Corticosteroid-induced differential regulation of β-adrenergic receptors in circulating human polymorphonuclear leukocytes and mononuclear leukocytes. J Clin Endocrinol Metab 1980; 51:599–605.

30. Stein M. Bereavement, depression, stress and immunity. In Guillemin R, Cohn M, Melnechah T, eds: Neural modulation of immunity. New York: Raven Press, 1985; 29–44.

31. Palmblad J. Malnutrition associated immune dysfunction syndrome. Acta Med Scand (in press).

32. Goetzl EJ, Payan DG, Goldman DW. Immunopathogenic roles of leukotrienes in human diseases. J Clin Immunol 1984; 4:79–84.

33. Rola-Pleszcynski M, Gagnon L, Sirois P. Leukotriene B$_4$ augments human natural cytotoxic cell activity. Biochem Biophys Res Commun 1983; 113:531–37.

34. Serhan CN, Fahlstadius P, Dahlen SE, Hamberg M, Samuelsson B. Biosynthesis and biological activities of lipoxins. Adv Prostagl Thrombox Leukotr Res 1985; 15:163–6.

35. Yue TL, Varma DR, Powell WS. Effects of protein deficiency on the metabolism of arachidonic acid by rat pleural polymorphonuclear leukocytes. Biochim Biophys Acta 1983; 751:332–9.

36. Lee TH, Hoover RL, Williams JD, Sperling RI, Ravalese J, Spur BW, Robinson DR, Corey EJ, Lewis RA, Austen KF. Effect of dietary enrichment with eicosapentaenoic and docosahexaenoic acids on in vitro neutrophil and monocyte leukotriene generation and neutrophil function. N Engl J Med 1985; 312:1217–24.

37. Kremer JM, Michalek AV, Lininger L, Huyck C, Bigaouette J, Timechalk MA, Rynes RI, Zieminski J, Bartholonew LE. Effects of manipulation of dietary fatty acids on clinical manifestations of rheumatoid arthritis. Lancet 1985; i:184–6.

38. Mertin J. Essential fatty acids and cell-mediated immunity. In: Holman R, ed. Progress in lipid research. New York: Academic Press, 1982; Vol 20, 851–6.

39. Hulting AL, Lindgren JA, Hökfelt T, Eneroth P, Werner S, Patrono C, Samuelsson B. Leukotriene C$_4$ as a mediator of LH release from rat anterior pituitary cells, Proc Natl Acad Sci USA 1985; 8Z:3834–8.

40. Bulloch K. Neuroanatomy of lymphoid tissue. In Guillemin R, Cohn M, Melnechuk T, eds: Neural modulation of immunity. New York: Raven Press, 1985; 111–41.

41. Payan DG, Goetzl EJ. Specific suppression of human T-lymphocyte function by leukotriene B$_4$. J Immunol 1983; 131:551–3.

42. Besedovsky H, del Rey A, Sorkin E. Immunological-neuroendocrine feed-back circuits. In: Guillemin R, Cohn M, Melnechuk T, eds. Neural modulation of immunity. New York: Raven Press, 1985; 163–78.

Cancer Detection and Prevention Supplement 1:65–71 (1987)

Antibody-Induced Modulation of H-2K^b Antigens on Mouse Tumor Cells In Vitro

Jan Stagsted
Lennart Olsson

Cancer Biology Laboratory, State University Hospital (Rigshospitalet), Copenhagen, Denmark.

ABSTRACT   Modulation of H-2K^b antigens on cells of a subline of the murine Lewis lung carcinoma was induced in vitro by a monoclonal antibody with specificity for H-2K^b antigens. High antibody concentrations resulted in a more spherical morphology of the cells, in a discrete loss of all antibody-antigen complexes within 4–6 hr, and in a corresponding maximal decrease in the total cellular antigen content 6–8 hr after antibody exposure. Restoration was complete within 2 hr after removal of the complexed antigen and occurred without any visible cap formation.

Key words: monoclonal antibody, mouse histocompatibility antigens, flow cytometry

INTRODUCTION

Antibody-induced antigenic modulation has been described in several independent cell and antigen-antibody systems [for review, see 1] and has in most cases been estimated by measuring resistance to complement-dependent antibody-mediated cytolysis [2–8]. However, it seems more appropriate to define antigenic modulation as an antibody-induced decrease of a specific membrane antigen density [1].

Divalent monoclonal anti-H-2K^b antibodies recognize only one epitope on each H-2K^b antigen and thus might not result in the extent of cross-linking required for capping. The present study was designed to evaluate modulation by following directly both the amount of

Abbreviations: Ag/Ab^c, antigen-antibody complexes; EDTA, ethylene diamine tetraacetic acid; FACS, fluorescence activated cell sorter; FACS buffer, 1 mg/ml bovine serum albumin, 15 mM NaN$_3$ in PBS; fau, FACS arbitrary units (logaritmic scale); FITC, fluorescein isothiocyanate; f-ram, FITC-conjugated rabbit antimouse immunoblobulin serum (Dakopatts); mAb, monoclonal antibody; PBS, phosphate-buffered saline; PEG 8000, polyethylene glycol with average polymeric MW of 8,000 dalton (stated percentages w/w PEG dissolved in distilled water; R medium, RPMI 1640 supplemented with 0.3% fresh L-glutamine and gentamycin; RF medium, R medium with 10% fetal bovine serum and complement inactivated by heating to 56°C for 3 hr; SDS-PAGE, polyacrylamide gel electrophoresis in 0.1% sodium dodecylsulphate.

Address reprint requests to Lennart Olsson, Cancer Biology Laboratory, State University Hospital (Rigs hospitalet), 9 Blegdamsvej, DK-2100 Copenhagen, Denmark.

antigen-antibody complexes (Ag/Ab^c) remaining on the cell surface as well as the total amount of H-2K^b antigen.

MATERIALS AND METHODS
Cells

The establishment and characterization of sublines of the Lewis lung carcinoma have been described elsewhere [9,10]. Briefly, sublines with different metastatic activities, including nonmetastatic lines, were established. One line, designated G$_2$, was chosen to study antibody-induced H-2K^b modulation, because it has elevated cell surface H-2K^b. The cells were grown at 37°C with RPMI 1640 supplemented with 10% fetal bovine serum (RF medium) in 5% CO$_2$, 95% humidity. Population doubling time was ~30 hours. The cell cultures were split and seeded at a density of 10^4 cells/cm^2 in 80 cm^2 tissue culture flasks 1 day prior to modulation experiments to ensure uniform exponential growth during modulation.

Hybridomas producing IgG$_1$ (κ) against H-2K^b were obtained from ATCC (Rockville, MD) and have been described elsewhere [11]. The hybridoma cells were cultured in vitro in RF medium or propagated as ascites cells in pristane-primed Balb/c mice.

Purification of Monoclonal Antibody

Hybridoma culture supernatants were concentrated 10–20-fold by ultrafiltration under nitrogen pressure using Amicon filters YM100 (~ 100 kD cut-off) and the resulting concentrate fractionated by precipitation in 4–8% PEG 8,000. The 8% PEG precipitate was washed once in 10% PEG and dissolved in PBS and soluble protein passed through a protein A sepharose column (Pharmacia). The column was washed thoroughly with PBS and bound IgG eluted with 100 mM glycine HCl, pH 3.0, and immediately neutralized in 1 M Tris HCl, pH 8.0. The IgG was finally dialyzed extensively against PBS and stored in aliquots at −20°C.

The purity of the antibody preparation was assured by SDS-PAGE, in which only heavy and light immunoglobulin chains were observed, and the IgG concentration was determined by absorbance at 280 nm. Alternatively, mAb was purified as above using ascitic fluid instead of culture supernatants and omitting the ultrafiltration step.

Antigenic Modulation

Culture flasks with ~ 10^6 cells were washed once in RPMI 1640 (R medium) to remove dead and floating cells and incubated with 10 ml of R medium supplemented with 100 μg anti-H-2K^b mAb for 30 min on ice.

The cells were then washed in R medium and incubated with 30 ml of RF medium at 37°C. Controls included G$_2$ cells incubated with an irrelevant monoclonal antibody [IgG$_2$b (κ)] that did not bind to the G$_2$ cells and was added in concentrations similar to the anti-H-2K^b mAb. The cells were harvested by detachment with Versene (0.5 mM EDTA in PBS) at various time intervals. The cells from each flask were split into three samples and processed for flow cytometry.

Flow Cytometry

The three cell samples from each time point were resuspended in FACS buffer and washed twice by centrifugation at 200g for 5 min. The cells were then processed according to scheme shown in Table I. The cells were analyzed on a fluorescence-activated cell sorter (FACS IV; Becton-Dickinson, Mt. View, CA).

RESULTS
Number of H-2K^b Antigens on G$_2$ Cells

Titration of G$_2$ cells with various concentrations of the mAb indicated a saturating concentration of 1–10 μg anti-H-2K^b mAb/ml (Fig. 1A); 10 μg/ml was consequently used as the standard mAb concentration to induce modulation. The fluorescence intensity of G$_2$ cells

TABLE I. Cell Processing Scheme for Flow Cytometry

Cell sample:	α	β	γ
	$\downarrow$	$\downarrow$	$\downarrow$
1 hr at 0–4°C with:	A*	A	B
	$\downarrow$	$\downarrow$	$\downarrow$
		Two washes in buffer A	
	$\downarrow$	$\downarrow$	$\downarrow$
1 hr at 0–4°C with:	A	C	C
	$\downarrow$	$\downarrow$	$\downarrow$
		Two washes in buffer A	
		fix all in buffer D	
	$\downarrow$	$\downarrow$	$\downarrow$
FACS analysis of:	α	β	γ

*A, 200 μl FACS buffer; B, 10 μg/ml anti-H-2K^b mAb in 200 μl FACS buffer; C, 500 μg/ml f-ram in 200 μl FACS buffer; D, 200 μl 1% paraformaldehyde in PBS.

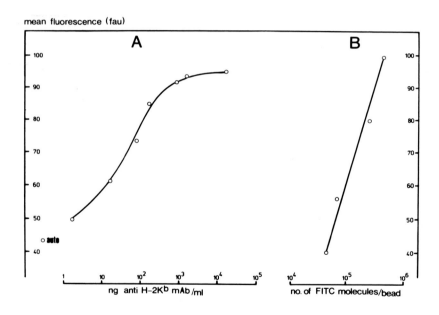

Fig. 1. Titration curve for G$_2$ cells with anti H-2K^b mAb. A, 5 × 10^5 G$_2$ cells from exponentially growing cultures (> 95% viability as judged by nigrosine dye exclusion) were harvested by Versene and incubated with the indicated concentrations of anti-H-2K^b mAb diluted in FACS buffer for 30 min at 0–4°C. The cells were washed twice and incubated with saturating amounts of f-ram (500 μg/ml in FACS buffer) for an additional 30 min at 0–4°C, washed twice, fixed, and analyzed on the FACS IV. Autofluorescence (auto) was defined as the nonspecific fluorescence measured on cells treated with f-ram only. fau, FACS arbitrary units (logaritmic). B, standard polystyrene beads with 4.2, 7, 28, and 43 × 10^4 FITC molecules per bead (±10%) were obtained from Becton-Dickinson and run parallel to the cell samples on the FACS IV. See text for calculations.

at saturating anti H-2K^b mAb concentrations may be used to estimate the number of H-2K^b antigens on the G$_2$ cell surface. A standard curve was established (Fig. 1B) by using fluorescent beads with a defined number of FITC molecules per bead. The anti-H-2K^b mAb-saturated fluorescence of G$_2$ cells (channel 95; Fig. 1A) was equivalent to ~3.8 × 10^5 FITC molecules/cell, and, with an autofluorescence of ~5.1 × 10^4 FITC molecules/cell (channel 43), the specific fluorescence could be determined as ~3.3 × 10^5 FITC molecules/cell. Setting the molecular ratio of H-2K^b antigen:anti-H-2K^b mAb to 1 and also the anti-H-2K^b mAb:f-ram ratio to 1 (the ratio may be less than one, since f-ram is a polyclonal antiserum) and knowing that the FITC/IgG molar ratio is 2.3 for the f-ram preparation, it could be calculated that the 3.3 × 10^5 FITC molecules/cell was equivalent maximally to 140,000 H-2K^b molecules/cell.

Modulation of H-2K^b Antigen

Modulation experiments were performed under sterile conditions. Modulating cells showed a marked change in morphology as they lost their flat and adherent phenotype and rounded up as modulation progressed (data not shown). A relatively large number of cells completely lost adherence to plastic.

Three parameter flow cytometric analyses of cells from each modulation time point allowed determination of both Ag/Ab^c and total surface H-2K^b antigen amount. A typical flow cytometric analysis is shown in Figure 2. The autofluorescence (α) served as an internal standard. The cell sample treated with f-ram only (β) indicated the amount of Ag/Ab^c remaining on the cell surface, whereas pretreatment for flow cytometry with additional saturating anti-H-2K^b mAb followed by f-ram (γ) revealed total H-2K^b antigen content per cell. Though the cells were originally incubated with saturating amounts of modulating mAb, a further amount of the mAb can apparently be bound during incubation for flow cytometry. This might be due to 1) minor differences in the exact conditions (time, temperature, etc) between the first modulating incubation and the subsequent flow cytometric incubation, 2) partial loss of complexed modulating antibody during the harvesting and washing procedures, 3) newly synthesized H-2K^b antigen appearing on the cell surface after incubation with modulating mAb (cellular metabolism of the "zero" time point sample was actually not blocked

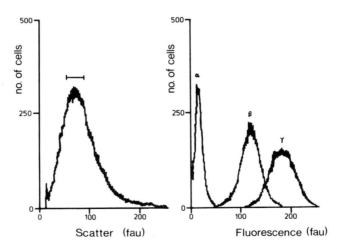

Fig. 2.   Flow cytometric profiles of modulating G$_2$ cells 2 h after addition of anti-H-2K^b mAb. Cells were processed as described in Materials and Methods. The histograms for the three cell samples are superimposed for comparison. The scattergate for sampling fluorescence is indicated on the left histogram by the bar above the scatterpeak. The fluorescent profiles are α, autofluorescence; β, complexed modulating mAb revealed by f-ram; and γ, total antigen revealed by additional anti-H-2K^b mAb + f-ram. fau, FACS arbitrary units (logaritmic).

by azide until about 30 min after the mAb incubation), or 4) modulation being biphasic, with an early (<30 min) modulation occurring before the cells were blocked with sodium azide. We consider 2) to be the most likely explanation.

Figure 3 shows the flow cytometric profiles of the cell samples treated to reveal total H-2K^b antigen content and harvested at the indicated time points relative to modulation start at 37°C. The fluorescence histogram profiles showed that it was the total cell population that changed during modulation.

The complete three parameter analyses of the modulating G$_2$ cells are shown in Figure 4. The autofluorescence mean distribution did not change in time, nor did the scatter signal (not shown). Control mean fluorescence intensity levels were determined for cells treated identically to the modulating cells but with an irrelevant mAb instead of the anti-H-2K^b mAb. The time course of the γ mean intensities (total surface antigen) showed a significant decrease between 6 and 8 hr after addition of antibody, but this was restored to normal 2 hr later. The initial surface Ag/Ab^c, as revealed by the β curve, was completely removed between 4 and 6 hr after addition of mAb. Examination of the modulating G$_2$ cells by fluorescence microscopy (results not shown) revealed that the initial uniform fluorescence at time 0 appeared finely punctuated after addition of the antibody and then suddenly disappeared in line with the flow cytometric analyses.

DISCUSSION

The pulselike experiments were performed to dissect out the modulating events in relation to time. The mAb pulse initially gave rise to a uniform population of cells with surface Ag/Ab^c and induced synchronous behavior of the total cell population. In fact, preliminary experiments performed with the mAb continuously present showed that a periodic modulation did occur. Eventually, the cells lost synchrony and modulation became invisible (results not shown).

Furthermore, the pulse experiments suggested that modulation was cell cycle-independent; the flow cytometric profiles would reveal any major subpopulation of cells in a certain cell cycle if these cells behaved differently than the rest of the population. The trivial explanations for the observed removal from the cell surface of complexed antibody are 1) antibody dissociates into the medium and 2) the antigen-antibody complexes are removed by the normal antigen turnover (shed or internalized). However, both seem unlikely in the present experiments because 1) removal of Ag/Ab^c resulted in a concomitant decrease of total antigen

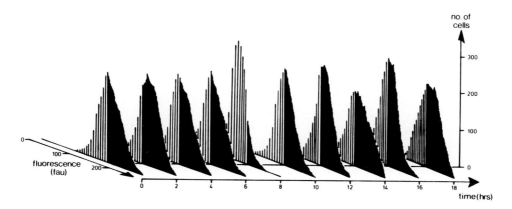

Fig. 3.   Fluorescence histograms (γ cell samples) are shown for the indicated time points. The part of the cell populations of less fluorescence intensity than the 0 time mean (channel no. 170) is represented by vertical lines, and the part of higher fluorescence by solid black. A decrease in the fluorescence intensity of a modulating cell population is shown by a higher proportion of vertical lines and vice versa.

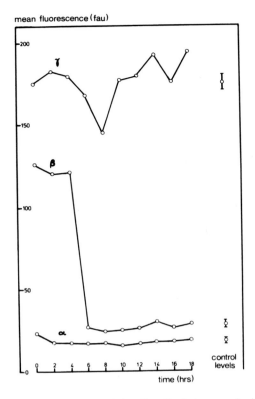

Fig. 4.   Mean fluorescence intensities of modulating G_2 cells that were pulsed with 10 µg/ml of anti-H-$2K^b$ mAb and harvested at the indicated time points relative to modulation start (time 0 as described in Material and Methods). Flow cytometric analysis was performed and the mean of the population fluorescence plotted as a function of time. α, β, and γ are explained in the legend to Figure 2. The control levels shown to the right were determined in parallel as described in text.

amount and 2) dissociation and a normal antigen turnover would be expected to result in a gradual loss of Ag/Ab^c from the cell surface and not abruptly as observed.

The absence of any visible cap formation during removal of complexed antigen antibody was striking and could be the result of the limited extent of cross-linking [12]. Apparently, the cells are able to free themselves of complexed H-2K^b antigen in a way distinct from capping. This might involve endo-/exocytosis of the small patches observed as a punctuated fluorescence [13]. The ultimate fate of the antigen-antibody complexes is presently unknown.

ACKNOWLEDGMENTS

Mr. J.P. Stenvang is thanked for his almost unlimited patience in performing flow cytometric analyses. This work was supported by PHS grant CA-35227, The Danish Cancer Society, and The Boel Foundation.

REFERENCES

1. Chatenoud L, Bach J-F. Antigenic modulation—A major mechanism of antibody action. Immunol Today 1984; 5:20–5.
2. Boyse EA, Stockert E, Old LJ. Modification of the antigenic structure of the cell membrane by thymus-leukemia (TL) antibody. Proc Natl Acad Sci USA 1967; 58:954–7.
3. Old LJ, Stockert E, Boyse EA, Kim JH. Antigenic modulation. Loss of TL antigen from cells exposed to TL antibody. Study of the phenomenon in vitro. J Exp Med 1968; 127:523–39.

4. Schlesinger M, Chaouat M. Modulation of the H-2 antigenicity on the surface of murine peritoneal cells. Tissue Antigens 1972; 2:427–35.

5. Lesley J, Hyman R. Antibody-induced changes in the expression of the H-2 antigen. Eur J Immunol 1974; 4:732–39.

6. Lesley J, Hyman R, Dennert G. Effect of antigen density on complement mediated lysis, T-cell-mediated killing, and antigenic modulation. J Natl Cancer Inst 1974; 53:1759–65.

7. Richards JM, Jacobson JB, Stackpole CW. Antigenic modulation in vitro. III. Failure to modulate H-2 antigens on several mouse tumors. J Natl Cancer Inst 1979; 62:825–32.

8. Gordon J, Anderson VA, Robinson DSF, Stevenson GT. The influence of antigen density and a comparison of IgG and IgM antibodies in the anticomplementary modulation of lymphocytic surface immunoglobulin. Scand J Immunol 1982; 15:169–77.

9. Olsson L, Kiger N, Kronstrøm H. Sensitivity of Lewis lung tumor cells derived from primary tumor site and from lung metastases to cytotoxic attack of syngeneic self-directed lymphoid spleen cells. Cancer Res 1981; 41:4706–9.

10. Olsson L, Forchhammer J. Induction of the metastatic phenotype in a mouse tumor model by 5-azacytidine, and characterization of an antigen associated with metastatic activity. Proc Natl Acad Sci USA 1984; 81:3389–93.

11. Köhler G, Lindahl KF, Heusser C. Characterization of a monoclonal anti-H-2K^b antibody. Immune System 1981; 2:202–8.

12. Schreiner GF, Unanue ER. Membrane and cytoplasmic changes in B lymphocytes induced by ligand-surface immunoglobulin interaction. Adv Immunol 1976; 24:37–165.

13. Willingham MC, Hanover JA, Dickson RB, Pastan I. Morphologic characterization of transferrin endocytosis and recycling in human KB cells. Proc Natl Acad Sci USA 1984; 81:175–9.

Cancer Detection and Prevention Supplement 1:73–79 (1987)

Cell Surface Glycoprotein Differences Between a Highly Malignant Murine Tumor Line and a Plastic-Adherent, Less Malignant Variant

Elke Lang, PhD
Peter Altevogt, PhD
Volker Schirrmacher, PhD

Institut für Immunologie und Genetik, Deutsches Krebsforschungszentrum, Heidelberg, Federal Republic of Germany

ABSTRACT A highly metastatic murine tumor line (ESb) and a plastic-adherent variant derived from it (ESb-M) were compared for expression of cell surface glycoproteins. Previous studies had shown that ESb-M cells were very similar to ESb cells in terms of cell surface marker expression and invasive capacity in vitro, but studies in vivo revealed that they exerted a decreased metastatic capacity. Syngeneic animals inoculated SC with ESb-M cells developed larger primary tumors and survived much longer than animals inoculated similarly with ESb cells. When using the lectin soybean agglutinin (SBA), distinct differences were observed in the glycosylation of a 220 kDa and a 80 kDa cell surface glycoprotein. Further differences in expression of cell membrane proteins were detected by means of variant-specific monoclonal antibodies. These specific ligands reacted with 65–75 kDa membrane glycoproteins, which were more prominent in ESb-M cells than in ESb cells. Apart from these differences, the two cell lines showed very similar profiles of membrane glycoproteins and lectin staining. Whether the structural differences seen in cell surface proteins can explain the changes in functional behavior (metastatic behavior and plastic-adhesive properties) of the cells remains to be investigated.

Key words: ESb, ESb variant, metastasis, plant lectins, monoclonal antibodies

INTRODUCTION

Many recent studies in which metastatic and nonmetastatic related tumor lines were compared have revealed subtle differences in certain cell surface components. These findings suggested that cell surface properties are of great importance in cancer metastasis. To obtain more information about cell surface molecules that might be of importance in cancer cell metastatic properties, we have performed a comparative biochemical analysis of two closely related well characterized tumor lines differing in adhesiveness and malignancy. Important tools in this analysis were plant lectins and monoclonal antibodies.

Address reprint requests to Prof. V. Schirrmacher, Institut für Immunologie und Genetik, Deutsches Krebsforschungszentrum, Im Neuenheimer Feld 280, D-6900 Heidelberg, Federal Republic of Germany.

The high metastatic tumor line ESb is a spontaneous variant of the chemically induced DBA/2-derived lymphoma L5178Y [1]. From this tumor line, which grows in suspension culture, we could select and isolate a plastic-adherent variant (ESb-M), which turned out to be still tumorigenic in syngeneic animals but to have marked decreased malignancy in terms of overall mortality [2]. ESb and ESb-M cells were shown to express similar differentiation antigens detected by monoclonal antibodies and tumor antigens detected by tumor-specific cytotoxic T lymphocytes [2] and were both highly invasive in in vitro assays [3]. No major differences were detected in immunogenicity (unpublished results). We now report on distinct, subtle structural differences of cell surface glycoproteins and their glycosylation between these cell lines that might be of importance in their changed functional behavior.

MATERIALS AND METHODS
Tumor Cell Lines

The ESb cell line is derived from the methylcholanthrene A-induced T-cell lymphoma L5178Y (Eb) and displays a highly metastatic behavior when injected into syngeneic DBA/2 mice [1]. A variant cell line, ESb-M, was isolated from ESb cells by repeated selection for plastic adherence [2]. Both cell lines were grown in RPMI 1640 culture medium (Gibco, Grand Island, NY) supplemented with glutamine (5 mM), 2-mercaptoethanol ($5 \times 10 - {}^5$M), Hepes (50 mM), and 5% FCS (Gibco).

Lectin Binding Assays

The staining of the tumor cells with FITC-conjugated lectins was performed as described previously [4]. For lectin binding studies with ^{125}I-iodinated lectins, 1×10^5 tumor cells were incubated with increasing concentrations of radiolabeled lectins (up to 200 μg/ml) in the presence of 1% bovine serum albumin for 30 min on ice. Cell-bound radioactivity was measured after washing the cells. The number of binding sites per cell was estimated by Scatchard plot analysis.

Iodination of Cell Surface Proteins and Solubilization

Cell surface proteins were ^{125}I-radiolabeled on intact cells by the lactoperoxidase procedure and solubilized as described elsewhere [5].

Isolation of Lectin Binding Glycoproteins

The ^{125}I-iodinated cell lysate (200 μl $= 5 \times 10^6$ cells) was mixed with 200 μl lectin-coupled Sepharose [25% suspension in PBS (Medac, Hamburg, Federal Republic of Germany)] and incubated for 2 hr at 4°C overend rotating. After washing, the bound glycoproteins were eluted from lectin Sepharose with the lectin-specific sugar (0.5 M in 0.5% NP40/PBS; conA-inhibitory sugar, α–methylmannoside; PNA-inhibitory sugar, galactose; SBA-inhibitory sugar, N-acetylgalactosamine). Controls for unspecific binding consisted of Sepharose conjugated with human serum albumin.

Immunoprecipitation With Monoclonal Antibodies

Anti-T200 monoclonal antibody was a gift from Dr. I. Trowbridge [6]. The monoclonal antibodies 18-9 and 12-15 have been prepared in our laboratory from immunization of Sprague-Dawley rats with ESb tumor cells.

For immunoprecipitation, 200 μl (5×10^6 cells) of the radiolabeled cell lysate was mixed with 800 μl hybridoma supernatant. After 1 hr at 4°C, 25 μl of protein A Sepharose (Pharmacia, Uppsala, Sweden) was added. The protein A Sepharose had been preincubated before with a protein A binding monoclonal antibody from mouse directed against rat κ light chain. The incubation was performed at 4°C overend rotating for 2–4 hr. The Sepharose was washed five times with 0.2% NP40/PBS, and bound proteins were eluted with twofold concentrated sample buffer for PAGE. Specificity of the binding was assured by precipitation with culture medium instead of hybridoma supernatant and by immunoprecipitation with a control antibody (anti-T200).

SDS-PAGE

SDS-PAGE was performed as described by Laemmli [7]. Proteins were mixed with sample buffer and analyzed under reducing conditions on 10% SDS-polyacrylamide gels, which were run at constant power of 15 mA.

After electrophoresis, gels were dried and exposed to Kodak X-Omat AR films for autoradiography. ^{14}C-radiolabeled molecular weight markers are myosin, 200,000; phosphorylase B, 92,500; bovine serum albumin, 69,000; ovalbumin, 46,000; carbonic anhydrase, 30,000; lysozyme, 14,000 (Amersham, Braunschweig, Federal Republic of Germany).

RESULTS
Differences Between ESb and ESb-M Detected With GalNac-Specific Lectins

The ESb-M cell line, which was generated spontaneously in vitro from ESb cells without any drug treatment, just by repeated selection for plastic adherence, was found to resemble ESb cells in growth behavior in vitro, cell surface markers, and protein profiles when total cellular protein or cell membrane proteins were analyzed by one-dimensional SDS-PAGE. Differences were, however, observed in the expression of lectin binding sites. Lectin binding was measured by staining the cells with various fluoresceine-conjugated lectins and analyzing them by flow cytofluorography. The adhesive variant ESb-M reacted with vicia villosa (VV) and soybean agglutinin (SBA), lectins that recognize preferentially terminal N-acetylgalactosamine (GalNac) residues. In contrast, when using conA, which reacts with the inner core of N-glycosidic oligosaccharides (mannose), very similar binding profiles were observed. When using peanut agglutinin (PNA), which is thought to recognize the sugar sequence Galβ-1.3-GalNac in 0-glycosidically linked carbohydrate side chains of glycoproteins, slightly higher binding values were observed for ESb-M cells than ESb cells.

Next we performed a quantitative analysis of lectin binding sites by means of ^{125}I-labeled lectins and determination of saturation binding curves. When this was performed with PNA, the Scatchard plot analysis of the binding data revealed two independent straight lines indicating two different binding molecules for PNA on the cell surfaces of both cell types. The number of binding sites and the affinity constant were similar on ESb and ESb-M cells for both binding molecules.

In contrast to this, the ^{125}I-SBA binding curves from ESb were found to be distinct from those of ESb-M cells. The number of binding sites for SBA was increased on the plastic-adherent ESb-M cells (2.3×10^6) compared to ESb cells (1.8×10^6) as calculated by Scatchard plot analysis. Furthermore, a drastic increase in the affinity of SBA binding was found on ESb-M cells. The association constant reveals the existence of a high-affinity binding site on ESb-M cells ($K_a = 1.5 \times 10^{-7}$ M) and a low-affinity one on ESb cells ($K_a = 0.5 \times 10^{-7}$ M). These results indicate an alteration in glycosylation of cell membrane molecules between the two cell lines leading to an increase in number of binding sites and binding affinity for the lectin SBA on the less malignant ESb-M cells.

Isolation of Lectin Binding Glycoproteins With Lectins Coupled to Sepharose

For identifying lectin binding cell surface glycoproteins, cell surface proteins were iodinated by the lactoperoxidase procedure and solubilized in 1% NP40 buffer. The solubilized proteins were then incubated with lectin Sepharose and bound glycoproteins eluted with 0.5 M inhibitory sugar. As negative control for unspecific binding we used Sepharose coupled to human serum albumin, and as positive control for detection of all glycoproteins carrying N-glycosidically linked oligo-saccharide side chains we used Sepharose coupled to conA (Fig. 1). Nothing or only weak bands was seen in the negative control, whereas many membrane glycoproteins could be detected with conA Sepharose. No differences were observed between ESb and ESb-M cells when using conA Sepharose.

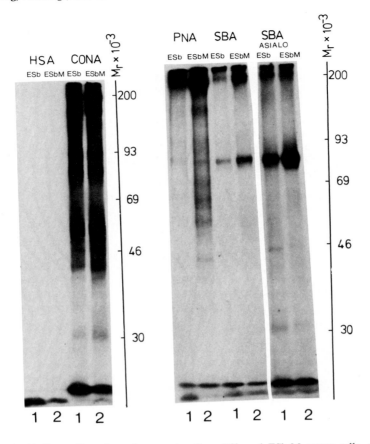

Fig. 1. Lectin binding cell surface glycoproteins from ESb and ESb-M tumor cells. Cell surface glycoproteins were ^{125}I-iodinated with lactoperoxidase, solubilized and isolated with lectins coupled to Sepharose, and analyzed by 10% SDS-PAGE. Elution was prepared with the lectin-specific competitive inhibitory sugar (see Materials and Methods). Lane 1, proteins derived from ESb cells; lane 2, proteins derived from ESb-M cells. HSA, human serum albumin coupled to Sepharose; ConA, concanavalin A coupled to Sepharose; PNA, peanut agglutinin coupled to Sepharose; SBA, soybean agglutinin coupled to Sepharose; SBA ASIALO, cells treated with neuraminidase [4] before radiolabeling and isolation of SBA binding glycoproteins.

When the lectin SBA, which reveals alterations in glycosylation of cell membrane components of the two cell lines, was coupled to Sepharose and used for the isolation, two major glycoproteins of 220 and 80 kDa were detected. The glycoproteins were present in lysates from both cell lines, but much more glycoprotein could be isolated from lysates from Esb-M cells. After removal of sialic acid by neuraminidase treatment of the cells, the amount of isolated 80 kDa glycoprotein was increased, but the quantitative difference between the cells still remained.

Differences Between ESb and ESb-M Cells Detected With Monoclonal Antibodies

To obtain monoclonal antibodies (mAb) that differentiate between the two cell lines, we immunized rats with the corresponding tumor cells and fused their spleen cells with mouse AG8 myeloma cells. After screening, selection, and subcloning, several interesting hybridomas could be isolated that produced antibodies that distinguish the adherent variant ESb-M from the parent ESb cell line. In Table I we have summarized the binding specificity on various cell

TABLE I. Binding Specificity of ESb-M-Selected Monoclonal Antibodies

Cell type tested	Control* (2nd antibody only) (%)	Monoclonal antibodies*		
		18-9-C2	12-15-B4	MP1-21
Thymus cells	2	1	6	3
Bone marrow cells	7	7	8	9
Lymph node cells	10	9	8	10
Spleen cells	25	27	25	27
Tumor lines				
Eb	3	12	10	30
ESb	5	32	28	87
ESb-MP	11	78	85	96

*Percent positive cells as analyzed by cytofluorography.

types of three selected monoclonals as tested in an indirect immunofluorescence assay and analyzed with cytofluorographic analysis.

All three monoclonal antibodies were nonreacting with normal lymphoid cells of different organs but reacted strongly with the adherent variant ESb-M and weakly with the ESb cell line. The nature of the antibody binding molecule was determined by immunoprecipitation of cell surface glycoproteins that had been labeled by lactoperoxidase catalyzed iodination and analyzed on SDS-PAGE. Figure 2 shows the results obtained with two monoclonals, 18-9 and 12-15, and in addition the molecules precipitated with an anti-T200 monoclonal antibody. The molecules recognized by MP1-21 were not precipitated. The precipitates with the mAb 18-9 showed a 67 kDa protein, and the protein isolated with mAb 12-15 revealed a broad band with a molecular weight of 65–75 kDa and an additional minor band at 220 kDa with autoradiography of SDS gels. Both monoclonals (18-9 and 12-15) distinguished ESb and ESb-M cells (see Fig. 2). The immunoprecipitates with the anti-T200 mAb demonstrated that similar amounts of T200 glycoproteins could be isolated from the lysates of ESb and ESb-M cells. These data show that in addition to differences in glycosylation the expression of a 65–75 kDa protein on the cell surface detected by a monoclonal antibody is altered on the two tumor cell lines with different metastatic capacities.

DISCUSSION

We have shown here that a plastic-adherent variant of a highly metastatic murine tumor line shows distinct but subtle differences in cell surface glycoproteins, which can be detected only by rather specific tools such as plant lectins or monoclonal antibodies. The changes detected were mostly quantitative. When using soybean agglutinin or ESb-M-selected monoclonal antibodies for isolation of cell surface glycoproteins, only very weak bands were detectable with ESb cells, whereas strong bands were seen with ESb-M cells. The most prominent bands were in the range of 220 and 80 kDa (SBA) and 65–75 kDa (12-15 monoclonal antibody). The 220 kDa molecule is likely to belong to the T200 family of lymphoid differentiation antigens, but the nature of the other molecules is not known.

As we reported previously, we have found quite a good correlation between expression of lectin binding sites for SBA and low metastatic capacity when comparing various pairs of highly and lesser metastatic tumor lines [8]. Similar findings have been obtained in other tumor models [9,10] (also, J.G. Collard, personal communication). In this particular study, we have identified the molecules carrying the SBA lectin binding sites. The 220 and 80 kDa molecules were also detected with another method, namely, reacting intact labeled cells with biotinylated lectins and then solubilizing them and isolating lectin bound molecules by means of avidine agarose. The major glycoprotein of ESb-M cell membranes, which showed strong SBA binding by this method, had a molecular weight of 220 kDa. It is likely that these molecules belong to

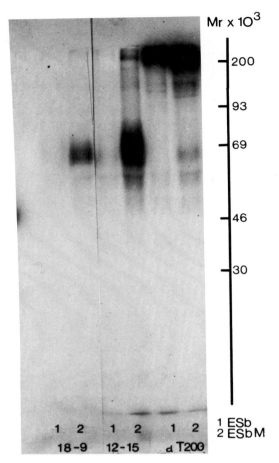

Fig. 2. Cell surface molecules from ESb and ESb-M cells detected by monoclonal antibodies and immunoprecipitation. ^{125}I-iodinated cell surface proteins were precipitated with mAb 18-9, mAb 12-15, or anti-T200 as indicated and analyzed by 10% SDS-PAGE under reducing conditions. Lane 1, proteins derived from ESb cells; lane 2, proteins derived from ESb-M cells.

the family of T200 glycoproteins, because very similar bands could be precipitated with monoclonal anti-T200 antibodies.

The structural basis for the observed changes in glycosylation of the two proteins of 220 and 80 kDa is unknown at present. One possibility is that the oligosaccharide side chains recognized by SBA are less accessible or decreased in number on the glycoproteins from ESb cells. Alternatively, the sugar sequence of the oligosaccharide side chain of these proteins is different and leads to a decreased binding affinity of the lectin.

It would be quite interesting to know whether these molecules have anything to do with the changed adhesiveness of the ESb-M cells. Could they represent adhesion molecules? The laminin receptor, for instance, has been reported to have a molecular weight of 69 kDa. Another possibility is that these glycoproteins are of viral origin. Recently, Hochmann et al [11] have shown that a plastic-adherent variant of a murine lymphoma cell line showed increased expression of viral antigens belonging to the mouse mammary tumor virus (MMTV) group. We are presently investigating these different possibilities.

REFERENCES

1. Schirrmacher V, Shantz G, Clauer K, Komitowski D, Zimmermann HP, Lohmann-Matthes ML. Tumor metastases and cell-mediated immunity in a model system in DBA/2 mice. I. Tumor invasiveness in vitro and metastases formation in vivo. Int J Cancer 1979; 23:233–44.

2. Fogel M, Altevogt P, Schirrmacher V. Metastatic potential severely altered by changes in tumor cell adhesiveness and cell surface sialylation. J Exp Med 1983; 157:371–6.

3. Waller CA, Braun M, Schirrmacher V. Quantitative analysis of cancer invasion in vitro: Comparison of two new assays and of tumor sublines with different metastatic capacity. Clin Exptl Met 1986; 4:73–89.

4. Altevogt P, Fogel M, Cheingsong-Popov R, Dennis J, Robinson P, Schirrmacher V. Different patterns of lectin binding and cell surface sialylation detected on related high- and low-metastatic tumor lines. Cancer Res 1983; 43:5138–44.

5. Altevogt P, Kurnick JT, Kimura AK, Bosslet K, Schirrmacher V. Different expression of Lyt differentiation antigens and cell surface glycoproteins by a murine T lymphoma line and its high metastatic variant. Eur J Immunol 1982; 12:300–7.

6. Trowbridge IS. Interspecies spleen-myeloma hybrid producing monoclonal antibodies against mouse lymphocyte surface glycoprotein, T200. J Exp Med 1978; 148:313–23.

7. Laemmli UK. Cleavage of structural proteins during the assembly of the head of bacteriophage T4. Nature 1970; 227:680–5.

8. Schirrmacher V, Altevogt P, Fogel M, Dennis J, Waller CA, Barz D, Schwartz R, et al. Importance of cell surface carbohydrates in cancer cell adhesion, invasion and metastasis. Does sialic acid direct metastatic behavior? Inv Met 1982; 2:313–60.

9. Yogeeswaran G, Salk PL. Metastatic potential is positively correlated with cell surface sialylation of cultured murine tumor cell lines. Science 1981; 212:1514.

10. Zvibel I, Raz A. The establishment and characterization of a new BALB/c angiosarcoma tumor system. Int J Cancer 1985; 36:261.

11. Hochmann J, Mador N, Panet A. Tubular structures in S49 mouse lymphoma are regulated through in vivo host-cell interaction and in vitro interferon treatment. J Cell Biol 1985; 100:1351–6.

Cancer Detection and Prevention Supplement 1:81–89 (1987)

The Tumor Promoter 12-O-Tetradecanoylphorbol-13-Acetate (TPA) Accelerates Expression of Differentiation Markers in Cultures of Rat Palatal Epithelial Cells

Dorthe Arenholt, DDS, PhD
Erik Dabelsteen, DDS, PhD

Department of Oral Pathology, Royal Dental College, Aarhus, (D.A.) and Department of Oral Diagnosis, Royal Dental College, Copenhagen, (E.D.), Denmark

ABSTRACT   Cultures of rat palatal epithelium grown on collagen rafts were treated with different doses of the potent tumor promoter 12-O-tetradecanoylphorbol-13-acetate (TPA). Sections from biopsies taken 1, 6, 24, and 48 hr after the addition of TPA were examined for the localization of staining by blood group antigen H antibody and antikeratin antibody AE1. In contrast to control cultures, where antigen H was seen exclusively at the cell membranes of the second and third cell layer, several antigen H-positive cells, some appearing in groups, were found in the basal cell layer of TPA-treated specimens. Staining for keratins with the AE1 antikeratin antibody showed no staining of basal cells but only suprabasal cells in controls, whereas several cells of the basal cell layer of TPA-treated cultures stained positively with this antibody. The results support the theory that TPA, by forcing a part of the basal cell population to terminal differentiation, strongly affects the composition of the basal cell population.

Key words: TPA, maturation, epithelium in vitro

INTRODUCTION

One of several effects of tumor promoters is the stimulation of proliferative and differentiative events [1]. A single application of TPA to the back skin of mice has been found to cause cytological and histological changes in the epidermis different from those produced by nonpromoting, hyperplasiogenic chemicals [2–4]. The findings in the epidermis were characterized as having an embryonic appearance along with induction of a phenotypically new, so-called dark cell population [4]. Recent in vivo reports have demonstrated that phorbol esters stimulate proliferation or accelerate differentiation in distinct subpopulations of epidermal basal cells [5].

Numerous in vitro studies using different cell types have also demonstrated that TPA either inhibits or enhances terminal differentiation [6]. In hamster and mouse epidermal cell

Address reprint requests to Dr. Dorthe Arenholt, Royal Dental College, Department of Oral Pathology, Vennelyst Boulevard, 8000 Aarhus, Denmark.

systems TPA was shown to inhibit differentiation [7–9]. In mouse epidermal basal cells a subset of cells was demonstrated to be resistant to both calcium-induced differentiation and TPA-induced transglutaminase elevation [10,11]; instead, they were stimulated to proliferate by the phorbol ester. In cultures of human epidermal cells TPA has been shown to induce differentiation of more than 90% of cells, while it may have stimulated growth of an unidentified subpopulation [12].

Studies of epithelial cell surface carbohydrates have demonstrated that these are related to cell differentiation and that the ABO blood group antigens and their structural precursors can be used as differentiation markers in both human and rodent stratified epithelia [13,14]. Histochemical studies of cellular keratins have demonstrated that these also can be used as markers, since a gradual change in the expression of keratin polypeptides takes place during cell differentiation [15].

In this report it is demonstrated that, by use of monoclonal antibodies to both cell surface carbohydrate and keratin polypeptides, TPA in cultures of stratified rat palate epithelium induce markers of terminal differentiation in one fraction of the basal cell population, leaving another fraction unaffected.

MATERIALS AND METHODS
Cell Cultures

Isolation, culture, and subcultivation of rat palatal squamous epithelial cells was performed as described previously [16]. Briefly, the cells were plated by crowding technique: 2×10^6 cells per milliliter in plastic culture flasks (Falcon 3013) coated with 0.6% collagen gels, allowing the cells to obtain a high degree of tissue organization in vitro [17]. After the cells were allowed to attach for 24 hr in a humidified atmosphere, growth medium consisting of minimal essential medium with Earle's salts (MEM), 5% fetal bovine serum, and 0.5% penicillin/streptomycin was added. The cultures were incubated at 30°C in a gasseous environment of 95% air and 5% CO_2.

From 20 days after subcultivation the cultures were divided into three groups, one receiving 0.2% DMSO alone and a second and a third receiving 1 ng and 100 ng TPA per milliliter medium, respectively. Biopsy specimens from each group were taken 1, 6, 24, and 48 h after the addition of TPA to the culture medium. Thereafter, biopsy specimens were taken every seventh day. Biopsies were fixed in 10% buffered formalin, embedded in paraffin, and cut at 4 μm. Culture medium was changed twice a week.

Tumor Promoter

12-O-tetradecanoylphorbol-13-acetate (TPA) was purchased from P-L Biochemicals Inc. (Milwaukee, Wisconsin), dissolved in dimethylsulphoxide (DMSO) from Pierce (Rockford, Illinois), and diluted in the medium to a final concentration of 0.2% DMSO.

Antigens and Antibodies

The chemical compositions of blood group antigen B and the precursor structures blood group H and N-acetyllactosamine have previously been described [14]. Two types of carbohydrate chains, type 1 and type 2, may carry the B and H antigens [18]. The type 2 chain has a repeating Gal 1–4 GluNAc structure (N-acetyllactosamine), and type 1 has a repeating structure Gal 1–3 GluNAc. Both chains carry B and H antigens as end structures. We used monoclonal antibodies prepared by the hybridoma technique directed to blood group H only when carried on type 2 chain and to its precursor carbohydrate structure N-acetyllactosamine.

The antibody against blood group antigen B was a human blood group test serum (Statens Seruminstitut, Copenhagen, Denmark) reacting with antigens carried on both type 1 and type 2 chains. The antibody production has previously been described [19].

Keratin expression was investigated by monoclonal antikeratin antibody AE1 (kindly provided by Dr. Tung-Tien Sun, New York University Medical School). The antibody was prepared against SDS-denaturated human epidermal keratins by the hybridoma techinque and characterized by immunofluorescence and immunoblot techniques [20].

Staining

Sections were cut from paraffin blocks at a thickness of 4 μm and mounted on gelatine-coated slides. Antigens were detected in the tissue by a double layer immunofluorescence technique. Paraffin sections were depraffinized and washed in phosphate-buffered saline at pH 7.4 (PBS). Sections were incubated with monoclonal antibodies anti-H and AE1, respectively, in a moist chamber for 20 h at 4°C, and, following three washes in PBS (5 min each), FITC-conjugated rabbit antimouse immunoglobulin diluted 1:20 (Dakopatt, Copenhagen, Denmark) was applied for 40 min. The sections were washed and mounted in a mountant made by adding 10 ml PBS containing 100 mg P-phenylene-diamine to 90 ml of glycerol [21]. The staining procedure using human anti-B serum followed the same schedule but used rabbit antihuman IgG 1:20 (Dakopatt) as the second layer. The monoclonal antibodies and the human serum were used in a working dilution of 1:100 and 1:50, respectively. Before staining sections with AE1 antibodies, the sections were pretreated with 0.4% pepsin (Sigma code P7000) disolved in distilled water adjusted to pH 2.5 with HC1. Incubation took place at 37°C for 1.5 hr. Following three washes in PBS (3 min each) monoclonal antibodies were applied as described above. The slides were examined with a Zeiss fluorescence microscope using EPI illumination. The microscope was equipped with FITC interference filters (The Optical Laboratory, Lyngby, Denmark) and a 50 W Zenon lamp. The control reactions consisted of 1) staining with conjugates alone and 2) substitution of the primary antisera with a mouse monoclonal antibody of an irrelevant specificity (OKT4, Ortho Pharmaceuticals, Raritan, New York) and use of absorbed human anti-B serum.

RESULTS

During the observation period the cultures exposed to TPA developed increasing amounts of squames compared to the controls (Figs 1, 2). Phase contrast microcsopy revealed that the

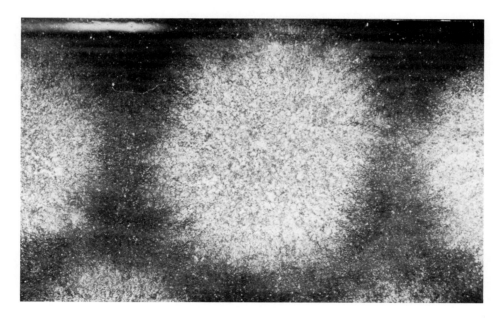

Fig. 1.   Rat palatal epithelium (RPE) control culture, day 20 in subculture. ×6.

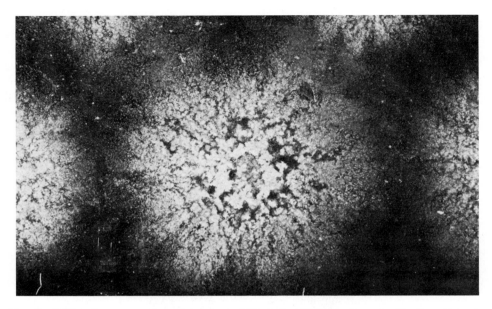

Fig. 2. RPE culture exposed continuously to TPA during 20 days after subcultivation. Extensive sloughing of squames. ×6.

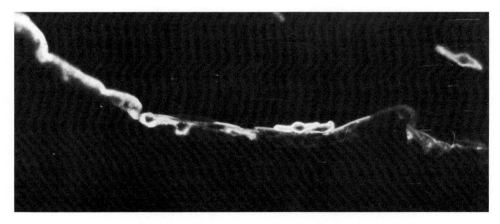

Fig. 3. RPE control culture, day 20 in subculture. Blood group antigen H present at the surface of cell membranes of the second and third cell layers. ×600.

squames in the TPA-treated cultures only differed quantitatively from the control cultures. The squames appeared as flattened cells containing either none or pycnotic nuclei.

In both controls and TPA-treated cultures all basal cells and the one to two cell layers above stained positively for antigen B. In specimens from cultures that had not received any treatment with TPA blood group antigen H was seen at the cell membranes of the second and third cell layer and was not expressed on the basal cells except on a few drop-shaped cells with the apex facing basement membrane (Fig. 3). These cells appeared to be in the process of leaving the basal cell layer and expressed H antigen as strongly as the second and third cell layers. In specimens treated for 1 hr with TPA several blood group antigen H-positive cells were found in the basal cell layer. The H-positive cells had a patchy distribution, appearing as small groups of positive cells in between a basal cell layer that did not react for the H antigen (Fig. 4). A similar pattern was seen in specimens treated for 6 hr with TPA (Fig. 5), whereas specimens having received TPA treatment for 24 hr showed a basal cell layer in which about half of the cells stained positively for blood group antigen H (Fig. 6). In specimens having received TPA treatment for another 24 hr, 1 week, 2 weeks, 3 weeks, or 4 weeks, there was no major difference in the distribution of H-positive cells. In all these specimens a few H-positive reacting basal cells were always seen. However, the majority of the cells in the basal cell layer reacted negatively, and the H antigen was normally found in the second and third cell layer as in the control specimens. When comparing the results in the TPA-treated cultures, there seemed to be no difference in results obtained when cell cultures were treated with 1 ng/ml culture medium or 100 ng/ml culture medium.

The staining with the AE1 antibody showed that specimens from cultures treated with DMSO alone stained positively in the second and third cell layers, leaving the basal cells negative (Fig. 7). In specimens treated with TPA for 6 and 24 hr, an irregular staining of basal

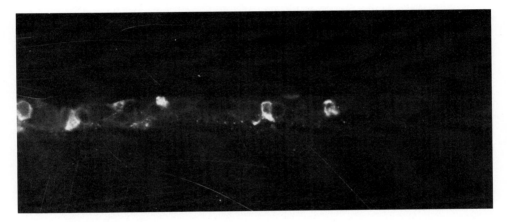

Fig. 4. RPE culture day 20, exposed to TPA for 1 hr. A few blood group antigen H-positive cells present in the basal cell layer. ×600.

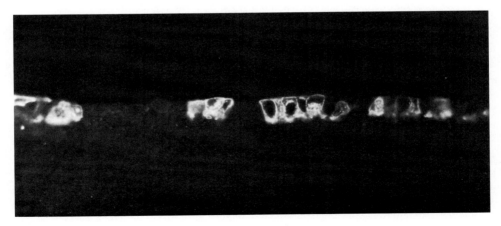

Fig. 5. RPE culture day 20, exposed to TPA for 6 hr. Several blood group antigen H-positive cells present in the basal cell layer. ×600.

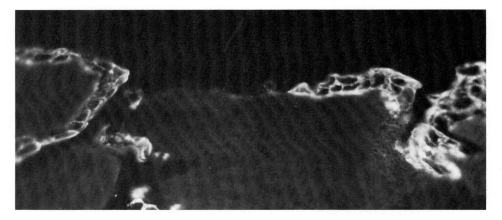

Fig. 6.   RPE culture day 21, exposed to TPA for 24 hr. About half of the cells in the basal cell layer show positive staining for blood group antigen H. ×600.

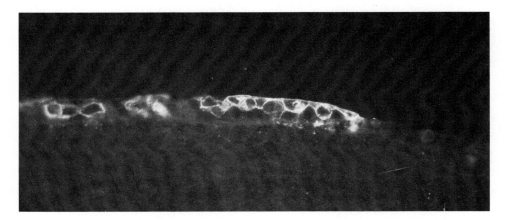

Fig. 7.   RPE control culture day 20. Staining of suprabasal cells with AE1 antikeratin antibody. ×600.

cells was seen with AE1 antibody (Fig. 8). The staining pattern was similar but not identical to the staining pattern obtained with the anti-H antibody. The staining with AE1 antibody was more irregular, and, based on serial sections, it seemed that they were not the same cells that stained with anti-H and AE1 antibodies. It also appeared that when the time for pepsin treatment was extended, all cells irrespective of TPA treatment stained positive with the AE1 antibody.

DISCUSSION

In the present study we have investigated the distribution of different cellular markers that in normal epithelium show an expression related to the stage of cellular differentiation [22]. The pattern of staining observed in the control cultures showed a distribution of the different markers similar to that seen in histological sections of normal epithelium. It is therefore tempting to anticipate that the distribution of these markers in cell cultures similar to the normal epithelium are linked to the stage of cellular differentiation. The antibodies to the blood group H antigen are specific for the type 2 chain H structure, whereas the AE1 antibodies have a broad specificity in that they are reacting with all acidic keratin polypeptides [23]. The

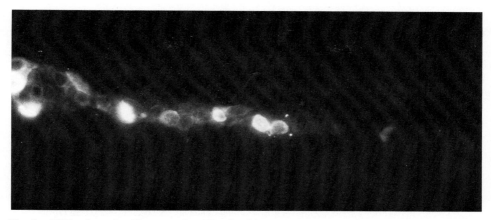

Fig. 8.   RPE culture day 20, exposed to TPA for 6 hr. Several basal cells show positive staining with AE1 antikeratin antibody. ×600.

staining patterns observed with the AE1 antibodies are therefore not related to the expression of a single keratin protein but may reflect the expression of several different keratin proteins. Also, keratin proteins may be present in biochemical analysis of the tissue but not stainable by immunofluorescence staining methods because of the masking of the antigen determinant. Therefore, the use of AE1 antibodies in the investigation of cellular differentiation may be expected to be less conclusive than the use of anti-H antibodies, which have been shown to possess high specificity for glycolipids carrying H antigen. This may explain the variable results obtained with the AE1 antibodies in comparison to the results obtained with the anti-H antibodies.

The results of our study support previous studies in mouse and human epidermal cell cultures that demonstrated the TPA induced, forced maturation of a part of the basal cell population [5,10,11]. The presence of H-positive cells in the basal cell layer may indicate that these basal cells do differentiate even before they move to the second cell layer. Also, the presence of the AE1-positive cells in the basal cell layer in contrast to the suprabasal expression seen in the control cultures suggest an early differentiation in the basal cell layer, although the interpretation of the staining reactions with AE1 antibodies should be done with some caution, as mentioned above. The basal cells apparently resistant to stimulated differentiation might be identical to the TPA-induced, transitional morphology (TT) cells observed in TPA-exposed cultures of human epidermis [12].

The in vitro demonstration of a TPA-induced, forced differentiation is supported by detailed cell kinetic studies following painting of hairless mouse back skin in vivo with TPA. These studies have shown that TPA causes an increased rate of normal maturation [24]. The time course for the increase in the number of maturing cells followed by a decline within 48 hr demonstrated in the present study also corresponds very well with findings following TPA painting of mouse back skin in vivo [5].

Data indicating TPA-induced inhibition of differentiation have been reported in a variety of cell culture systems [6] including cultures of hamster epidermal cells [7]. The latter result might be a reflection of the fact that hamster epithelium in vivo does not undergo promotion with TPA following a two-stage carcinogenesis protocol [25].

The present work is part of a study elucidating the effects of TPA on stratifying rat epithelial cells in vitro. Previously it was demonstrated that TPA at the same time exerted an effect on intercellular communication [26] and mitotic activity [27]. Taken together, our studies lend support to the papers emphasizing the importance of the induction of terminal differentiation in epidermis as a permissive environment for clonal expansion of initiated cells [10,28].

Furthermore, the present study suggests that blood group antigens, which are not commonly used as cell maturation markers in vitro, are a useful tool in determining cell maturation changes in epithelial cell cultures.

ACKNOWLEDGMENTS

The authors thank Dr. Arne Jepsen for providing the cells used in this study. This study was supported by grants from the Danish Cancer Society.

REFERENCES

1. Schweizer J. Modification of epithelial cell differentiation in vivo by tumor-promoting diterpene esters. In Hecker E, Fusenig NE, Kunz W, Marks F, Thielmann HW, eds: Carcinogenesis and biological effects of tumor promoters. New York: Raven Press, 1982; 285–304.
2. Raick AN. Ultrastructural, histological and biochemical alterations produced by 12-O-tetradecanoylphorbol-13-acetate on mouse epidermis and their relevance to skin tumor promotion. Cancer Res 1973; 33:269–86.
3. Raick AN, Burdzy K. Ultrastructural and biochemical changes induced in mouse epidermis by a hyperplastic agent, ethylphenylpropiolate. Cancer Res 1973; 33:2221–30.
4. Klein-Szanto AJP, Major SK, Slaga TJ. Quantative evaluation of dark keratinocytes induced by several promoting and hyperplasiogenic agents: Their use as an early morphological indicator of tumor-promoting action. In Hecker E, Fusenig NE, Kunz W, Marks F, Thielmann HW, eds: Carcinogenesis and biological effects of tumor promoters. New York: Raven Press, 1982; 305–9.
5. Reiners JJ, Slaga TJ. Effects of tumor promoters on the rate and commitment to terminal differentiation of subpopulations of murine keratinocytes. Cell 1983; 32:247–55.
6. Yamasaki H, Drevon C, Martel N. In vitro studies on the mechanism of tumor promoter mediated inhibition of cell differentiation. In Hecker E, Fusenig NE, Kunz W, Marks F, Thielmann HW, eds: Carcinogenesis and biological effects of tumor promoters. New York: Raven Press, 1982: 359–77.
7. Sisskin EE, Barrett JC. Inhibition of terminal differentiation of hamster epidermal cells in culture by the phorbol ester 12-O-tetradecanoylphorbol-13-acetate. Cancer Res 1981; 41:593–603.
8. Fusening N, Samsel W. Growth-promoting activity of phorbol ester TPA on cultured mouse skin keratinocytes, fibroblasts and carcinoma cells. In Slaga TJ, Sivak A, Boutwell RK, eds: Mechanisms of tumor promotion and carcinogenesis. New York: Raven Press, 1978: 203–20.
9. Yuspa SH, Ben T, Patterson E, Michael D, Elgjo K, Hennings H. Stimulated DNA-synthesis in mouse epidermal cell cultures treated with 12-O-tetradecanoylphorbol-13-acetate. Cancer Res 1978; 36:4062–8.
10. Yuspa SH, Ben T, Hennings H, Lichti V. Divergent responses in epidermal basal cells exposed to the tumor promoter 12-O-tetradecanoylphorbol-13-acetate. Cancer Res 1982; 42:2344–9.
11. Kawamura H, Strickland JE, Yuspa SH. Inhibition of 12-O-tetradecanoylphorbol-13-acetate induction of epidermal transglutaminase activity by protease inhibitors. Cancer Res 1983; 43:4073–7.
12. Hawley-Nelson P, Stanley JR, Schmidt J, Guillino M, Yuspa SH. The tumor promoter, 12-O-tetradecanoylphorbol-13-acetate accelerates keratinocyte differentiation and stimulates growth of an unidentifeid cell type in cultures of human epidermis. Exp Cell Res 1982; 137:155–76.
13. Hakomori S. Glycosphingolipids in cellular interaction, differentiation and oncogenesis. Annu Rev Biochem 1980; 50: 733–64.
14. Reibel J, Dabelsteen E, Hakomori S, Young WW, Mackenzie IC. The distribution of blood group antigens in rodent epithelia. Cell Tissue Res 1984; 237:111–6.
15. Cooper D, Schermer A, Sun TT. Classification of human epithelia and their neoplasms using monoclonal antibodies to keratins: Strategies, applications, and limitations. Lab Invest 1985; 52:243–56.
16. Jepsen A, MacCallum D, Lillie J. Fine structure of subcultivated stratified squamous epithelium. Exp Cell Res 1980; 125:141–52.
17. Lillie J, MacCallum D, Jepsen A. Fine structure of subcultivated stratified squamous epithelium grown on collagen rafts. Exp Cell Res 1980; 125:153–65.
18. Watkins WM. Biochemistry and genetics of the ABO, Lewis, and the P blood group systems. Adv Hum Genet 1980; 10:1–136.
19. Young WW, Portoukalian J, Hakomori S. Two monoclonal anticarbohydrate antibodies directed to glycosphingolipids with a lacto-N-glycosyl type II chain. J Biol Chem 1981; 256:10967–72.

20. Woodcock-Mitchell J, Eichner R, Nelson WG, Sun TT. Immunolocalization of keratin polypeptides in human epidermis using monoclonal antibodies. J Cell Biol 1982; 95:580–8.
21. Johnson GD, Nogueira-Araujo GMC. A simple method of reducing the fading of immunofluorescence during microscopy. J Immunol Methods 1981; 43:349–50.
22. Reibel J, Dabelsteen E. Staining patterns of rodent squamous epithelia by monoclonal antikeratin antibodies. Scand J Dent Res 1986; 94:38–46.
23. Sun TT, Eichner R, Nelson WG et al. Keratin classes: Molecular markers for different types of epithelial differentiation. J Invest Dermatol 1983; 81:109s–15s.
24. Astrup EG, Iversen OH. Cell population kinetics in hairless mouse epidermis following a single topical application of 12-O-tetradecanoylphorbol-13-acetate II. Virchows Arch (Cell Pathol) 1983; 42:1–18.
25. Goerttler K, Loehrke H, Schweizer J, Hesse B. Two-stage tumorigenesis of dermal melanocytes in the back skin of the Syrian golden hamster using systematic initiation with 7, 12-dimethylbenz (a) anthracene and topical promotion with 12-O-tetradecanoylphorbol-13-acetate. Cancer Res 1980; 40:155–61.
26. Arenholt D, Philipsen HP, Nikai H, Andersen L, Jepsen A. Chemically unrelated tumorpromoters induce identical morphological changes in cultured rat oral epithelium. Eur J Cancer Clin Oncol 1987; 23:19–29.
27. Arenholt D. Tumorpromoters in epithelial cell cultures. Ph.D. Thesis, Royal Dental College, Aarhus, Denmark, 1984.
28. Yuspa SH, Hennings H, Lichti V. Initiation and promotor induced specific changes in epidermal function and biological potential. J Supramol Struct 1981; 17:245–57.

Cancer Detection and Prevention Supplement 1:91–96 (1987)

Escape of Hybridomas From Cellular Defense Mechanisms:
An In Vitro Study Using Autologous and Allogeneic Lymphocytes

K.S. Zänker, MD
G. Blümel, MD
J. Lange, MD
J.R. Siewert, MD

Institute for Experimental Surgery (K.S.Z., G.B.), and Surgical Clinic (J.L., J.R.S.), Technical University Munich, Munich, Federal Republic of Germany

ABSTRACT   This study revealed that a hybridoma cell line made from an adenocarcinoma of the colon and autologous enucleated peripheral lymphocytes shared antigenicity of the fusion partners. The hybrid cells could be grown in BALB c nu/nu mice, forming a solid tumor. Gating out hybridoma cells with both CEA and T3 antigens by means of cytofluorometer cell sorting and using them as target cells in a cytotoxicity assay against autologous and allogeneic lymphocytes, the susceptibility for cell-mediated lysis within the cultured hybridoma cells was already lost. These findings suggest that transferred membrane component(s) (T3 antigen) from enucleated lymphocytes are candidates for functional regulator(s) in cell-mediated lysis.

Key words: enucleated lymphocytes, cytoplasts, whole cell fusion, antigenicity sharing, immune escape

INTRODUCTION

Recently Leu-7–positive cells were found in nonhemopoietic tissues [1–3] and tumors of neuroectodermal origin [4,5]. Leu-7 is a human differentiation antigen present on a subpopulation of morphologically homogenous large granular lymphocytes that have natural killer cell and antibody-dependent cell-mediated cytolytic functions. This Leu-7–positive subpopulation comprises about 15% of peripheral blood lymphocytes and is responsive to interferon [6]. Furthermore, Cole et al [7] reported on differential expression of Leu-7 antigen on human tumor cells. Their results indicated that the degree of expression of Leu-7 antigen may be under the control of differentiation-related events and useful in studying heterogeneity within and among tumor cells.

Attention has been turned to those host cells that infiltrate tumors, although for some time their presence has been taken as a good prognostic sign. Work on human tumors in which

Address reprint requests to Prof. Dr. K.S. Zänker, University of Witten, Herelecke Stockumerstr 10 5180 Witten, GFR.

immunological reactivity of lymphocytes is studied is hindered by the unavailability of target cells possessing the relevant tumor-specific antigens, because the presence of the latter in human tumors is sometimes doubtful.

The function of tumor-invading lymphocytes is, again, under discussion, because experimental and clinical results show that tumor-specific reactivities only seldom bear correlation to the tumor-host relationship as reflected in the persistence and growth of the tumor.

It is hypothesized that tumor-infiltrating lymphocytes fuse spontaneously, on rare occasions, with certain tumor cells. This event may lead to tumor cell clones, carrying surface cell markers, like the described Leu antigens, which operate as "stop signals" for attacking lymphocytes.

In the present study the susceptibility of a human adenocarcinoma of the colon and the hybridoma was examined in respect to cellular lysis in vitro by allogeneic and autologous lymphocytes.

MATERIALS AND METHODS
Cell Lines

Unless otherwise specified, tumor cell lines were routinely cultured in RPMI 1640 medium supplemented with 10% heat-inactivated fetal bovine serum (FBS), 2 mM L-glutamine, and 50 μM 2-mercaptoethanol. Cultures were checked for mycoplasma using the 4′,6-diamidino-2-phenylindole DNA binding assay [8] and found to be negative. hAd/13-84 is a cell line started in our laboratory in 1984 from a biopsy sample from a woman with a poorly differentiated adenocarcinoma of the sigmoid. The line had been in suspension culture 32 weeks at the time of testing and fusion with autologous lymphocytes.

Preparation of Peripheral Blood Lymphocyte (PBL)

Heparinized blood was taken from the patient and from healthy donors, and PBL were isolated from a Ficoll-Paque gradient. Blood was diluted 1:2 with RPMI medium (Seromed, Munich, FRG) and centrifuged for 20 min at 900g on a cushion of Ficoll-Paque. The lymphocyte band was collected, washed, and suspended in RPMI 1640 medium.

Enucleation of Lymphocytes and Fusion With Tumor Cells to Obtain Hybrid Cells

The autologous lymphocytes were enucleated with cytochalasin B by a method modified from that of Wigler and Weinstein [9]. In brief, suspension lymphocytes on cover glasses were placed into tubes for centrifugation in an upside-down position. Then medium containing 10 μg/ml of cytochalasin B was poured slowly into the tubes. After centrifugation at 10,000g for 7 minutes at 37°C, nucleoplasts at the bottom of the tubes were separately collected from cytoplasts (enucleated lymphocytes), which were still attached to the cover glasses. Samples from both fractions were stained with lactopropionic orcein to determine the efficiency of enucleation; the yield of enucleated lymphocytes was approximately 95%.

Hybrid cells were formed by the fusion of cytoplasts with whole cells of the adenocarcinoma line hAd/13-84 by 500 hemagglutinating units of β-propiolactone–inactivated Sendai virus/10^5 cell fragments. Colonies arising in the culture flasks were counted as soon as their presence was noted macroscopically. Further cloning was carried out by limiting dilution using irradiated human T-cell feeder layers seeded at 2×10^5 cells/well in 96-well microtiter dishes. After 4 to 6 weeks arising clones were isolated with Pasteur pipettes and transferred to 25 cm^2 flasks containing modified Iscove's medium supplemented with 5% FBS, pyruvate (1 mM), 2-mercaptoethanol (50 μM), bombesin (50 μM), hydrocortisone (10 μg/ml), insulin (0.01 IU/ml), transferrin (10 μg/ml), arginine vasopression (0.1 IU/ml), L-glutamine (4 mM), and ehtanolamine (0.2 μM). All biochemical supplements were obtained from Sigma Chemical Co. (St. Louis, MO) except for bombesin, which was obtained from Peninsula Laboratories Inc. (Belmont, CA). Colcemid-arrested cells were spread on microscopic slides, and chromosomes were stained to study general morphology by the standard Giemsa technique.

Xenotransplantation of Hybrid Cells

Solid tumors (hybridomas) in nude mice were obtained by SC inoculation of hybrid cells (5×10^5) in a volume of 0.2 ml into the left upper groin of 6-week-old BALB c nu/nu female mice. Tumor growth was grossly apparent after 18 to 23 days; 35 days after inoculation, tumor specimens were harvested for further processing in cell culture.

Tumorigenicity

The ability of the cells (parental line and hybrid cells) to form tumors was measured by recording growth curves and survival times of the xenotransplanted animals.

Cellular Cytotoxicity

To determine the susceptibility of the various cell lines to cellular cytotoxicity, the appropriate target cells were seeded in RPMI medium at a density of 1×10^5 cells/ml and labeled with ^{75}Semethionine (20 μl) (Amersham-Buchler, Braunschweig, FRG; total activity at time of delivery, 25 mCi/ml). After thorough washings, autologous or allogeneic PBL were added to give target:effector cell ratios of 1:10, 1:25, and 1:50. After 4 hours incubation of 37°C the supernatant was counted for released radioactivity. Medium release was determined by omitting effector cells; total release was counted after adding 2% (v/v) Triton X-100 to the labeled target cells. Cellular cytotoxicity was calculated by the formula:

$$\% \text{ cytotoxicity} = \frac{\text{experimental}_{\text{release}} - \text{medium}_{\text{release}}}{\text{Triton X-100}_{\text{release}} - \text{medium}_{\text{release}}} \times 100.$$

Flow Cytometry Analysis and Cell Sorting

Stable hybridoma cells were incubated for 30 min with fluorescein isothiocyanate-conjugated anti-CEA (Bio-Yeda, Rehovot, Israel) and phycoerythrin-labeled anti-Leu-4 (Becton and Dickinson, Mountain View, CA) antibodies. After repeated washings in phosphate-buffered saline, the cells were resuspended in PBS, 5% FBS, and 0.01 M NaN$_3$ and analyzed using the FACS 420 (Becton and Dickinson). Ten thousand cells were analyzed using a laser output of 400 mV and fluorescence gain 8. Each analysis was performed in triplicate, and the binding experiments were repeated at least twice. The cell fractions that expressed both epitopes for the tracing antibodies were sorted out and used as target cells for cellular cytotoxicity.

RESULTS

A cell culture was established from a human adenocarcinoma of the colon and propagated in vitro (parental line hAd/13-84). The glandular structure of the tumor was almost completely gone, the cells grew in solid masses, and the cell polarity was lost; mitoses were numerous, and there was an accumulation of mucin in individual cells. The established cell line was highly susceptible for cellular cytotoxicity mediated by autologous or allogeneic PBL. Furthermore, subcutaneously injected tumor cells could be passaged as a solid tumor in nude mice, indicating that the subsequent experiments were performed with autonomously growing tumor cells. The parental cell line could be fused in the presence of attenuated Sendai virus with autologous PBL to obtain hybrid cells. The analysis indicated that the hybrid cells contained only one parental nuclear genome, and the cells were able to form hybridomas in nude mice. Table I summarizes the survival and chromosomes of the parental and hybridoma cells. Three out of 512 clones were stable and could be used in cytofluorometric and cytotoxicity experiments. These clones were kept in culture for about 12 passages in vitro. The contour plot in Figure 1 shows that a bulk of the hybridoma cells carried the epitopes both for anti-CEA and anti-T3 antibodies. This result is in agreement with the E-rosetting of the hybridoma

TABLE I. Tumorigenicity and Cellular Markers of Parental and Hybridoma Cells

Cell lines	Survival (days)	No. of chromosomes	
		Modal	Range
Parental cells hAd/13–84	72 ± 12	42	40–48
Hybridoma cells	112 ± 21	42	41–45

Six BALB c nu/nu mice were xenografted with each cell line.

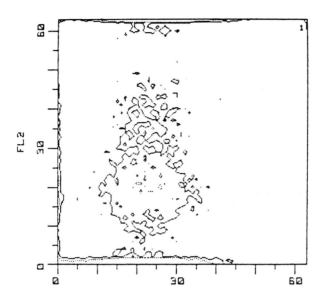

Fig. 1.   Dual parameter contour plot of hybridoma cells incubated with fluorescence-labeled anti-CEA (Fl 1) and anti-Leu-4 (Fl 2) antibodies.

cells. Cells positively stained for CEA and T3 antigen were gated and sorted out by means of FACS 420. A very limited amount of cells from the three stable clones showed reactivity with only one of the markers by gating out cells with signals at vertical and horizontal axes of the fluorescence region. The fluorescence intensity profile observed with peripheral blood lymphocytes was consistent with the fact that 78% of these cells were Pan-T cells, and the parental cells only reacted strongly with the FITC-conjugated anti-CEA antibody. In Figure 2, the susceptibility for cell-mediated cytotoxicity at different target:effector cell ratios are compared for the parental and the hybridoma cells. Using allogeneic lymphocytes from healthy donors where about 15% of these cells were natural killer cells as monitored by anti-Leu-7 antibody staining, the level of cytotoxicity was markedly reduced when hybridoma cell were used as target cells. In another set of experiments we used autologous PBL as effector cells and obtained similar results, with the minor exception that the parental line as target was slightly less susceptible for these effector cells than it was for allogeneic PBL. We found that virtually all susceptibility for cytolysis of immune competent cells could be removed when the fused target cells presented T3 antigen.

DISCUSSION

The lymphocyte plasma membrane plays a key role in the functions of the immune system. Both humoral and cell-mediated immune phenomena depend on the presence of specific membrane components and receptors located at the surface of the lymphocyte.

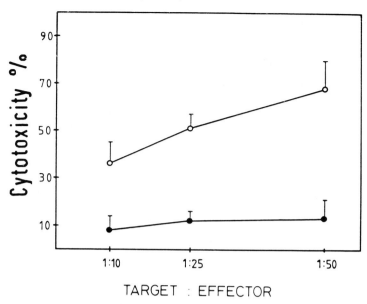

Fig. 2. Cell-mediated cytotoxicity of allogeneic PBL against hybridoma cells (filled circles) and parental cell line (hAd/13-84; open circles) at different target:effector ratios.

A new and promising approach involves the transfer of membrane components from one cell type (the donor), in our PBL experiments, to another (the acceptor), here the hAd/13-84 cell line, to study the effect of the new membrane composition on the ability of the acceptor cell to respond to the cell-mediated immune system. To test the effects of foreign cytoplasmic and/or membrane component regulators on an established human tumor cell line, we prepared cytoplasts (enucleated PBL) as one fusing partner. Several studies on other cell types have suggested that differentiated functions and tumorigenicity can be influenced by cytoplasmic factors and that the regulatory elements in the cytoplasm can remain active in the absence of nuclear genes [10–12].

We investigated the immune escape with hybridomas made from enucleated PBL and human adenocarcinoma of the colon. The hybrid cells showed the ability to form solid tumors in nude mice, like the parental line. The hybridoma cell still carried an antigenic determinant for CEA, but also shared antigenicity for T3 antigen, which was not detectable on cells of the parental line. The hybrid cells grew as heterotransplants in nude mice, and the harvested hybridoma cells did not lose the antigens, demonstrating that the fusion procedure succeeded in membrane constituent(s) transfer of enucleated PBL. Concomitant with the expression of the T3 antigen the susceptibility for cell-mediated lysis decreased. This observation might suggest that attacking lymphoid cells in vitro regarded the hybridoma cells as "self," in contrast to the parental cell line. It is a rationale to argue that the transfer to T3 antigen from enucleated PBL is somewhat associated with the diminished cytotoxicity seen for the hybridoma cells; the influence of cytoplasmic factor(s) on this described phenomenon could not be ruled out completely. However, based on the morphological appearance of the hybridoma cells, which closely resembled the parental line, and on the nuclear/cytoplasmic ratio of the nonstimulated PBL, it is suggested that we have transferred lymphoid plasma membrane components, as reflected by T3 antigen.

Our results provide additional evidence supporting the results on the shared antigenicity of tumor cells and PBL [7]. Moreover, the reported findings and their functional properties support the view of tumor escape phenomena in respect to cell-mediated cytotoxicity.

REFERENCES

1. Ilyas A, Quarles RH, Brady RO. The monoclonal antibody HNK-1 reacts with a human peripheral nerve ganglioside. Biochem Biophys Res Commun 1984; 122:1206–11.
2. McGarry RC, Helfand SL, Quarles RH, Roder J. Recognition of myelin-associated glycoprotein by the monoclonal antibody HNK-1. Nature 1983; 306:376–8.
3. Schuler-Petrovic S, Gebhart W, Lassmann H, Rumpold H, Kraft D. A shared antigenic determinant between natural killer cells and nervous tissue. Nature 1983; 306:179–81.
4. Caillaud JM, Benjelloun S, Bosq J, Braham K, Lipinski M. HNK-1 defined antigen detected in paraffin-embedded neuroectoderm tumours and those derived from cells of the amine precursor uptake and decarboxylation system. Cancer Res 1984; 44:4432–9.
5. Lipinski M, Braham K, Caillaud JM, Carlu C, Tursz T. HNK-1 antibody detects an antigen expressed on neuroectodermal cells. J Exp Med 1983; 158: 1775–80.
6. Abo T, Balch CM. Characterization of HNK-1$^+$ (Leu 7) human lymphocytes. III. Interferon effects on spontaneous cytotoxicity and phenotypic expression of lymphocyte subpopulations delineated by the monoclonal HNK-1 antibody. Cell Immunol 1982; 73:376–84.
7. Cole SPC, Mirski S, McGarry R, Cheng R, Campling BG, Roder JC. Differential expression of the Leu-7 antigen on human lung tumour cells. Cancer Res 1985; 45:4285–90.
8. Russel WC, Newman C, Williamson DH. A simple cytochemical technique for demonstration of DNA in cells infected with mycoplasmas and viruses. Nature 1975; 253:461–2.
9. Wigler MH, Weinstein IB. A preparative method for obtaining enucleated mammalian cells. Biochem Biophys Res Comm 1975; 63:247–58.
10. Gopalakrishnan TV, Anderson WF. Epigenetic activation of phenylalanine hydroxylase in mouse erythroleukemia cells by the cytoplast of rat hepatoma cells. Proc Natl Acad Sci USA 1979; 76:3932–6.
11. Lipsich LA, Kates JR, Lucas JJ. Expression of a liver-specific function by mouse fibroblast nucleus transplanted into rat hepatoma cytoplasts. Nature 1979; 281:74–6.
12. Jonasson J, Harris H. The analysis of malignancy by cell fusion. VIII. Evidence for the intervention of an extra-chromosomal element. J Cell Sci 1977; 24:255–64.

Cancer Detection and Prevention Supplement 1:97–102 (1987)

Relevance of Aging Research for Cancer

P. Ebbesen, MD

The Institute of Cancer Research, The Danish Cancer Society, Radiumstationen, Aarhus, Denmark

ABSTRACT   Experimental studies of the survival curves of different species and of in vitro cell culture survival point to normal aging as a largely preprogrammed process. Reciprocal skin grafting among syngeneic young and old animals further demonstrates autonomous aging of this organ independent of the remainder of the body. This compartmentalization of change with age is also suggested when immune functions of various lymphoid organs are compared at different ages. Experimental studies also show that for some organs their susceptibility to certain carcinogens is diphasic, high early in life and high in senescence. A major question now is if preprogrammed age changes at the molecular level have steps in common with carcinogenetic processes.

Key words: carcinogen susceptibility, immune system, programmed aging, oncogenes

INTRODUCTION

Cancer is primarily a disease of the old both in humans and in all other mammalian species. For theoretical and practical reasons, therefore, it is necessary to get an understanding of the interrelationship between these two entities. In particular, some light may be shed on areas of cancer research from studies in genontology, which have made important progress especially since the establishment of the U.S. National Institute of Aging more than a decade ago.

Normal aging is a gradual change in time that occurs in all members of a species and enhances the risk of dying. In this definition, cancer is not part of normal aging, but there is partial overlapping of the two processes.

The finite and species-dependent number of cell divisions available for at least some types of normal cells in vitro [1] represents one of the fundamental observations that seems relevant to normal aging and at the same time presents a major difference between normal and malignant phenotype. Fusion experiments revealed that in vitro senescence resides in the nucleus [2] and that senescence is dominant versus youth when normal cells are studied in vitro [3]. When incompletely differentiated cells that are immortal but not tumorigenic are fused with in vitro-aged normal cells the senescent nucleus is still dominant [4]. The genome of fully differentiated cells, however, seems able to overrule the block on cell division exerted by senescent cells [5].

Address reprint request to P. Ebbesen, The Institute of Cancer Research, The Danish Cancer Society, Radiumstationen, DK-8000 Aarhus C, Denmark.

The maximum number of in vitro doubling of fibroblasts correlates with the maximum survival time of each mammal species. In keeping with our studies in mice [6], the male-female difference in mean survival time is not reflected in the in vitro doubling potential.

In vivo aging of postmitotic cells like neurons of the brain and heart muscle cells is associated with a loss of a majority of the DNA templates necessary for ribosomal RNA production [7]. Cancer rarely develops in such tissue, but there is evidence that a somewhat similar phenomenon may take place in dividing cells.

During the replicative postmitotic life span of human fibroblasts, highly repetitious DNA sequences are depleted from the fibroblast genome leading to progressive diminution in functions such as the initiation of DNA replication [8]. At the same time the expression of the c-Ha-ras protooncogene is enhanced [9]. A sorting out of the relative importance of these two genomic alterations for aging is an important task. Likewise the possible importance of loss of DNA sequences for oncogene activation is an interesting problem.

From studies of immunoglobulin gene ontogeny [10] it is known that gene rearrangements can play a role in the differentiation of immune cells, but this has not been shown to be the case in other developmental processes, and its possible importance for normal aging is also unknown.

Aging of somatic cells thus might proceed along the line of terminal differentiation with progressive restriction of options, which would fit a deterministic molecular mechanism. However, more stochastically occurring events also are statistically correlated with aging. Extrachromosomal DNA circles have been observed in leukocytes of the old, and Shmookler Reis and Goldstein [11] speculate that these DNA sequences may integrate at random. Furthermore, the progressive DNA demethylation may enhance the risk of random expression of otherwise silent genes. Such events may predispose to the benign focal hyperplasias that are characteristic of normal aging [12]. In rare cases these foci are the site of malignant transformation.

INFLUENCE OF HOST AGE ON TUMOR INDUCTION AND INDIVIDUAL AND RACIAL DIFFERENCES IN SUSCEPTIBILITY

That differences in susceptibility to carcinogens in humans may reside in genetic differences is suggested by migrant studies of humans. Cancer of the nasopharynx, a rare tumor in most parts of the world, is known to be frequent among Chinese, in particular the Cantonese. Cancer of the nasopharynx remains frequent after migration of Cantonese to Singapore or to the United States [13]. Certain Chinese genotypes are now suspected to be important in increasing the susceptibility to nasopharyngeal cancer development [14]. Furthermore, susceptibility to ultraviolet light-mediated induction of skin carcinomas and melanomas is dependent on skin color and thus on genetics [13].

There is an age-dependent change in susceptibility to cancer induction in humans. Fetuses that have completed organogenesis, children, and adolescents are more susceptible to cancer induction by some agents than are adults. Examples are adenocarcinomas of the vagina in offspring of mothers treated with stilbestrol during pregnancy [15], leukemia after X-ray irradiation of children [16], and breast cancer as a consequence of irradiation, where the adolescent girl is most at risk [17]. In these age groups cell proliferation related to organ growth is likely to be a major reason for the high susceptibility to carcinogens.

It is less obvious whether normal aging of the adult influences susceptibility to the tumor-inducing effect of a carcinogen to which one has not been previously exposed. Human environments are complex and do not permit conclusively ascertaining nonexposure to certain chemicals. Most studies indicate that the risk of cancer development increases in relation to a person's age at first exposure to a carcinogen; such examples are bladder cancer in dyestuff workers [18], skin warts after tar exposure [19,20], lung cancer in asbestos workers [21], and sinus cancer in nickel workers [22]. The same relation of age to cancer development is reported for adult humans exposed to irradiation. The number of cancer cases caused by irradiation increase with age at first treatment. The ratio of observed cancer cases to expected incidence, however, does not necessarily change with age, because the spontaneous incidence of many tumors also increases with age. Examples are cancer following treatment of ankylosing spondylitis [23,24] and uterine cancer after irradiation treatment of metropathia hemorrhagica [25]. Jablon and Kato [26] and Beebe et al [27] found an increased risk of leukemia in A-bomb survivors with increase in age at time of detonation. An example of another age-susceptibility relationship is the incidence of cancer of the lung in nickel workers, which increases with age at first exposure up to 25 years of age and then, for unknown reasons, decreases again [22].

ANIMAL EXPERIMENTAL EVIDENCE

In animal experiments, the conditions are fairly well defined in regard to the type of chemical and the doses employed. However, it is important to keep in mind that the dosage necessary to induce a few tumors using a large number of animals far exceeds the exposure of humans to carcinogens. The high carcinogen doses used in the animal experiments may easily conceal what differences in susceptibility there may be when using doses more manageable by detoxification and/or repair processes [28].

When senescent BALB/c mouse skin is exposed to small doses of carcinogens one finds an increase in susceptibility compared to younger adult skin. This is the case both when tumors are induced with a small dose of 7-12-dimethylbenz(α)anthracene, β-irradiation, and UV light [29]. Skin grafted from middle-aged to young recipients developed the same increased susceptibility to carcinogens with further aging as did nongrafted skin. The high susceptibility to carcinogens of senescent skin thus must derive from local, autonomously developing alteration in the skin itself.

More abnormalities of chromosomes are produced by in vitro carcinogen treatment of leukocytes from old than from young human donors [30]. Summerhayes and Franks [31] found in vitro transformation of bladder epithelium easier with bladder epithelium cultures that were established from old than from young mouse donors. Furthermore, in vitro aging may be accompanied by increased susceptibility to a transforming chemical [32].

THE IMMUNE SYSTEM

The role of immunity in normal development of the growing organism is largely unknown. It has been proposed that the recognition sites on normal lymphocytes may influence the development of nonlymphoid organs [33]. Presence of receptors shared by lymphoid cells and brain cells [34,35] suggests a possible interaction of both.

A declining capacity for T cell-dependent immune responses is one of the most apparent features of aging of the organism. Most studies on immunological aging have for obvious practical reasons been performed in rodents. Such studies have shown that aging of the immune system is not an entirely irreversible process. It may be influenced temporarily by the administration of substances such as thymic factors and lymphokines and by grafting of syngeneic bone marrow. Its possible effect on tumor development is not well known. Other important aspects are the different patterns of immunologic aging that exist within different compartments of the organism [36] similar to the previously described aging of skin. This compartmentalization certainly limits the interpretations that can be made from human studies, which mostly consist of tests on cells from peripheral blood.

Attempts to demonstrate if the age-related decline in immune reactivity and its relationship to the development of malignant neoplasms has met with limited success. But nature's cruel experiment with AIDS is strong evidence of the enhanced risk of cancer development following immunosuppression. Work from our own group showed that endemic Kaposi sarcoma in eastern Zaire occurs independently of infection with HTLV-III/LAV, and Baley et al [37] have demonstrated that the aggressive form of Kaposi sarcoma in Africa, as elsewhere, is associated with HTLV-III/LAV infection.

TABLE I. Cromium 51 Release From Labeled Syngeneic Fibroblasts and YAC Cells

Strain	Attacking spleen cells	Target cells	
		Fibroblasts	YAC cells
CBA	Young	Baseline	Baseline
	Old	10	19
	Old-dying	15	32
DBA	Young	Baseline	Baseline
	Old	5	5
	Old-dying	10	41

Fibroblasts and cells were incubated in vitro with unfractionated spleen cells from young healthy, old healthy, and like-aged old dying mice. The values given are percentage increase above that obtained with attacking cells from young donors (baseline).

Lifelong chronic social stress will in experimental animals at least accelerate development of changes characteristic of normal aging [38], including depression of cellular immune functions [39]. Its role in oncogenesis has been demonstrated for virus-induced tumor by facilitated tumor induction [40] and by accelerated growth of the virus-induced tumor [41].

Longevity of mice in captivity, which have a survival curve very similar to that of humans, seems to be genetically controlled [42]. Furthermore, there is some evidence that the genetic control of longevity may be associated with the major histocompatibility complex—the H-2 region of the mouse [43]. Decline in immune capacity and occurrence of autoimmune processes is the one objective parameter that has shown the most predictive value with respect to the remaining life span [44]. Our preliminary work, furthermore, suggests that autoimmune reactions may be acutely involved in the very process of spontaneous death in mice [45] (Table I).

The death certificates of most countries require the physician to state the primary cause of death, and cancer often is reported as such. Experimental studies suggest that this procedure may lead to some misinterpretation. In a previous experiment [46], 213 untreated (CBA/DBA/2)F_1 female mice had been followed throughout life. The detectable cause of death was classified as leukemia, other malignancy, or degenerative lesion such as amyloidosis; for some no evidence of disease was detectable clinically or histologically upon death. The mean and median survival times for the three groups were to our surprise nearly identical, and we speculated that an underlying cause common to most mice in all groups was responsible for most deaths. Studies of normal aging thus already have offered some information for cancer research, and it is anticipated that further progress may be made in the decade ahead.

REFERENCES

1. Hayflick L, Moorhead PS. The serial cultivation of human diploid cell strains. Exp Cell Res 1961; 25:585–621.
2. Wright WE, Hayflick L. Contributions of cytoplasmic factors to in vitro cellular senescence. Fed Proc 1975; 34:76–9.
3. Littlefield JW. Attempted hydribidizations with senescent human fibroblasts. J Cell Physiol 1973; 82:129–32.
4. Stein GH, Yanishevsky RM. Entry into S phase is inhibited in two immortal cell lines fused to senescent human diploid cells. Exp Cell Res 1979; 120:155–65.
5. Rabinovitch PS, Norwood JH. Comparative heterokaryon study of cellular senescence and the serum-deprived state. Exp Cell Res 1980; 130:101–9.
6. Ebbesen P. No male-female difference in in vitro lifespan of skin fibroblasts from humans and mice. Exp Gerontol 1983; 18:323–4.
7. Strehler BL, Chang MP. Loss of hybridizable ribosomal DNA from human postmitotic tissues during aging: II. Age-dependent loss in human cerebral cortex-hippocampal and somatosensory cortex comparison. Mech Ageing Dev 1979; 11:379–82.

8. Schmid CW, Jelinek WR. The Alu family of dispersed repetitive sequences. Science 1982; 216:1065–70.

9. Shih C, Weinberg RA. Isolation of a transforming sequence from a human bladder carcinoma cell line. Cell 1982; 29:161–9.

10. Tonegara S, Sakano H, Mati R, Traunecker A, Heinrich G, Roeder W, Kurosawa Y. Somatic reorganisation of immunoglobulin genes during lymphocyte differentiation. Cold Spring Harbor Symp Quant Biol 1981; 46:839–58.

11. Shmookler Reis RJ, Goldstein S. Mitochondrial DNA in mortal and immortal human cells. J Biol Chem 1983; 258:9078–85.

12. Martin GM. Proliferative homeostatis and its age-related aberrations. Mech Ageing Dev 1979; 9:385–91.

13. Waterhouse J, Muir CS, Correa P, Powel J, eds. Cancer, Incidence in Five Continents, Vol III. Lyon: International Agency for Research on Cancer, 1976 (IARC Sci Publ No. 15).

14. Simons MJ, Wee GB, Chan SH, Shanmugaratnam K. Probable identification of an HL-A second-locus antigen associated with a high risk of nasopharyngeal carcinoma. Lancet 1975; 1:142–5.

15. Herbst AL, Poskanzer DC, Robboy SJ, Friedlander L, Scully RE. Prenatal exposure to stilbestrol. A prospective comparison of exposed female offspring with unexposed controls. N Engl J Med 1975; 292:334–9.

16. Schwartz EE, Upton AC. Factors influencing the incidence of leukemia: Special consideration of the role of ionizing radiation. Blood 1958; 13:845–64.

17. McGregor DH, Land CE, Chor K, Tokvuku S, Liv PI, Watabayashi T, Beebe GW. Breast cancer incidence among atomic bomb survivors, Hiroshima and Nagasaki, 1950–1969. JNCI 1977; 59:799–811.

18. Case RAM, Hoster ME, McDonald DB, Pearson JT. Tumours of the urinary bladder in workmen engaged in the manufacture and use of certain dyestuff intermediates in the British chemical industry. Br J Ind Med 1954; 11:75–104.

19. Fisher REW. The effect of age upon the incidence of tar warts. In: 12th Int Congr Occupational Health, Valtaneuvoston Kirjapaino, Helsinki, 1958, p 402.

20. Doll R. Epidemiological observations on susceptibility to cancer in man with special reference to age. Acta Unio Int Contra Cancrum 1964; 20:747–52.

21. Knox JF, Holmes S, Doll R, Hill ID. Mortality from lung cancer and other causes among workers in an asbestos textile factory. Br J Ind Med 1968; 25:293–303.

22. Doll R, Morgan L, Speitzer FE. Cancers of the lung and nasal sinuses of nickel workers. Br J Cancer 1970; 24:623–32.

23. Court BWM, Doll R. Mortality from cancer and other causes after radiotherapy for ankylosing spondylitis. Br Med J 1965; 2:1327–32.

24. Smith PG, Doll R. Age- and time-dependent changes in the rates of radiation-induced cancers in patients with ankylosing spondylitis following a single course of X-ray treatment. IAEA-SM 1982; 224:205–18.

25. Smith PG, Doll R. Late effects of X irradiation in patients treated for metropathia hemorragica. Br J Radiol 1976; 49:224–32.

26. Jablon S, Kato H. Studies of the mortality of A-bomb survivors. Radiat Res 1972; 50:649–98.

27. Beebe GW, Kato A, Land CE. Studies on the mortality of A-bomb survivors. 8. Mortality experience of A-bomb survivors 1950–1974. Hiroshima: Radiation Effects Research Foundation, 1977; 1–77 (RERF Tech Rep).

28. Pegg AE, Nicoll JW, Magee PN, Swann PF. Importance of DNA repair in an organ. Specificity of tumour induction by N-nitroso carcinogens. Proc Eur Soc Toxicol 1976; 17:39–54.

29. Ebbesen P, Kripke ML. The influence of age and anatomical site on ultraviolet carcinogenesis in BALB/c mice. JNCI 1982; 68:691–4.

30. Bochov MP, Kulestrov NP. Age sensitivity of human chromosomes to alkylating agents. Mutat Res 1972; 14:345–53.

31. Summerhayes IC, Franks LM. Effects of donor age on neoplastic transformation of adult mouse bladder epithelium in vitro. JNCI 1979; 62:1017–23.

32. Lasne C, Gentil A, Chouroulinkov I. Two-stage malignant transformation of rat fibroblasts in tissue culture. Nature 1974; 247:490–1.

33. Burch PRJ. The biology of cancer. A new approach. Lancaster: MTP Press Ltd, 1976.

34. Besedovsky HO, del Rez AE, Sorkin E. What do the immune system and the brain know about each other? Immunol Today 1984; 4:342–6.

35. Renoux G. Brain neocortex and the immune system. Immunology Today 1984; 5:318.
36. Steinmann GG, Klaus G, Gillis S, Müller-Hermelink HK. Thymic and splenic IL 2-production and response during aging and correlations with immunohistologic studies. In de Weck AL, (ed): Lymphoid cell functions in aging, 3. 1984; 161–9.
37. Baley AC, Downing RG, Cheigson-Pau R, Tedder RS, Dalgleish AG, Weiss RA. HTLV-III serology distinguishes atypical and endemic Kaposi's sarcoma in Africa. Lancet 1985; 1:359–61.
38. Ebbesen P. Spontaneous amyloidosis in differently grouped and treated DEA/2, BALB/c, and CBA mice and thymus fibrosis in estrogen-treated BALB/c males. J Exp Med 1968; 127:387–96.
39. Monjan AA. Effects of acute and chronic stress upon lymphocyte blastogenesis in mice and humans. In Cooper EL, ed: Stress, immunity and aging. New York: Marcel Dekker, Inc., 1984; 81–108.
40. Amkraut A, Solomon GF. Stress and murine sarcoma virus (Moloney)-induced tumors. Cancer Res 1972; 32:1428–33.
41. Justice A. Review of the effects of stress on cancer in laboratory animals: Importance of time of stress application and type of tumor. Psychol Bull 1985; 98:108–38.
42. Popp DM, Popp RA. Genetics. In: Kay MM, Makinodan T, eds: Handbook of immunology in aging. Boca Raton, FL: CRC Press, 1981; 15.
43. Ohno S, Nagai Y. Genes in multiple copies as the primary cause of aging. Birth Defects 1978; 14:501.
44. Bender BS, Nagel JE, Adler WH, Andres R. The prognostic significance of a declining lymphocyte count in elderly men: Relation to subsequent mortality. Submitted, 1986.
45. Ebbesen P, Faber T, Fuursted K. Dying old mice: Occurrence of non-viable lymphocytes and autoaggressive cells. Exp Gerontol 1982; 17:425–8.
46. Rask-Nielsen R, Ebbesen P. Spontaneous reticular neoplasms in (CBA × DBA/2)F$_1$ mice, with special emphasis on the occurrence of plasma cell neoplasms. JNCI 1969; 43:553–64.

Cancer Detection and Prevention Supplement 1:103–109 (1987)

Phenotypic and Functional Analyses of Tumour-Infiltrating Leu 7 + Natural Killer-Like Cells in Non-Hodgkin Lymphomas

Diponkar Banerjee, MB, ChB, PhD

Department of Pathology, St. Joseph's Health Centre and the University of Western Ontario, London, Canada

ABSTRACT Biopsy specimens of lymphoid tissues were analysed by two-colour flow cytometry to determine the proportions and phenotypes of natural killer-like cells present in the lesions. No significant difference was found between the proportions of Leu 7+ cells in reactive and malignant nodes. Low numbers of Leu 11+ cells were found in both benign and malignant nodes. The most common phenotype among the tumour-infiltrating Leu 7+ cells in the malignant nodes was Leu 7+OKT3+OKM1−. Only low numbers of Leu 7+ cells in malignant nodes coexpressed OKM1.

Isolated Leu 7+ cells from four out of five malignant nodes were unable to lyse autologous B lymphoma cells in vitro. However, in one of five malignant nodes tested, autologous B lymphoma cells were lysed by isolated tumour-infiltrating Leu 7+ cells but not by Leu 7− cells. These observations indicate that tumour-infiltrating Leu 7+ cells are infrequently capable of lysing autologous lymphoma cells.

Key words: monoclonal antibodies, panning, flow cytometry

INTRODUCTION

In a previous study from this laboratory it was shown that lymph node cells expressing Leu 7 antigen, a marker expressed by a subpopulation of human natural killer (NK) cells, are located almost exclusively within B cell compartments and coexpress pan-T antigens Leu 1 and OKT3 but not myeloid antigen OKM1 [1]. This is in contrast to circulating or splenic red pulp Leu 7+ cells, which predominantly coexpress OKM1 [1, 2]. It was also demonstrated that Leu 7+ cells are found not only in normal B cell compartments but can also infiltrate malignant lymphomas of both T and B cell orgin [1]. The Leu 7+OKM1+ subset has more potent NK activity than the Leu 7+ OKT3+ subset against K562 cells, a standard in vitro target for NK cells [2]. Whether the same holds true for autologous tumour cell lysis is not known. Preliminary results are reported here from a prospective study to determine the major phenotype of NK-like cells infiltrating lymphomas and the ability of isolated Leu 7+ cells to

Address reprint requests to Dr. D. Banerjee, Department of Pathology, St. Joseph's Health Centre, 268 Grosvenor Street, London, Ontario, Canada N6A 4L6.

lyse autologous lymphoma cells and K562 cells in vitro. Since there is recent evidence that the most active NK cells express Leu 11 and do not coexpress Leu 7 [3], the presence of Leu 11 + cells was also determined.

MATERIALS AND METHODS
Preparation of Cell Suspensions

The use of human tissues obtained for diagnostic purposes in investigative tests was approved by the University of Western Ontario Health Sciences Standing Committee on Human Experimentation. Biopsy specimens of lymph nodes or masses in patients clinically suspected to have malignant lymphomas were obtained and divided into two portions under aseptic conditions. One portion was processed for routine histological examination, and the other was placed in sterile phosphate-buffered saline (PBS) containing penicillin and streptomycin. The latter portion was chopped with a pair of fine-tipped scissors to obtain a cell suspension. The suspension was filtered through two layers of sterile gauze to remove large clumps and layered on Ficoll Hypaque gradients. The gradients were centrifuged for 20 min at 18°C at 400g. Interface cells were collected, washed three times, and resuspended in PBS at a concentration of 10^6 cells per millilitre.

Labeling of Cells With Monoclonal Antibodies

One hundred microlitres of the suspension were placed in Eppendorf microcentrifuge tubes, and each tube was incubated with a 50 μl volume of prediluted monoclonal antibody at 4°C for 30 min. The antibodies used were as follows: anti-OKT3, anti-OKM1 (Ortho Diagnostics, Willowdale, Ontario), anti-Leu 7 biotin, and Leu 11 (Becton Dickinson, Sunnyvale, CA), all at a dilution of 1:10 in AB serum. Samples for two colour analysis were incubated with mixtures of anti-OKT3 FITC and anti-Leu 7 biotin or anti-OKM1 and anti-Leu 7 biotin at final dilutions of 1:10 in AB serum. Following the incubation, the cells were washed three times and then incubated with affinity-purified goat antimouse γ-chain FITC (Jackson Laboratories, Hornby, Ontario) and/or avidin-phycoerythrin (Becton Dickinson) at final dilutions of 1:10 in AB serum at 4°C for 30 min.

Flow Cytometry

The cells were washed three times and analysed, using an EPICS C flow cytometer (Coulter Electronics, Haileah, FL). The laser was tuned to a wavelength of 488 nm, with a power setting of 500 mW. Filters used were 1) a 488 nm dichroic filter, 2) a 515 nm long pass interference filter, 3) a 560 nm short pass dichroic filter placed before the green PMT, and 4) a 590 nm long pass filter placed before the red PMT. Unlabeled cells were analysed first by simultaneous sensing of log 90° light scatter and forward light scatter. By displaying a two parameter histogram, it was possible to resolve the light scatter signals into two main clusters, one representing lymphocytes and the other macrophages. A bit map was drawn around the lymphocyte cluster, and labeled samples were then analysed for fluorescence with reference to cells whose light scatter characteristics matched the lymphocyte bit map. Both log-red fluorescence and log-green fluorescence were simultaneously detected and displayed as a two parameter histogram. Single-labeled cells were analysed first to set the lower thresholds so that no spectral overlap could occur in the red and green emissions. Minor adjustments of the colour subtraction module were needed to resolve the red and green signals as scattergrams perpendicular to one another. The percentages of cells showing positive red or green fluorescence were recorded. Dual-labeled cells were then analysed, and the percentages of cells showing only red fluorescence, only green fluorescence, or both were recorded.

Separation of Lymphocyte Subpopulations

Ficoll Hypaque-separated mononuclear cells were incubated in fetal calf serum-coated petri dishes for 45 min to remove adherent cells and then passed through nylon wool columns to separate T and B cells. The T cell fraction was then incubated on anti-Leu 7-coated petri dishes for 2 hr at 4°C. Nonadherent (Leu 7−) and adherent (Leu 7+) fractions were harvested by panning as described by Wysocki and Sato [4]. Purity of the Leu 7+ fraction was in general between 70 and 86%, while the Leu 7− fraction usually contained less than 3% Leu 7+ cells.

Cytotoxicity Assay

K562 cells were labeled with ^{51}Cr for 1 hr at 37°C as described previously [5]. Nylon wool-separated B cells from lymph node biopsy specimens were labeled with 200 μCi of ^{51}Cr per 10^6 cells for 5 hr. Labeled cells were distributed in 96 well round-bottomed microtitre plates (10^4 cells per well) and mixed with effector cells at various ratios. The plates were incubated for 18 h at 37°C in a humidified CO_2 incubator. Supernatants were harvested and radioactivity determined by γ-counting. Percentage of corrected ^{51}Cr release was calculated as previously described [5].

Histological Diagnosis

Diagnoses were based on routinely stained paraffin sections in all cases.

Lymphoma Phenotyping

Cell suspensions were labeled with FITC-conjugated antibodies to T cell differentiation antigens (T3, T4, T8), B cell differentiation antigens (B1, B2, B4), HLADR antigen, and κ and λ light chains and analysed by flow cytometry.

RESULTS
Histological Diagnoses and Phenotypes of the Lymphomas

Of the ten cases of non-Hodgkin lymphoma studied, five were of the follicular small, cleaved cell type, two were of the diffuse small, cleaved cell type, two were of the diffuse large noncleaved type, and one was an immunoblastic sarcoma of T cell origin. Of the nine reactive lymph nodes studied, six showed follicular hyperplasia, two showed sinus hyperplasia, and one showed paracortical hyperplasia. The phenotype of each lymphoma is indicated in Table I.

Percentage of Tumour-Infiltrating Leu 7+ and Leu 11+ Cells

In the reactive nodes, the proportion of Leu 7+ cells ranged from 0 to 10.4%, with a mean of 4.5% (SD 3.8%). In the lymphoma cases, the proportion of Leu 7+ cells ranged from 0.7 to 40% of total lymphocytes, with a mean of 11.95% (SD 5.2%). The mean was not significantly higher than in the control cases (P = 0.056). Only low numbers of Leu 11+ cells were found in controls (range 0 to 5.9%, mean 1.9%, SD 1.9%) and even lower numbers in the malignant nodes (range 0 to 2.1%, mean 0.9%, SD 0.7%), although this difference was not statistically significant. The number of Leu 7+ cells was significantly higher than the number of Leu 11+ cells in both malignant (P = 0.008) and reactive (P = 0.04) nodes (Table I).

Phenotypes of Leu 7+ Cells

Of the Leu 7+ cells present in the reactive nodes, 63 to 100% coexpressed pan-T antigen OKT3 (mean 84.7%, SD 12.2%), while those in the malignant nodes showed a similar proportion of Leu 7+ cells coexpressing this marker (range 26 to 100%, mean 82.0%, SD 25.6%; P = 0.4). Only a minority of the Leu 7+ cells coexpressed myeloid antigen OKM1 in the reactive nodes (range 0 to 40%, mean 11.1%, SD 13.3%) as well as the malignant nodes (range 0 to 23%, mean 5.0%, SD 6.9%; P = 0.1) (Table I).

Lytic Activity of Leu 7+ and Leu 7− Fractions

Of the ten lymphomas studied, lytic activity of isolated Leu 7+ and Leu 7− fractions against autologous B cells and K562 cells could be tested in five cases from which sufficient

TABLE I. Results of Phenotypic and Functional Analyses

Diagnosis	Phenotype	Percent Leu 7+ cells	Percent Leu 11+ cells	Percent Leu 7+ cells expressing	
				OKT3	OKM1
Non-Hodgkin lymphoma					
IBS-T	T	10.0	ND	90	0
SCC, FOLL	B	2.4	1.4	100	23
SCC, FOLL	B	8.4	2.1	45	9
LNCC, DIFF	B	40.0	0.8	90	2
SCC, FOLL	B	25.7	1.5	81	4
SCC, FOLL	B	18.7	0.9	26	2
LNCC, DIFF	B	5.2	0.7	92	6
SCC, FOLL	B	4.5	ND	96	4
SCC, DIFF	B	3.2	0	100	0
SCC, DIFF	B	0.7	0	100	0
Mean ± SD		11.88 ± 5.19*,‖	0.93 ± 0.73†	82.0 ± 25.6‡	5.0 ± 6.9§
Benign cases					
PH		0	0.6	ND	ND
FH		8.0	1.6	89	4
FH		4.8	3.5	63	19
SH		1.0	2.0	100	0
FH		0.7	0.3	100	14
FH		6.1	2.4	89	5
SH		2.0	5.9	85	40
FH		7.8	0	ND	3
FH		10.4	1.0	82	4
Mean ± SD		4.53 ± 3.77¶	1.92 ± 1.86	84.7 ± 12.2	11.1 ± 13.3

NHL, non-Hodgkin lymphoma; IBS-T, immunoblastic sarcoma of peripheral T cell origin; SCC, small cleaved cell lymphoma; FOLL, follicular; DIFF, diffuse; LNCC, large, noncleaved cell lymphoma; PH, paracortical hyperplasia; FH, follicular hyperplasia; SH, sinus hyperplasia; ND, Not done.
*P = 0.056, NHL vs benign cases, t test.
†P = 0.09, NHL vs benign cases, t test.
‡P = 0.04, NHL vs benign cases, t test.
§P = 0.1, NHL vs benign cases, t test.
‖P = 0.008, Leu 7 vs Leu 11 in NHL cases.
¶ = 0.04, Leu 7 vs Leu 11 in benign cases.

cells were recovered. Four of the five cases showed no detectable lysis of autologous B lymphoma cells. All of these lymphomas were of the small, cleaved cell, follicular type. Figure 1A shows the absence of detectable lysis of autologous B lymphoma cells by isolated Leu 7+ or Leu 7− cells in one of these four cases. The Leu 7+ cells had no activity against K562 cells, whereas Leu 7− cells had a low level of lytic activity (Fig. 1B). The lack of lytic activity against autologous B cell targets was probably not due to resistance of these targets to NK-mediated lysis, because they could be effectively lysed by normal peripheral blood lymphocytes from a healthy donor (Fig. 1A). One of the five cases, a large, noncleaved, diffuse lymphoma, however, yielded Leu 7+ cells that, although only modestly active against K562 cells (Fig. 2A), could kill autologous B cells (Fig. 2B). Leu 7− cells from this case had lytic activity against K562 cells similar to Leu 7+ cells but no activity against autologous B cells (Fig. 2B).

DISCUSSION

The results presented here indicate that the major phenotype of tumour-infiltrating Leu 7+ cells is Leu 7+OKT3+, identical to that in reactive nodes and normal B cell compartments

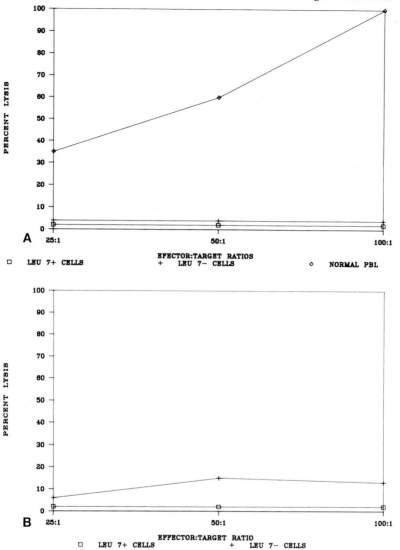

Fig. 1 **A:** Lytic activity of isolated Leu 7+ and Leu 7− tumour-infiltrating cells against autologous B lymphoma cells from a small, cleaved cell, follicular lymphoma. To demonstrate that the tumour cells were not resistant to NK-mediated lysis, allogeneic peripheral blood lymphocytes (PBL) were also used as effector cells. Whereas the tumour cells were not killed by autologous effector cells, they were killed by normal allogeneic PBL. **B:** Lytic activity of isolated Leu 7+ and Leu 7− tumour-infiltrating cells against K562 targets. The effector cells were from the same case as those in A.

[1]. This suggests that tumour-infiltrating Leu 7+ cells originate from within B cell compartments and are not recruited from circulating Leu 7+ cells, which are predominantly of the phenotype Leu 7+OKT3−OKM1+ [2]. The very low numbers of Leu 11+ cells in the malignant lymph nodes do not give much support to the idea that these cells, which are highly lytic toward K562 cells in vitro [3], have a major role in the host response to malignant lymphomas. Since the physiological role of intrafollicular Leu 7+OKT3+ cells in normal B cell compartments is, as yet, not established, the presence of these cells within malignant

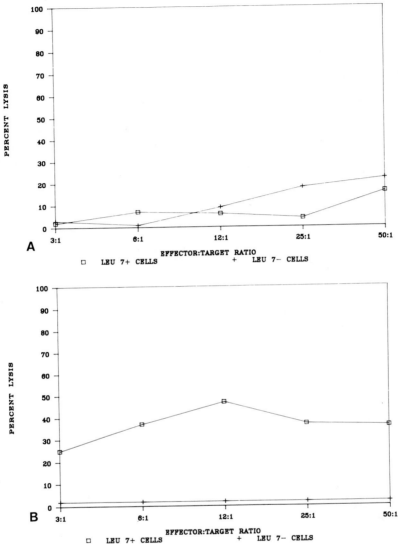

Fig. 2. **A:** Lytic activity of isolated tumour-infiltrating Leu 7+ and Leu 7− cells from a large, noncleaved cell diffuse lymphoma against K562 targets. **B:** Lytic activity of Leu 7+ and Leu 7− cells, from the same case as in A, against autologous B lymphoma cells.

lymph nodes is of unknown significance. Recent publications have documented that the concentration of Leu 7+ cells in lymph nodes is higher in low grade lymphomas compared to higher grade lymphomas [6, 7]. It is tempting to speculate that such observations point toward a role of these cells in influencing the biological behaviour of malignant lymphomas. However, functional studies of isolated Leu 7+ cells from lymph node biospy material do not support such a speculation. Of the four low grade lymphomas from which Leu 7+ cells were isolated, not one yielded cells capable to lysing autologous lymphoma cells, and, at most, modest lysis was observed against K562 cells, which are highly susceptible to NK-mediated lysis. B cell targets from a low grade, small, cleaved cell lymphoma were highly susceptible to lysis by allogeneic normal peripheral blood lymphocytes despite the lack of lytic activity by autologous

Leu 7+ cells (Fig. 1A, B), providing good evidence that the lack of autologous in vitro killing was not due to target cell resistance to lysis but due to a lack of lytic activity in the effector cells. On the contrary, lysis of tumour cells was demonstrated in a large cell lymphoma, generally considered to be of intermediate grade. This was not associated with concurrently high lytic activity against K562 cells, indicating that conventional NK cells are not involved in the autologous lytic reaction (Fib. 2A, B).

Clearly, there is a potential for tumour-infiltrating Leu 7+ cells to lyse autologous lymphoma targets, but, in most cases, this cannot be demonstrated. Whether the lack of autologous lytic activity is due to a defect in this subset of NK cells or to suppression of killing by other host cells or factors released by the tumour cells remains to be established. It is known, for example, that monocyte-derived soluble factors can suppress the lytic activity of peripheral blood NK cells and that by depleting monocytes and enriching NK cells followed by short-term culture, enhanced lysis of autologous targets can be demonstrated [8]. The role of tumour-infiltrating macrophages and other host cells in the suppression of NK activity in non-Hodgkin lyphomas requires investigation. Such lines of investigation may reveal methods of enhancing the lytic ability of tumour-infiltrating NK cells.

ACKNOWLEDGMENTS

The author thanks Judy Elliott and Dave McFarlane for technical assistance and Drs. K.L. Turner and R. Armstrong for submitting samples for the study. This study was supported by a grant from the National Cancer Institute of Canada and was presented in part at the Symposium on the Immunobiology of Cancer and Allied Immune Dysfunctions, Copenhagen, Denmark, November 4–7, 1985.

REFERENCES

1. Banerjee D, Thibert RF. Natural killer-like cells found in B cell compartments of human lymphoid tissue. Nature 1983; 304:270–2.
2. Abo T, Cooper MD, Balch CM. Characterisation of HNK-1+(Leu 7+) human lymphocytes. I. Two distinct phenotypes of human NK cells with different cytotoxic capability. J Immunol 1982; 129:1752–7.
3. Perussia B. Trinchieri G, Jackson A, et al. The Fc receptor for IgG on human natural killer cells. Phenotypic, functional and comparative studies with monoclonal antibodies. J Immunol 1984; 133:180–90.
4. Wysocki LJ, Sato VL. "Panning" for lymphocytes: A method for cell selection. Proc Natl Acad Sci USA 1978; 75:2844–8.
5. Banerjee D, Fernando L, Sklar S, Richter M. The antibody independent cytotoxicity activity of normal circulating human leucocytes. Lysis of target cells by monocytes and neutrophils in a non phagocytic pathway. Immunology 1981; 44:97–107.
6. Mori S. Yamaguchi K, Morita H, Mohri N. Distribution of HNK-1+ cells in malignant lymphomas. Acta Pathol Jpn 1985; 35:339–50.
7. Gattringer C, Radaskiewicz T, Pfaller W, Huber H. Infiltration density of HNK-1 positive cells in non-Hodgkin's lymphomas depends on histologic subtype: An in situ morphometric analysis. Immunobiology 1985; 169:280–91.
8. Oshimi K. Oshimi Y, Satake M, Mizoguchi H. Natural killer-mediated lysis of normal and malignant target cells, and its regulation by monocytes. J Exp Med 1985; 162:472–86.

Cancer Detection and Prevention Supplement 1:111–120 (1987)

Novel Tumor-Specific Antigen(s) Response Observed in a Syngeneic Lymphoma-Bearing Host

Lionel A. Manson

The Wistar Institute of Anatomy and Biology, Philadelphia, PA

ABSTRACT Immunoglobin (Ig) has been found to accumulate on P815Y (H-2^d) and L5178Y (H-2^d) tumor cells during progressive growth in syngeneic host DBA/2 mice. Density of the accumulated Ig per cell increases as the tumor grows while the tumor cells become resistant to lysis by ascitic syngeneic cytotoxic cells. Tumor cells grown in vivo coated with this specific Ig no longer bind significant amounts of antibodies against H-2D and H-2K antigens. The membrane-bound Ig reacts with a rabbit antimouse Fab and a rabbit antimouse IgM reagent, but it does not react with a rabbit antimouse IgG or IgA reagent. It binds specifically to tumor cell lines that are sensitive to the ascitic cytotoxic cells but not to resistant tumor cell lines. The membrane-bound Ig can be eluted from tumor cells with 3 M NaSCN or 0.2 M acetic acid. Binding studies indicate that this eluted Ig is not an anti-H-2D/K antibody, yet it immunoprecipitates H-2D/K antigens from NP40 lysates of P815Y cells. It is proposed that the Ig is directed against a tumor antigen that is physically associated with the H-2D/K antigens of the tumors.

Key words: MHC, tumor immunity, antibody, immunomodulation

INTRODUCTION

A question that dominates the study of tumor immunobiology is why and how tumors can grow progressively and overwhelm a host despite the immune response of the host to the tumor. Because early efforts to obtain evidence of immune responses in serum (antitumor antibody) and in spleen and lymph nodes to growing lymphoid tumors were inconclusive, we focused on the tumor mass itself as the major site for host-tumor interaction. In a previous study of P815Y mastocytoma cells growing as ascites in syngeneic host DBA/2 mice [1,2], cytotoxic lymphoid cells were detected and isolated from ascites as early as 8 days after intraperitoneal injection of 10^3 P815Y cells. These cytotoxic cells resembled T-cytotoxic cells [2]; in addition, they were able to lyse not only P815Y but also L-5178Y cells, another DBA/2 lymphoma. Two DBA/2 leukemias, P815-X2 and L-1210, were resistant to these cytotoxic cells. P815Y cells isolated from the tumor mass on day 10 after inoculation were sensitive to these effectors, as were cultured P815Y and L-5178Y cells, whereas the tumor cells isolated 16 days after inoculation, when tumor load was 10–20-fold higher, were completely resistant to these cytotoxic cells. Cold target inhibition studies with these day 16 tumor cells showed

Address reprint requests to Lionel A. Manson, The Wistar Institute of Anatomy and Biology, 36th Street at Spruce, Philadelphia, PA 19104.

that they did not inhibit the lysis of cultured P815Y target cells. When the day 16 tumor cells were put into tissue culture, they recovered their sensitivity to the cytotoxic cells. It was concluded that the tumor-specific antigen(s) of the tumor had undergone antigenic modulation [1] during progressive growth in the syngeneic host.

Recently, the role of Ig as the possible modulating agent has been reinvestigated. We present evidence here indicating that a humoral response to a tumor-associated antigen(s) occurs in the tumor-bearing animal during early tumor growth. Ig can be detected accumulating on the multiplying tumor cells in the animal with a number of iodinated antimouse Igs. This antitumor Ig can be eluted from the in vivo grown tumor cells, and the tumor eluates have been used in immunoprecipitation protocols in attempts to identify the putative tumor antigen(s).

MATERIALS AND METHODS
Mice

Female DBA/2J mice were obtained from The Jackson Laboratories (Bar Harbor, ME) at 10 weeks of age.

Tumors

The P815Y (DBA/2, H-2^d) and P815-X2 (DBA/2, H-2^d) mastocytomas and L-5178Y (DBA/2, H-2^d) and L-1210 (DBA/2, H-2^d) leukemias were maintained as ascites tumors in the syngeneic host and cultured in vitro. All four cell lines were positive when tested for gp69/71 murine leukemia virus antigens [2].

Assay for Cell Surface Ig

Cell surface Ig was detected by the binding of ^{125}I-labeled rabbit antimouse Fab. In some experiments, a ^{125}I-labeled rabbit antimouse μ reagent, a rabbit antimouse γ reagent, and a rabbit antimouse α reagent were also used. These reagents were prepared [3] and kindly provided by Dr. Michael Cancro (Department of Pathology, University of Pennsylvania School of Medicine).

Cells were removed from animals or from tissue culture media and washed twice in phosphate-buffered saline. They were then incubated for 1 hr at 4°C in 1% paraformaldehyde, 0.05 M Na_2HPO_4, 0.85% NaCl, pH 8.3, a treatment that does not affect the H-2 antibody-binding capacity of cells [4,5]. The cells were washed three times in IB$^+$ (0.01 M Tris or phosphate buffer, pH 8.0, 0.15 M NaCl, 0.05% sodium azide, 0.25% bovine serum albumin, and 2% calf serum) and suspended at 10^6 cells/0.1 ml in IB$^+$ and incubated either in this buffer or in antiserum dilutions made in IB$^+$ for 2 hr at 4°C. After washing three times in IB$^+$, cells (10^6/0.1 ml IB$^+$) were incubated with iodinated reagent for 18 hr at 4°C, washed three more times in IB$^+$, and suspended in 0.4 ml. Triplicate 0.1 ml aliquots were then counted in a γ-spectrometer. The SD of the mean was always less than $\pm 10\%$ for triplicate determinations. Control experiments showed that overnight incubation and an input greater than 5×10^5 cpm/10^6 cells/0.1 ml were necessary for optimal reactivity.

Sera

Normal sera were obtained from untreated DBA/2 and C57BL/6 mice. The C57BL/6 anti-L-5178Y serum, M67E (anti-H-2^d), was obtained from five C57BL/6 mice immunized at monthly intervals for 6 months with 10^7 L-5178Y cells (an H-2^d-positive, Ia-negative tumor line [6]). One month after the last injection, the animals were bled and the sera pooled. This serum had an end point titration in a complement-dependent cytotoxic assay against L-5178Y cells of 1:10,000. When this serum was absorbed 12 times with packed DBA/2 red cells, the cytolytic titer was reduced to 1:4, and no H-2K/D gene product could be immunoprecipitated from H-2^d cell lysates, indicating that most of the antibodies in this serum were directed against H-2K and H-2D antigens.

The other sera used in this study, D-4, D-13, and D-31, were obtained from the Transplantation Immunology Branch of the National Institute of Allergy and Infectious Diseases (Table I). These are relatively monospecific sera directed against the numbered specificity encoded by the H-2K or H-2D region of the H-2 complex. These sera, made by immunizing appropriately bred mice with spleen cells from an allogeneic source, are not likely to contain antibodies against tumor antigens but reportedly contain antibodies against viruses [7].

H-2K/D Antigens Displayed by Tumor Cell Lines

Paraformaldehyde-treated cells were incubated with the appropriate monospecific sera at a 1:50 or a 1:100 dilution. In a previous study, we found that all cell lines adsorbed Ig nonspecifically when treated with normal sera [8]. Thus H-2K and D antigen expression on the cell surface was taken as the amount of iodinated reagent bound to the cells after incubation with immune sera minus the amount bound to the cells after incubation with normal sera. These values are indicated in the tables in italics.

Radioimmunoassay

Antibody preparations were assayed in a disc radioimmunoassay as previously described [9]. Antigen discs were made by binding the microsomal lipoprotein fraction (MLP) of the various cell lines used [7] to cyanogen bromide-activated filter-paper discs. The cells used for MLP isolation were grown in tissue culture. Antibody bound to the discs was detected with a ^{125}I-labeled rabbit antimouse Fab or a ^{125}I-labeled rabbit antimouse IgM. The reagents were used within 3 weeks of their preparation.

Tumor Antibody Elution Procedure

Immunoglobulin eluates were made from solid tumors obtained from mice inoculated subcutaneously 2–3 weeks earlier with 10^6 tumor cells. By this time, the tumors weighed 2–4 g. After surgically removing the tumors and trimming off fatty tissue, they were washed in phosphate-buffered saline, suspended in 3 vol of 3 M NaSCN with a ground-glass hand homogenizer, and allowed to stand for 30 min at room temperature. The mixture was centrifuged at 100,000 g for 1 hr. The clarified supernatant fluid was dialyzed overnight against 2 liters of 0.15 M NaCl, 0.05% sodium azide, or 0.05% merthiolate at 4°C. The dialyzate was again centrifuged at 100,000g for 30 min and concentrated by vacuum dialysis to 1 ml/g of original tumor.

Tumor Cell Separation Procedure

Tumor cells grown for 10 or 16 days were separated as previously described [1,2] from the ascites on the Sta-Put apparatus. Briefly, 10^8 ascitic cells in 20 ml RPMI-1640 were layered over a 1500 ml linear gradient of RPMI-1640 varying from 5% to 25% calf serum. After 3 hr, 50 ml fractions were collected. The tumor cells were generally found in fractions 15–20, whereas the cytolytic effector host cells were found in fractions 28–30 (sedimentation rate 2–6 cm/hr).

TABLE I. Antisera Used in This Study

Designation	Animals immunized	Source
D4	(B10.AKM × 129) anti-B10.A	Jackson Laboratories
D13	(B10 × LP.RIII) anti-B10.A (5R)	Jackson Laboratories
D31	(B10 × A) anti-B10.D2	Jackson Laboratories
M67E*	C57BL/10 anti-L-5178Y	This laboratory

*When tested against P815Y in a ^{51}Cr-release assay, this antiserum had an end point titer of 1:10,000. It was absorbed ten times with purified DBA/2 erythrocytes; thus the majority of the antibodies were classified as anti-H-2^d.

Labeling of Cells

Tumor cells were grown in tissue culture media (Fischer's leukemia cell media [GIBCO, Grand Island, NY] plus 10% fetal calf serum). ^{3}H-glucosamine was added to cultures when the cell concentration was 3–5 $\times$ 10^5 cells per ml. Cells were harvested 48 hr later by centrifugation. During this period, 35–60% of the isotope was incorporated into the cells. Ascitic or cultured tumor cells were iodinated by a modification of the lactoperoxidase procedure [10]. Both iodinated and tritium-labeled cells were suspended at 5 $\times$ 10^7 per ml in PBS and stored frozen.

Cells in suspension were solubilized with an equal volume of lysis buffer (0.15 M NaCl, 0.01 M phosphate buffer, pH 7.5, 0.5% Nonidet P40 [Shell International Chemical Co., London, England], and 0.2 mM phenylmethylsulfonyl fluoride). After 1 hr, in an ice bath, the supernatant fluid was separated in a Beckman microfuge centrifuge after a 5 min spin. The supernatant fluid contained 60–90% of the isotope present in the cells and was subsequently used in immunoprecipitation studies.

Immunoprecipitation

An antigen-antibody mixture was prepared by adding to an aliquot of isotopically labeled cell lysate (2–4 $\times$ 10^7 cells, 1–5 $\times$ 10^6 cpm) either 0.5 μl of an antiserum or 5 μl of tumor antibody eluate. This antigen-antibody mixture was added to a 50 μl pellet of goat or rabbit antimouse IgG-coated *Staphylococcus aureus* Cowan I (SacI) [11] (15 μl of goat or rabbit antimouse IgG was used per 50 μl of a 10% [m/v] of SacI in PBS). After incubation for 2 hr at 37°C or overnight at 4°C, the pellets were collected in a Beckman microfuge B, washed three times in PBS, then suspended in 50–100 μl of sample buffer (2% sodium dodecylsulfate [NaDod SO$_4$] and 2% mercaptoethanol in PBS) and placed in a boiling water bath for 3 min.

Gel Electrophoresis

Dissolved and reduced immunoprecipitates were electrophoresed on 0.6 $\times$ 20 cm 10% polyacrylamide gels [12] at 7 mA per gel until the dye front (bromophenol blue) reached the end of the gel. Gels were calibrated by the addition of reduced fluorescent complexes of bovine serum albumin, egg albumin, and trypsinogen. The positions of the standards were determined by scanning the gel while still in the tube using a Gilford fluorescence gel accessory with a Gilford spectrophotometer [13]. The gels were then sliced into 2 mm slices. For the ^{3}H-labeled samples, each slice was incubated overnight in 4 ml of scintillation fluid (6% protosol; New England Nuclear, Boston, MA) and 10% water in Econofluor (New England Nuclear) at 37°C and then counted in an Intertechnique SL4000 scintillation counter. Samples labeled with ^{125}I were counted in a γ-counter immediately after slicing.

RESULTS

The level of H-2 antibody binding to the tumor cells appeared to decrease as the tumors grew in vivo. Table II shows the results of three experiments carried out with the protocol used by Biddison and Palmer [1] to isolate anti-P815Y ascitic cytotoxic cells. Ascites were harvested from seven mice on day 10 after inoculation of 1,000 cells, and from the other three mice on day 16, and processed on the Sta-Put gradient. The tumor targets were removed from the gradient and fixed with paraformaldehyde, and the cell-bound Ig was assayed. In experiments 2 and 3, only five animals were inoculated and the ascites harvested and pooled within each experiment on day 16. Aliquots of the tumor cells as well as cultured P815Y controls were assayed for their capacity to bind H-2 antibody. In experiments 1 and 3, data were obtained from tumor cells isolated from DBA/2 mice inoculated with P815Y. In experiment 2, L-5178Y was inoculated at 1,000 cells per DBA/2 mouse and ascites harvested on day 16. There was a decrease in apparent H-2 antibody-binding capacity in part because of the increase with time of the background binding capacity of in vivo-grown tumor cells themselves (cells incubated

TABLE II. Cell-Bound Ig of P8157 and L5178Y Grown in DBA/2 as Ascites

Exp. No.	Tumor	Antiserum*	Cultured cell controls	Day 10	Day 16
1	P815Y	Buffer	754 ± 80†	4,742 ± 455	11,550 ± 489
		Normal	2,593 ± 232	5,186 ± 272	10,034 ± 309
		M67E	14,619 ± 482 *12,026*‡	12,902 ± 271 *7,716*	15,219 ± 429 *5,185*
		D31 + D13	13,869 ± 224 *11,276*	13,849 ± 493 *8,663*	16,190 ± 599 *6,156*
2	L-5178Y	Buffer	208 ± 18		3,415 ± 75
		Normal	1,290 ± 18		4,113 ± 110
		M67E	4,934 ± 85 *3,640*		6,458 ± 175 *2,342*§
		D31 + D13	3,843 ± 65 *3,843*		6,191 ± 150 *2,079*§
3	P815Y	Buffer	348 ± 13		1,554 ± 6
		Normal	4,352 ± 149		4,782 ± 125
		M67E	10,585 ± 115 *6,233*		6,285 ± 317 *1,503*
		D4 + D31	12,982 ± 177 *8,630*		7,333 ± 272 *2,551*

*Antisera were used at a 1:100 dilution.

†Data are given as cpm ± SD per 0.25 × 10⁶ cells. The detecting reagent was ¹²⁵I-anti-Fab; input in Exp. 1 was 4×10^5 cpm/0.1 ml, in Exp. 2 7.7×10^4 cpm/0.1 ml, and in Exp. 3 8.1×10^5 cpm/0.1 ml.

‡The values in italics were obtained by subtracting the radioactivity bound to cells treated with normal serum from that found after immune serum treatment.

§These values were significantly lower (P = 0.02) than those obtained with cultured cells in the same experiment.

TABLE III. H-2 Antibody Binding Capacity of P815Y Cells Pretreated With Normal Serum or Ascitic Fluid

Pretreatment*	Second incubation†	cpm/0.25 × 10⁶ cells ‡
Buffer	Buffer	2,394 ± 197
	Normal serum	18,950 ± 677
	D4 + D31	40,293 ± 1,674 *21,343*§
Normal DBA/2 serum	Buffer	16,304 ± 1,045
	Normal serum	28,052 ± 2,141
	D4 + D31	55,553 ± 3,742 *27,501*§
L-5178Y Ascitic fluid	Buffer	8,843 ± 467
	Normal serum	26,113 ± 1,284
	D4 + D31	52,389 ± 993 *26,276*§

*Cultured P815Y were pretreated in buffer or in undiluted serum or ascitic fluid for 2 hr at 4°C on a rotator. They were washed, fixed with paraformaldehyde, and assayed for their H-2 antibody binding capacity.

†Sera were used at a 1:50 dilution.

‡Input of anti-Fab was 1.3×10^6 cpm/0.1 ml.

§The values in italics were obtained by subtracting as described in the legend of Table II. These values did not differ significantly from each other.

in buffer), although in experiment 3 there also appear to be fewer binding sites for the anti-Fab.

To determine whether the Ig present in normal mouse sera or in ascitic fluid might account for the diminished capacity to bind anti-H-2 antibody, we examined the effect of this Ig on tissue culture-grown P815Y cells (Table III). Although relatively large amounts of Ig were absorbed by the cells from the normal serum and from the ascitic fluid, H-2 antibody binding ability was not affected significantly by pretreatment of the tumor cells with either normal DBA/2 serum or L-5178Y ascitic fluid.

Growing L5178Y as a solid subcutaneous tumor rather than as ascites did not appear to influence the rate of formation of the cell-bound Ig in vivo. Table IV shows data obtained when L-5178Y were grown as subcutaneous tumors in their syngeneic hosts. Large amounts of Ig bound to the L-5178Y cells obtained from the tumors, and the capacity of the cells to bind additional H-2 antibody was diminished, more so when tested with the D4-D31 antiserum mixtures than with our own M67E.

If the Ig was bound to the tumor cells as an antigen-antibody complex, it should be possible to elute it with 3 M NaSCN. Table V shows typical results using the disc radioimmunoassay to measure binding activity of the 3 M NaSCN eluate of P815 and P815Y-X2 tumors grown in vivo. At all dilutions, but most markedly at the 1:100 dilution of the P815Y eluate, there is a component that binds P815Y and L-5178Y at twice the level found with P815-X2. No such component was found in the P815-X2 eluate. From these values, it is estimated that the eluate contains 2.8 μg of specific antibody per milliliter. With this elution procedure, the eluate obtained has retained its activity when stored at 4°C for over 1 year. Acid eluates also demonstrate a specific anti-P815Y component, but the activity is lost after several weeks of storage.

The surface Ig bound to the cells during in vivo growth was found to react with a ^{125}I-anti-Fab and a ^{125}I-anti-IgM but not with a ^{125}I-anti-IgG reagent (not shown). Table VI shows reactivity of the specific binding material eluted from in vivo-grown P815Y in the radioimmunoassay with a number of iodinated antimouse Ig reagents. The P815Y tumor eluate contained Ig that bound to P815Y discs and that reacted with anti-Fab and anti-IgM but not with an anti-IgG nor an anti-IgA reagent.

Figure 1 shows the immunoprecipitates obtained from a lysate of ^{3}H-glucosamine-labeled P815Y cells treated with either the anti-P815Y eluate or a specific anti-H-2[d] antiserum

TABLE IV. H-2 Binding Activity of L-5178Y Grown In Vivo as a Solid Subcutaneous Tumor in DBA/2 Mice*

Antiserum	Cultured cells	Day 15
Buffer	803 ± 103	17,735 ± 726
Normal	8,667 ± 211	16,182 ± 844
M67E	32,418 ± 227 *23,751*	24,964 ± 591 *7,782*
D4 + D31	31,709 ± 1,132 *23,042*	19,358 ± 462 *3,176*

*Two female DBA/2 mice were injected SC with 0.5×10^5 cultured L5178Y cells. Fifteen days later, the tumors (1 cm in diameter) were removed surgically and suspended by syringing. All subsequent treatments were similar to those used with ascitic cells. All antisera were used at a 1:50 dilution. Values are cpm/0.25×10^6 cells. The input of ^{125}I-anti-Fab was 7.0×10^5 cpm/0.1 ml. The values in italics were obtained by subtracting the radioactivity bound to cells treated with normal serum from that found after immune serum treatment.

TABLE V. Binding Activity of 3 M KSCN Eluate of In Vivo-Grown P815Y and P815-X2 Tumors as Measured in the Disc RIA*

Tumor	Dilution	L-5178Y discs (cpm)	P815Y discs (cpm)	P815-X2 discs (cpm)
	Buffer	1,315 ± 297	1,376 ± 110	1,222 ± 230
P815Y	1:50	3,577 ± 263 *2,262*	5,260 ± 308 *3,884*	2,782 ± 158 *1,560*
	1:100	3,463 ± 632 *2,148*	4,672 ± 146 *3,296*	2,516 ± 145 *1,294*
	1:200	2,613 ± 394 *1,298*	3,370 ± 191 *1,994*	2,170 ± 133 *948*
P815-X2	1:50	2,643 ± 205 *1,328*	2,878 ± 96 *1,502*	2,145 ± 519 *923*
	1:100	1,981 ± 311 *666*	1,957 ± 293 *581*	1,543 ± 258 *321*
	1:200	1,466 ± 363 *151*	1,657 ± 125 *281*	1,466 ± 332 *244*

*Values are cpm ± SD. Values in italics were obtained by subtracting the binding found with buffer from the binding found with the eluate dilution. Input was 7.8×10^4 of ^{125}I-rabbit antimouse Fab/well.

TABLE VI. Reactivity of the Antitumor Ig Eluted From In Vivo-Grown P815Y Cells in an
RIA With P815Y Discs

	^{125}I-anti-Fab*	^{125}I-anti-μ*	^{125}I-anti-γ*	^{125}I-anti-α*
	(cpm)	(cpm)	(cpm)	(cpm)
Control†	1,565	1,520	1,429	1,239
TE‡	4,329 *2,764*§	3,501 *1,981*	1,629 *220*	1,478 *239*

*Input radioactivity was 1.2×10^5 cpm per well. The preparations had been iodinated over a period of 3 weeks, so the specific activities were comparable.
†cpm from discs incubated in IB$^+$ alone.
‡Tumor eluate from P815Y cells grown subcutaneously in DBA/2 mice (1:50 dilution).
§Values in italics are the difference between cpm of IB$^+$ and cpm of tumor eluate.

D4. The lysate had been pretreated with an eluate of P815-X2 (emergence-associated tumor immunogen [EATI]-negative); the gp69/71 of MuMTV was removed from the lysate in this step. The pattern of peaks obtained in both cases is very similar; major peaks appeared at approximately 35,000, 45,000, and 62,000–68,000 daltons with the D4 antiserum, and 23,000–25,000, 48,000, 62,000, and 71,000–78,000 daltons with the eluate obtained from in vivo-grown P815Y cells. Peaks similar to those found with D4 serum were also seen with the D31 serum.

The supernatant fluids of the P815Y eluate and the H-2 antiserum treatments were then sequentially treated with the same anti-H-2 antiserum. No peaks were found in the immunoprecipitates obtained from the D4 treatment supernatant fluid (data not shown), and a single small peak was seen in the anti-P815Y supernatant fluid at 68,000 daltons (Fig. 1). The other peaks, including the 48,000 dalton peak, were completely removed by the anti-P815Y eluate. Similar results were obtained when the experiment was carried out with the D31 antiserum instead of the D4 antiserum (data not shown).

DISCUSSION

The ability of a sensitized syngeneic host to reject a tumor challenge requires that the animal be capable of mounting a secondary immune response. Such a response has been induced in vivo and in vitro against both P815Y and L-5178Y cells [14,15]. Thus these tumors are considered positive for a tumor-associated transplantation antigen (TATA). When effector spleen populations were induced by culturing immune DBA/2 cells with mitomycin C-treated L-5178Y, they were H-2-restricted and able to lyse P815Y and L-5178Y but not L-1210 or P815-X2 cells. We have also found that DBA/2 mice sensitized with mitomycin C-treated P815Y or L-5178Y cells rejected either P815Y or L-5178Y cells, suggesting the presence of a common transplantation antigen(s) in both cell lines [15]. L-1210 and P815-X2 have been found to be TATA-negative in inducing an in vivo response in DBA/2 mice.

We have observed in this study a humoral immune response to a tumor antigen(s) shared by P815Y and L-5178Y cells. We designate this antigen(s) "emergence-associated tumor immunogen" (EATI), since, unlike TATA, it is observable as a primary immune response, and the cytotoxic cells induced are primary peritoneal effector cells and are not H-2-restricted [1,2]. It is not clear as yet whether the EATI and TATA systems are identical but with different effector systems or whether these two responses involve two different antigens.

Little is known about the properties of the surface-bound Ig detected in this study. No such Ig can be detected in the sera of tumor-bearing animals, since every experiment involving measurement of the cell-bound Ig indicated an excess of available binding sites on the tumor cells for Ig. The tumor multiplies and induces a suppressed state only when the tumor load exceeds 10^8 cells per animal [15]; thus the amount of specific antibody produced by the triggered B cells might always be less than the number of available binding sites. This Ig is not present in normal sera (Table III), so its production must be the result of an immune response triggered by the growing tumor.

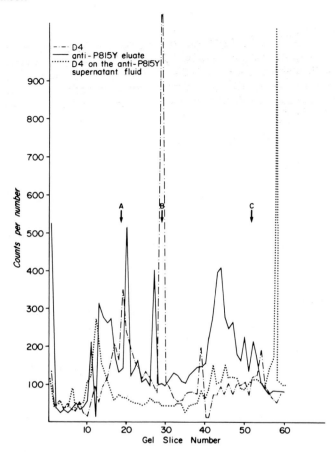

Fig. 1. Gel electrophoresis of immunoprecipitated ^{3}H-glucosamine-labeled P815Y cells. NP-40 solubilized extract was first reacted with a tumor eluate of P815-X2 to remove nonspecific labeled material. The supernatant fluid was divided in two portions, one treated with D4 serum and the other treated with the anti-P815Y eluate. Both supernatant fluids were again treated with D4 antiserum. The arrows indicate the positions at which bovine serum albumin (A), egg albumin (B), and trypsinogen (C) were found as molecular weight markers.

We do know that the eluted Ig binds to EATI-positive cells and not to EATI-negative cells nor to spleen cells. It reacts with the ^{125}I-anti-Fab and a ^{125}I-anti-IgM but does not react with an anti-IgG nor an anti-IgA reagent. It therefore appears to be an IgM, consistent with its kinetics of appearance in response to a primary immunization stimulus.

The tumor cells during in vivo growth appear to lose their capacity to bind additional amounts of H-2K and D antibodies gradually as the Ig accumulates on the cells. One possibility is that specific anti-EATI is an H-2D/K antibody. It is clear from binding studies such as those shown in Table V that the Ig eluted from in vivo-grown P815Y has a specific component that binds to L5178Y discs and P815Y discs and not to P815-X2 discs. Similar results have been obtained when whole cells were used to absorb the eluates (data not shown). Since all the cell lines originated in DBA/2 mice, they are H-2^d in origin and therefore express the H-2D^d and H-2K^d antigens on their surface membrane. These tumor lines do not express Ia antigens and are frequently used to remove H-2D/K antibodies to generate Ia-specific antisera. Other experiments (data not shown) demonstrate that this antibody also binds to EL4, which is H-2^b

in origin, yet contains a cross-reactive tumor antigen to P815Y and L-5178Y [2]. We therefore conclude that anti-EATI antibody in the tumor eluate is not an anti-H-2D/K antibody.

One possibility is that the EATI substitutes for the H-2K and D antigens in the membrane; another is that the EATI is sufficiently close to the H-2K and D antigens so that anti-EATI antibody sterically blocks H-2D/K antibody uptake. This latter possibility is supported by the immunoprecipitation data. First, from detergent solubilized extracts of P815Y, in addition to the H-2D/K gene products (a 48,000 dalton glycoprotein), several peaks are precipitated with anti-H-2 antisera D4 and D31. In other immunoprecipitation studies, using all the antisera in Table I with ^{3}H-glucosamine-labeled spleen cells, only the 48,000 dalton glycoprotein is revealed on the gels. Thus one or more of the additional peaks seen here may be EATI. This possibility is strengthened by the fact that the anti-P815Y eluate precipitates the H-2D/K gene products and other similar peaks from the same extract, because the supernatant fluid from the anti-P815Y eluate precipitation no longer contains these substances (as demonstrated by the sequential precipitation with the D4 antiserum shown in Fig. 1). Since the binding studies indicate that the P815Y eluate does not contain anti-H-2D/K antibody, we suggest that the anti-P815Y antibody is directed against and is precipitating a glycoprotein associated with the H-2D/K gene product in the cell membrane. Whether the additional peaks seen on these gels are the only candidates for EATI requires further experimentation. Most likely, EATI is a gene product encoded in some region of the genome other than the H-2D/K regions and is found associated hydrophobically or covalently with the H-2D/K antigens in the cell membrane. An example of such a substance is already known, since β2-microglobulin is encoded on chromosome 2 of the mouse genome yet is found on the cell membrane hydrophobically associated with the H-2D/K antigens.

A reciprocal relationship has been observed with other tumors between the appearance of new antigens on ascitic tumor cells growing in vivo and an apparent loss of H-2 antigen sites. The BALB/c tumor LPC-1, for example, loses its sensitivity to cytotoxic T cells and develops a 160,000 dalton membrane glycoprotein that is associated with the H-2 antigen sites of the tumor line [16].

Our preliminary data [17] suggest that anti-EATI is important in progressive tumor growth. In those experiments, DBA/2 mice immunized with the anti-EATI rejected a tumor challenge of P815Y cells, consistent with the notion of an antiidiotype response to anti-EATI in these mice.

In recent years, much effort has focused on the evaluation of the role of immunosuppression, either specific or nonspecific, in progressive tumor growth. We observed immunosuppression in our systems only when the tumor load per animal reached 1×10^8 cells [15]. Both in the present analysis and in the previous studies [1,2], the immune responses observed had already been triggered and were fully expressed before the tumor load had reached this level. Recently, Dye and North [18] reported that infusion of immune spleen cells into immunocompetent tumor-bearing mice did not lead to tumor regression, whereas infusion into thymectomized and γ-irradiated tumor-bearing animals did lead to tumor regression. The active component in the immune spleen preparation was sensitive to treatment with anti-Thy 1.2 serum plus complement. Those authors concluded that immunosuppression and T suppressor cells are responsible for progressive tumor growth of P815 cells in DBA/2 mice. An alternative explanation to their results is that P815 and Meth A tumor had become resistant to the cytotoxic cells in the immune spleen preparations used. In the present and previous studies [1,2], we have found that P815 cells undergo an antigenic modulation to become effector cell resistant when growing in vivo in immunocompetent mice so that further infusion of immune spleen cells into such tumor-bearing mice should have no effect on the progressively growing tumor. Further, if the modulating agent in in vivo conversion is a blocking antibody, then thymectomized and γ-irradiated animals would be severely handicapped in producing such an antibody. Thus the growing tumors in such immunologically deprived animals would be sensitive to passively infused cytotoxic cells, as Dye and North observed [18].

Our working hypothesis is that production of a blocking antibody is required for progressive growth of immunogenic tumors in immunocompetent animals and that this production is a T-dependent response. A general conclusion that we have reached based on this study and the previous ones [1,2] is that immunogenic tumors can grow in the immunocompetent syngeneic host from very small inocula even though they trigger both humoral and cell-mediated responses. It is in understanding the interrelationships between the two responses that we may be able to explain how tumors appear to evade immune surveillance.

ACKNOWLEDGMENTS

Some of the early experiments were carried out by a predoctoral student, Lee A. Fleisher. We are indebted to the assistance of Ms. Anita Guarini, Betty van Dyke, Leslie Ferron, and Nancy Guy. These studies were supported in part by USPHS Research Grants CA-07973, CA-10815, and CA-34654 from the National Cancer Institute. We are indebted to Ms. Marina Hoffman for editorial assistance.

REFERENCES

1. Biddison WE, Palmer JC. Development of tumor cell resistance to syngeneic cell-mediated cytotoxicity during growth of ascitic mastocytoma P815Y. Proc Natl Acad Sci USA 1977; 74:329–33.
2. Biddison WE, Palmer JC, Alexander MA, Cowan EP, Manson LA. Characterization and specificity of murine antitumor cytotoxic effector cells within an ascitic tumor. J Immunol 1977; 118:2243–53.
3. Cancro MP, Klinman NR. B cell repertoire ontogeny: heritable but dissimilar development of parental and F_1 repertoires. J Immunol 1981; 126:1160.
4. Parr EL, Oei JS. Immobilization of membrane H-2 antigens by paraformaldehyde fixation. J Cell Biol 1973; 59:537–42.
5. Flaherty L, Zimmerman D. Surface mapping of mouse thymocytes. Proc Natl Acad Sci USA 1979; 76:1990–3.
6. Manson LA. Intracellular localization and immunogenic capacities of phenotypic products of mouse histocompatibility genes. In Manson LA, ed: Biomembranes. New York: Plenum Press, 1976; 47–88.
7. Wettstein PJ, Krammer P, Nowinski RC, David CS, Frelinger JA, Shreffler DC. A cautionary note regarding Ia and H-2 typing of murine lymphoid tumors. Immunogenetics 1976; 3:507–16.
8. Tax A, Manson LA. Immunologic analysis of A strain mice bearing the A-10 mammary adenocarcinoma. Cancer Res 1979; 39:1739–47.
9. Manson LA, Verastegui-Cerdan E, Sporer R. A quantitative disc radioimmunoassay for antibodies directed against membrane-associated antigens. In Melchers F, Potter M, Warner N, eds: Current topics in microbiology and immunology. Berlin: Springer-Verlad, 1978; 232–4.
10. Jones PP. Analysis of radiolabeled lymphocyte proteins by one- and two-dimensinal polyacrylamide gel electrophoresis. In Mishell BB, Shiigi SM, eds: Selected methods in cellular immunology. San Francisco: WH Freeman & Co, 1980; 398–440.
11. Cullen SE, Schwartz BD. An improved method for isolation of H-2 and Ia alloantigens with immunoprecipitation induced by protein A-bearing staphylococci. J Immunol 1976; 117:136–42.
12. Laemmli UL. Cleavage of structural proteins during the assembly of the head of bacteriophage T4. Nature 1970; 227:680–5.
13. Weigle M, DeBernardo S, Leingruber W, Cleeland R, Grunberg E. Fluorescent labeling of proteins. A new methodology. Biochem Biophys Res Commun 1973; 54:899–906.
14. Goldstein LT, Klinman NR, Manson LA. A microtest radioimmunoassay for noncytotoxic tumor-specific antibody to cell-surface antigens. J Natl Cancer Inst 1973; 51:1713–5.
15. Mason LA. The role of cell-surface antigens in progressive tumor growth (Immunological surveillance re-visited). In Reisfeld RA, Ferrone S, eds. Current Trends in Histocompatibility, Vol. 2, New York: Plenum Press, 1981; 105–12.
16. Celis E, Eisen HN. Interactions between a novel cell surface glycoprotein and H-2K and H-2D antigens on myeloma tumor cells. Eur J Immunol 1980; 10:455–61.
17. Manson LA. The role of anti-tumor antibody in progressive tumor growth. Transplant Proc 1984; 16:524–7.
18. Dye ES, North RJ. T cell-mediated immunosuppression as an obstacle to adoptive immunotherapy of the P815 mastocytoma and its metastases. J Exp Med 1981; 154:1033–42.

Cancer Detection and Prevention Supplement 1:121–125 (1987)

High Incidence of Stomach Cancer in Relatives of Patients With Malignant Lymphoproliferative Disorders

A. Genčík, MD, PhD, CSc
M. Buser, PhD
B. Temminck, PhD

J.P. Obrecht, MD
W. Weber, MD
Hj. Müller, MD

Laboratory of Human Genetics (A.G., B.T., W.W., Hj.M), Department of Research of the University Clinics and Division of Oncology (J.P.O.), Department of Medicine, Cantonal Hospital, CH-4031 Basel, and University Computer Center and Institute for Informatics, CH-4056 Basel, Switzerland (M.B.)

ABSTRACT   Family histories of 189 patients with lymphomas and leukemias and 14 patients with stomach cancer were used in this study. Controls consisted of family histories of 391 patients with other tumors. In the 189 probands with lymphoproliferative disorders stomach cancer accounted for 17.3% of the total cancers in the relatives, whereas in the probands with breast and other types of cancer the corresponding figures were 8.1% and 8.3% as against an incidence of 5.9% of stomach cancers in Basel. In first-degree relatives, the incidence of stomach cancer was higher than expected in the families of probands with malignant lymphoma and stomach cancer. It is suggested that an inherited subclinical disturbance of the immune system is involved in familial association of stomach cancer with malignant lymphoproliferative disorders.

Key words: stomach cancer lymphomas, leukemias, family histories, subclinical immunodeficiency

INTRODUCTION

Many associations of tumor diseases have been reported in the literature, either in the form of multiple primary neoplasms in a single patient [1] or in the form of increased occurrence in close relatives. In some cases the cause of the association is known; for instance, there are certain syndromes for which gene mutations are responsible (MEN syndromes) [6]. In other cases it is thought that common pathogenetic factors are responsible, eg, hormonal mechanisms in the association of breast and ovarian cancer [7,8] or faulty nutritional habits in the association of breast and colon cancer [9].

Many results suggest that subclinical immunodeficiency plays a role in the pathogenesis both of cancer of the stomach and of leukemias and lymphomas. Kinlen et al [10] have recently

Address reprint requests to Dr. A. Genčík, Laboratory of Human Genetics, Department of Research of the University Clinics, Cantonal Hospital, CH-4031 Basel, Switzerland.

reported a 47-fold excess of stomach cancer and a 30-fold excess of lymphoma in patients with hypogammaglobulinaemia. If common factors are involved in the pathogenesis of these tumor diseases, lymphomas and cancer of the stomach should occur more often than usual in members of the same family. In this paper we attempt to prove the truth of this hypothesis.

MATERIALS AND METHODS

The family histories of 189 patients with lymphomas and leukemias (non-Hodgkin lymphoma, Hodgkin disease, multiple myeloma, leukemia) and of 14 patients with stomach cancer were collected. As controls, we used the family histories of 391 patients with other tumor diseases (211 with breast cancer, 180 with solid tumors of different sites). The probands with lymphoproliferative disorders included practically all the patients being treated or under observation at the Department of Oncology, Cantonal Hospital (the children at the Children's Hospital), Basel, and in a private practice between April 1, 1982, and December 31, 1984. The probands with other cancer types (control group) were randomly selected. The families were divided into groups according to the cancer site of the proband. All members of each family with and without cancer were noted and pedigrees constructed. The number of relatives in each group who had had stomach cancer was calculated as a percentage of the total number of relatives with cancer.

The detected number of relatives with cancer was compared with the expected number calculated by the age-standardized mortality method or the Markow procedure. Using the age-standardized mortality method, the cumulative incidence of stomach cancer can be calculated taking into account the age-specific mortality of the total population. The Markov procedure takes into account in addition the expected (increased) mortality caused by illness, so that the expected frequency decreases and differences that would remain unnoticed using the age-standardized mortality method become significant.

The various malignant lymphoproliferative diseases were analyzed separately. Lymphomas were subdivided into four types: histiocytic, lymphocytic, lymphohistiocytic, and others. As controls, we took first 211 families of probands with breast cancer and second 180 families of probands with 60 other different types of cancer (excluding stomach cancer). The significance of any differences was determined with the χ^2 test (Fischer).

RESULTS

Table I shows the occurrence of stomach cancer in the relatives of cancer patients divided according to the cancer sites of the probands. For the 189 probands with lymphoproliferative disorders, stomach cancer accounted for 17.3% of the total cancers in the relatives, whereas, in the probands with breast cancer and other cancer types, the corresponding figures were 8.1% and 8.3%. Population incidence for stomach cancer in Basel is 5.9% of all malignancies.

Table II shows the results of the two statistical analyses we used applied to first-degree relatives. Using the Markov procedure, we found that the detected incidence of stomach cancer

TABLE I. Occurrence of Stomach Cancer in Relatives of 594 Cancer Patients

Malignancy of probands	No. of families	No. of relatives with cancer	Relatives with stomach cancer	
			No.	Percent
Malignant lymphoma and leukemia	189	423	73	17.3*
Stomach cancer	14	22	7	31.8*
Breast cancer	211	469	38	8.1
Solid tumors of different sites	180	361	30	8.3

*Statistically significant.

TABLE II. Occurrence of Stomach Cancer in First-Degree Relatives of Cancer Patients: Statistical Analysis

Malignancy of proband	No. of families	No. of relatives	No. of relatives detected with	Age-standardized mortality		Analysis with Markow procedure	
				No. expected	P%	No. expected	P%
Malignant lymphoma	63	416	4	2.73		1.78	3.36
Morbus Hodgkin	32	180	1	0.71		0.48	
Stomach cancer	13	97	3	0.82	0.05	0.54	0.22
Breast cancer	163	1,045	5	6.16		4.07	

TABLE III. Occurrence of Stomach Cancer in Second-Degree Relatives of Cancer Patients: Statistical Analysis

Malignancy of proband	No. of families	No. of relatives	No. of relatives detected with	Age-standardized mortality		Analysis with Markow procedure	
				No. expected	P%	No. expected	P%
Malignant lymphoma	59	499	11	6.91	4.86	4.30	0.05
Morbus Hodgkin	25	214	5	2.42	3.97	1.58	1.22
Stomach cancer	9	66	1	0.98		0.60	
Breast cancer	153	1,176	11	16.25		10.11	

was higher than expected in the families of probands with malignant lymphoma and stomach cancer. Corresponding results for second-degree relatives are shown in Table III. In this case, the incidence of stomach cancer was higher than expected in the families of probands with Hodgkin disease and malignant lymphoma; the number of probands with stomach cancer was too small for significance. In both first- and second-degree relatives, no significant differences were found in the group of breast cancer probands.

Table IV shows the probands with malignant lymphoma subdivided according to histological type. The high occurrence of stomach cancer was found only for the histiocytic and lymphohistiocytic types of malignant lymphoma. In families of probands with multiple myeloma, there were seven cases of stomach cancer out of 23 tumors, that is, 30% of all the cancer cases in relatives.

DISCUSSION

Congenital and acquired immune defects play an important role in the genesis of malignant lymphomas and leukemias [11–13]. Recent publications show that immune defects are also involved in stomach cancer [14]. Stomach cancer is the most common epithelial tumor in the Immunodeficiency Cancer Registry [15]. Stomach cancer occurred 70 times more frequently in ataxia teleangiectasia females than in females of the general cancer population [15]. The stomach is also the most frequent carcinoma site among ataxia teleangiectasia heterozygotes [16].

TABLE IV. Stomach Cancer in Relatives of Patients With Malignant Lymphoma and Multiple Myeloma

Histological type	No. of families	No. of relatives with cancer	Relative with stomach cancer	
			No.	Percent
Histological	14	18	5	28
Lymphohistiocytic	11	39	6	15
Lymphocytic	16	43	2	5
Others	12	23	1	4
Multiple myeloma	12	23	7	30

Tables II and III show that the number of relatives detected with stomach cancer among relatives of probands with malignant lymphoma is significantly higher than the expected number calculated from the population incidence using the two methods described. In the control group, no such difference was found in either first- or second-degree relatives.

The lymphomas and leukemias are a heterogenous group of malignancies. Therefore, it was necessary to divide the group into its different histological types. Table IV shows that the increased incidence of stomach cancer in relatives does not hold for all these types but only for the lymphohistiocytic and lymphocytic types and for multiple myeloma. A significant difference between the histological types of malignant lymphoma is the 350-fold excess of the diffuse histiocytic type following renal transplantation [17]. In conclusion, we suggest that an inherited subclinical disturbance of the immune system is involved in familial association of stomach cancer with malignant lymphoproliferative disorders.

ACKNOWLEDGMENTS

The authors are grateful to Dr. H. Langemann for her help with this manuscript. This work was supported by the Swiss National Fund No. 3.868.0.81.

REFERENCES

1. Schoenberg BS. Multiple primary malignant neoplasms. Rec Results Cancer Res (Berlin: Springer Verlag) 1977; 58:103–19.
2. Albano WA, Lynch HT, Recabaren JA, et al. Familial cancer in an oncology clinic. Cancer 1981; 47:2113–8.
3. Lynch HT, Follett KL, Lynch PM, Albano WA, Mailliard JL, Pierson RL. Family history in an oncology clinic. JAMA 1979; 242:1268–72.
4. Organ CH. A new horison for surgeons: Genetics and cancer control. Am J Surg 1977; 134:685–90.
5. Harnden DG. Familial susceptibility to cancer. Br Med J 1983; 286:1531–2.
6. Knudson AG. Hereditary cancer of man. Cancer Invest 1983; 1:187–93.
7. Henderson BE, Pike MC, Gerkins VR, Casagrande JT. The hormonal basis of breast cancer: Elevated plasma levels of oestrogen, prolactin and progesterone. In: Hiatt HH, Watson JD, Winston JA, eds. Origins of human cancer. Cold Spring Harbor, NY: Cold Spring Harbor Laboratory, 1977; 77–86.
8. Green MH, Clark JW, Blayney DW. The epidemiology of ovarian cancer. Semin Oncol 1984; 11:209–26.
9. Bremond A, Collet P, Lambert R, Martoin JL. Breast cancer and polyposis of the colon. Cancer 1984; 54:2568–70.
10. Kinlen LJ, Webster ADB, Bird AG, et al. Prospective study of cancer in patients with hypogamma-globulinaemia. Lancet 1985; 8423:263–6.
11. Louie S, Schwatz RS. Immunodeficiency and the pathogenesis of lymphoma and leukemia. Semin Hematol 1978; 15:117–38.
12. Hermans PE, Huizenga KA. Association of gastric carcinoma with idiopathic late-onset immunoglobulin deficiency. Ann Intern Med 1972; 76:605–9.

13. Toge T, Tanada M, Yajima K, Kohno H, Itagaki E, Hattori T. Induction of suppressor cell activities in normal lymphocytes by sera from gastric cancer patients. Clin Exp Immunol 1983; 54:80–6.

14. Creagen ET, Fraumeni J. Familial gastric cancer and immunologic abnormalities. Cancer 1973; 32:1325–31.

15. Spector BD, Filipovich AH, Perry GS, Kersey JH. Epidemiology of cancer in ataxia teleangiectasia. In: Bridges BA, Harbden DG, eds. Ataxia-teleangiectasia. A cellular and molecular link between cancer, neuropathology and immune deficiency. Chichester: John Wiley, 1982; 103–38.

16. Daly MB, Swift M. Epidemiological factors related to the malignant neoplasms in ataxia-teleangiectasia families. J Chronic Dis 1978; 31:625–34.

17. Hoover R, Fraumeni JF. Risk of cancer in renal transplant recipients. Lancet 1973; 2:55–57.

Cancer Detection and Prevention Supplement 1:127–135 (1987)

Lectin Binding Pattern of Hodgkin Disease-Derived Cell Lines in Comparison to Other Human Cell Lines

Marin Schwonzen
Gerhard Uhlenbruck
Michael Schaadt

Detlev Funken
Heinz Burrichter
Volker Diehl

Medizinische Klinik I der Universität zu Köln, Köln, Federal Republic of Germany

ABSTRACT The three Hodgkin disease-derived cell lines L 428, L 540, and L 591 were characterized in their carbohydrate epitope composition by a panel of lectins. Nine other human cell lines were tested in comparison to the Hodgkin (H) and Sternberg Reed (SR) cells: promyelocytic (HL 60), lymphoblastoid, myeloma, histiocytic lymphoma (U 937), and other non-Hodgkin lymphoma cell lines. Twenty-four different fluoresceinated lectins bound to the Hodgkin and other cell lines in different percentages of positive cells and with varying intensities. Lotus lectin and a monoclonal anti-Lewis blood group X antibody showed very similar binding patterns (L 428, L 540, HL 60, U 937). Soybean agglutinin stained only L 428 and L 540, although nearly all were positive after neuraminidase treatment. Cell lysis of the three H cell lines resulted in a very similar electrophoretic mobility pattern of proteins. In addition, staining of transblotted glycoproteins with biotinylated concanavalin A by avidin peroxidase reaction revealed corresponding bands. Differences were seen with Lotus staining. In summary, the origin of H cells is still unknown, but there is obviously some relationship in the glycoconjugate profile to the myelohistiocytic lineage.

Key words: lymphoma cell lines, promyelocytic, histiocytic; glycoproteins

INTRODUCTION

The uncertain nature of Hodgkin (H) and Sternberg Reed (SR) cells has stimulated decades of research despite the characteristic and striking morphological features. In recent years Diehl and coworkers [1, 2] have established long-term cultures from tumor material of Hodgkin disease. Meanwhile, there is no doubt that the in vitro cells represent the counterpart of in vivo H and SR cells as shown by the identity of multiple characteristic properties. However, these intensive investigations could not identify a relationship of H and SR cells with a known cell type.

We tried to classify the three Hodgkin disease-derived cell lines L 428, L 540, and L 591 in comparison to promyelocytic, histiocytic, lymphoblastoid, B, T, and Burkitt lymphoma

Address reprint requests to Gerhard Uhlenbruck, Medizinische Klinik I der Universität zu Köln, Joseph-Stelzmann straße 9, D-5000 Köln 41, Federal Republic of Germany.

cell lines with a panel of fluoresceinated lectins. Lectins are glycoproteins known to bind specifically to simple or complex carbohydrates. The changes in glycosylation of glycoproteins and membrane glycolipids occur as quickly and as dramatically as the process of phosphorylation at all stages of differentiation, development, and oncogenesis, as Hakomori [5] has pointed out. Accordingly, stage specific, tissue-specific, or tumor-associated carbohydrate antigens are expressed.

MATERIALS AND METHODS
Cells

Establishment of the Hodgkin disease (HD)-derived in vitro cell lines and culture conditions are described elsewhere [1, 2]. Cell lines were maintained in RPMI-1640 medium with 5–10% fetal calf serum, glutamine, and penicillin/streptomcyin in a 5% CO_2 atmosphere.

Lectin Binding of Cell Surface Carbohydrates

Cells were washed three times in 10 mM Tris-buffered saline (TBS; 154 mM NaCl, 5 mM $CaCl_2$, 2 mM $MgCl_2$, 0.01% NaN_3, pH 7.2) and counted. Cells (10^6/0.1 ml) were incubated with 0.1 ml lectin-FITC conjugates (50 μg/ml) for 30 min at 4°C with intermittent shaking. *Geodia cydomium* was purified and FITC-labeled as previously described [6]. *Geodia* and other FITC-conjugated, affinity-purified lectins (Medac, Hamburg, Federal Republic of Germany) were stored in aliquots at -20°C and diluted in TBS before use. After incubation, excess lectin was removed by washing in TBS two times. Sedimented cells were examined with a Leitz fluorescence microscope equipped with appropriate filters. Two hundred cells were counted in each assay, and the percentage of cells demonstrating membrane fluorescence was determined.

A similar procedure was used for *monoclonal antibody Leu M1 and FH6 staining.* Leu M1 was purchased from Becton Dickinson, (Heidelberg, Federal Republic of Germany) and diluted 1:100 in PBS supplemented with 1% bovine serum albumin (BSA). The FH6 monoclonal antibody was kindly provided by S.I. Hakomori, University of Washington, Seattle. Secondary fluoresceinated antibody (antimouse Ig; Medac) was used in a working dilution of 1:400 in PBS containing 5% BSA.

Pretreatment of Cells With Neuraminidase or Pronase

Before incubation with lectin or antibody, 0.1 ml neuraminidase (0.1 U/ml) from *Vibrio cholera* (Behringwerke AG, Marburg, Federal Republic of Germany) or 0.1 ml pronase (0.1 mg/ml; Calbiochem, Frankfurt, Federal Republic of Germany) was added to sedimented cells (10^6/0.1 ml) for 30 min at 37°C and the cells were washed twice.

Sodium Dodecyl Sulfate-Polyacrylamide Gel Electrophoresis (SDS-PAGE) and Transblot of Cell Lysates

Cells (10^7) were washed four times with cold PBS, and then 0.1 ml lysis buffer (2% Triton X, 2 mM $MgCl_2$, 2 mM phenylmethysulfonylfluoride, glycine buffered 50 mM Tris, pH 8.9) was added on ice. After a 20 min incubation, the tubes were centrifuged in an Eppendorf microfuge and the supernatant was recovered. Sample buffer (4% SDS, 6M urea) was added in the same volume. SDS-PAGE was run under reducing conditions according to the method of Laemmli [7] using a linear acrylamide gradient concentration of 7.5% to 15% with a 3% stacking gel.

Electrophoretically separated samples were transferred to nitrocellulose sheets as described by Towbin et al [8]. Sheets were stained for protein by Ponceau S or were blocked with 5% BSA for 6 hr at room temperature (RT) and stained by a 3 hr incubation at RT with biotin conjugated lectins in a concentration of 0.1–0.2 mg/ml TBS supplemented with 1% BSA. Washing was done four times in TBS for 10 min each time. The transfers were treated subsequently with a 5 μg/ml avidin-conjugated horseradish peroxidase (Sigma, Deisenhofen,

TABLE I. Lectin Binding Patterns of Cell Lines Before (b) and After (a) Neuraminidase Treatment

Cell line	DSA		ECA		PHA		VFA		GSA		Geodia	
	b	a	b	a	b	a	b	a	b	a	b	a
L 428	++100*	+++100	+++100	+++100	++90	+++100	+++100	+++100	+30	+80	++80	++100
L 428 KSA	+90	++100	+++100	+++100	++90	+90	+100	+90	—	+30	+50	++80
L 540	+90	+++100	++90	+++100	—	—	++100	++90	+50	++90	+80	++100
L 591	++100	++100	++100	+++100	++90	+++100	+100	+100	+80	++100	—	+70
HL 60	++80	++100	+60	+++100	+90	++100	+100	+80	NT	NT	—	+70
U 937	+80	++100	—	+100	+90	+100	+80	+80	NT	NT	NT	NT
LCL 725	++100	++100	+80	++100	++90	++90	—	+100	—	+50	—	+70
LCL 660	+80	+80	++100	+++100	++80	++90	++90	+100	—	++50	+100	++100
CEM	+100	+100	+100	+++100	+90	++90	+100	+80	++100	++100	+50	+50
L 662	—	+100	+100	+++100	NT	NT	+90	+70	+50	NT	NT	NT
L 363	+80	+100	+10	+++100	+90	++90	—	—	NT	+80	+100	++100
U 266 H	+100	+100	+90	+++100	+10	+80	+100	+100	+80	++80	—	+80
RAJI	+90	+90	++100	++100	+90	+100	+90	+30	+10	+80	+90	++100

*+−+++, Intensity of positive membrane fluorescence; numbers designate percent of cells counted with positive membrane fluorescence; NT, not tested.

TABLE II. Lectin Binding Patterns of Cell Lines Before (b) and After (a) Neuraminidase Treatment

Cell line	HPA		MPA		SJA		VVA		VAA		PWM	
	b	a	b	a	b	a	b	a	b	a	b	a
L 428	+20*	++90	+90	+100	–	++100	–	–	–	+50	++100	+++100
L 428 KSA	–	–	–	–	+90	+++100	–	+80	–	+100	+60	+60
L 540	+60	++90	+30	++70	–	++90	+50	–	–	++90	++100	+40
L 591	–	–	+100	+90	+30	+90	+100	++100	–	–	–	+100
HL 60	–	+80	+90	+100	NT	NT	–	+80	–	+90	–	+90
U 937	–	–	–	+90	NT	NT	–	++100	–	–	+5	+90
LCL 725	–	–	–	+++90	+50	++100	–	–	++100	++100	–	–
LCL 660	–	–	+100	+++100	–	+++100	–	–	–	–	+90	+100
CEM	–	+100	+100	+100	++70	++80	–	++100	+100	++90	–	–
L 662	+20	++80	–	+100	NT	NT	–	+100	+80	+70	+100	++90
L 363	–	–	+50	+90	+50	++100	–	++100	–	–	–	–
U 266 H	–	+100	+100	+100	–	–	+100	++100	+90	+80	–	+100
RAJI	–	+100	+100	+80	–	+70	–	++80	–	–	+100	+80

*+–+++, Intensity of positive membrane fluorescence; numbers designate percent of cells counted with positive membrane fluorescence; NT, not tested.

TABLE III. Lectin Binding Patterns of Cell Lines Before (b) and After (a) Neuraminidase Treatment

Cell line	PNA b	PNA a	TKA b	TKA a	WFA b	WFA a	SBA b	SBA a	Lotus b	Lotus a	Leu M1	FH6
L 428	++10*	++100	+80	+90	+100	+100	+30	+100	+90	+100	++70	—
L 428 KSA	+5	+100	+80	+80	+50	+50	+30	++100	—	++80	—	—
L 540	++10	+++100	+70	+10	+5	+70	++70	+++100	+30	++80	+50	—
L 591	+100	++100	+80	+100	—	—	—	+++100	—	—	—	++80
HL 60	—	+++100	—	+50	—	+90		+++100	—	—	—	++80
U 937	—	+++100	—	+80	—	+90	—	+++100	+50	+90	+70	NT
LCL 725	+30	++100	+70	+80	+40	+80	—	+100	—	+80	+80	NT
LCL 660	—	+100	—	NT	—	—	—	—	—	—	—	NT
CEM	+40	+++100	+50	+80	—	—	—	++100	—	—	—	NT
L 662	—	++100	—	—	—	+80	—	+100	—	—	NT	NT
L 363	—	+100	—	—	—	—		+100	—	—	—	NT
U 266 H	—	++100	+100	+90	—	—	—	++100	—	—	—	NT
RAJI	+70	+++100	+80	+80	—	—	—	++90	—	—	—	NT

*+–++++, Intensity of positive membrane fluorescence; numbers designate percent of cells counted with positive membrane fluorescence; NT, not tested.

Federal Republic of Germany) containing 1% BSA for 40 min and washed again. Specific lectin binding bands were detected after a 5 min incubation with 0.5 μg/ml 3,3'-diaminobenzidine (4HCl) as substrate in a 100 mM citric acid-ammonium acetate buffer, pH 6.5, containing 0.015% hydrogen peroxide.

RESULTS AND DISCUSSION

The origin of H and SR cells is still controversial. To obtain some information as to this question, we used fluoresceinated lectins as tools in preliminary studies of epitope carbohydrate structures of H and SR cells in comparison to other human cell lines.

Native con A, succinylated con A, *Lens culinaris* (LCA), *Ricinus communis I* (RCA I), RCA II, wheat germ (WGA), and *Pisum sativum* (PEA) strongly stained all cell lines tested even at a concentration of 5 μ/ml. Most of the other lectins (Tables I–III) also showed no differences in typing a sort or subclass of cells. DSA (for abbreviations see Tables IV and V), for example, reacts quantitatively with glycoproteins, and ECA detects predominantly glycolipids of most cell lines as revealed by proteolytic digestion.

As a common finding, the HD-derived cell lines L 428 and L 540 share many similarities in glycoconjugate composition in contrast to L 591 (Lotus, SBA, PWM, WFA, PHA, Leu Ml, FH6). However, cell lysis of the three HD cell lines showed similarities in their electrophoretic mobility patterns of proteins (Fig. 1). L 428 KSA, a calf serum-adapted subline derived from L 428 by a single exposure to phorbolester (TPA), which shows a different growth pattern (plastic adherent monolayer), did not express HPA or MPA receptor (Table II).

SBA only stained L 428 and L 540, although nearly all lines were positive after neuraminidase treatment. Normal peripheral blood lymphocytes were also shown to be stained

TABLE IV. Origin of Agglutinins and Monoclonal Antibodies Shown in Tables I–III

DSA, *Datura stramonium*	PWM, *Pokeweed mitogen*
ECA, *Erythrina cristagalli*	SBA, *Soybean*
FH6, Monoclonal antibody defining a sialyldifucoganglioside [5]	SJA, *Saphora japonica*
	TKA, *Trichosantes kinlowii*
Geodia, *Geodia cydonium*	VAA, *Viscum album*
GSA, *Griffonia simplicifolia* I	VFA, *Vicia faba*
HPA, *Helix pomanita*	VVA, *Vicia villosa*
Leu M1, Monoclonal antibody defining lacto-N-fucopentaose III (X-hapten, myelomonocytic antigen CD 15)	WFA, *Wistaria floribunda*
Lotus, *Lotus tetragonolobus*	
MPA, *Maclura pomifera*	
PHA, *Phaseolus vulgaris*	
PNA, *Arachis hypogaea (Peanut)*	

TABLE V. Origin of Cell Lines Tested

L 428, L 540, L 591	Hodgkin's disease [1,2]
L 428 KSA	Calf serum-adapted variant of L 428 growing as an adherent monolayer after exposure to phorbolester TPA [2]
HL 60	Acute promyelocytic leukemia
U 937	Histiocytic lymphoma
LCL 725, LCL 660	Epstein-Barr virus-transformed lymphoblastoid cell lines
CEM	T-cell acute lymphatic leukemia
L 662	B-cell acute lymphatic leukemia
RAJI	Burkitt lymphoma

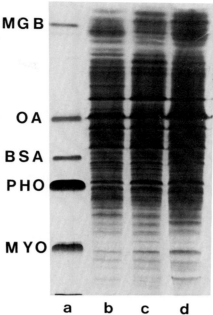

Fig. 1. Coomassie blue stain of cell lysates (b, L 428; c, L 540; d, L 591) after SDS-PAGE. a, Molecular weight standards. MGB, horse myoglobin (18 kD); OA, ovalbumin (43 kD); BSA, bovine serum albumin (68 kD); PHO, phosphorylase b (97 kD); MYO, myosin (205 kD).

by SBA only after neuraminidase treatment [10]. Cytoplasmic binding of SBA to macrophages and histiocytes in histological sections has been reported [11]. It was proposed by Altevogt et al [9] that the difference in positioning sialic acid on the cell surface, leading to masking or unmasking of the SBA-receptor, could influence the metastatic potential of tumor cells. This corresponds to the low metastatic potential of these HD cell lines after heterotransplantation in nude mice. Lack of metastatic potential, however, is a common feature of heterotransplanted lymphoma cell lines.

In a prior study, the lectins from peanut and Lotus were reported to bind only weakly or not at all to H and SR cells in histological sections [12], but Möller [13] found a prominent, constant, and characteristic pattern in cytoplasmatic staining of H and SR cells. Our results agree with the data of Hsu et al [14], who showed a nonconstant reaction of PNA with H and SR cells in biopsies.

Although fucose is an important determinant of PEA and LCA binding [15], and all cell lines were stained, differences were seen with the fucose binding lectin from Lotus tetragono-lobus (Table III). In a previous study Elias and Elias [16] noted a correlation between the reactivity of Lotus lectin, DR, and Fc receptor expression. An increasing intensity of Lotus binding has also been reported to parallel the normal myeloid maturation sequence [17]. Enhancing of binding after neuraminidase treatment in our results might be due to steric effects.

Con A, LCA, and WGA attached to more than 25 transblotted glycoproteins after SDS-PAGE of all HD cell lines, showing corresponding bands. This result is not unexpected [18], but the Lotus lectin may be suitable for further characterization of HD cells; only a few Lotus binding glycoproteins were seen: 236 kD, 220 kD, 100–110 kD, 62 kD, and 37 kD (Fig. 2).

The monoclonal and anti-Lewis blood group X antibody (anti-Leu Ml) showed a binding pattern very similar to that of Lotus lectin (Table III). However, anti-Leu Ml staining of histiocytes and interdigitating reticulum cells requires pretreatment of sections with neuramin-

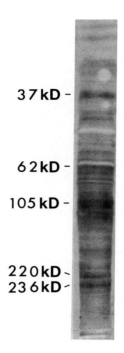

37 kD -

62 kD -

105 kD -

220 kD -
236 kD -

Fig. 2. Transblot following the SDS-PAGE of L 540 cell lysate stained by Lotus biotin conjugate and avidin peroxidase.

idase [14]. This is not true for the HD cell lines. L 591 remains negative for Leu Ml staining also after neuraminidase treatment but shows a positive reaction with the FH6 antibody.

Recent work has shown an identical population of round and branched cells in four histiocytic lymphomas possessing a lectin staining pattern similar to that of lines L 428 and L 540; they were positive for SBA, PNA, and Lotus [19]. Reactivity of these lymphomas to monoclonal antibody Ki-1 should be determined [4]. In summary, the origin of the H and SR cells is still unknown, but there is obviously some relationship to the myelohistiocytic lineage in the glycoconjugate profile.

ACKNOWLEDGMENTS

This work has been supported by the Minister für Wissenschaft und Forschung des Landes Nordrhein-Westfalen. M. Schwonzen is a stipendiate of the Deutsche Forschungsgemeinschaft.

REFERENCES

1. Diehl V, Kirchner H, Schaadt M, Fonatsch, C, Stein H, Gerdes J, Boie C. Hodgkin's disease: Establishment and characterisation of four in vitro cell lines. J Cancer Res Clin Oncol 1981; 101:111–24.
2. Diehl V, Kirchner HH, Burrichter H, Stein H, Fonatsch C, Gerdes J, Schaadt M, Heit W, Uchanska-Ziegler B, Ziegler A, Heintz F, Sueno K. Characteristics of Hodgkin's disease-derived cell lines. Cancer Treat Rep 1982; 65:615–32.
3. Schwab U, Stein H, Gerdes J, Lemke H, Kirchner H, Schaadt M, Diehl V. Production of a monoclonal antibody specific for Hodgkin and Sternberg Reed cells of Hodgkin's disease and a subset of normal lymphoid cells. Nature 1982; 299:65–7.
4. Schaadt M, Burrichter H, Stein H, Pfreudschuh M, Fonatsch C, Diehl V. The cell of origin in Hodgkin's disease: Conclusions from in Vivo and in Vitro studies. Int Exp Pathol 1985; 2:185–202.

5. Hakomori S-I. Aberrant glycosylation in cancer cell membranes as focused on glycolipids: Overview and perspectives. Cancer Res 1985; 45:2405–14.
6. Hanisch FG, Saur A, Müller WEG, Conrad J, Uhlenbruck G. Further characterization of a lectin and its in vivo receptor from Geodia cydonium. Biochim Biophys Acta 1982; 801:388–95.
7. Laemmli UK. Cleavage of structural proteins during the assembly of the head of bacteriophage T4. Nature 1970; 227:680–5.
8. Towbin H, Staehelin T, Gordon J. Electrophoretic transfer of proteins from polyacrylamide gels to nitrocellulose sheets: Procedure and some applications. Proc Natl Acad Sci USA; 76:4350–4.
9. Altevogt P, Fogel M, Cheingsong-Popov R, Dennis J, Robinson P, Schirrmacher V. Different patterns of lectin binding and cell surface sialylation detected on related high and low metastatic tumor lines. Cancer Res 1983; 43:5138–44.
10. Newman RA, Uhlenbruck G, Schumacher K, van Miel A, Karduck D. Interaction of peanut agglutinin with human lymphocytes. Binding properties and topology of the receptor site. Z Immunol Forsch 1978; 154:451–62.
11. Wirbel R, Möller P, Schwechheimer K. Lectin binding spectra in the hyperplastic human tonsil. Histiochemistry 1984; 81:551–60.
12. Strauchen JA. Lectin receptors as markers of lymphoid cells. Am J Pathol 1984; 116:370–6.
13. Möller P. Peanut lectin: A useful tool for detecting Hodgkin cells in paraffin sections. Virchows Arch Pathol Anat 1982; 396:313–7.
14. Hsu S-M, Yang K, Jaffe E. Phentotypic expression of Hodgkin's and Reed-Sternberg cells in Hodgkin's disease. Am J Pathol 1985; 118:209–17.
15. Kornfeld K, Reitman ML, Kornfeld R. The carbohydrate-binding specificity of pea and lentil lectins. J Biol Chem 1981; 256:6633–40.
16. Elias L, Elias D. Analysis of myelomonocytic leukemic differentiation by a cell surface marker panel including a fucose binding lectin from Lotus tetragonolobus. Blood 1984; 63:1285–90.
17. Nicola NA, Morstyn G, Metcalf D. Lectin receptors on human blood and bone marrow cells and their use in cell separation. Blood Cells 1980; 6:563–79.
18. Gürtler LG, Sramota B, Cleve H. The lectin binding sites on the plasma membrane components of human lymphoblastoid cell lines. Hoppe-Seyler Z Physiol Chem 1979; 360:1819–28.
19. Freemont AJ, Matthews S, Stoddart RW, Jones CJP. The distribution of cells of the monocytic-lineage in relative lymph nodes and non-Hodgkin's lymphomata. Characterization using protein histiochemistry, lectin binding and monoclonal antibodies. J Pathol 1985; 146:139–50.

Production of Interleukin-2 and Expression of Tac Antigen in Hodgkin Disease

Narendra N. Joshi, PhD
Rabindranath Mukhopadhyay, PhD
Suresh H. Advani, MD
Sudha G. Gangal, PhD

*Immunology Division, Cancer Research Institute (N.N.J., R.M., S.G.G.)
and Department of Medicine, Tata Memorial Hospital (S.H.A.), Parel,
Bombay-400 012, India*

ABSTRACT Phytohemagglutinin (PHA)- induced Interleukin-2 (IL-2) production by peripheral blood mononuclear cells was studied in 28 untreated patients with Hodgkin Disease (HD). A group of 28 patients were also investigated for the expression of Tac antigen in the resting stage of lymphocytes and after activation with PHA and mixed leukocyte culture (using anti-Tac monoclonal antibody). The blastogenic response to PHA and IL-2 production by lymphocytes of HD patients was significantly lower than that of normal lymphocytes. Production of IL-2 appeared to be severely affected in 14 of 28 HD patients who also showed PHA response less than the normal range. The Tac antigen expression was found to be lower in PHA-stimulated but not alloantigen-stimulated lymphocytes from the HD patients. No correlation was observed between the levels of IL-2 production, Tac antigen expression, and blastogenic response to PHA or allogeneic cells and the stage of disease when tested in the same patients.

Key words: Interleukin-2, Tac antigen, Hodgkin Disease

INTRODUCTION

Patients with active Hodgkin disease (HD) exhibit significant depression in their cell-mediated immunity [1,2]. In our earlier studies [3,4,] we have shown the existence of soluble inhibitory factors that influence the T cell responses of HD patients to the mitogen phytohemagglutinin (PHA). We also found partial recovery of mitogen-induced blastogenic potential of peripheral blood mononuclear cells by exogenous supplementation of cultures with crude Interleukin-2 (IL-2)- containing medium [5]. It is now well established that after recognition of antigen or mitogen, the proliferation of activated T lymphocytes requires the synthesis of IL-2 as well as the synthesis of specific membrane receptors for IL-2 [6,7]. Recently a number of workers have studied either or both of these requirements for T cell expansion in several pathological conditions to determine the level at which the T cell defect may exist [8–13]. In

Address reprint requests to Dr. Sudha G. Gangal, Head, Immunology Division, Cancer Research Institute, Tata Memorial Centre, Parel, Bombay-400 012, India.

this article, we report experiments conducted to assess the production of IL-2 by mitogenic stimulation and the expression of IL-2 receptors following mitogenic or allogeneic stimulation by lymphocytes from untreated HD patients.

MATERIALS AND METHODS
Patients and Controls

The lymphocyte response of 44 untreated HD patients of both sexes, with ages ranging between 10 to 55 years, were investigated. Clinically 15 patients were in stage IA/B, 18 in stage II A/B, eight in stage III A/B, and three in stage IV A/B [14]. Histologically 13 patients showed lymphocyte predominance, 19 showed mixed cellularity, eight had nodular sclerosis, and one was of the lymphocyte depletion type [15]. Histological classification of three patients was not available. Sixteen controls used in the study were healthy donors of both sexes (either patients' relatives or laboratory volunteers) aged between 20 to 50.

PHA-Induced Blastogenesis

Peripheral blood mononuclear cells (PBMNC) separated on Ficoll-Hypaque density gradient [16] were suspended at a concentration of 1×10^6 cells/ml of complete medium (CM) consisting of RPMI 1640 (Gibco, Grand Island, NY) with 10% heat-inactivated human AB group serum, 25mM HEPES (Sigma, St. Louis, MO), 2 mM glutamine, 40 μg/ml gentamicin, and 5 IU/ml nystatin. The PHA response of PBMNC was assessed as described earlier [3].

Mixed Leukocyte Culture

Mixed leukocyte culture (MLC) was established in bulk using siliconized glass tubes by culturing together 1×10^6/ml responder PBMNC and 1×10^6/ml allogeneic stimulator PBMNC (irradiated with 2,500 rads) in equal volume of CM. The cultures were harvested at the end of 144 hours. Control cultures consisted of responders alone in CM.

IL-2 Production and Assay

IL-2 production was carried out by stimulation of 1×10^6 cells/ml of CM with 10 μg/ml PHA-P for 24 hours at 37°C in humidified 5% CO_2 atmosphere. Control cultures were incubated without PHA. At the end of the incubation period cell-free supernatant was collected and stored at −20°C until use. Supernatants from PHA-stimulated PBMNC obtained from normal healthy donors and untreated HD patients were compared for IL-2 production. The level of IL-2 in conditioned medium was tested on proliferation of the IL-2 dependent mouse CTLL cell line maintained in our laboratory [17]. CTLLs suspended at 1×10^5/ml were plated in 0.1 ml volume/well in a 96-well tissue culture plate. Equal volumes of test supernatants were added to replicate cultures and incubated at 37°C in 5% CO_2 containing humidified atmosphere for 24 hours. Four hours before termination, cultures received ^{3}H-TdR and its incorporation was measured.

Immunofluorescence With Anti-Tac Antibody

For immunofluorescence study both the mitogen and MLC stimulation were conducted using bulk cultures of 1×10^6 cells/ml of CM, which were harvested after 72 hours and 144 hours, respectively. Anti-Tac monoclonal antibody, which is known to recognize the receptor for IL-2 on both activated human T and B cells [18–20], was kindly donated by Dr. T. Waldman, NIH (Bethesda, MD). Cells activated by PHA and MLC were suspended at the concentration of 1×10^6 cells/ml of balanced salt solution (BSS) supplemented with 10% FCS (Difco, Detroit, MI) and 0.2% sodium azide. They were incubated for 45 minutes at 4°C with saturating amounts of anti-Tac (final dilution 1:6,000) monoclonal antibody. The cells were washed twice in cold BSS and were further incubated for 30 minutes at 4°C with a 1:30 dilution of fluorescein-conjugated antimouse immunoglobulin reagent (Zymed, San Francisco, CA). After three washes the cells were resuspended in 10 μl of 0.1% P-phenylene-diamine in

PBS-glycerol and analyzed for membrane immunofluorescence. In controls, treatment with anti-Tac monoclonal was omitted and there was no nonspecific staining seen. Also, cells from unstimulated cultures kept as negative controls did not show immunofluorescence. Results were expressed as percentage of Tac-positive cells.

RESULTS
PHA-Induced Blastogenesis

The blastogenic response of PBMNC from HD patients to 10 μg/ml of PHA was significantly lower ($P < 0.001$) than that of the normal control (Fig. 1). The net CPM values were 23,494 $\pm$ 3,435 in HD and 46,051 $\pm$ 3,264 in controls. In addition, it was observed that 14 of 28 HD patients showed a PHA response below the 95% confidence limit (ie, 2 SD below the mean) of the normal response. Thus the HD patients could be categorized into two groups of low responders and normal responders on the basis of their proliferative response pattern. However, the pattern of normal or low responses had no correlation with the clinical stage of the disease (Fig. 1).

IL-2 Production

The production of IL-2 by PBMNC in response to stimulation by PHA in 28 HD patients and 16 controls is shown in Figure 2. IL-2 activity is expressed in terms of ^{3}H-TdR incorporation by the indicator CTLL cells. Mean IL-2 production in healthy donors (CPM 12,345 $\pm$ 1,589) was significantly higher ($P < 0.01$) than that of the HD patients (CPM 6,615 $\pm$ 1,109). PBMNC from some HD patients could produce IL-2 in the normal range. Also, in these experiments no correlation between IL-2 production and the stage of disease progression was seen.

Since PHA-induced blastogenesis was significantly lower in some HD PBMNC while in others it overlapped the normal range, we compared the IL-2 production by both normal and

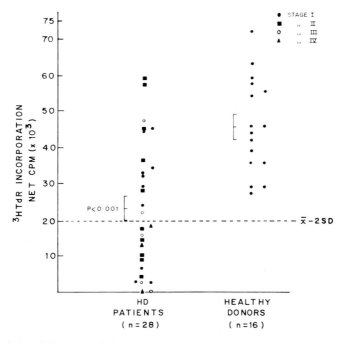

Fig. 1. PHA-induced blastogenesis by PBMNC from healthy controls and untreated HD patients in relation to clinical stage of the disease. The dotted line represents the mean of the control value −2 SD.

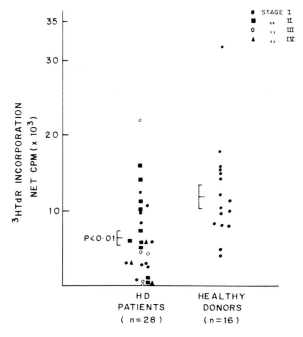

Fig. 2.   Production of IL-2 by PHA-activated PBMNC from healthy controls and untreated HD patients in relation to clinical stage of the disease. IL-2 production measured in terms of ^{3}H-TdR incorporation by mouse CTLL.

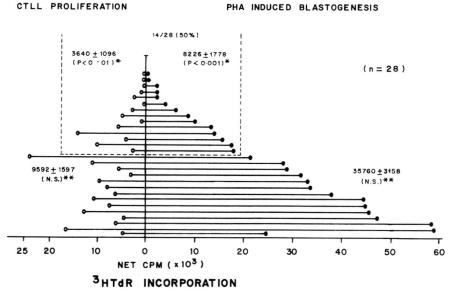

Fig. 3.   The relationship of IL-2 production to PHA response of PBMNC from individual Hodgkin disease patients. The low PHA responders producing low IL-2 are shown within the upper boxed area. *P value compared to high responders/high producers. **P value compared to healthy controls.

low PHA responders (Fig. 3). Patients who were low PHA responders were usually also significantly low producers of IL-2. On the other hand, the normal responders produced a fairly good amount of IL-2. The mean IL-2 production level of low responders was lower than that of the normal responder group (CPM $3,640 \pm 1,096$ and $9,592 \pm 1,597$ respectively, P < 0.01). It was also found that the lower residual IL-2 in conditioned medium did not result from utilization of IL-2 by cells for their own proliferation especially in normal HD responders (Fig. 3).

Expression of Tac Antigen

The resting cell populations from both healthy controls and HD patients did not express significant differences in the number of IL-2 receptor-bearing cells as reflected by Tac-positive cells (Table I). PBMNC from HD patients and normal controls, when stimulated with PHA, exhibited differences in percentage of Tac-positive cells. The overall mean percentage of Tac-positive cells in HD was less than that of the controls ($42.3 \pm 11.2\%$ and $52.2 \pm 14.1\%$, respectively, $P < 0.05$). However, when PBMNC from 26 HD patients and 11 normal controls were studied with allogeneic stimulation, a comparable number of IL-2 receptor-bearing cells (16.2 ± 5.8 and $18.5 \pm 6.1\%$ respectively) were noted. Stage of disease had no bearing on the expression of IL-2 receptors by stimulated cells (data not shown).

Correlation Between IL-2 Production and Tac Expression in HD Patients

The data on IL-2 production and expression of IL-2 receptors by the same PBMNC samples from 12 HD patients is demonstrated in Table II. There was no conclusive correlation

TABLE I. Tac Antigen Expression by PBMNC From HD Patients and Healthy Donors

Lymphocyte population tested	% Tac-positive cells $\pm$ SD	
	Control (N = 11)	HD (N = 28)
Resting cells	0	$0.7 \pm 1.3^*$
PHA-stimulated cells	52.2 ± 14.1	$42.3 \pm 11.2\dagger$
MLC-stimulated cells	18.5 ± 6.1	16.2 ± 5.8

*Six of 28 samples showed Tac-positive cells.
$\dagger P < 0.05$.

TABLE II. IL-2 Production and IL-2 Receptor Expression by PBMNC From HD Patients (N = 12)

Clinical stage and pathological grade	Net CPM IL-2 production (mean $\pm$ SE)	% Tac-positive cells		
			Stimulated with	
		Resting	PHA	MLC
IIA, LP	$5,973 \pm 378$	2	42	14
IA, LP	$3,031 \pm 654$	0	51	21
IIIA, LP	$4,681 \pm 879$	2.5	29	15
IA, MC	$8,251 \pm 232$	4	53	12
IIA, LP	$6,015 \pm 208$	0	52	16
IA, LP	$12,515 \pm 710$	0	30	18
IA, MC	$2,844 \pm 376$	0	48	22
IIA, MC	$16,194 \pm 2,109$	2.5	31	10
IB, LP	$5,880 \pm 1,080$	0	41	11
IIB, LP	$11,073 \pm 1,087$	0	36	23
IIA, LP	$5,162 \pm 168$	0	43	21
IIIB, MC	503 ± 91	0	44	19

between the level of IL-2 activity and the receptor expression and between the clinical stage and pathological grade of the disease.

DISCUSSION

Although the primary activating signal produces specificity to the immune response, the secondary lymphocyte proliferation signal is a nonspecific event in terms of IL-2 production and response [6,7]. In HD, the decreased response to mitogen is a well-known observation. In the present study we have attempted to evaluate the possible level of deviation in the central regulatory mechanism that is involved in the mitogen-induced proliferation phenomenon of untreated HD patients. Our observations of hyporesponsiveness to the mitogen PHA by HD PBMNC is in keeping with earlier observations [3]. Following identification of the central regulatory role of IL-2 on mitogen-induced proliferation, in several diseases including HD the production of IL-2 and the expression of IL-2 receptors have been studied. Our present finding of depressed IL-2 production by peripheral blood lymphocytes in HD confirms the recent observations in other laboratories [12, 21, 22]. However, we were able to deliniate the normal and hyporesponsive HD patients and have demonstrated that PBMNC from HD patients had comparatively low responsiveness to the mitogen and were also low producers of the lymphokine. Although a large number of patients investigated by us represents a wide clinical spectrum of the disease, it was not possible to correlate anomalies in IL-2 production and response by HD patients with other cellular or molecular events such as PGE2 production by HD monocytes [21,23,24] or deficiency in IL-1 production [12,21]. Further studies are needed to determine IL-2 regulation in HD by other possible agents and mechanisms.

Our finding of a lower number of IL-2 receptor-bearing cells in PHA-stimulated PBMNC in HD is similar to the results reported by Zamkoff et al [21]. However, we did not observe any difference in Tac antigen-bearing cells after MLC stimulation as an indication of a specific stimulus for IL-2 receptor expression. Contrary to reports that IL-2 regulates the expression of its own receptors on activated cells [25], our test system failed to reveal any correlation between IL-2 activity and Tac antigen expression in the same PBMNC samples. Our findings suggest that production of both IL-2 and its receptor expression are defective in a large number of HD patients irrespective of clinical stage, which may be partially responsible for the cell-mediated immune deficiency characteristic of this disease.

REFERENCES

1. Kaplan HS. Hodgkin's disease: Biology, treatment, prognosis. Blood 1981; 57:813–22.
2. Kumar R, Penny R. Cell-mediated immune deficiency in Hodgkin's disease. Immunol Today 1982; 3:269–73.
3. Moghe MV, Advani SH, Gangal SG. Demonstration of inhibitory factors affecting cell mediated immunity in patients with Hodgkin's disease. Eur J Cancer 1980; 16:937–43.
4. Mukhopadhyaya R, Advani SH, Gangal SG. Impairment of T lymphocyte colony formation in Hodgkin's disease: Effect of soluble inhibitory factors on normal T lymphocytes colony formation potential. Acta Haematol 1983; 70:357–63.
5. Mukhopadhyaya R, Advani SH, Gangal SG. Effect of exogenous interleukins on in vitro responses of T lymphocytes from patients with Hodgkin's disease. Cancer Detect Prevent 1987; (in press).
6. Robb RJ. Interleukin-2: The molecule and its function. Immunol Today 1984; 5:203–9.
7. Sarin PS, Gallo RC. Human T cell growth factor (TCGF) CRC Crit Rev Immunol 1984; 4:279–305.
8. Paganelli R, Aiuti F, Beverley PCL, Levinsky RJ. Impaired production of interleukins in patients with cell mediated immunodeficiencies. Clin Exp Immunol 1983; 51:338–44.
9. Nakayama E, Asano S, Takuwa N, Yokota J, Miwa S. Decreased TCGF activity in the culture medium of PHA stimulated peripheral mononuclear cells from patients with metastatic cancer. Clin Exp Immunol 1983; 51:511–6.
10. Ebert EC, Wright SH, Lipshutz WH, Hauptman SP. T-cell abnormalities in inflammatory bowel disease are mediated by Interleukin-2. Clin Immunol Immunopathol 1984; 33:232–44.

11. Prince HE, Kermani-Arab V, Fahey JL. Depressed interleukin-2 receptor expression in acquired immune deficiency and lymphadenopathy syndromes. J Immunol 1984; 3:1313–7.

12. Ford RJ, Tsao J, Kouttab NM, Sahasrabuddhe CG, Mehta SR. Association of an interleukin abnormality with the T cell defect in Hodgkin's disease. Blood 1984; 64:386–92.

13. de Faucal P, Godard A, Peyrat MA, Moreau JF, Soulillou JP. Impaired IL-2 production by lymphocytes of patients with systemic lupus erythematosus. Ann Immunol (Inst. Pasteur) 1984; 135 D:161–72.

14. Carbone PP, Kaplan HS, Musshoff K, Smithers DW, Tubiana M. Report of the committee on Hodgkin's disease staging. Cancer Res 1971; 31:1860–1.

15. Lukes RJ, Craver LF, Hall TC, Rappaport H, Rubin P. Report of the nomenclature committee. Cancer Res 1966; 26:1311.

16. Boyum A. Isolation of mononuclear cells and granulocytes from human blood. Scan J Clin Lab Invest 1968; 21 [Suppl 97]:77–89.

17. Baker PE, Gillis S, Smith KA. Monoclonal cytolytic T-cell lines. J Exp Med 1979; 149:273.

18. Leonard WJ, Depper JM, Uchiyama T, et al. A monoclonal antibody that appears to recognize the receptor for human T-cell growth factor: partial characterization of the receptor. Nature 1982; 300:267–9.

19. Muraguchi A, Kehrl JH, Longo DL, Volkman DJ, Smith KA, Fauci AS. Interleukin-2 receptors on human B cells: Implications for the role of Interleukin-2 in human B cell function. J Exp Med 1985; 161:181–97.

20. Tsudo M, Uchiyama T, Uchino H. Expression of Tac antigen on activated normal human B cells. J Exp Med 1984; 160:612–7.

21. Zamkoff KW, Reeves WG, Paolozzi FP, Poiesz BJ, Comis RL, Tomar RH. Impaired interleukin regulation of the phytohemagglutinin response in Hodgkin's disease. Clin Immunol Immunopathol 1985; 35:111–24.

22. Soulillou JP, Douillard JY, Vie H, et al. Defect in lectin induced Interleukin-2 (IL-2) production by peripheral blood lymphocytes of patients with Hodgkin's disease. Eur J Cancer Clin Oncol 1985; 21:935–9.

23. Goodwin JS, Ceuppens J. Regulation of the immune response by prostaglandins. J Clin Immunol 1983; 3:295–315.

24. Honda M, Steinberg AD. Effects of prostaglandin E_2 on responses of T-cell subsets to mitogen and autologous non-T-cell stimulation. Clin Immunol Immunopathol 1985; 33:111–22.

25. Welte K, Andreeff M, Platzer E, et al. Interleukin-2 regulates the expression of Tac antigen on peripheral blood T lymphocytes. J Exp Med 1984; 160:1390–403.

Cancer Detection and Prevention Supplement 1:145–148 (1987)

Correlative Studies on Antigenicity of Pancreatic Cancer and Blood Group Types

Eiji Uchida, MD
Margaret A. Tempero, MD
David A. Burnett, MD
Zenon Steplewski, MD
Parviz M. Pour, MD

The Eppley Institute for Research in Cancer and Allied Diseases (E.U., P.M.P.), Department of Internal Medicine (M.A.T., D.A.B.) and Department of Pathology and Microbiology (P.M.P.) University of Nebraska Medical Center, Omaha NE; The Wistar Institute of Anatomy and Biology, Philadelphia, PA (Z.S.)

ABSTRACT Blood group-related antigenicity in 14 pancreatic cancer patients was examined by immunohistological method using monoclonal antibodies (MoAbs) against A, B, H, Le^a, Le^b, and CA 19-9 and compared with the phenotypic expression of the individuals' blood groups. MoAb-A reacted strongly with tumor tissue in four of five blood group A patients. Two of two patients with blood type B showed a weak, focal reactivity of their cancer with MoAb-B. H antigen was found in four of five patients from blood group A, while it was present in only one blood group O person and absent in B-type individuals. B antigen was inappropriately expressed in one person with type A blood and in two with type O. Le^a antigen was expressed in all but two tumor tissues and Le^b antigen in all tumorous tissues, irrespective of Le blood group status. MoAb 19-9 reacted with 11 of 14 cases.

Key words: neoplasia, Lewis antigen, blood group types, pancreatic cancer

INTRODUCTION

Carbohydrate antigen 19-9 (CA 19-9), a sialosylated Lewis^a (Le^a) antigen [1], has been identified in cases of colorectal and pancreatic carcinoma and regarded as a tumor marker [2,3]. A relationship between the expression of CA 19-9 and host Le blood groups has been noticed [4]. However, little detailed information is available on the relationship between tumor-associated antigens and the blood group types of individuals [4,5].

The purpose of this study was to examine the expression of blood group antigens, including ABH, Le^a, Le^b, and CA 19-9, in adenocarcinomas of the exocrine pancreas and to correlate these findings with blood group antigen phenotypes.

Address reprint requests to Dr. Margaret A. Tempero, Department of Internal Medicine, University of Nebraska Medical Center, 42nd & Dewey Avenue, Omaha, NE 68105.

MATERIALS AND METHODS
Patients

Fourteen patients with clinically proven pancreatic cancer were selected for study at University Hospital, University of Nebraska Medical Center (Omaha, NE). The patients consisted of six males and eight females and had an average age of 62 years (range 42–82 years).

Samples

Formalin-fixed and paraffin-embedded biopsy material from 14 pancreatic cancer patients was cut into serial sections. In some cases, only a metastatic site was available for analysis. Blood samples from all cases were available for typing.

Monoclonal Antibodies

Commercially available monoclonal antibodies (MoAbs) against ABH blood group antigens, produced by the hybridoma technique (DAKO Corp., Santa Barbara, CA), were used. Le-related monoclonal antibodies were generated and characterized as previously reported [6,7].

Immunoperoxidase Procedure (IP)

Indirect IP staining was performed by a modified method of Primus and Goldenberg [8].

Scoring of Slides

In individual tumors the intensity of staining in positive cells was estimated by the method of Brown et al [9], with slight modifications.

Determination of the ABO and Le Phenotypes

The ABO and Le phenotypes of red blood cells in each patient were determined by the conventional hemoagglutination technique from blood grouping sera, anti-ABH, anti-Le^a, and anti-Le^b (American Dade, Miami, FL).

RESULTS

The results of the immunohistochemical localization of blood group antigens in pancreatic cancerous tissue in comparison with host blood group phenotypes on red blood cells are summarized in Table I. MoAb-A reacted strongly with tumor tissue from four of five blood type A patients. Two of two patients with type B had weak and focal reactivity with MoAb-B. H antigen was found in four of five samples of blood type A, was present in only one type O individual, and was absent in all patients of type B. B antigen was inappropriatey expressed in a patient with type A (B.R.) and in two of the type O patients (H.M. and J.K.).

Le^a antigen was expressed in all of the tumor tissues except two. Irrespective of ABH blood types, eight of nine Le^b patients expressed Le^a antigen.

Le^b antigen was found in all tumorous tissues, irrespective of the Le blood group status of the individuals.

MoAb 19-9 reacted with tumor tissues in 11 cases. In three cases in which the 19-9 reaction was negative, the Le types differed (Le^{a-b-}, Le^{a-b+}, and Le^{a+b-}, respectively).

DISCUSSION

Davidsohn et al [10] reported that ABH blood group antigens could not be demonstrated in over 80% of all pancreatic tumors by the Coomb's mixed-cell agglutination reaction. Our results showed that all five patients having blood type A and two patients with type B expressed their corresponding blood group antigens in these tumors. The difference between the two studies might well be due to the differing sensitivities of the methods used. Inappropriate

TABLE I. Blood Group Antigens in Pancreatic Cancer

Patients	Tumor*						RBC		
	Le^a	Le^b	A	B	H	19–9	Le^a	Le^b	ABO
1. F.E.1	−	+ + + +	+ + +	−	+ + + +	+	−	+	A
F.E.2	+	+ + + +	+ + + +	−	+ + + +	+ + + +	−	+ + + +	
2. G.B.	−	+	+ + + +	−	+ + + +	−	−	−	A
3. E.J.	+ + + +	+ + + +	+	−	−	+ + + +	+	−	A
4. B.R.1	+ +	+ + + +	+ + + +	−	+ + + +	+ +	−	+	A
B.R.2	+ + + +	+ + +	+ +	+	+	+			
B.R.3	+ + + +	+ + + +	+ + + +	−	+ + + +	+ + + +			
B.R.4	+ + + +	+	+	−	−	+			
5. K.W.	+ +	+ +	+ + +	−	ND	+ +	−	+	A
6. J.G.	+ + + +	+ + + +	−	+ +	−	+ + + +	−	+	B
7. M.E.	+ + + +	+ + + +	−	+	−	+ + + +	−	+	B
8. H.M.	+ +	+ + + +	−	+	−	+ + + +	+	−	O
9. R.L.	+ + + +	+ + + +	−	−	−	−	−	+	O
10. J.K.	+ + + +	+ + + +	−	+ +	−	+ + + +	+	−	O
11. L.H.	+ + + +	+ + + +	−	−	−	+ + + +	+	−	O
12. A.B.	+ + + +	+ + + +	−	−	+	+ + + +	−	+	O
13. E.S.	+ +	+	−	−	−	−	+	−	O
14. V.D.	+ + + +	+ + + +	−	−	−	+ + + +	−	+	O

*+, <5% cells stain positive; + +, <5–30%; + + +, 30–70%; + + + +, >70%; −, negative.

expression of blood group antigen was found in one person with type A and in one with type O, while five of six patients with type O blood lacked the appropriate antigenicity. Such an inappropriate antigen expression or the loss of ability to secrete the antigen by tumor cells have been observed in a variety of tumors [11] and have been considered to be due to the changes in carbohydrate structures in malignant cells as an expression of functional dedifferentiation [10] and possibly due to an alteration of glycosyl transferases or to a failure of their coordinated action [11]. Apparently no correlation exists between the expression of blood group antigens and the malignant degree of tumors.

As for Le-related antigens, apparently inappropriate antigen expression occurred in almost all patients. All five patients with Le^a type expressed Le^b antigen and seven out of eight Le^b patients expressed Le^a antigen. The question as to whether the expression of Le^b in Le^a persons is inappropriate remains presenty unknown, because we did not have information on the Le antigenicity of the normal pancreatic tissue of the individuals.

CA 19-9 has been found in up to 90% of persons with pancreatic adenocarcinoma [12]. This correlates with our findings. However, we have shown that CA 19-9 antigen is also present in the normal pancreatic ductal cells from 12 of 18 normal individuals we previously examined [13]. Bara et al [4] showed that CA 19-9 antigen is similarly expressed in the normal adult colon in about the same frequency. Consequently this antigen cannot strictly be regarded as a tumor-associated antigen, although it is possible that the distribution and level of its expression vary following malignant transformations.

In our study tumors expressing Le^a antigen demonstrated CA 19-9 antigen reactivity with almost the same staining intensity in all but two patients. Although the sample number is too small to reach a definite conclusion, it appears that patients with Le^a phenotype may fail to express CA 19-9 antigen in pancreatic malignancy. This finding contrasts with the hypothesis that only patients who belong to the Le^{a-b-} blood group type will fail to express CA 19-9 antigen in tumor tissue [14]. It is possible that our failure to detect 19-9 in both Le^{a+} patients was due to antigen heterogenicity. In both these cases only a metastatic tissue was available for examination. Further studies of blood group antigenicity in primary and metastatic pancreatic cancer and in normal pancreas will be required to clarify the relationship between Le antigenicity and CA 19-9. Since "inappropriate" Le antigen expression appeared in almost all cases, it is possible the Le antigen serologies using sensitive assays with MoAbs may prove to be a useful biomarker in patients with known Le antigen phenotypes.

REFERENCES

1. Koprowski H, Herlyn M, Steplewski Z, Sears HF. Specific antigen in serum of patients with colon carcinoma. Science 1981; 212:53–5.
2. Herlyn M, Sears HF, Steplewski Z, Koprowski H. Monoclonal antibody detection of a circulating tumor-associated antigen. I. Presence of antigen in sera of patients with colorectal, gastric, and pancreatic carcinoma. J Clin Immunol 1982; 2:135–40.
3. Sears HF, Herlyn M, Villano BD, Steplewski Z, Koprowski H. Monoclonal antibody detection of a circulating tumor-associated antigen. II. A longitudinal evaluation of patients with colorectal cancer. J Clin Immunol 1982; 2:141–9.
4. Bara J, Herrero Z, Mollicone R, Nap M, Burtin P. Distrubution of GICA in normal gastrointestinal and endocervical mucosae and in mucinous ovarian cysts using antibody NS 19-9. Am J Clin Pathol 1986; 85:152–9.
5. Brockhaus M, Wysocka M, Magnani JL, Steplewski Z, Koprowski H, Ginsburg V. Normal salivary mucin contains the gastrointestinal cancer-associated antigen detected by monoclonal antibody 19-9 in the serum mucin of patients. Vox Sang 1985; 48:34–8.
6. Steplewski Z, Koprowski H. Glycolipid and glycoprotein markers of gastrointestinal cancers. In H Koprowski, S Ferrone, A Albertini, eds: Biotechnology in Diagnostics. New York: Elsevier, 1985: 117–21.
7. Steplewski Z, Sears HF, Koprowski H. Monoclonal antibodies against gastrointestinal tumor-associated antigens. In Immunity to cancer. Mitchell M, eds: New York: Academic; 1985: 97–107.
8. Primus FJ, Goldenberg DM. Functional histopathology of cancer. A review of immunoenzyme histochemistry. Methods Cancer Res 1982; 20:139–82.
9. Brown A, Ellis IO, Embleton MJ, Baldwin RW, Turner DR, Hardcastle JD. Immunohistochemical localization of Y hapten and the structurally related H type-2 blood-group antigen on large-bowel tumors and normal adult tissues. Int J Cancer 1984; 33:727–36.
10. Davidsohn I, Ni LY, Stejskal R. Tissue isoantigens A, B, and H in carcinoma of the pancreas. Cancer Res 1971; 31:1244–50.
11. Feizi T. Blood group antigens and gastric cancer. Med Biol 1982; 60:7–11.
12. Herlyn M, Sears HF, Steplewski Z, Koprowski H. Monoclonal antibody detection of a circulating tumor-associated antigen. J Clin Immunol 1982; 2:135–40.
13. Uchida E, Steplewski Z, Mroczek E, Büchler M, Burnett D, Pour PM. Presence of two distinct acinar cell populations in human pancreas based on their antigenicity. Int J Pancreatol 1986; 1:213–25.
14. Koprowski H, Brockhaus M, Blaszczyk M, Morgani J, Steplewski Z, Ginsburg V. Lewis blood-type may affect the incidence of gastrointestinal cancer. Lancet 1982; 1:1332–3.

Neoplastic Consequences of Transplantation and Chemotherapy

Israel Penn, MD

*Department of Surgery, University of Cincinnati Medical Center, and
Cincinnati Veterans Administration Medical Center, Cincinnati, OH*

ABSTRACT An increased incidence of certain neoplasms occurs in immunodeficiency states. The incidence of cancer in organ transplant patients is approximately 4%. The predominant tumors are lymphomas, carcinomas of the skin and lips, carcinomas of the vulva/perineum, in situ carcinomas of the uterine cervix, and Kaposi sarcoma (KS). Tumors appear a relatively short time after transplantation. Unusual features of the lymphomas are the high incidence of non-Hodgkin lymphomas, frequent involvement of extranodal sites, and marked predilection for the brain. Skin cancers present unusual features: predominance of squamous cell carcinomas, young age of the patients, and a high incidence of multiple tumors. Cancers of the vulva/perineum occur at a younger age than in the general population and may be preceded by condyloma acuminatum or herpes genitalis.

Lymphomas, leukemias, and skin cancers are increased in nontransplant patients who receive immunosuppressive therapy for nonmalignant diseases. Second tumors that develop in cancer patients, after treatment with cytotoxic therapy, are mainly leukemias, lymphomas, and bladder carcinomas.

Key words: cancer, immunodepression, cytotoxic therapy, lymphoma, Kaposi sarcoma

INTRODUCTION

Any condition causing profound and prolonged suppression of immunity may be complicated by the development of an increased incidence of certain cancers [1–3]. For example, patients with congenital immunodeficiency disorders have a high incidence of lymphomas, leukemias, and certain carcinomas. In addition, the acquired immunodeficiency syndrome (AIDS) is associated with a high incidence of Kaposi sarcoma and lymphomas. In this report those types of malignancies will be considered that have developed following the use of immunosuppressive or cytotoxic agents in three groups of patients, namely, organ transplant recipients, nontransplant patients given immunosuppressive therapy, and cancer patients given cytotoxic drug therapy.

MALIGNANCIES IN ORGAN TRANSPLANT RECIPIENTS
Immunosuppressive Agents Used

Organ transplant recipients, excluding those receiving bone marrow transplants, are given immunosuppressive therapy for many months or years to prevent or treat rejection of

---

Address reprint requests to Dr. Israel Penn, Department of Surgery, MSB 558, University of Cincinnati Medical Center, 231 Bethesda Avenue, Cincinnati, OH 45267-0558.

the grafts [1,2,4–6]. Most patients have been treated with a combination of azathioprine and prednisone. Other frequently used medications include antilymphocyte or antithymocyte globulin (ALG or ATG), cyclophosphamide, and, recently, cyclosporine, OKT$_3$, and other anti-T cell monoclonal antibody preparations. Other immunosuppressive measures used in some patients are splenectomy, thoracic duct fistula, and local irradiation of the graft. The immunosuppressive regimen used in bone marrow transplantation is mentioned below.

Incidence of Tumors

From 1968 to August 1985, the Cincinnati Transplant Tumor Registry (CTTR) accumulated data on 2,435 types of neoplasia that arose in 2,278 organ transplant recipients [1–9]. The patients included 2,216 who received kidney, 43 heart, eight bone marrow, six liver, three pancreas, and two combined heart and lung transplants. Of several tens of thousands of renal transplant recipients at risk, the incidence of cancer at several major transplant centers has ranged from 1 to 16% with an average of 4% [9]. The differences in incidence may reflect variations in the intensity of immunosuppressive therapy given at various centers. Another explanation is that some centers report all malignancies, no matter how trivial, while others report only the more florid types of cancers. The true incidence of tumors is greater than the 4% figure noted above, as many centers include individuals treated in the pioneering years of transplantation when patient survival often was brief. The statistics also include recipients with short lengths of follow-up.

The incidence of cancer was 10% in a series of 182 cardiac transplant recipients who underwent 199 transplantations [10]. The small numbers of liver or bone marrow transplant recipients in this series may reflect the short survival of many patients who undergo these procedures. A more important factor may be the markedly different immunosuppressive regimen used in bone marrow recipients compared to that used in renal, hepatic, pancreatic, or cardiac allograft patients. The recipients of solid organs are given immunosuppressive therapy more or less continuously for many months or years, whereas bone marrow patients receive very intensive immunosuppressive therapy (usually with a large dose of cyclophosphamide or total body irradiation) for several days prior to transplantation, followed by a course of immunosuppression given over a period of several months, to prevent or treat graft versus host disease. Once this dangerous period has passed no further immunosuppressive therapy is given.

Types of Malignancies

The neoplasms that frequently occur in the general population, including carcinomas of the lung, prostate, colon and rectum, female breast, and invasive carcinoma of the uterine cervix, are not increased in incidence in transplant recipients [1–9]. Instead, the CTTR data show that certain cancers appear with remarkable frequency. Skin and lip cancers are the most common [7]. Their incidence varies with the amount of exposure to sunshine. In areas with restricted sunlight, there is a four- to seven fold increase, but in regions with plentiful exposure there is an almost 21-fold increase above the already high incidence seen in the local control population [1,2,7]. A study of 934 renal transplant recipients from a Swedish center shows that lip cancers are increased 29-fold in incidence compared with controls [11]. Two epidemiologic studies indicate that the incidence of non-Hodgkin lymphomas is 28- to 49-fold higher than in age-matched controls [12,13]. In situ carcinomas of the uterine cervix have a 14-fold increase over controls [14]. Nonmelanoma skin cancers and in situ carcinomas of the uterine cervix are usually excluded from cancer statistics. If we omit them from the CTTR data then several other tumors show a substantial increase in incidence. Kaposi sarcoma (KS) then makes up 5.3% of cancers in the CTTR compared to its incidence in the general population of the United States (before the AIDS epidemic started), where it comprised only 0.02 to 0.07% of all tumors [3,8]. The high incidence of KS in this worldwide collection of patients is comparable to that seen in areas of the world where it occurs with greatest frequency, namely, in the rain forest areas of Africa, where it makes up 3 to 9% of all malignancies [15]. These observations are in keeping with a report of a 400–500-fold increase in the incidence of KS in renal transplant recipients compared to a control population of the same ethnic origin [16]. Carcinomas of the vulva and perineum comprise 4.0% of tumors in the CTTR data, a much higher figure than in the general population [1–3]. This finding is in keeping with a 100-fold increase in the incidence of carcinomas of the vulva and anus in renal transplant patients compared to controls [11]. Transplant patients also are prone to small increases in the incidence of leukemia, carcinomas of the kidney, and carcinomas of the liver and biliary passages [13].

Time of Appearance of the Tumors

As the length of follow-up of organ transplant recipients has increased it has become evident that certain cancers manifest themselves at fairly distinct intervals after transplantation [1–9]. In contrast to other known oncogenic stimuli in man, which often take 15 to 20 years or more before they cause overt cancers, neoplasms appear a relatively short time after transplantation [1–9,12,13]. KS is the first to appear, at an average of 23 (range 2.5–225.5) months after transplantation. Lymphomas appear at an average of 36 (range 1–154) months after transplantation. Other tumors (excluding carcinomas of the vulva and perineum) appear at an average of 61 (range 1–221.5) months following transplantation. Carcinomas of the vulva and perineum appear at the longest interval after transplantation, at an average of 90 (9–215) months.

The incidence of cancers increases with length of follow-up after transplantation [1–5]. Twenty-six percent of 418 renal transplant patients who survived at least 1 year had neoplasms, while at 10 years 14 of 30 survivors (47%) were so affected [17]. Similarly, in 124 cardiac transplant recipients the actuarial risk of developing cancer was $2.7 \pm 1.9\%$ at 1 year and $25.6 \pm 11.0\%$ at 5 years [13]. These statistics underscore the need to follow transplant patients indefinitely [1–9].

Age and Sex of Patients

The tumors occurred in a relative young group of patients, whose average age at the time of transplantation was 40 years (range 7 months to 72 years) [1–9]. Forty-nine percent were under the age of 40 years at the time of transplantation. Sixty-four percent of patients were male and 36% female, in keeping with the 2:1 ratio of male to female patients who undergo renal transplantation.

Cancers of the Skin and Lips

The most common neoplasms were those of the skin and lips [1–9,19]. They comprised 944 of 2,435 (39%) cancers in the CTTR. Their incidence increased with duration of follow-up after transplantation. In an Australian study skin cancers occurred in 8% of patients who survived 1 year or more after transplantation, but they affected 17% of those who lived 4 years or longer [20]. In addition, premalignant keratoses occurred in 28% of the 4 years survivors.

Skin cancers in transplant patients show several unusual features compared to their counterparts in the general population [1–9,17,19,20]. Basal cell carcinomas (BCCs) outnumber squamous cell carcinoma (SCCs) in the general population, but the opposite is true in transplant patients, in whom SCCs comprised 52% and BCCs 28%. (Another 13% of patients have both types of malignancy.) Another difference is the age of the transplant patients, whose average age was 30 years younger than persons with similar tumors in the general population [7,21]. In addition, the incidence of multiple skin cancers, which were present in at least 410 of 944 patients (43%), is remarkably high and is comparable to that seen only in areas of plentiful exposure to sunlight [7]. Several individuals each had more than 100 skin tumors. Malignant melanomas comprised 5% of the skin neoplasms in this series in contrast to an incidence of 2.7% in the general population of the United States [22].

Most skin cancers were of low-grade malignancy but a number were very aggressive [1–3,7]. Metastases to lymph nodes occurred in 73 patients (8%), 61 of whom had SCCs, 10 of whom had malignant melanoma, and two of whom had Merkel cell tumors. Of the SCCs with lymph node metastases, 41 involved the skin, 12 affected the lips, and eight were cases with skin and lip involvement. In the last group, metastases probably arose from skin lesions in four patients, from lip lesions in two, and in another two the origin was unclear.

Sixty-five patients (7%) died of their skin cancers, 42 with SCCs, 21 with malignant melanomas, one with BCC, and one with Merkel cell tumor. Of the lethal SCCs 30 arose from skin, four from the lips, and eight from lesions involving the lips and skin, with the skin lesions apparently responsible for fatal metastases in four patients, the lip lesions in three, and in one it was not clear which lesions caused the lethal outcome. Not included in the above figures are seven patients, all with SCCs, who are alive with metastases, and two patients who died of complications of chemotherapy given for treatment of an advanced SCC and Merkel cell tumor, respectively. All these findings are in keeping with a more than 10-fold increased mortality from SCCs of the skin observed in Australian renal transplant recipients [12]. The behavior of skin tumors in the present series is in marked contrast with that seen in the general population, in whom they cause only 1 to 2% of all cancer deaths, the great majority of which are from malignant melanomas [23].

Lymphomas

In transplant patients lymphomas show several unusual features compared to their behavior in the general population [1–6,8,9,13]. They comprise 3 to 4% of all neoplasms in the community at large [23], but make up 331 (330 patients of whom one had two distinct types of lymphoma that occurred at different times) of 2,435 neoplasms (14%) in the CTTR. If we exclude nonmelanoma skin malignancies and in situ carcinomas of the uterine cervix, the incidence is 20%.

It would be preferable to classify lymphomas according to the cell of origin, such as T cell, B cell, null cell, and so forth. However, many lymphomas in the present series were reported before immunologic methods of identifying lymphocyte markers became available [1–6,8,9]. Of the cases studied, 44 lymphomas and seven lymphoproliferations, which were suspected to be lymphomas, were of B cell origin. In several other lymphomas the cells did not demonstrate cellular immunoglobulin and could not be characterized further. Thus far, five T-cell lymphomas have been reported, including one case of mycosis fungoides. There has been one case of null cell lymphoma.

An unusual feature of the lymphomas is the rarity of Hodgkin disease [1–6,8,9]. There were only 13 cases among 330 patients (4%) with lymphomas. This is much lower than its incidence in the general population, where it comprises at least 18% of lymphomas. If we excludes the 13 patients with Hodgkin disease and another 10 with myelomas (plasma cell lymphomas), we are left with 307 patients with non-Hodgkin lymphomas (NHL). These tumors differed markedly from those seen in the general population in several respects [1–3,9]. Extranodal involvement was reported in from 24 to 48% of NHL patients in the general population [24,25]. In the present series, the distribution of NHL was unknown in two patients, and extranodal disease occurred in 229 (75%) of the remaining 305 patients. Most of the 76 patients with nodal involvement had widespread disease, involving mainly the liver, lungs, spleen, bone marrow, renal allograft, and brain. A single organ was affected in 154 of the 229 recipients (67%) with extranodal disease. The organ most often involved was the central nervous system (CNS), which was affected in 86 of 154 patients (56%). Overall, 111 of the 305 patients (36%) had CNS involvement. Patients with meningeal involvement were not included in these statistics. Lesions of the CNS almost always occurred in the brain and frequently had a multicentric distribution. Spinal cord involvement was rare. The remarkably high incidence of brain involvement contrasts with a 1% incidence of focal cerebral involvement by NHL in a series of 1,039 patients in the general population (meningeal involvement occurred in 3.7%) [26].

The gastrointestinal tract is frequently involved by NHL in transplant patients. A quite common presentation is acute perforation of an intestinal lymphoma with resultant peritonitis.

A remarkable finding in the 307 recipients with NHL was the frequency of lymphomatous involvement of the allograft, which occurred in 43 recipients (14%); 38 renal, two cardiac, two pancreatic, and one hepatic [1–3,9]. Another unusual feature was that NHL presented in the soft tissues at the sites of injection of antilymphocyte or antithymocyte globulin in at least four patients.

The mortality of lymphomas in renal transplant recipients is 48-fold greater than that observed in age-matched controls in the general population [12].

Kaposi Sarcoma

Of 90 patients with KS, 63 were male and 27 female. The 2:1 male to female ratio is the same as that seen in transplant patients having other neoplasms but is much less than the 9:1 to 15:1 ratio seen with KS in the general population [8]. KS was most common in transplant patients who were Jewish, black, or of Mediterranean ancestry [8]. Seven of the 90 patients (8%) had other cancers, an incidence similar to that seen in the general population [27]. Sixty of the 90 patients (67%) had "benign" KS involving the skin, conjunctiva, or oropharyngolaryngeal mucosa, and 30 (33%) had the "malignant" variety with involvement of the internal organs. With treatment complete remissions occurred in 32 of the 60 patients (53%) with "benign" disease. Six of the remissions (19%) occurred when the *only* treatment was a drastic reduction of immunosuppressive therapy [1–3,8]. The other 26 remissions followed surgery, radiotherapy, or chemotherapy. In the malignant group five of the 30 patients (17%) had complete remissions after chemotherapy or radiotherapy together with alteration of immunosuppressive therapy. Twenty of the 60 patients with nonvisceral KS died, usually of causes unrelated to the KS, whereas 21 of the 30 patients with visceral KS are dead, the major cause being the malignancy.

Carcinomas of the Uterus

Carcinomas of the cervix occurred in 144 of the 812 women in this series (18%) [1–5]. At least 79% were in situ lesions. These tumors are probably more common than is realized. It is, therefore, advisable that all postadolescent female patients have pelvic examinations and cervical smears done on a regular basis [1–5].

Carcinomas of the body of the uterus are uncommon. Perhaps this is because most transplant patients are young; these tumors occur mainly in postmenopausal women [1–15].

Carcinomas of the Vulva and Perineum

Carcinomas of the vulva, perineum, scrotum, penis, perianal skin, and anus occurred in 67 patients; 50 women and 17 men [1–3]. The patients were surprisingly young compared to persons with similar lesions in the general population. The average age of the women at the time of transplantation was 30 years (range 15–55 years) and of the men 39 (range 25–60) years. In women there was sometimes a "field effect" with involvement by cancer of the vulva and vagina and/or the cervix of the uterus. In some cases there was a preceding history of condyloma acuminatum or herpes genitalis, suggesting that oncogenic viruses may cause at least some of the tumors in these immunosuppressed patients [1–3].

CANCERS IN NONTRANSPLANT PATIENTS GIVEN IMMUNOSUPPRESSIVE THERAPY

Immunosuppressive drug therapy has been used to suppress immunity or inflammatory responses in a large number of autoimmune disorders, collagen-vascular diseases, and disorders of obscure etiology [1–3,5,6,12,28]. These include glomerulonephritis, nephrotic syndrome, rheumatoid arthritis, systemic lupus erythematosus, psoriasis, chronic cold agglutin disease, dermatomyositis, ulcerative colitis, hepatitis, idiopathic thrombocythemia, primary amyloidosis, Wegener granulomatosis, multiple sclerosis, and other disorders. The agents used include the adrenal corticosteroids, azathioprine, cyclophosphamide, methotrexate, chlorambucil, and other cytotoxic drugs. Cancers have occurred following the use of these agents in the disorders listed above. A problem in determining their incidence is that some autoimmune disorders per se are associated with an increased frequency of tumors. Despite this, several studies show an increased incidence of certain cancers in this category of patients. Azathioprine, cyclophosphamide, or chlorambucil were administered to 1,349 patients for at least 3 months as treatment for the disorders mentioned above [12]. The types of malignancies that subsequently developed were similar to those seen in transplant patients. There was an increased incidence of NHL (four cases observed compared with 0.34 expected), SCCs of the skin (two observed against 0.38 expected), bladder cancer (four observed against 1.00 expected), and other neoplasms (29 observed compared with 20.74 expected) [12]. In another study 15 of 1,853 patients (0.85%) with rheumatoid arthritis, treated mainly with chlorambucil or cyclophosphamide, developed acute leukemia [28]. The malignancy was not observed in patients treated for less than 6 months or in those who received a total dose of less than 1 g of chlorambucil or 50 g cyclophosphamide. In addition, four of 35 patients (11.4%) treated with chlorambucil for severe psoriatic arthropathy developed acute leukemia. In another study of 54 patients treated with cyclophosphamide for systemic lupus erythematosus or rheumatoid arthritis, two cases of bladder cancer were observed compared to 0.02 expected [29]. In addition to these series there are numerous isolated case reports of cancers after the use of immunosuppressive therapy in nontransplant patients. The author collected data on 149 cancers that developed in 143 such patients. Thirty percent were leukemias and 20% were lymphomas, the majority of which were reticulum cell sarcomas [1,2,4–6]. In a separate study, the author collected 16 cases of KS in this category of patients [8]. The overall impression is that cancer following immunosuppressive therapy has been less of a problem in nontransplant patients than in organ transplant recipients or in patients who developed second neoplasms following chemotherapy for their original malignancies. Perhaps this is because dosage was usually smaller and duration of treatment shorter than is used in the management of organ transplant recipients or in treating cancer.

SECOND NEOPLASMS IN PATIENTS GIVEN CANCER CHEMOTHERAPY

Most cancer chemotherapeutic agents have immunosuppressive side effects [1–6,30]. As a result, patients may develop infections and, paradoxically, new tumors. While the latter probably result from direct oncogenic or cooncogenic effects of the drugs used, we cannot excluded immunosuppression as a possible etiologic factor.

The most common new malignancies were acute leukemias, lymphomas, and carcinomas of the urinary bladder [1–6]. Most leukemias were preceded by a period of therapy-induced marrow depression and by a preleukemic phase. The mean interval from diagnosis of the primary cancer to development of acute leukemia was 4–6 years. In some instances leukemias appeared after chemotherapy had been discontinued for some months or even years.

The incidence of acute myeloid leukemia (AML) in treated Hodgkin disease (HD) ranged from 0.9 to 2% of patients [31–34]. The risk of developing AML was increased five- to 75-fold. In treated multiple myeloma the incidence of AML was 0.6 to 7.0%, and the risk was increased 100-fold [3,33,34]. Patients treated with chlorambucil for polycythemia rubra vera had a 2.3 times higher incidence of acute leukemia compared with individuals treated with P^{32} and a 13 times greater incidence than persons treated by phlebotomy [33]. An increased frequency of AML has also been noted in treated NHL [35], acute lymphoblastic leukemia, and chronic lymphocytic leukemia [33]. Three of 13 patients given adjuvant chemotherapy with chlorambucil for breast cancer developed acute leukemia [36]. In another study four of 1,460 breast cancer patients treated with cyclophosphamide developed acute leukemia [37]. In nine randomized trials evaluating flourouracil plus methyl CCNU as adjuvant therapy for gastrointestinal cancers leukemia occurred in 14 of 2,067 patients given chemotherapy but in only one of 1,566 untreated "controls." The relative risk for the development of leukemia was 12.4, with a cumulative 6 year risk of approximately 4% [38]. The incidence of acute leukemia in treated ovarian cancer was 0.2 to 1.4% [39]. The risk increased 21- to 26-fold within 2 years of treatment, but rose to 66- to 170-fold in patients who survived more than 2 years. The question has been raised whether the development of acute leukemia in the above diseases represents part of their natural history in patients who were kept alive sufficiently long by chemotherapy or by chemotherapy combined with radiotherapy. This viewpoint is enhanced by the occasional simultaneous appearance of leukemia in untreated patients with HD or multiple myeloma [33]. However, as AML was rarely seen in patients with these two diseases before the era of intensive therapy, it seems highly likely that the patient's treatment played a major role in the development of the hematologic malignancy. Furthermore, there has been an increase in the incidence of acute leukemia following chemotherapy of ovarian, breast, and colon cancers, diseases in which leukemia is not considered to be part of the natural history [2,3,33,39].

There are conflicting opinions about the incidence of NHL after treatment of HD. In 1,222 HD patients treated with chemotherapy, radiotherapy, or combined modality therapy the actuarial risk at 10 years for the development of subsequent second neoplasms was 9.9%. Leukemias made up 3.5%, lymphomas 0.5%, and solid tumors 5.9% [31]. The latent period from HD to the development of second lymphomas was as long as 15.5 years. In another study of 579 HD patients treated with chemotherapy, six subsequently developed NHL [40]. The actuarial risk of developing the second tumor was approximately 4.5% at 10 years. In these two series the development of NHL appears to be related to the potentially carcinogenic treatments that were used. However, in another series of 51 HD patients, five developed NHL 4 to 11 years after the onset of HD, but four of the five had received no treatment, and the investigators concluded that, in some patients with the lymphocytic predominance nodular variety of HD, the disorder may spontaneously evolve into a more malignant NHL [41].

There have been at least 38 cases of bladder cancer reported following the use of cyclophosphamide therapy for various malignancies [42]. Another alkylating agent, chlornaphazine, is metabolized to yield B-naphthylamine, which is known to be a carcinogen in the human bladder. After several bladder carcinomas developed in patients following its administration [43], chlornaphazine was withdrawn from clinical use.

A variety of other second neoplasms have been reported following the treatment of various primary malignancies [1,2,4,6,31,32,44]. Most common were carcinomas of the lung, skin, bladder, breast, colon, pancreas, Kaposi sarcoma and soft tissue sarcomas. In one study the observed versus expected cases per 100,000 people were lung, 309.4 vs 43; colon, 265.2 vs 27.8; stomach 176.8 vs 10.6; bladder, 132.6 vs 12.7; esophagus, 132.6 vs 3.4; anorectal, 88.4 vs 13.9; and pancreas, 44.2 vs 8.1 [44].

CAUSES OF CANCER FOLLOWING TRANSPLANTATION AND CHEMOTHERAPY

The causes of cancer following transplantation and chemotherapy have been discussed in detail elsewhere [1–6,32,34,45]. The malignancies probably arise from a complex interplay of multiple factors including depression of immunity, liberation or activation of oncogenic viruses, oncogenic or cooncogenic effects of the immunosuppressive or cytotoxic agents, or of other treatments such as radiotherapy and variations in individual susceptibility to carcinogenic stimuli.

The discovery that immunosuppression is associated with an increased incidence of certain neoplasms emphasizes the importance of the immune system in host defenses against cancer. It is curious that the various states of immunodeficiency described above have in common an increased incidence of malignancies arising from the immune cells themselves, namely, lymphomas. If Kaposi sarcoma is a variety of lymphoreticular tumor, as some investigators believe, the situation becomes even more intriguing.

We should try to use immunosuppressive therapy as little as possible. In autoimmune and other disorders such treatment should be reserved for severe cases that fail to respond to other forms of treatment. However, immunosuppressive therapy is essential for the survival and function of organ transplants. Attempts are being made to modify the present blunderbuss assault on the immune system with more specific methods of control of certain components of the immune system. Eventually, it is hoped that states of immune unresponsiveness directed specifically, and only, at the foreign antigens of the transplanted organ will be produced. In the field of cytotoxic drug treatment attempts are being made to develop less immunosuppressive and less carcinogenic forms of therapy.

We need to study the various groups of immunosuppressed patients, including those with and without tumors, to obtain clues to the etiology of the cancer. This information may shed light on the causes of similar neoplasms seen in the control of cancer. Hopefully such knowledge may provide immunological methods for the prevention and cure of cancer.

ACKNOWLEDGMENTS

The author thanks the numerous colleagues, working in transplant and cancer therapy centers throughout the world, who have generously contributed data concerning their patients to the Cincinnati Transplant Tumor Registry. This work was supported in part by Veterans Administration grant 6985.

REFERENCES

1. Penn I. The price of immunotherapy. Curr Probl Surg 1981; 18(11):682–751.
2. Penn I. The occurrence of cancer in immune deficiencies. Curr Probl Cancer 1982; 6(10):1–64.
3. Penn I. The occurrence of malignant tumors in immunosuppressed states. In Klein E ed: Acquired immunodeficiency syndrome. Progress in allergy series, Basel: S. Karger, 1986; 37:259–300.
4. Penn I. Chemical immunosuppression and human cancer. Cancer 1974; 34:1474–80.
5. Penn I. Tumors arising in organ transplant recipients. In Klein G, Weinhouse S, eds: Advances in cancer research. New York: Academic Press, 1978; 28:31–61.
6. Penn I. Malignancies associated with immunosuppressive or cytotoxic therapy. Surgery 1978; 83:492–502.
7. Penn I. Immunosuppresion and skin cancer. Clin Plastic Surg 1980; 7:361–8.
8. Penn I. Kaposi's sarcoma in immunosuppressed patients. J Clin Lab Immunol 1983; 12:1–10.
9. Penn I. Allograft Transplant Cancer Registry. In Purtilo DT, ed: Immune deficiency and cancer: Epstein-Barr virus and lymphoproliferative malignancies. New York: Plenum Publishing Corp., 1984; 281–308.
10. Weintraub I, Warnke RA. Lymphoma in cardiac allograft recipients. Clinical and histological features and immunological phenotype. Transplantation 1982; 33:347–51.
11. Blohme I, Brynger H. Malignant disease in renal transplant patients. Transplantation 1985; 39:23–5.
12. Kinlen LJ, Sheil AGR, Peto J, Doll R. Collaborative United Kingdom–Australasian study of cancer in patients treated with immunosuppressive drugs. Br Med J 1979; 2:1461–6.
13. Kinlen L. Immunosuppressive therapy and cancer. Cancer Surv 1982; 1:565–83.
14. Porreco R, Penn I, Droegemueller W, Greer B, Makowski E. Gynecologic malignancies in immunosuppressed organ homograft recipients. Obstet Gynecol 1975; 45:359–64.
15. Templeton AC. Kaposi's sarcoma. In Andrade R, Gumport SL, Popkin GL, Rees TD, eds: Cancer of the skin. Biology–diagnosis–management. Philadelphia: W.B. Saunders Co., 1976; 1183–225.
16. Harwood AR, Osaba D, Hofstader SL, Goldstein MB, Cardella CJ, Holecek MJ, Kunynetz R, Giammarco RA. Kaposi's sarcoma in recipients of renal transplants. Am J Med 1979; 67:759–65.
17. Sheil AGR, Mahony JF, Horvath JS, Johnson JR, Tiller DJ, Stewart JH, May J. Cancer following successful cadaveric renal transplantation. Transplant Proc 1981; 13:733–5.
18. Krikorian JG, Anderson JL, Bieber CP, Penn I, Stinson EB: Malignant neoplasms following cardiac transplantation. JAMA 1978; 240:639–43.
19. Koranda FC, Dehmel EM, Kahn G, Penn I. Cutaneous complications in immunosuppressed renal homograft recipients. JAMA 1974; 229:419–24.

20. Marshal V. Premalignant and malignant skin tumors in immunosuppressed patients. Transplantation 1974; 17:272–5.

21. Mullen DL, Silberberg SG, Penn I, Hammond WS. Squamous cell carcinoma of the skin and lip in renal homograft recipients. Cancer 1976; 37:729–34.

22. Sober AJ. Diagnosis and management of skin cancer. Cancer 1983; 51:2448–52.

23. Silverberg E. Cancer statistics, 1985. CA 1985; 35:19–35.

24. Freeman C, Berg JW, Cutler SJ. Occurrence and prognosis of extranodal lymphomas. Cancer 1972; 29:252–60.

25. Reddy S, Pellettiere E, Saxena V, Hendrickson FR. Extranodal non-Hodgkin's lymphoma. Cancer 1980; 46:1925–31.

26. Herman TS, Hammond N, Jones, SE, Butler JJ, Byrne GE, Jr., McKelvey EM. Involvement of the central nervous system by non-Hodgkin's lymphoma. The Southwest Oncology Group Experience. Cancer 1979; 43:390–7.

27. Safai B, Miké V, Giraldo G, Beth E, Good RA. Association of Kaposi's sarcoma with second primary malignancies. Possible etiopathogenic implications. Cancer 1980; 45:1472–9.

28. Kahn MF, Arlet J, Bloch-Michel H, Caroit M, Chaouat Y, Renier JC: Leucémies aiguës après traitement par agents cytotoxique en rhumatologie. 19 observations chez 2006 patients. Nouv Presse Med 1979; 8:1393–7.

29. Plotz PH, Klippel JH, Decker JL, et al. Bladder complications in patients receiving cyclophosphamide for systemic lupus erythematosus or rheumatoid arthritis. Ann Intern Med 1979; 91:221–3.

30. Harris J, Sengar D, Stewart T, Hyslop D: The effect of immunosuppressive chemotherapy on immune function in patients with malignant disease. Cancer 1976; 37:1058–69.

31. Coleman CN, Kaplan HS, Cox R, Varghese A, Butterfield P, Rosenberg, SA: Leukaemias, non-Hodgkin's lymphomas and solid tumours in patients treated for Hodgkin's disease. Cancer Surv 1982; 1:733–744.

32. Some antineoplastic and immunosuppressive agents. IARC Monogr Eval Carcinog Risk Chem Hum 1981; 26:1–411.

33. Rosner F, Grunwald HW, Zarrabi HM. Cancer after the use of alkylating and nonalkylating cytotoxic agents in man. Cancer Surv 1982; 1:599–612.

34. Sieber SM. Cancer chemotherapeutic agents and carcinogenesis. Cancer Chemother Rep 1975; 59:915–8.

35. Zarrabi MH. Association of non-Hodgkin's lymphoma (NHL) and second neoplasms. Semin Oncol 1980; 7:340–51.

36. Lerner H. Second malignancies diagnosed in breast cancer patients while receiving adjuvant chemotherapy at the Pennsylvania Hospital. Proc Am Assoc Cancer Res 1977; 18:340.

37. Portugal MA, Falkson HC, Stevens K, Falkson G. Acute leukemia as a complication of long-term treatment of advanced breast cancer. Cancer Treat Rep 1979; 63:177–181.

38. Boice JD, Jr., Greene MH, Killen JY, Jr., et al. Leukemia and preleukemia after adjuvant therapy of gastrointestinal cancer with semustine (methyl-CCNU). N Engl J Med 1983; 309:1079–84.

39. Reimer RR, Hoover R, Fraumeni JF, Jr., Young RC. Acute leukemia after alkylating-agent therapy for ovarian cancer. N Engl J Med 1977; 297:177–81.

40. Krikorian JG, Burke JS, Rosenberg SA, Kaplan HS. The occurrence of non-Hodgkin's lymphoma following therapy for Hodgkin's disease. N Engl J Med 1979; 300:452–8.

41. Miettenen M, Franssila KO, Saxen E. Hodgkin's disease, lymphocytic predominance nodular. Increased risk for subsequent non-Hodgkin's lymphomas. Cancer 1983; 51:2293–300.

42. Seo IS, Clark SA, McGovern FD, Clark DL, Johnson EH. Leiomyosarcoma of the urinary bladder. 13 years after cyclophosphamide therapy for Hodgkin's disease. Cancer 1985; 55:1597–603.

43. Thiede T, Christensen BC. Bladder tumors induced by chlornaphazine. Acta Med Scand 1969; 185:133–7.

44. Krause JR, Ayuyang HQ, Ellis LD: Secondary non-hematopoietic cancers arising following treatment of hematopoietic disorders. Cancer 1985; 55:512–5.

45. Harris CC. The carcinogenicity of anticancer drugs: A hazard in man. Cancer 1976; 37:1014–23.

Cancer Detection and Prevention Supplement 1:159–164 (1987)

Malignant Lymphoproliferative Disorders of Viral Origin in Transplant Patients Undergoing Immunosuppressive Therapy

J.L. Touraine, MD
J. Traeger, MD

Transplant Unit and INSERM U80, Hôpital Edouard Herriot, Lyon, France

ABSTRACT   Although no case of lymphoproliferative syndrome occurred among our first 680 transplant patients, 13 cases developed in a subsequent series of 170 patients. This severe condition involved a proliferation of B cells and/or plasma cells that invaded a number of organs, resulting in the deaths of eight patients. Early tapering off of immunosuppressive therapy enabled five patients to recover without loss of the transplant. The factors likely to be involved in the occurrence of malignant lymphoproliferation are immunosuppressive drugs, and introduction of allogeneic EBV-infected cells or reactivation of EBV.

Key words: lymphomas, EBV infections, immunosuppressive therapy, transplant patients

INTRODUCTION

In our transplant center, no case of lymphoproliferative disorder had been observed for 16 years, a period during which 680 patients were transplanted. However, in a recent period of 18 months, 13 of 170 patients developed a severe condition associated with B-cell and/or plasma-cell proliferation. All patients had received kidney or kidney plus pancreas transplants a few weeks or months previously, and they were under one of two immunosuppressive regimens: nine patients were treated with cyclosporine A (CsA), antilymphocyte globulins (ALG), and corticosteroids; four patients were treated with ALG, azathioprine (Az), and corticosteroids (Table I). The outcome was death in eight cases and complete recovery without loss of the transplant(s) in five cases following early tapering off of immunosuppression. The case reports of the initial eight patients and the immunoglobulin (Ig) abnormalities in a group of 227 transplant patients have previously been reported [1].

MATERIALS AND METHODS

The immunosuppressive treatments were given at the following dosages: In the first group, CsA 12 mg/kg/day orally then adapted to maintain a plasma level of CsA between 100 and 200 ng/ml indefinitely, ALG 10 mg/kg/day for 1–3 months, prednisone 1 mg/kg/day tapered off after 2 weeks; some patients had initially received azathioprine, then CsA in

Address reprint requests to Prof. J.L. Touraine, Pavillon P, Hôpital Edouard Herriot, 69374 Lyon Cedex 08, France.

**TABLE I. Infectious Lymphoproliferative Syndrome in 13 Patients:
Predisposing Therapy and Outcome**

Immunosuppressive treatment
CsA + ALG + steroids (±Az): 9 patients
ALG + steroids + Az: 4 patients
Outcome
Death: 8 patients
Recovery: 5 patients (following discontinuation of immunosuppressive therapy);
all 5 patients still have a functional transplant

substitution for azathioprine due to leukopenia. In the second group: ALG 10 mg/kg/day for 1–2 months, azathioprine 1.5–2.5 mg/kg/day indefinitely, prednisone 1 mg/kg/day for 2 weeks and then indefinitely maintained at a lower dose.

Immunoglobulin heterogeneity was investigated by isoelectric focusing on thin-layer (500 μm) acrylamide gel (T4C3) in a 3.5–9.5 pH gradient [2]. B lymphocytes and plasma cells were studied for surface or intracytoplasmic Ig by immunofluorescence with monospecific antibodies. T-lymphocyte subsets were repeatedly determined in the peripheral blood of four patients, using monoclonal antibodies of the OKT series (Ortho Pharmaceuticals, Piscataway, NJ). Cytomegalovirus (CMV) was searched for weekly in the urine. CMV, herpes simplex virus (HSV), herpes zoster virus (HZV), parainfluenza virus, influenza virus, adenovirus, and Epstein-Barr virus (EBV; VCA, EA, and EBNA serologies were also routinely performed). The serologies for human T-cell lymphoma-leukemia virus (HTLV-I) and for lymphadenopathy associated virus (LAV/HTLV-III) were carried out retrospectively on frozen sera drawn from the patients during the acute episode of infectious lymphoproliferative syndrome (ILPS). Autopsies were performed on three patients, and pathology investigations were limited to multiple biopsies in the others.

RESULTS
Infectious Lymphoproliferative Syndrome

Clinical and laboratory findings were homogeneous in most patients with ILPS. Fever and leukopenia first developed as well as labial vesicles (without HSV in the vesicles). At this stage, all ILPS patients had a significant restriction of Ig heterogeneity or even well character-ized oligoclonal Ig components. The onset of clinical and laboratory abnormalities was between 11 and 125 days after the transplant.

In a period of 1–3 weeks, the picture was completed with abdominal pain, liver and spleen enlargement, respiratory distress, hepatic failure, and rapidly deteriorating general condition. Uricemia and lactic dehydrogenase were increased; lactic acidosis was present. Despite intensive care for all patients, eight died in a few weeks. In the five surviving patients, ALG, CsA, and/or azathioprine had been withdrawn as soon as fever and Ig abnormalities were noted. In these patients, clinical symptoms initially proceeded as in the other cases, then progressively disappeared. Acyclovir treatment proved to be ineffective even in large doses (15 mg/kg/8 hr) given IV. In two patients, ILPS actually occurred several days after initiation of acyclovir given prophylactically at the dose of 5 mg/kg/8 hr.

Pathological Findings

Biopsies and postmortem investigations revealed a massive infiltration of oligoclonal B cells and plasma cells in the liver, spleen, bone marrow, transplant organs, and lung (Table II). In contrast, lymph nodes and the CNS were not invaded. By immunofluorescence analysis with antiheavy- and antilight-chain antisera, it was shown that there were several cell clones, some of which were secreting clones, the other nonsecreting clones (Fig. 1).

TABLE II. Pathological Findings in ILPS

Infiltration with:
   B lymphocytes (several clones)
   Plasma cells
   (There are secreting and nonsecreting clones, as shown by immunofluorescence analysis with
      antiheavy- and antilight-chain antisera)

Invasion of the following organs:
   Spleen   Bone marrow
   Liver   Kidney transplant
   Lung   Pancreas transplant

Noninvasion of:
   Lymph nodes
   Central nervous system

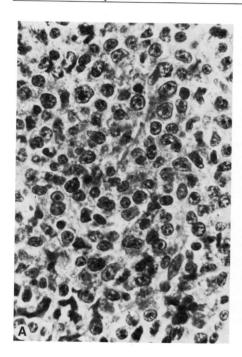 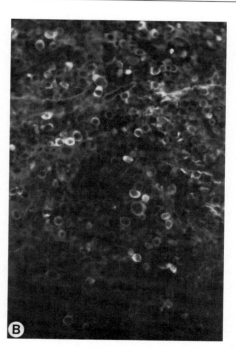

Fig. 1. Lymphocyte infiltration of the liver of a patient with ILPS. Photonic microscopy (A) and immunofluorescence microscopy (B) with anti-μ antiserum. Analysis of the same specimen with anti-γ antiserum revealed some IgG-bearing B cells in smaller amounts.

Immunological Abnormalities

The most precocious manifestation of the disease was the appearance of a restriction of Ig heterogeneity in the serum. In many cases, this Ig abnormality proceeded up to oligoclonal or monoclonal serum Ig component(s). However, comparable findings were noted in 45% of patients treated with CsA and ALG and in 21.5% of patients treated with Az and ALG (Table III). No significant difference in the Ig pattern was seen between most patients who developed ILPS and those who had asymptomatic Ig abnormalities. Only the rapid constitution of large oligoclonal components, illustrated in a previous publication [1], can be used as a warning in patients monitored for Ig heterogeneity. In one patient, the amount of Ig thus produced became so high that it accounted for a gammaglobulin serum level of 50 g/liter (Fig. 2).

TABLE III. Immunoglobulin Abnormalities in Transplant Patients Undergoing Immunosuppressive Therapy

CsA treatment:
  27 abnormalities in 60 patients
    11: restriction of heterogeneity
    16: mono- or oligoclonal component

Conventional treatment:
  21.5 % of abnormalities
  (lower frequency and delayed appearance)

In vitro, CsA may help B-cell transformation into lymphoblasts under EBV influence

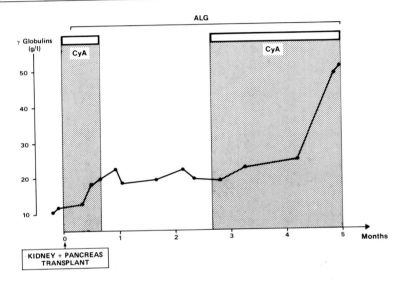

Fig. 2. Rapid and high production of gammaglobulins in a patient with a form of ILPS resembling multiple myeloma (large and diffuse infiltration of plasma cells, in addition to B cells).

The analysis of T-cell subsets in peripheral blood demonstrated levels of OKT4[+] lymphocytes as low as in AIDS patients: 16% as a mean. The absolute numbers were even more significantly decreased because of lymphopenia. The percentage of OKT8[+] lymphocytes was increased up to a mean of 58%. Correction of these abnormalities required 2 months in the surviving patients (Fig. 3). During this time, the proliferative responses of lymphocytes to phytomitogens in vitro remained extremely low.

Virological Findings

CMV was repeatedly isolated in the urine of six patients. CMV serology switched from negative to positive in one patient. HSV seroconversion was found in one patient and parainfluenza seroconversion in three patients. EBV serology was suggestive of reactivation (especially manifested by a significant increase of anti-VCA antibodies) in six patients. However, in two of the patients with unmodified EBV serology, EBNA was clearly present in cells from the bone marrow and the liver biopsies (Table IV); in addition, a very rapid and spontaneous development of EBV-positive cell lines was readily obtained from those bone marrow cells. HTLV-I serology was midly positive in three cases and LAV/HTLV-III in seven cases by ELISA assay. When the sera were studied with a competition technique or a Western blotting technique, no specific reaction was found for either HTLV-I or LAV/HTLV-III.

% Positive cells

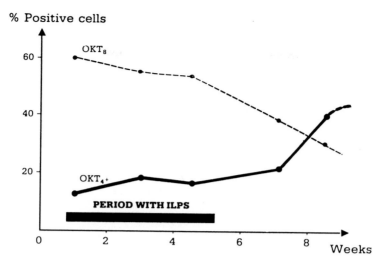

Fig. 3.   Decreased percentage of OKT4$^+$ cells and increased percentage of OKT8$^+$ cells during ILPS and slow correction of the abnormalities after disappearance of the syndrome.

TABLE IV. EBV Serology and EBV Antigens in Patients With ILPS

EBV serology strongly suggestive of reactivation:
 6 patients
EBNA positive in cells infiltrating the bone marrow and the liver:
 2 additional patients

DISCUSSION

ILPS appears to be a condition involving several sequential stages: (1) moderate proliferation of many B-cell clones, several of which retain their capacity to differentiate into Ig-secreting plasma cells; then (2) oligoclonal proliferation of B cells and plasma cells, up to a large number of cells, and organ infiltration; finally (3) oligoclonal or monoclonal proliferation of B cells and plasma cells, in enormous amounts, with escape from all regulatory influences. The two initial stages are reversible, provided that immunosuppression is reduced and T-cell functions are regained. The latter stage presently appears to be almost irreversible even with the more aggressive therapies usually given in lymphomas.

Early diagnosis of this condition is therefore crucial for a complete recovery. ILPS can be anticipated when a patient presents with both Ig abnormalities and an unexplained infectious syndrome. Tapering off of immunosuppressive drugs results in cure of this condition. Ig abnormalities are frequent in immunosuppressed patients [1], as they are in congenital immunodeficiencies or in aging [3]. They cannot therefore be, by themselves, the diagnostic criterion, but they can raise the awareness threshold. Using this Ig monitoring (and reduction of immunosuppressive drugs in patients with a restriction of Ig heterogeneity), we have avoided any new case of ILPS for the last 18 months.

The causative agent responsible for ILPS may well be EBV. This virus is known to induce B-cell transformation in vitro and in vivo. CsA can help B-cell transformation into lymphoblasts under EBV influence. Other immunosuppressive drugs may also favor such a phenomenon by reducing T-cell "surveillance" onto B cells. The batches of ALG that we used were shown to be devoid of any viral material and of reverse-transcriptase activity but the potent immunosuppression provided by the addition of ALG and CsA may depress all the various defense mechanisms against EBV and EBV-transformed cells.

CsA has been shown to inhibit the production of IL2, γ-IFN, and possibly other interleukins [4]. This agent, as well as most immunosuppressive drugs or factors, can decrease the activity of cytotoxic T lymphocytes and NK cells. The control of virus-infected cells may thus be hindered. Reactivation of EBV is possible. In addition, infection brought by donor cells may represent some hazard to the patient. EBV-infected donor cells can hardly be eliminated by the host due to the "allogeneic restriction" of T-cell functions, to the polyclonal activation resulting from the "allogeneic effect," and to the decreased T-cell and NK-cell activities.

Oncogenes (c-myc and B-lym), which become activated in Burkitt lymphoma, may also be involved. It will be important to determine whether some gene rearrangements or some chromosomal translocations occur in lymphomatous cells from these patients. It will also be useful to ascertain, with the utmost precision, the donor or host origin of transformed cells. By HLA typing, in a few studied cases, the oligonal proliferation was found to be of host type. This does not, however, rule out the possibility of a smaller and early proliferation of EBV-infected donor B cells nor the transmission of EBV from donor cells to host B cells in some patients.

The occurrence of 13 cases of ILPS in a short period suggests a role for an agent less ubiquitous than EBV and that would further decrease defense capacities against EBV-infected B cells. No direct evidence for a "two-virus model," however, has been obtained, and, in particular, HTLV infection has not been substantiated.

Analysis of cancer in transplant patients has been extremely valuable in the understanding of relationships between some malignancies, immune disturbances, genetic phenomena, and possibly viral infections [5]. Similarly, the study of ILPS and lymphomas developing in transplant patients [5–9] should provide useful information in this field as well as in the definition of early stages of B-cell lymphomas and myelomas. Finally, these conditions give evidence that an oligoclonal lymphocyte proliferation, considered to be malignant by most investigators, can be eliminated by the immune system provided that restoration of immune defense mechanisms does not occur at a very late stage of tumor development. The target of the involved immune phenomena has not yet been conclusively established; it may be EBV-associated antigens expressed by the EBV-infected tumor cells.

ACKNOWLEDGMENTS

We thank Drs. M. Aymard, N. Blanc, E. Bosi, J. Bosshard, C. Chapuis-Cellier, M. Chevallier, R. Creyssel, G.B. De Thé, J.M. Dubernard, M.S. El Yafi, J. Gazzolo, A. Gelet, G. Lenoir, P.M. Piatti, C. Pouteil-Noble, F. Touraine, and C. Trepo for their help during these investigations. Parts of the text have been reproduced from "Revue de l'Institut Pasteur de Lyon" [1985; 18:109–15] with permission.

REFERENCES

1. Touraine JL, El Yafi S, Bosi E, et al. Immunoglobulin abnormalities and infectious lymphoproliferative syndrome (ILPS) in Cyclosporine-treated transplant patients. Transplant Proc, 1983; 15[suppl I]:2798–804.
2. Chapuis-Cellier C, Francina A, Arnaud P. In Radola BJ, ed: Electrophoresis 79, Berlin: Walter de Gruyter, 1980; 711.
3. Radl J. In Adler WH, Nordin AA, Adelman RC, et al, eds: Immunological techniques applied to aging research, Boca Raton, FL. CRC Press, 1981; 121.
4. Reem GH, Cook LA, Palladino MA. Cyclosporine inhibits interleukin-2 and interferon gamma synthesis by human thymocytes. Transplant Proc, 1983; 15[suppl I]:2837–9.
5. Penn I. Tumor incidence in human allograft recipients. Transplant Proc 1979; 11:1047–51.
6. Calne RY, Rolles K, White DJG, et al. Cyclosporin A initially as the only immunosuppressant in 34 recipients of cadaveric organs: 32 kidneys, 2 pancreases and 2 livers. Lancet 1979;ii:1033–36.
7. Crawford DH, Thomas JA, Janossy G, et al. Epstein-Barr virus nuclear antigen positive lymphoma after cyclosporin A treatment in patient with renal allograft. Lancet 1980ii:1355–7.
8. Jacobs P, Gordon-Smith EC. Cyclosporin A, transplantation, and lymphoma. Lancet 1980;ii:1296.
9. Hanto DW, Gajl-Peczalska KI, Frizzera G, et al. Epstein-Barr (EBV) induce polyclonal and monoclonal T cell lympho-proliferative diseases occurring after renal transplantation. Clinical, pathological and virological findings and implication for therapy. Ann Surg 1983; 198:356–68.

Cancer Detection and Prevention Supplement 1:165–172 (1987)

Difficulty in Establishing Diagnosis From Lung Biopsies and Bronchial Washing Analysis in Children With Leukemia Following Bone Marrow Transplantation

Thomas Miale, MD
Nat Mody, MD
Barrett Dick, MD
Parashar Nanavati, MD
Lilly Mathew, MD

R. Frederick Boedy, MD
Michael Steinberg, MD
Diane Davis, MT (ASCP)
Subhash Chaudhary, MD
L. Gilbert Thatcher, MD

Departments of Pediatrics (T.M., L.W., R.F.B., M.S., D.D., S.C., L.G.T.), Radiation Therapy (P.N.), and Pathology (N.M., B.D.), Southern Illinois University School of Medicine, Springfield, IL

ABSTRACT   Three children developed severe respiratory distress at days +12, +11, and +11 following allogeneic bone marrow transplantation from donors. The first child was a 13-year-old Hispanic boy transplanted in relapse of Philadelphia chromosome-positive acute lymphoblastic leukemia (ALL). At day −14, a bronchial washing done for a streaky pulmonary infiltrate was negative for acid-fast bacilli. Miliary tuberculosis was discovered at postmortem examination. A second child, transplanted in remission of null-cell ALL, developed severe hypoxia and hypercarbia on day +11 but recovered fully following prolonged mechanical ventilation. An open-lung biopsy showed a pattern of nonspecific, diffuse alveolar damage compatible with respiratory distress syndrome. The third child was transplanted in remission of B-cell ALL and developed fatal fungal and cytomegalovirus pneumonia on day +12. In these latter two cases, it is likely that open-lung biopsy would have missed the diagnosis because of the uneven pulmonary involvement and multiple etiologies observed. All three children received cyclosporine, granulocyte transfusions, and multiple antimicrobials, including amphotericin B. Hyperfractioned total-body irradiation with lung shielding was used in the latter two patients.

Key words: amphotericin B, cytomegalovirus, tuberculosis, pneumonitis, radiation, cyclosporine

INTRODUCTION

The lung is a crucial target organ for a variety of pathologic processes following allogeneic bone marrow transplantation. The acute mortality for such processes approaches 50% [1, 2]. The chest X-ray is almost never diagnostic of a single etiology. Even at postmortem

Address reprint requests to Dr. Thomas D. Miale, Department of Pediatrics, Southern Illinois University School of Medicine, P.O. Box 3926, Springfield, IL 62708

examination, the exact diagnosis remains doubtful in 20% of cases [3]. Any report of a specific diagnosis in cases of transbronchoscopic or open-lung biopsy should be questioned. Furthermore, establishing a precise cause of the pulmonary disease with an invasive procedure does not necessarily alter or improve the clinical outcome. With these problems in perspective, we present three cases illustrating the critical diagnostic challenges associated with the clinical management of pneumonia following allogeneic bone marrow transplantation for leukemia in children.

PATIENTS, MATERIALS, AND METHODS
Patients

Three patients who were treated with allogeneic bone marrow transplantation for acute lymphoblastic leukemia (ALL) and developed severe pulmonary complications that were fatal in two of these patients are the subjects of this report. All specimens and participation of these patients were obtained after written parental consent in accordance with a protocol approved by the Institutional Review Board for the Protection of Human Subjects. This was done in accordance with the bioethical standards established in the Helsinki Declaration of 1975. Brief case reports are given below.

Case No. 1. The patient was a 13-year-old Hispanic boy who was diagnosed with ALL in January, 1982, after symptoms of recurrent epistaxis and gingival and subconjunctival hemorrhages prompted medical evaluation. He complained of lethargy, myalgia, and anorexia. Significant findings included bilateral subconjunctival and retinal hemorrhage, mucocutaneous purpura, tender axillary and inguinal lymphadenopathy, and moderate hepatosplenomegaly. Significant laboratory findings included a hyperleukocytosis with a total white blood count of $312,000/mm^3$, of which 80% were malignant lymphoblasts. Bone marrow aspiration also showed a predonderance of lyphoblasts of a predominantly L-2 morphology according to the French-American-British classification system [4]. Immunologic surface markers for detection of E-rosetting and surface immunoglobulin were negative. Cytochemical strains for myeloperoxidase and Sudan black B were also negative, with 10% of the peripheral and bone marrow blasts positive for the PAS strain.

Initial supportive care included leukopheresis to lower the white blood count to $42,000/mm^3$, platelet transfusions, and antibiotics. He was treated according to protocol #193P of the Children's Cancer Study Group, with induction therapy consisting of vincristine, prednisone, daunomycin, and asparaginase plus intrathecal methotrexate. After 4 weeks, he entered a partial remission and then received CNS treatment with both radiation therapy (2,400 cGy to whole brain and cervical segments 1 and 2), and intrathecal methotrexate, and systemic cyclophosphamide and 6-mercaptopurine. He then entered complete remission with a second course of vincristine, asparaginase, daunomycin, and prednisone, which persisted until October, 1982, when he developed an isolated CNS relapse, which was successfully treated with intrathecal cytosine arabinoside, methotrexate, and hydrocortisone. He was also given intensive reinduction therapy with vincristine, dexamethasone, and prednisone. A second isolated CNS relapse was controlled similarly in February, 1983. The Philadelphia chromosome was then detected.

He was maintained in remission with systemic methotrexate and asparaginase supplemented with triple intrathecal chemothereapy until May 26, 1985, when he received an allogeneic bone marrow transplant from a histoincompatible brother. Two weeks before, he had developed a streaky pulmonary infiltrate with a negative bronchial washing for pathogens including fungi and acid-fast microorganisms and a negative tuberculin skin test. He was prepared for transplant with both fractionated total-body irradiation (eight fractions of 165 cGy each, twice daily for 4 days, 6 MV X-rays compensated with lead shadow shields to produce +6% dose rate over the total body; on the fourth day, the thorax was irradiated with 6 MeV electrons for two fractions of 350 cGy each). Following the bone marrow infusion, he was treated with high-dosage cyclosporine according to the protocol of R. Powles and colleagues

[5]. He developed progressive precipitous pulmonary problems 5 days later and died of this complication 12 days after the marrow infusion despite mechanical ventilation and all resucitative measures. He received broad-spectrum antibiotic coverage including amphotericin B and granulocyte transfusions. At autopsy, he was found to have both disseminated fungal and tuberculous infection (Fig. 1).He had associated stomach hemorrhage, left-side pleural adhesions with pleural effusions bilaterally, ascites, and hepatomegaly. There was no evidence of persistent leukemia, renal disease, or graft-versus-host reaction.

Case No. 2. This 7-year-old white girl was given the diagnosis of ALL at age 4 years and remained in complete remission until December, 1984. After initial induction therapy, she had received 2,400 cGy whole-brain irradiation and intrathecal methotrexate. She was reinduced into a second remission with vincristine, asparaginase, and prednisone and received intrethecal methotrexate for CNS retreatment. Subsequently, she received IV methotrexate and IM asparaginase as maintenance chemotherapy with teniposide (VM-26), cytosine arabinoside, vincristine, asparaginase, daunomycin, and prednisone as consolidation and periodic reinduction chemotherapy. On April 30, 1985, she received 1,320 cGy total-body irradiation via 11 fractions in 3 days with lung shielding with half-layer blocks [6]. She also received electron beam chest wall irradiation (a total of 600 cGy, calculated at the 100% isodose line via a 9 MeV electron beam cone) [6]. The total-body irradiation was delivered on the 18 MeV linar accelerator with a 10 MeV photon beam. She then received two dosages of cyclophosphamide (30 mg/kg/dosage) followed by an allogeneic marrow graft from her histocompatible 9-year-old sister. On day +11, after transplant, she developed sudden pulmonary infiltrates (Fig. 2),which were treated with broad-spectrum antibiotic coverage, including amphotocericin B, and granulyocyte transfusions. Alpha-streptococcus was cultured from her central venous access line. She recovered fully following mechanical ventilation for 2 weeks. A right open-lung biospy (Fig. 3) showed interstitial and intraalveolar edema and hemorrhage with focal hyaline membrane formation with no microorganisms demonstrated on special and routine strains and cultures. She suffered an episode of sudden blindness and disorientation soon after being weaned from the respirator with improvement to total recovery in 1 day's time. A

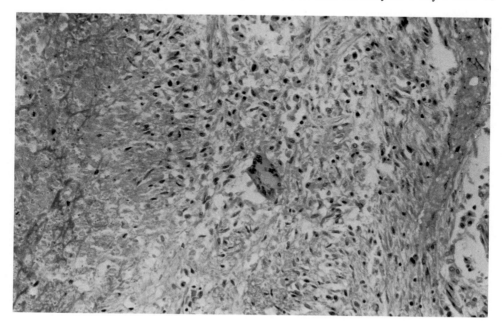

Fig. 1. Pulmonary granuloma in Case No. 1.

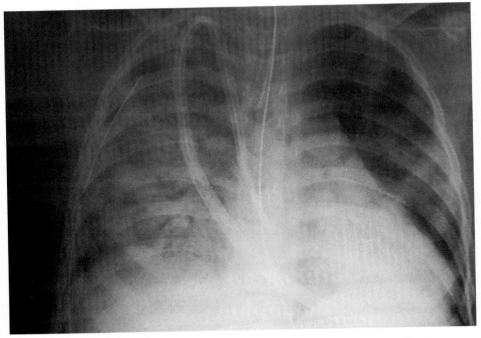

Fig. 2.   Chest X-ray (PA view) demonstrating severe pneumonitis in Case No. 2.

computer scan of the head showed bilateral occipital lesions of low density, suggesting edema with hemorrhage present on the right. Spinal fluid was normal, examination including routine and special cultures for fungi, protozoans, and viruses. India ink preparation was negative also. The patient has suffered recent memory losses and decreased school performance, but has remained in remission for 6 months after transplantation, remaining on maintenance chemotherapy with teniposide (VM-26), cytosine arabinoside, vincristine, asparaginase, and prednisone.

Case No. 3. In January, 1985, this 6-year-old white boy was evaluated for recurrent joint pains, swollen gums, and zyogma and found to have ALL with L-3 morphology according to the French-American-British classification system [4]. Immunologic studies revealed that surface IgM was present on 72% of bone marrow cells, κ chain, on 65%, whereas only 3% were positive for T-11 antigen. Seventy-eight percent of bone marrow cells at diagnosis were positive for the B-1 antigen. The patient was induced into complete remission with vincristine, prednisone, and methotrexate and maintained in remission with cyclophosphamide, vincristine, methotrexate, and corticosteroids. He also received reinduction pulses of vincristine, asparaginase, daunomycin, and prednisone and was maintained with teniposide (VM-26) and cytosine arabinoside. He remained in remission until May 28, 1985, when 53 leukemic blast cells were discovered in the cerebrospinal fluid with a normal bone marrow aspirate and peripheral blood findings. The patient had no other sign of relapse except moderate splenomegaly and was treated with triple intrathecal therapy (hydrocortisone, methotrexate, and cytosine arabinoside) and with 2,400 cGy total-brain and upper cervical spine radiation therapy. Immediately following this treatment, the patient received the identical preparative regimen for bone marrow transplantation as described for Case No. 2. [6]. He developed a "skin tunnel" infection along the subcutaneous course of his central venous catheter and a cerebrospinal fluid leak at the site of his lumbar punctures. He was placed on broad-spectrum antibiotic coverage

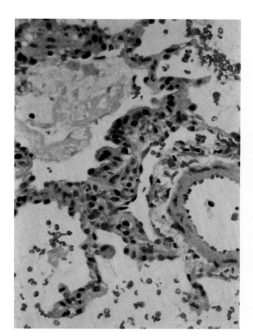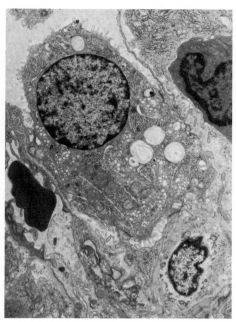

Fig. 3.   Left, light microscopy; right, electron microscopy. Both illustrate marked diffuse hyperplasia of type II pneumocytes lining the alveolar septae in Case No. 2, with diffuse alveolar damage. Case No. 3.

with the addition of acyclovir, amphotericin B, and vancomycin. His central venous line was replaced, and his lumbar leak stopped spontaneously. He developed bone marrow recovery on about day +8, and by day +11 the absolute neutrophil count had increased to 1,924/mm^3. Despite this, he developed rapidly progressive pulmonary infiltrates and received granulocyte transfusions daily from day +2 to day +6. As preparations for open-lung biospy were being completed, he developed ventilatory collapse suddenly and died. Postmortem findings showed pulmonary congestion and edema with evidence of fungal infection of the lungs (Fig. 4),minimal involvement of the lungs by cytomegalovirus (Fig. 5), and evidence of respiratory distress syndrome including hyaline membrane formation (Fig. 5).The bone marrow was normocellular with no evidence of residual leukemia here or in other organs, including the spleen. Histopathologic evidence of cytomegalovirus involvement of the bladder epithelium was also present. Postmortem cultures were negative for pathogens, including viruses and fungi.

Electron Microscopy

The tissues were postfixed in osmium tetraoxide in cacodylate buffer for 60 min. Dehydration was through graded alcohol. The tissues were stained en bloc in 2% uranyl acetate. Blocks were sectioned by the Dupont MT 5000 ultramicrotome. The sections were stained with uranyl acetate and lead citrate. The material was examined with Hitachi H-600 electron microscope.

RESULTS AND DISCUSSION

The role and timing of open-lung biopsy procedures in bone marrow transplant recipients with various pulmonary infiltrates remains controversial. Although less invasive procedures are available and have been utilized frequently, open-lung biopsy remains the "gold standard" to which the clinical accuracy and utility of other procedures are generally compared [1, 2].

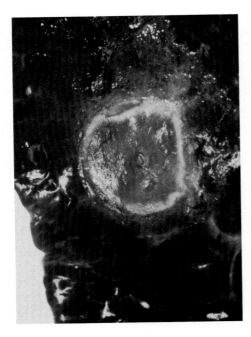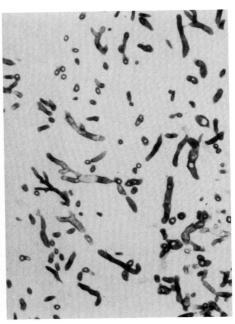

Fig. 4.   Left, white-tan plaque on pleural surface with underlying infract. Right, branching hyphae stained with Grocott methenamine silver, indicative of one of the higher fungi, possibly *Aspergillus* sp.

The sample of lung tissue obtained, however, is necessarily limited, and this can lead to a missed diagnosis. This is especially true when many separate pathologic processes are present simultaneously. The procedure is hazardous in that pneumothorax and accelerated pulmonary failure, with need for mechanical ventilation often supervene. Mechanical ventilation may lead to further compromise of pulmonary function and enhanced entry of pathogenic micro-organisms.

Many alternative procedures have proposed to evaluate these pneumonias more safely and yet establish a tissue- and/or culture-proven diagnosis. The most effective have been high-volume bronchopulmonary lavages [7] supplemented with enhanced detection of cytomegalovirus by centrifugation and monoclonal antibody staining [8]. This has been most commonly applied to the discovery of the etiology of interstitial pneumonia in the acquired immunodeficiency syndrome but, of course, can easily be applied also in the marrow transplant setting. An alternative procedure has been the use of thoracoscopy with biopsy in the diagnosis of peripheral lung lesions in children with cancer [9].

Our three patients illustrate difficulties in establishing the accurate diagnosis of severe lung disorders following allogeneic bone marrow transplantation. The first patient died of lung failure secondary to disseminated fungal and tuberculous infections despite a negative tuberculin skin test and bronchial washing performed 2 weeks before transplant. Fungal disease advanced while the patient was being treated with amphotericin B and granulocyte transfusions. Postmortem cultures were positive for *M. tuberculosis* and negative for fungi and other microbial pathogens. Lung sections showed multiple granulomas (Fig. 1).

The second patient suffered sudden and severe pneumonia 11 days after transplantation (Fig. 2). An open-lung biopsy led to the diagnosis of acute respiratory distress syndrome (Fig. 3), from which the patient slowly recovered with vigorous supportive care, including prolonged mechanical ventilation. The third patient developed three different processes in various lung regions including fungal pneumonia (Fig. 4), presumed cytomegaloviral disease (Fig. 5), and

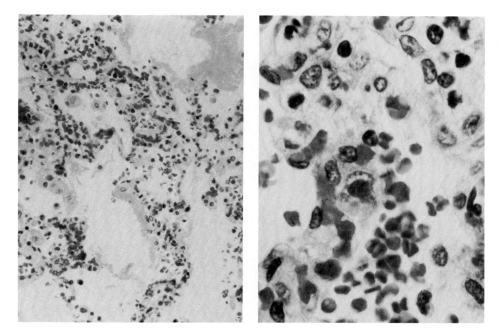

Fig. 5. Left, hyaline membrane formation in Case No. 3. Right, large eosinophilic inclusion in another area of lung tissue in Case No. 3.

acute respiratory distress syndrome (Fig. 5). Since the pathologic processes were multifactorial in Cases 1 and 3, it is possible that open-lung biopsy findings would have lead to inappropriate management depending on the site biopsied.

D. Wright and colleagues [10] reported lethal pulmonary reactions following the combination of amphotericin B and granulocyte transfusions. This might explain a component of the respiratory compromise in all three of our patients. However, this toxicity was absent in another comparable group of 144 patients [11]. R.S. Weiner and colleagues [12] found that a lower risk of interstitial pneumonitis following allogeneic bone marrow transplant was statistically associated with the following features in the International Bone Marrow Transplant Registry patient group: 1) younger age, 2) higher pretransplant Karnofsky performance scores, 3) cyclosporine as opposed to methotrexate as the drug used to prevent graft-versus-host disease, 4) lower dose rate of total body irradiation, 5) female donor to female recipient transplants.

R. Kurzrock and coworkers [13] have recently reported particular difficulty in establishing the diagnosis of severe mycobacterial pulmonary infections following allogeneic bone marrow transplantation. The general current approach appears to be empirical antibiotic therapy, perhaps including amphotericin B, erythromycin, trimethoprim-sulfamethoxazole for 48–72 h. If clinical improvement occurs, treatment is continued for 10–14 days [1,2,14]. If no improvement occurs, then open-lung biopsy is performed [1,2,14]. However, it should be realized that some patients' care, such as for those described here, might be compromised unless it is realized that a single-site biopsy can miss essential diagnostic features. This may make therapy too narrow in scope to encompass the multiple lung problems that can be present in a given transplant patient.

ACKNOWLEDGMENTS

We thank the critical care nursing and paramedical teams of the Memorial Medical Center and St. John's Hospital of Springfield, Illinois. We also thank Mrs. June Auvil for her able editorial assistance.

REFERENCES

1. Rosenow EC, Wilson WR, Cockerill FR. Pulmonary disease in the immunocompromised host (First of two parts). Mayo Clin Proc 1985; 60:473-87.
2. Wilson WR, Cockerill FR, Rosenow EC. Pulmonary disease in the immunocompromised host (Second of two parts). Mayo Clin Proc 1985; 60:610-1.
3. Singer C, Armstrong D, Rosen PP, Walzer, PD, Yu B. Diffuse pulmonary infiltrates in immunosuppressed patients: Prospective study of 80 cases. Am J Med 1979; 66:110-20.
4. Bennett JM, Catovsky D, Daniel MT, Flandrin G, Galton DAG, Gralnick HR, Sultan C. Proposals for the classification of the acute leukemias. Br J Haematol 1976; 33:451-8.
5. Powles R, Pedrazzini A, Crofts M, Clink H, Millar J. Bhatti G, Perez D. Mismatched family bone marrow transplantation. Semin Hematol 1984; 21:182-7.
6. Shank B, Hopfan S, Kim JH, Chu FCH, Grossbard E, Kapoor N, Kirkpatrick D, Dinsmore R, Simpson L, Reid A, Chui C, Mohan R, Finegan D, O'Reilly RJ. Hyperfractionated total body irradiation for bone marrow transplantation: I. Early results in leukemia patients. Int J Radiation Oncol Biol Phys 1983; 7:1109-15.
7. Stover DE, White DA, Romano PA, Gellene RA. Diagnosis of pulmonary disease in acquired immunodeficiency syndrome (AIDS). Role of bronchoscopy and bronchopulmonary lavage. Annu Rev Resp Dis 1984; 130:659-62.
8. Gleaves CA, Smith TF, Shuster EA, Pearson GR. Rapid detection of cytomegalovirus in MRC-5 cells innoculated with urine specimens using low speed centrifugation and monoclonal antibody to early antigen. J Clin Microbiol 1984; 19:917-9.
9. Rodgers BM, Talbert JL. Thoracoscopy for diagnosis of intrathoracic lesions in children. J Pediatr Surg 1976; 11:703-8.
10. Wright DG, Robichaud KJ, Pizzo PA, Deisseroth AB. Lethal pulmonary reactions associated with the combined use of amphotericin B and leukocyte transfusions. N Engl J Med 1981; 304:1185-9.
11. Dana BW, Durie BGM, White RF, Heustis DW. Concomitant administration of granulocyte transfusions and amphotericin B in neutropenic patients: Absence of significant pulmonary toxicity. Blood 1981; 57:90-4.
12. Weiner RS, Bortin MM, Gale RP, Gluckman E, Kay HEM, Kolb H-J, Hartz AJ, Rimm AA. Risk factors associated with interstitial pneumonitis following allogeneic bone marrow transplantation for leukemia. Transplant Proc 1985; 17:470-4.
13. Kurzrock R, Zander A, Vellekoop L, Knojia M, Luna M, Dicke K. Mycobacterial pulmonary infections after allogeneic bone marrow transplantation. Am J Med 1984; 77:35-40.
14. Quinn JJ. Bone marrow transplantation in the management of childhood cancer. Pediatr Clin North Am 1985; 32:811-34.

Cancer Detection and Prevention Supplement 1:173–181 (1987)

Flow Cytofluorometric Analysis of Choriogonadotropin-Like Material on the Surface of Human and Mouse Malignant Cells

Radmila B. Raikow, PhD
Hernan F. Acevedo, PhD
Alexander Krichevsky, DVM
Mary Jo Buffo, BS
Patricia Fogarty, BS

Department of Laboratory Medicine, Allegheny-Singer Research Institute Allegheny General Hospital, Pittsburgh, PA (R.B.R., H.F.A., M.J.B., P.F.); Department of Medicine, College of Physicians and Surgeons, Columbia University, New York, NY (A.K.)

ABSTRACT   Quantitation by flow cytofluorometry of the distribution of human choriogonadotropin (hCG)-like material on the surface of various human and mouse tumor cells grown in tissue culture and as solid tumors has been done using fluorescein-tagged rabbit antisera (IgG fraction) to intact hCG and, in one experiment, by use of two monoclonal antibodies specific for hCG. Fibroblasts were used as a negative (nontumorigenic) cell control, and a rabbit antiserum to human hemoglobin was used as reagent control. All malignant cells tested stained more intensely with the anti-hCG serum than with the antihuman hemoglobin serum. Positive reaction with the monoclonal antibodies specific for hCG provided strong evidence that the material stained was identical to hCG. Heterogeneity of the expression of the hCG-like material was notable both within each cell line and between different cell lines. This heterogeneity was not associated with cell-cycle phase. 3T3 fibroblast-like cells in vitro were originally negative for hCG but acquired reactivity with anti-hCG serum after ten passages.

Key words: tumor cell marker, IgG, monoclonal antibodies, human and mouse tumors, 3T3 fibroblasts

INTRODUCTION

Material similar to human choriogonadotropin (hCG), a trophoblastic hormone, has been identified on various cancer cells of different species [1–11], and it has been hypothesized that hCG expression on the cancer cell surface is a universal characteristic of malignancy [4,5]. There is evidence that hCG protects cells from attack by immune killer cells [12–22] and that hCG may act as a growth promoter of malignant cells [23,24]. Thus, the production of hCG-

Address reprint request to Dr. Radmila B. Raikow, Allegheny-Singer Research Institute, 320 E. North Avenue, Pittsburgh, PA 15212.

like material by cancer cells may be a key feature conferring malignancy characteristics on these cells, ie, nonimmunogenicity (in spite of tumor-associated antigens), uncontrolled growth, and even invasiveness, since the latter is also a characteristic of the trophoblast. The hypothesis that hCG-like material with a high sialic acid content, and consequently high negative charge [18], is an invariable feature of the malignant cell surface [4,5] has been supported by data obtained with hybrids between HeLa cells and normal fibroblasts in which the malignant phenotype was suppressed [10]. The reappearance of malignancy in these experiments, measured by the ability to produce tumors in nude mice after random chromosome loss, was invariably associated with the reappearance of the expression of hCG-like material. In contrast, other phenotypic features thought to be characteristic of malignancy, such as anchorage-independent growth, were not so correlated.

When normal cells were examined for hCG on their surfaces by immunocytochemistry, only trophoblastic cells, trophoblast-derived placental cells, and sperm cells reacted positively [25–27]. Malignant cells, however, including human and experimental neoplasms of various histological types and origins, were found to display small and variable quantities of surface membrane-associated antigens with epitopes that reacted with hCG antibodies [2,3,5–9]. It was also reported that the expression of hCG-like material occurs very early in the process of malignant transformation [7].

Although there is immunocytochemical evidence for the presence of hCG-like material on the surface of cancer cells [1–12], the potential importance of this observation, which points to a possible single basis for malignancy that may be exploitable in diagnosis, prophylaxis, and therapy, makes it necessary to expand the available evidence and to determine under what conditions the hCG-like material is expressed. This report is a contribution to this end. The detection of hCG-like material using flow cytofluorometry combines the advantage of microscopic analysis (ie, individual cell readings) with the accuracy of bulk measurements on large numbers of cells. Experiments using two-well characterized monoclonal antibodies against hCG [28] provide strong evidence for the hypothesis that the material demonstrated on HeLa cells is the human trophoblastic hormone.

MATERIALS AND METHODS
Cell Lines and Experimental Tumors

Cell lines, obtained from the American Type Culture Collection (ATCC, Rockville, MD) unless otherwise specified, were grown in RPMI 1640 medium (MA Bioproducts, Baltimore, MD) supplemented with fetal calf serum (10% v/v) and gentamicin (10 μg/ml) (both from K.C. Biologicals, Inc., Lenexa, KS). Tumors grown in mice were obtained by injecting 10^6 cells/mouse into the gastrocnemius, and cells were harvested when the tumors were between 0.5 and 1.0 cm^3. Mice were purchased from Jackson Laboratories (Bar Harbor, ME) and kept in standard conditions as described previously [29] unless otherwise specified.

Each cell line was made into a single cell suspension with minimum manipulation before reaction with antibodies. Cells grown in suspension culture were HeLa S3 (ATCC CCL 2.2) and a HeLa S3 variant, obtained from Dr. M. Edmonds at the University of Pittsburgh, where it has been maintained in continuous spinner culture for over fifteen years. Cells that grew in loose monolayers were detached by scraping with a cotton swab. These were S180-II mouse sarcoma (ATCC CCL 8), Lewis lung carcinoma, colon 26 carcinoma No. 8414 (Mason Tumor Repository, Worcester, MA), and untransformed Balb/c 3T3 fibroblasts obtained from Dr. M. Snyder [30]. HeLa ATCC CCL 2.0 had to be detached with trypsin by exposing the cells for 1 minute to 0.25% trypsin (Gibco, Grand Island, NY) at room temperature. The trypsin was decanted, and the flasks were incubated upside down at 37°C for an additional 5 minutes. Cells from solid tumors were dispersed by forcing the tissue through metal sieves (No. 3435-B95, Arthur H. Thomas Co., Philadelphia, PA). These were S180-II sarcoma in SJL/J mice, Lewis lung carcinoma in C57BL/6J mice, colon 26 carcinoma in Balb/cByJ mice, a spontaneous mammary carcinoma of RIII/Imr mice (Institute for Medical Research, Camden, NJ), and HeLa CCL 2.0 cells growing as solid tumors in Balb/c-derived athymic (nu/nu) mice (Harlan Sprague-Dawley Inc., Madison, WI). Viability of cells in all experiments was determined by Trypan blue assessment.

Antibody Reactions

All dilutions and washes were made with Dulbecco's phosphate-buffered saline (PBS) containing 0.5% bovine serum albumin and 0.1% NaN_3. A 1:10 dilution of polyclonal reagents consisting of fluorescein isothiocyanate-conjugated (FITC) IgG fractions of sera from rabbits immunized against hCG or human hemoglobin (hHb) was used in most experiments. Both were purchased from Cooper Biomedical Inc. (Malvern, PA). In one experiment two mouse monoclonal antibodies (MAb) specific for hCG, B107, and B108 (supernatants from hybridoma cultures) were used [28]. After reaction with the MAb the cells were incubated with FITC-labeled goat antimouse serum, F(ab)$_2$ fragments (Cooper Biomedical). All FITC-labeled reagents were centrifuged at 400 g for 7 minutes before use to eliminate unconjugated dye. Incubations were carried out in glass vessels at 0°C for 30 minutes. Two washes with PBS were used between each incubation.

Flow Cytofluorometry

The stained cells were resuspended to 10^6 cells/ml in either the diluent described above and analyzed immediately or in 0.9% NaCl with 1% paraformaldehyde and stored at 0°C for analysis at a later date. A Coulter Epics C flow cytofluorometer with an argon laser and standard settings and filters for FITC was used. When the resulting cell preparation had low viability, as was the case with most of those derived from solid tumors, propidium iodide (PI; 5.0 μg/ml final concentration) was added to the unfixed cell samples suspended in PBS. The samples were then reanalyzed immediately using settings for FITC alone. Under these conditions only dead cells are stained by PI, and these become much more fluorescent than those stained with FITC, even when viewed with FITC settings.

HeLa ATCC 2.2 cells were also stained with PI for total DNA content after they were reacted with the rabbit anti-hCG and hHb, FITC-tagged IgGs, to determine whether expression of the hCG-like material is correlated with any phase of the cell cycle. For this purpose the cells were fixed in cold 95% ethanol after the FITC antibody reactions. They were then resuspended in PBS, digested with RNAse, stained with PI (20 μg/ml), and analyzed on the Coulter Epics C flow cytometer in a standard two-color analysis. (See Coulter Epics System Product Reference Manual, Appendix PN42365 for details).

RESULTS
HeLa, Human Cervical Carcinoma

Use of the polyclonal rabbit antiserum to stain hCG-like material on the surface of the two ATCC HeLa cell strains (Fig. 1 A–D) resulted in large differences in fluorescence intensity between the control and experimental profiles. Moreover, this pattern was consistently seen even after months of culture, during which each strain was tested at least four times. In contrast, the HeLa S3 variant from the University of Pittsburgh was less positive and somewhat more variable (Fig. 1E, F). The two experiments shown for each cell strain in Figure 1 are the one showing the greatest and the one showing the least difference in fluorescence intensity between the hCG and the control hHb reaction of all the trials run. HeLa ATCC strain CCL 2.0 cells were also positive when MAbs for hCG were used (Fig. 2). A greater intensity of staining was obtained when a mixture of the two MAbs was used even though the total amount of antibody in the mixture was the same as when a single MAb was used.

Attempts to correlate hCG expression with cell cycle phase were negative. Thus, HeLa 2.2 cells with G1, S, and G2 amounts of DNA were all equally stained with the anti-hCG serum (profiles not shown).

HeLa CCL 2.0 cells taken from a tumor growing in a nu/nu Balb/c-derived mouse stained less intensely with rabbit anti-hCG than the same cells growing in tissue culture (Fig.

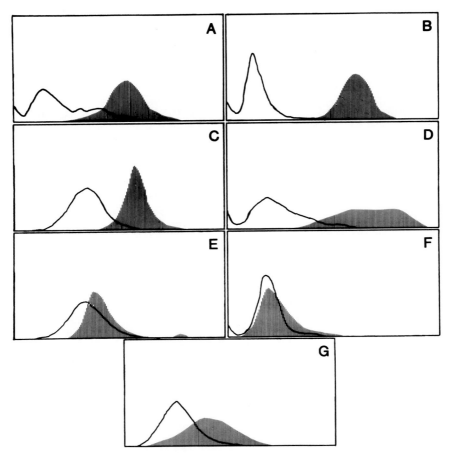

Fig. 1. Fluorescence profiles of three HeLa cell strains. **A,B:** ATCC strain CCL 2.0. **C,D:** HeLa strain S3 (ATCC CCL 2.2). **E,F:** HeLa strain S3, University of Pittsburgh variant. **G:** Variant from HeLa strain 2.0 derived from a solid tumor growing IM in a Balb/c-derived nu/nu mouse. IgG fractions of sera from rabbits immunized with human hemoglobin (control) and human choriogonadotropin (test) were used. The protein concentrations of the test and control reagents were equivalent. The control profiles are outlined with a solid line and the test profiles are shaded. Fluorescence intensity is on each abscissa, and cell number is on each ordinate. Log amplification was used, and 50,000 cells were counted in each sample.

1G). The viability of the cells derived from the solid tumor was only 11.1%, while all the HeLa cells in tissue culture were more than 90% viable.

Lewis Lung, Mouse Carcinoma

Lewis lung cells were either obtained from solid tumors growing in C57BL/6J mice (Fig. 3A–D) or from tissue culture (Fig. 3 E). Although some positivity for hCG was observed in each case, the amount varied in different preparations. This was not related to cell viability, which varied between 20 and 40% in the Lewis lung preparations from solid tumors.

S180-II, Mouse Sarcoma

S180-II cells were obtained either from tissue culture or from solid tumors growing in SJL/J mice. The cultured cells (viability >90%) were either totally negative or only slightly

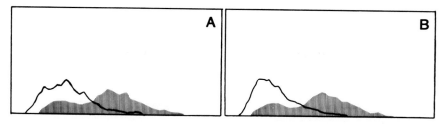

Fig. 2.   Fluorescence profiles of HeLa cell ATCC strain CCL 2.0. Two monoclonal antibodies against hCG (B107 and B108) were used as reagents. In each panel the fluorescent profiles obtained with only one MAb (B107 in **A** and B108 in **B**) are outlined with a solid line and compared to the profile obtained with both of the antibodies, used simultaneously. Equal volumes of each antibody preparation were mixed to obtain the reagent containing both antibodies. Fluorescence intensity is on each abscissa, and cell number is on each ordinate. Amplification and number of cells counted as in Figure 1.

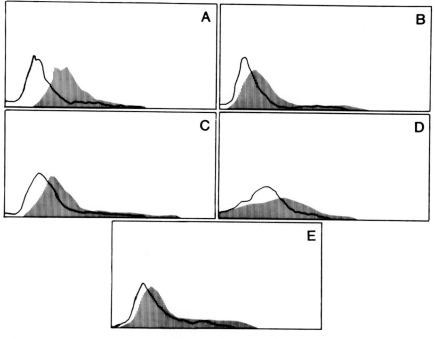

Fig. 3.   Fluorescence profiles of Lewis lung carcinoma cells obtained from solid tumors growing in different C57BL/6J mice **(A–D)**. Lewis lung cells growing in vitro **(E)**. See Figure 1 for further details.

positive for hCG. Two experiments are shown where the most (Fig. 4B) and the least (Fig. 4A) positivity for hCG was observed in four trials using 3 months of continuous culture. Cells obtained from a solid tumor (viability 24%) were more positive than the cultured tissue cells (Fig. 4C). When PI was used as a vital dye the heterogeneity of the staining intensity was reduced, while the percentage of cells staining more intensely with hCG antiserum than with control antiserum was not affected (Fig. 4D).

RIII/Imr, Spontaneous Mammary Carcinoma

Cells from RIII/Imr were also positive for hCG (Fig. 5A). The viability of the preparation was only 7% (Fig. 5), and when PI was added most of the cells were stained, but the percentage of cells positive for hCG was not affected (Fig. 5B).

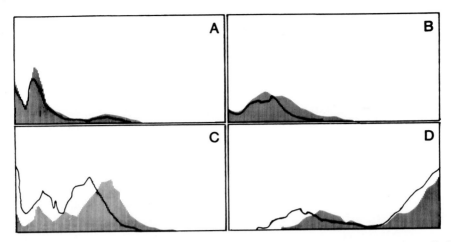

Fig. 4. Fluorescence profiles of S180-II mouse sarcoma cells. **A–B:** Cells from tissue culture. **C:** Cells obtained from a solid tumor growing in a SJL/J mouse. **D:** Same sample as in C, but after PI was added as a vital dye. See Figure 1 for further details.

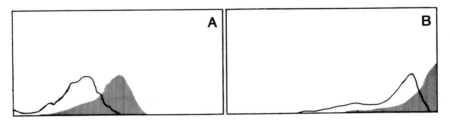

Fig. 5. Fluorescence profiles of carcinoma cells obtained from spontaneous mammary tumor of RIII/Imr mouse. **A:** Cells without PI treatment. **B:** Same cell sample of A to which PI was added. See Figure 1 for further details.

Colon 26 Carcinoma

The colon 26 mouse carcinoma cells were negative for hCG when grown in tissue culture (viability >90%) (Fig. 6A) but were positive for hCG when taken from a solid tumor growing in Balb/cByJ mice (viability 14%) (Fig. 6B). The fluorescence profiles in Figure 6B indicate the presence of two subpopulations: one totally negative and one somewhat positive for hCG. Adding PI as a vital dye (Fig. 6C) eliminated the positive subpopulation, showing that it contained most of the nonviable cells in this preparation.

3T3, Mouse Fibroblasts

3T3 cells were grown in tissue culture and tested at various passages. The viability of all 3T3 preparations was >90%. Cells were negative for hCG the first time they were tested (Fig. 7A) and became increasingly more positive with passage in culture (Fig. 7B–E). Figure 7F shows a direct comparison of the earlier passage (preserved by freezing) run simultaneously with the cells of a later passage (Fig. 7E).

DISCUSSION

Using flow cytofluorometry, some hCG-like material was found on all of the various tumor cells tested, which included various strains of HeLa cells and four different murine neoplasms. No hCG-like material was found on early passage mouse fibroblasts. The amount

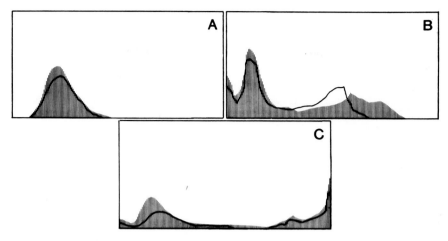

Fig. 6. Fluorescence profiles of colon 26 carcinoma cells obtained from a solid tumor growing in a Balb/cByJ mouse. **A:** From in vitro culture. **B:** Cells obtained directly from the solid neoplasm and processed without PI. **C:** Same cells as in B to which PI was added as a vital dye. See Figure 1 for further details.

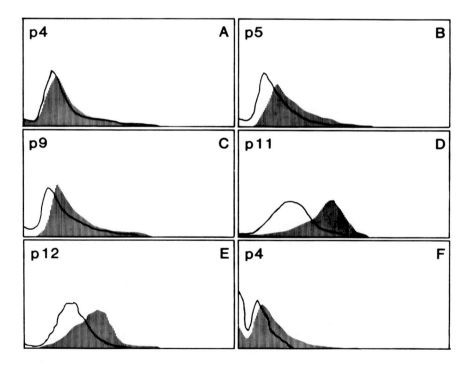

Fig. 7. Fluorescence profiles of Balb/c 3T3 fibroblasts. P refers to passage number. **A–E** show different passages as indicated. **F:** Cells taken from a frozen aliquot of an earlier passage and reacted at the same time as the cells in **E.** The frozen cells were passaged once before reacting them with the antibodies to eliminate any possible effects of the freezing. See Figure 1 for further details.

of hCG-like material varied between different tumor cell lines and, with one established tumor cell line, the HeLa S3 variant from the University of Pittsburgh, was found to vary over culture time. A wide heterogeneity was seen in the intensity of staining with the polyclonal anti-hCG reagent relative to staining with the control anti-hHb reagent in cells derived from solid tumors. This heterogeneity was decreased in most cases when dead cells were eliminated from consideration by using PI as a vital dye. In colon 26 cells growing in Balb/c mice this use of PI indicated that hCG-positive cells were less viable than the hCG-negative cells in the preparation. However, in S-180 II mouse sarcoma cells growing in SJL/J mice both live and dead cells were positive for hCG. The significance of cell viability in cell preparations after several hours of manipulations is debatable and may relate more to their fragility than to their ability to survive in vivo.

Reaction with the two monoclonal antibodies against hCG was done with HeLa ATCC CCL 2.0 cell cultures. Greater staining on the cell surfaces was obtained with a mixture of the two antibodies than with either one used alone. The observed effect was at least additive, showing the presence of the two epitopes identified by these antibodies [28]. The monoclonal antibody B107 has been shown to bind only with intact hCG with no significant cross-reactivity with the most closely related hypophyseal hormone human luteinizing hormone (hLH), and it does not bind to free β-subunit of hCG (hCGβ). It appears to be conformational, binding an epitope available only when the native quarternary structure of hCG is present. Antibody B108 binds hCGβ both free and as part of the intact hCG molecule, also without significant cross-reactivity with hLH. Thus, the results obtained indicate the presence of a molecule very similar to intact hCG on the surface of cultured HeLa CCL 2.0 cells. The presence of free hCGβ-like molecules in addition to intact hCG-like material cannot be ruled out. These results confirm and expand the report by Chou [31] showing that cultured HeLa CCL 2.0 cells synthesize and release hCGβ into its media.

Balb/c fibroblasts (3T3) are known to have the capacity to transform spontaneously in culture [32]. We have observed that they can express surface hCG-like material with passage in culture.

It remains to be determined whether differences in the amount of hCG-like material found on different cells can be correlated with differences in their tumorigenicity and/or metastatic potential.

ACKNOWLEDGMENTS

This work was supported in Pittsburgh by a donation to H.F.A. in memory of B.D. Cadwallader and by research grants from the Cancer Federation, Inc. and the Allegheny-Singer Research Institute. In New York it was supported by NIH grant HD-15454.

REFERENCES

1. Rabson AS, Rosen SW, Tashjian AH Jr, Weintraub BD. Production of human chorionic gonadotropin in vitro by a cell line derived from a carcinoma of the lung. JNCI 1973; 50:669–74.
2. Naughton MA, Merrill DA, McManus LM, et al. Localization of the β chain of human chorionic gonadotropin on human tumor cells and placental cells. Cancer Res 1975; 35:1887–90.
3. McManus LM, Naughton MA, Martinez-Hernandez A. Human chorionic gonadotropin in human neoplastic cells. Cancer Res 1976; 36:3476–81.
4. Odell WD, Wolfson AR, Yoshimoto Y, et al. Ectopic peptide synthesis. A universal concomitant of neoplasia. Trans Assoc Am Physicians 1977; 90:202–27.
5. Acevedo HF, Slifkin M, Pouchet GR, Rakhshan M. Human chorionic gonadotropin in cancer cells. I. Identification in in vitro and in vivo cancer cell systems. In Nieburgs HE, ed: Cancer Detection and Prevention, Vol 1, Part 2. New York: Marcel Dekker, 1978; 937–63.
6. Slifkin M, Acevedo HF, Pardo M, Pouchet GR, Rakhshan M. Human chorionic gonadotropin in cancer cells. II. Ultrastructural localization. In Nieburgs HE, ed: Cancer Detection and Prevention, Vol 1, Part 2. New York: Marcel Dekker, 1978: 965–79.
7. Malkin A, Kellen JA, Kolin A, Cameron R, Farber E. The immunohistochemical detection of chorionic gonadotropin in experimental rat hepatomas. Scand J Immunol 1978; [Suppl]8:603–7.

8. Acevedo HF, Campbell-Acevedo EA, Pardo M, Slifkin M. Immunohistochemical localization of choriogonadotropin-like antigen in animal malignant cells. In Burchiel SW, Rhodes BA, Eds: Tumor imaging. The radio-immunochemical detection of cancer. New York: Masson, 1981: 73–88.

9. Wilson TS, McDowell EM, McIntyre KR, Trump BF. Elaboration of human chorionic gonadotropin by lung tumors. Arch Pathol Lab Med 1981; 105:169–73.

10. Stanbridge EJ, Rosen SW, Sussman HH. Expression of the α subunit of human chorionic gonadotropin is specifically correlated with tumorigenic expression in human cell hybrids. Proc Natl Acad Sci USA 1982; 79:6242–5.

11. Cowley G, Smith JA, Ellison M, Gusterson B. Production of β-human chorionic gonadotropin by human squamous carcinoma cell lines. Int J Cancer 1985; 35:575–9.

12. Patillo RA. Trophoblastic cancers: Chorionic gonadotropin hormone production, antigenic expression, and trophoblast redifferentiation in multiple forms of malignancy. IN Ioachim HL, ed: Pathobiology annual. New York: Appleton-Century Crofts, Meredith Corp, 1973: 241–68.

13. Fauve RM, Hevin B, Jacob H, Gailland JA, Jacob F. Antiinflammatory effects of murine malignant cells. Proc Natl Acad Sci USA 1974; 71:4052–6.

14. Patillo RA. Tumor immunology. Obstet Gynecol 1976; 48:374–80.

15. Loke, YW, Immunology and immunopathology of the human foetal-maternal interaction. 2. Special surface properties of human trophoblast cell. New York: Elsevier-North Holland, 1978:15–26.

16. Hammarstrom L, Fuchs T, Smith CIE. The immunodepressive effect of human glucoproteins and their possible role in the nonrejection process during pregnancy. Acta Obstet Gynaecol Scand 1979; 58:417–22.

17. Yorde DE, Hussa RO, Garancis JC, Patillo RA. Immunocytochemical localization of human chorionic gonadotropin in human malignant trophoblast. Model for human chorionic gonadotropin secretion. Lab Invest 1979; 40:391–8.

18. August CS, Cox ST, Naughton MA. Interaction of choriocarcinoma cells to cell-mediated cytotoxicity by mitogen-activated lymphocytes. J Clin Invest 1979; 63:428–36.

19. Fuchs T, Hammarstrom L, Smith CIE, Brudin J. In vitro induction of human suppressor T cells by a chorionic gonadotropin preparation. J Reprod Immunol 1981; 3:75–84.

20. Yamauchi S, Shiotsuka Y, Kobayashi K, Ozawa A. Relationship between human chorionic gonadotropin and behavior of T cell populations in early pregnancy. Am J Reprod Immunol 1981; 1:340–4.

21. Bartocci A, Papademetriou V, Schlick E, Nisula BC, Chirigos MA. Effect of crude and purified human chorionic gonadotropin on murine delayed-type hypersensitivity: A role for prostaglandins. Cell Immunol 1982; 71:326–33.

22. Bartocci A, Welker RD, Schlick E, Chirigos MA, Nisula BC. Immunosuppressive activity of human chorionic gonadotropin preparations in vivo: Evidence for gonadal dependence. Cell Immunol 1983; 82:334–42.

23. Melmed S, Braunstein GD. Human chorionic gonadotropin stimulates proliferation of Nb2 rat lymphoma cells. J Clin Endocrinol Metab 1983; 56:1068–70.

24. Kellen JA, Acevedo HF, Fogarty PA, Raikow RB. Growth effects of human choriogonadotropin on malignant cells. In Anon: Abstracts, Proceedings of the International Symposium Immunobiology of Cancer and Allied Immune Dysfunctions, Copenhagen, Nov 4–7, 1985. Cancer Detect Prevent 1985; 8(5/6): Abstract 024.

25. Hussa RD. Biosynthesis of human choriogonadotropin. Endocrinol Rev 1980; 1:268–94.

26. Acevedo HF, Slifkin M, Pouchet GR, Rakhshan M. Identification of the β-subunit of choriogonadotropin (CG) in human spermatozoa. In Troen P, Nankin HR, eds: The testes in normal and infertile men. New York: Raven Press, 1977: 1985–92.

27. Asch RH, Fernandez EO, Siler-Khodr TM, Pauerstein CJ. Presence of hCG-like substance in human sperm. Am J Obstet Gynecol 1979; 135:1041–7.

28. Ehrlich PH, Moustafa ZA, Krichevsky A, Birken S, Armstrong EG, Canfield RE. Characterization and relative orientation of epitopes for monoclonal antibodies and antisera to human chorionic gonadotropin. Am J Reprod Immunol Microbiol 1985; 8:48–54.

29. Raikow RB, OKunewick JP, Buffo MJ, Kociban DL. Effect of cyclophosphamide on Friend leukemogenesis in virus sensitive and virus resistant mice. Cancer Res 1985; 45:555–7.

30. Snyder MA, Bishop JM, Colby WW, Levinson AD. Phosphorylation of tyrosine-416 is not required for the transforming properties and kinase activity of pp60^{v-src}. Cell 1983; 32:891–901.

31. Chou JY. Regulation of the synthesis of human chorionic gonadotropin by strains of HeLa cells in culture. In Vitro 1978; 14:775–8.

32. Rubin H, Chu BM, Arnstein P. Heritable variation in growth potential and morphology within a clone of Balb/3T3 cells and their relation to tumor formation. JNCI 1983; 71:365–75.

Cancer Detection and Prevention Supplement 1:183–188 (1987)

A Subset of Normal Human B Lymphocytes Expresses an Antigen Cross-Reactive With gp52 of Murine Mammary Tumor Virus

Anne Tax
Lionel A. Manson

Wistar Institute of Anatomy and Biology, Philadelphia, PA 19104

ABSTRACT   Three monoclonal antibodies (MAbs), VE7, VIG3, and IXF9, that detect the 52-kd glycoprotein (gp52) of murine mammary tumor virus (MMTV) were tested for reactivity on normal human tonsillar lymphoid cells in an indirect immunofluorescence assay. Two of the MAbs, VE7 and VIG3, reacted with subpopulations of B cells, whereas the third MAb, IXF9, showed only very low-level reactivity with human lymphoid cells. VE7 and VIG3 also reacted with small populations of peripheral blood lymphocytes, and all three MAbs reacted with some transformed human cell lines. The data suggest that subpopulations of normal human lymphocytes express antigens that are cross-reactive with the MMTV gp52, although not all of the viral gp52 epitopes are expressed on the surface of these cells.

Key words: MMTV, membrane glycoprotein

INTRODUCTION

We have shown by fluorescence microscopy that monoclonal antibody (MAb) VE7, which detects the major 52-kd glycoprotein (gp52) of mouse mammary tumor virus (MMTV) [1], reacts with a small subpopulation of B cells (2.5–4.5%) in C57B1/6 and C3H/He mice. In our most recent experiments (unpublished) using the same MAb but employing the fluorescence-activated cell sorter, we have detected 30–40% positive mouse spleen cells.

Reports from another laboratory have suggested that an antigen similar to that detected in our studies is present in human malignant mammary tissues [2,3]; those investigators detected an antigen immunologically related to gp52 in paraffin sections of human mammary tumors by means of peroxidase immunocytochemistry. The polypeptide rather than the polysaccharide portion of the human antigen is responsible for the immunological reactivity [3]. Furthermore, sequences related to the MMTV genome have been detected in fragments of restricted human cellular DNA isolated from normal spleen as well as from a mammary adenocarcinoma using blot hybridization under low-stringency conditions [4,5]. Although the sequences detected are related to the *gag*, *pol*, and *env* regions of recombinant MMTV proviral DNA, the origin of these sequences is as yet unknown.

Address reprint requests to Lionel A. Manson, The Wistar Institute of Anatomy and Biology, 36th Street at Spruce, Philadelphia, PA 19104.

These reports prompted us to investigate the possible expression by normal human lymphoid cells of the gp52-cross-reactive antigen using VE7 and other MAbs that detect gp52 [6,7]. We demonstrate here that a large subpopulation of normal human tonsillar lymphocytes and a small population of peripheral blood lymphocytes as well as some transformed human cell lines express antigens cross-reactive with gp52. The expression of gp52-cross-reactive antigens on both normal murine and human cells and on transformed human cells suggests a common ontogeny for the gp52 antigen in the two species.

MATERIALS AND METHODS
Cell Lines

All human cell lines used in this study (Table I) were provided by Dr. Giorgio Trinchieri of The Wistar Institute.

Antibodies

The preparation of biotinylated F(ab')$_2$ fragments of IgG$_3$ MAb VE7 (BIOT VE7,) which binds to gp52 of MMTV, and biotinylated F(ab')$_2$ fragments of J606 (BIOT J6O6), an IgG$_3$ myeloma (control), has been described previously [1]. Two IgM MAbs against gp52 of MMTV, VIG3 and IXF9 [7], were also used in these studies. The IgM fractions from the ascites fluid of these hybridomas and from the ascites fluid of antiphosphorylcholine (anti-PC) hybridoma, an IgM control (obtained from David Hilbert, University of Pennsylvania), were isolated by precipitation with 50% $(NH_4)_2SO_4$. These IgM fractions were biotinylated as described previously [8]. Fluoresceinated F(ab')$_2$ fragments of antihuman IgG (heavy and light chain-specific) preabsorbed on a mouse Ig-Sepharose 4B column to eliminate antibodies cross-reactive with mouse immunoglobulin were provided by Dr. Giorgio Trinchieri.

Competition Assay

MAb IXF9 or VIG3 was used to compete with the binding of MAb VE7 to YAC-1 cells, a tissue culture line derived from a Moloney virus-induced lymphoma of A/SN origin [9]. Because ^{125}I-labeled protein A binds to MAb VE7 but not to IXF9 or VIG3 (not shown), a decrease in binding of ^{125}I-labeled protein A was taken as an indicator of competition between VE7 and IXF9 or VIG3. YAC-1 cells were washed three times in phosphate-buffered saline (PBS) with gelatin and NaN$_3$. These cells were subsequently incubated for 30 min at 4°C with predetermined optimal dilutions of MAb alone or VE7 plus a competing MAb. After three washes with the PBS-gelatin solution, ^{125}I-labeled protein A (55,000 cpm; New England Nuclear, Boston, MA) was added to the cells, which were incubated for 15 min at 4°C, washed, and counted in a gamma counter.

TABLE I. Reactivity of Human Cell Lines With MAb to gp52

Cell line	Cell type	VE7*	VIG3†	IXF9†
Raji	Burkitt lymphoma	41.5‡	31.0	1.6
Daudi	Burkitt lymphoma	14.5	25.6	2.3
8866	B-cell line	3.5	2.6	6.7
MOLT4	T-cell acute lymphocytic leukemia	5.5	2.6	1.4
KGI-a	Acute myeloid leukemia	6.6	8.0	5.8
U937	Histiocytic lymphoma	7.2	22.1	29.8
K562	Erythroleukemia cell line	9.6	6.0	20.9
HL-60	Promyelocytic leukemia	5.5	13.2	11.6

*Control for VE7 was J606 (IgG$_3$ myeloma).
†Control for VIG3 and IXF9 was anti-PC (IgM).
‡Percent positive.

Human Peripheral Blood Lymphocyte and Tonsillar Lymphocyte Preparations

Mononuclear cells were obtained from heparinized venous peripheral blood of normal donors by Ficoll-Hypaque gradient centrifugation. The monocytes were partially depleted from these cells by two successive incubations on plastic flasks at 37°C for 1 hr. Nonadherent cells are referred to as peripheral blood lymphocytes.

Human tonsils were obtained after routine tonsillectomies from Children's Hospital of Philadelphia. These tissues were immediately submerged in cold saline after the surgery. Single cell suspensions were prepared by first cutting small pieces of tonsil with fine scissors and then extruding these pieces through a metal tissue sieve. Mononuclear cells were obtained from the washed tonsil cells by Ficoll-Hypaque gradient centrifugation. The monocytes were partially depleted from the mononuclear cells as described above. The remaining cells are referred to as tonsillar lymphocytes.

Indirect Immunofluorescence Assays

Cell preparations were washed three times before assay in PBS containing 0.1% gelatin and 0.1% NaN_3. Cell viability was greater than 90% as determined by erythrosin B dye exclusion.

Cells were incubated with biotinylated MAb preparations for 30 min at 4°C. After three washes in PBS with gelatin and NaN_3, the cells were incubated with fluorescein avidin DCS3 (Vector Laboratories, Burlingame, CA) for 15 min at 4°C. In dual immunofluorescence assays, the cells were first incubated with BIOT VE7 and subsequently incubated with fluoresceinated $F(ab')_2$ fragments of antihuman IgG and rhodamine 600 avidin D (Vector Laboratories). Fluorescent cells were analyzed by means of an Ortho Cytofluorograf System H50 connected to a Data General MP/200 microprocessor (Ortho Instruments, Westwood, MA).

RESULTS

Yac-1 cells were incubated with VE7 alone or VE7 plus VIG3, IXF9, or anti-PC (control). ^{125}I-labeled protein A was then added to detect the VE7 bound to the cells. YAC-1 cells were chosen for the competition assays because all three MAb against gp52 bind to the majority of the cells in this line, as shown by immunofluorescence analysis (Table II). The results of the competition experiment are presented in Table III.

The IgM control (anti-PC) or VIG3 did not interfere with the binding of VE7 to YAC 1 cells, suggesting that VE7 binds to a different epitope than does VIG3. In contrast, IXF9 partially blocked the binding of VE7 to YAC cells. Thus IXF9 and VE7 might bind to cross-reactive epitopes or to different epitopes located in close proximity on the YAC cell surface, where binding of VE7 to YAC might be prevented sterically.

We have shown previously in the mouse system that a subpopulation of B cells expresses an antigen cross-reactive with gp52 of MMTV [1]. We have now extended these results to the

TABLE II. Immunofluorescence Analysis of the Reactivity of MAb Against gp52 With YAC-1 Cells

Monoclonal antibody	Percent positive cells
J606* (control)	1.1
VE7*	71.2
Anti-PC (control)†	1.5
VIG3†	81.3
IXF9†	91.5

*BIOT VE7 and BIOT J606 were used at a 1:5 dilution.
†BIOT anti-PC, BIOT VIG3, and BIOT IXF9 were used at a 1:20 dilution.

**TABLE III. Competition of MAbs VIG3 and IXF9
With MAb VE7 for Binding to
YAC-1 Cells**

Antibodies*	cpm† (mean ± SE)
VE7 + buffer	1,171 ± 137
VE7 + anti-PC (control)	1,135 ± 39
VE7 + VIG3	1,249 ± 97
VE7 + IXF9	574 ± 18

*Final concentration of VE7, anti-PC, VIG3, and IXF9
was 1:16.
†Triplicate determinations.

**TABLE IV. Reactivity of Normal Human Peripheral Blood Lymphocytes and Tonsil Cells With
MAb Against gp52**

	J606* (IgG₃ control)	VE7	Anti-PC† (IgM control)	VIG3	IXF9
Peripheral blood lymphocyte (donor 1)	2.5‡	10.2	0.9	1.9	2.4
Peripheral blood lymphocyte (donor 2)	1.7	13.0	0.6	2.7	2.1
Tonsil cells	9.5	61.3	2.3	54.7	8.7

*Biotinylated J606 (IgG₃) and VE7 were diluted 1:5.
†Biotinylated anti-PC (IgM control), VIG3, and IXF9 were diluted 1:16.
‡Percent positive.

**TABLE V. Dual Immunofluorescence Analysis of the Reactivity of Monoclonal Antibody VE7 and
Antihuman IgG for Normal Human Tonsillar Lymphocytes**

Experiment	J606* (IgG₃ control)	VE7	VE7-positive cells staining with antihuman IgG
1	1.1†	39.8	99.1
2	1.7	34.6	97.0

*Biotinylated J606 (IgG) and VE7 were diluted 1:5. Fluoresceinated F(ab')₂ antihuman IgG was diluted
1:20.
†Percent positive.

human system. As listed in Table IV, VE7 binds to 10–13% normal peripheral blood lymphocytes and 61% of tonsillar lymphocytes. VIG3 binds to a smaller percentage of peripheral
blood lymphocytes and also of tonsillar lymphocytes. IXF9 binds less than 15% of the number
of tonsillar lymphocytes bound by VE7. These data, consistent with the data in Table III,
suggest that VE7, VIG3, and IXF9 bind to different epitopes on the cell surface. They further
suggest that subpopulations of normal human lymphocytes express antigens that are cross-
reactive with gp52 of MMTV, although not all of the epitopes present on the viral gp52 are
expressed on the surface of these cells.

Dual fluorescence labeling experiments were carried out to determine as to whether VE7
detects a B-cell subset among tonsil cells (Table V). More than 95% of the tonsil cells that
bound BIOT VE7 also bound antihuman IgG, suggesting that most of the VE7-positive cells
are B cells.

The results of an immunofluorescence experiment in which the three anti-gp52 MAb
were reactive with various human cell lines are shown in Table I. In general, VE7 and VIG3

bound to a larger proportion of Burkitt lymphoma (B cells) cells as compared to other cell lines with the exception of U937 histiocytic lymphoma cells.

DISCUSSION

The results of this study are consistent with those of Callahan et al [4] and May et al [5], who showed that normal human tissue DNA contained sequences that annealed to MMTV probes under low-stringency conditions. It is possible that our MAbs are detecting the proteins encoded by these sequences.

Studies in other retrovirus systems suggest a relationship between retrovirus expression and B-cell function. For the mouse system, there have been reports of inhibitory effects on the immune responses in mice after exposure to antisera against murine leukemia viruses [10.11], a mitogenic effect of certain goat and rabbit antileukemia virus antisera on B lymphocytes of most conventional mouse strains [12], and the induction of endogenous retrovirus synthesis and viral antigen expression in mouse spleen cells exposed to LPS [13,14]. In addition, mitogen stimulation of chicken lymphocytes increases the expression of retroviral envelope protein [15]. These studies suggest that retroviral sequences in DNA might influence normal lymphocyte maturation and/or function.

ACKNOWLEDGMENTS

We express our appreciation to Dr. William Potsic of the Children's Hospital of Philadelphia for providing us with tonsils and to Dr. Giorgio Trinchieri for his helpful advice. We also appreciate the technical assistance of Ms. Jennifer Kennedy and the editorial assistance of Ms. Marina Hoffman. This work was supported by USPHS grant CA-10815 awarded by the National Cancer Institute, NHHS, and grant IM-309 awarded by the American Cancer Society.

REFERENCES

1. Tax A, Ewert D, Manson LA. An antigen cross-reactive with gp52 of mammary tumor virus is expressed on a B cell subpopulation of mice. J Immunol 1983; 130:2368–71.
2. Mesa-Tejada R, Keydar I, Ramanarayanen M, Ohno T, Fenoglio C, Spiegelman S. Detection in human breast carcinomas of an antigen immunologically related to a group-specific antigen of mouse mammary tumor virus. Proc Natl Acad Sci USA 1978; 75:1529–33.
3. Ohno T, Mesa-Tejada R, Keydar I, Ramanarayanan M, Bausch J, Spiegelman S. Human breast carcinoma antigen is immunologically related to the polypeptide of the group-specific glycoprotein of mouse mammary tumor virus. Proc Natl Acad Sci USA 1978; 76:2460–4.
4. Callahan R, Drohan W, Tronick S, Schlom J. Detection and cloning of human DNA sequences related to the mouse mammary tumor virus genome. Proc Natl Acad Sci USA 1982; 79:5503–7.
5. May FEB, Westley BR, Rochefort H, Buetti E, Diggelmann H. Mouse mammary tumor virus related sequences are present in human DNA Nucleic Acids Res 1983; 11:4127–39.
6. Tax A, Manson LA. Monoclonal antibodies against antigens displayed on a progressively growing mammary tumor. Proc Natl Acad Sci USA 1981; 78:529–33.
7. Tax A, Manson LA. Monoclonal antibodies directed against epitopes of the gp52 of mouse mammary tumor virus. Fed Proc 1982; 41:521.
8. Godding JW. Antibody production by hybridomas. J Immunol Meth. 1980; 39:285–306.
9. Cikes M, Firber S, Klein G. Progressive loss of H-2 antigens with concomitant increase of cell-surface antigen(s) determined by Moloney leukemia virus in cultured murine lymphomas. JNCI 1973; 50:347–62.
10. Moroni C, Schumann G. Are endogenous C-type viruses involved in the immune system? Nature 1977; 269:600–1.
11. Wecker E, Schimple A, Hunig T. Expression of MuLV GP71-like antigen in normal mouse spleen cells induced by antigenic stimulation. Nature 1977; 269:598–600.

12. Moroni C, Forni L, Hunsmann G, Schumann G. Antibody directed against Friend leukemia virus stimulates DNA synthesis in a subpopulation of mouse B lymphocytes. Proc Natl Acad Sci USA 1980; 79:1486–90.

13. Moroni C, Schumann G. Lipopolysaccharide induces C-type virus in short-term cultures of Balb/c spleen cells. Nature 1975; 254:60–1.

14. Alberto BF, Callahan LF, Pincus T. Evidence that retrovirus expression in mouse spleen cells result from B cell differentiation. J Immunol 1982; 129:2768–72.

15. Ewert DL, Vainio O, Halpern MS. Increased endogenous retroviral gene expression is a consequence of lymphocyte activation. J Immunol 1983; 131:3036–41.

Cancer Detection and Prevention Supplement 1:189–205 (1987)

Monoclonal Antibody to HSV$_2$ Protein as an Immunodiagnostic Marker in Cervical Cancer

Silvano Costa, MD
Antonia D'Errico, MD
Walter F. Grigioni, MD
Camillo Orlandi, MD

Cinthya C. Smith, PhD
Antonio M. Mancini, MD
Laure Aurelian, PhD

Departments of Obstetrics and Gynecology (S.C., C.O.) and Pathology (A.D'E., A.M.M., W.F.G.), University of Bologna Medical School, Bologna, Italy; Divisions of Biophysics (C.C.S., L.A.) and Comparative Medicine (C.C.S., L.A.), The Johns Hopkins Medical Institutions, Baltimore, MD; Department of Pharmacology and Experimental Therapeutics, The University of Maryland School of Medicine, Baltimore, MD (L.A.)

ABSTRACT   The present study was designed to evaluate the possible use of monoclonal antibodies (mAbs) as diagnostic adjuncts to exfoliative cytology and tissue sections in intraepithelial (CIN) and invasive cervical cancer. Specimens were collected from 42 patients with various degrees of CIN, 15 patients with invasive cancer and two patients with condylomatous changes only. mAb H17, that recognizes a herpes simplex virus protein (ICP) representing a component of the viral ribonucleotide reductase, stained atypical exfoliated cells from 55% of patients with mild dysplasia and 100% of those with more severe lesions. The mean percentage of positive atypical cells increased as a function of the grading of CIN (32.6 $\pm$ 6.3%, 63.5 $\pm$ 2.7%, 67.9 $\pm$ 8.1%, 81.4 $\pm$ 10.1%, and 85.6 $\pm$ 2.0% for mild, moderate, and marked dysplasia, CIS, and invasive cancer, respectively). Only a very small proportion of atypical cells from only two patients stained with a mAb to another herpes simplex virus protein (gA/B). Normal squamous, metaplastic, inflammatory, or koilocytotic cells did not stain with the mAbs. Of the 15 cases examined by cryostatic fresh sections with immunohistochemical techniques, only one case of invasive cancer did not stain with mAb anti-ICP, and all controls were negative. The high specificity and sensitivity of MAbH17 suggests that it may be a useful diagnostic/prognostic marker in CIN.

Key words: cancer immunology, HSV$_2$ antigen, tumoral markers

INTRODUCTION

The progression of precancerous cervical lesions to invasive cancer is unpredictable and cannot be prognosticated on morphology alone. For the clinician and the pathologist, who

Address reprint requests to Dr. S. Costa, Virology Immunology Lab, Department of Pharmacology and Experimental Therapeutics, University of Maryland School of Medicine, 10 S. Pine Street, Rm. 500F, Baltimore, MD 21201.

every day face crucial prognostic decisions relating to patient management, recent viral etiology studies hold the promise of identifying biologically significant (viral) markers capable of defining those cytologically identified atypias that will progress to more severe (CIS/ invasive cancer) lesions.

Two viral infections [Herpes simplex (HSV$_2$) and human papillomavirus (HPV)] have been associated with squamous cervical carcinoma. Serological and epidemiological studies have shown that (1) HSV$_2$-infected women are at a significantly higher risk for developing cervical cancer than uninfected ones, (2) HSV$_2$ infection precedes the development of the cervical intraepithelial (CIN) or invasive neoplasia, and (3) the rate of CIN is two-to eight-fold higher in virus-infected than uninfected women. Furthermore, inactivated HSV$_2$ causes neoplastic transformation of normal diploid cells in vitro and CIN and invasive cancer in cervically infected mice. The transforming functions are mediated by viral genetic information as evidenced by the findings that (1) transforming potential is localized within specific HSV$_2$ DNA sequences and (2) HSV$_2$ immunization protects mice from HSV$_2$-induced cervical neoplasia [reviewed in 1]. Hybridization studies have revealed the presence of sequences homologous to invasive cervical cancer tissue [2], but the virus has not yet been shown to cause neoplastic transformation in vitro.

For the clinician interested in a rapid, simple, and reproducible marker of CIN cells destined to progress to invasive cancer, either one of these viruses holds promise. However, in the case of HPV, antigen expression decreases with the progression of atypical lesion [3], and DNA hybridization is a relatively complex assay that destroys cellular morphology, thereby precluding pathological staging of the individual DNA-positive cells.

In this paper, we describe the staining of exfoliated cervical CIN and invasive cancer cells with monoclonal antibodies (mAb) to a protein (ICP10) encoded by one set of transforming HSV$_2$ DNA sequences [4].

MATERIALS AND METHODS
Cells and Virus

Human epidermoid carcinoma No. 2 (HEp-2) cells were grown in medium 199 with 10% calf serum. The G strain of HSV$_2$ was used as previously described [5].

Production of Hybridomas

The method of production and culturing of the hybridomas was essentially as described by Oi and Herzenberg [6]. Briefly, BALB/c mice were injected in the footpad with soluble extracts of HEp-2 cells infected with HSV$_2$ for 12 hr (containing virtually all viral proteins [5]) emulsified in complete Freund adjuvant. After 4 weeks, the mice were primed (IP injection) with the extract in incomplete Freund adjuvant, and then an aqueous antigen boost was given intravenously 4 weeks later. After 3 days, the spleen cells were fused with an equal number of NS-1 cells with polyethylene glycol 1,000 (Sigma, St. Louis, MO). The cultures were subjected to a 2 week regime with culture medium containing hypoxanthine, aminopterine, and thymidine [7]. For screening the viable hybrids for production of the desired antibody, the culture fluids were tested by indirect immunofluorescent (FA) staining of murine L cells infected with HSV$_2$ for 12 hr (to avoid reactivity with host cell antigens). A hybridoma culture (designated H17) that secreted a sufficient amount of antibody to stain 100% of the infected cells (and did not stain the uninfected ones) was cloned by limiting dilution in the presence of BALB/c thymocytes. Ascitic fluid with antibody was obtained by injecting hybrid clones that continued to produce antibody IP into pristane-treated mice.

Antibodies

Antiserum to ICP10 was prepared in BALB/c mice with ICP10 obtained from HEp-2 cells infected with HSV$_2$ for 4 hr and purified to radiochemical homogeneity as previously described [8]. Antiserum to total soluble HSV$_2$ proteins was also prepared in BALB/c mice using extracts from 18 hr-infected HEp-2 cells prepared as previously described [5,9]. mAb 48S was obtained from Dr. M. Zweig (Laboratory of Molecular Virology, NCI, Frederick, MD). It recognizes type-common determinants on the HSV$_1$-encoded protein ICP6 [10] and precipitates the HSV$_1$- and HSV$_2$-induced ribonucleotide reductase activity [11]. mAb 20αD4 precipitates glycoprotein gA/B from HSV$_2$-infected cells [12]. It was obtained from Dr. W. Rawls (McMaster University, Ontario, Canada).

SDS-Acrylamide Gel Electrophoresis

Electrophoretic staining and autoradiography were as described previously [5,8]. The polyacrylamide gel electrophoresis was done in a discontinuous buffer system with 0.1% SDS. The separation gel contained 8.5% acrylamide cross-linked with N,N-diallyltartardiamide (Aldrich Chemical, North Chicago, IL) in an amount corresponding to 4% of the weight of acrylamide as described by Heine et al [13].

Radioimmunoprecipitation

To prepare radiolabeled infected cell proteins (ICP) HEp-2 cells were exposed to 20 plaque-forming units (PFU)/cell of HSV$_2$ for 12 hr and labeled with ^{35}S-methionine (20 μCi); Amersham, Arlington Heights, IL; sp. act. 200 C/mM). The medium for labeling the ICP was minimal essential medium (MEM) with 0.1$\times$ the normal concentration of L-methionine and 1% dialyzed fetal calf serum (FCS). Cell pellets were resuspended in one part Buffer A [10 mM Tris HCl, pH 7.8, 0.8 M KCl, 1 mM phenylmethilsulfonyl fluoride (PMSF) and 1% Triton] followed by four parts Buffer B (Buffer A free of KCl). Extracts were clarified by centrifugation for 1 hr at 190,000 g and the supernatants filtered through a 0.22 μm Millipore filter. The reaction mixtures contained 500 μl of cell extract (antigen) and 25 μl of the respective antibody. They were incubated for 1 hr at room temperature and then with 100 μl of a 50% v/v suspension of protein A-Sepharose Cl-4B for 15 min. At this time, the beads were washed three times in NET buffer (50 mM Tris HCl, pH 7.4, 150 mM NaCl, 5 mM EDTA, 0.02% sodium azide) with 0.5 M lithium chloride and 0.05% Triton. They were resuspended in 70 μm of denaturing solution, boiled for 5 min, and centrifuged at 4,500 g, and the supernatants were analyzed by SDS-acrylamide gel electrophoresis.

Immunocytohistochemical Procedures

Immunofluorescent staining. Indirect immunofluorescent (FA) staining was done as previously described [5] with fluorescein-conjugated goat anti mouse IgG (Cappel, Cochranville, PA). Slides were examined using a Zeiss microscope with epillumination (HBO 100 W lamp, KP 490 exciter, and KP 510 barrier filters). Documentation was done using Kodak 200 ASA daylight-type color film.

Immunoperoxidase staining. The immunohistochemical method employed was avidin-biotin-peroxidase complex [14,15]. Sections were rinsed in Tris-hydroximethyllamminomethane HCl buffer (TBS), pH 7.4, for 5 min, and treated in a 0.3% solution of 30% H$_2$O$_2$ in TBS for 30 min to inhibit endogenous peroxidase activity and washed in TBS for 20 min. Sections were then incubated with nonimmune horse serum (1:60) for 30 min and subsequently with mAb Hl7 overnight (we did not test the tissues with the others mAbs). After three washings in TBS for 20 min, the sections were incubated with biotynilated antimouse immunoglobulin for 30 min, washed in TBS for 20 min, reincubated with avidin-biotin-peroxidase complex for 1 hr at dark, and again washed in TBS for 20 min. The peroxidase reaction was developed for 3 min in a fresh solution of 0.02% 3,3'-diaminobenzidine-tetrahydrochloride in TBS with 0.12% H$_2$O$_2$. Next followed the counterstaining in Mayer's hematoxylin and the mounting in Eukitt.

Specimen Collection

Exfoliative cytology. Exfoliated cervical cells were collected by scraping the cervix with an Ayre spatula. They were washed three times in PBS by centrifugation at 3,000 rpm for 10 min and resuspended in PBS, and slides were prepared as previously described [5]. The slides were air dried, fixed in acetone, and stored at 4°C until stained. At least three slides were obtained for each patient.

All slides were examined with cell-by-cell analysis to establish the FA-positive/total atypical cell ratios. A cell was accepted as positive if it was sufficiently bright to be clearly visible against the dark background of the smear. The coordinates of all atypical cells (FA-positive or -negative), and those of 100 FA-negative normal squamous cells were established and the slides restained by the Papanicolau procedure. All the cells were relocated in order to classify them according to morphological criteria. The FA reading and the determination of the cell coordinates were done by one observer. The relocated cells were classified by an independent cytopathologist as previously described [5].

Histological section. Biopsy specimens for immunohistochemical study were taken under colposcopic vision and stored in liquid nitrogen. Four micrometer frozen sections were cut in a cryostat at −20°C, immediately fixed in cold acetone for 10 min, and stained using an avidin-biotin-peroxidase complex. Moreover, a fragment of a pathological tissue was used for histological diagnosis using the hematoxylin-eosin procedure.

Study population. Thirty-four patients (nine with mild dysplasia, 11 with moderate dysplasia, seven with marked dysplasia, four with carcinoma in situ (CIS), one with invasive cancer, and two (Nos. 821 and 828) with condylomatous features only), as well as 20 women with normal cytology, were seen in the outpatient cervical clinic of The Johns Hopkins Hospital. Among the patients with cervical dysplasia, two (Nos. 829, mild dysplasia, and 827, marked dysplasia) also had condylomatous features. Eleven patients with invasive cancer (identified by initials) were seen in the Obstetrics and Gynecology Clinic of the University of Bologna, Bologna, Italy. Cervical tissue samples were obtained by punch biopsy in 11 Italian patients with various degrees of CIN (one moderate, five marked dysplasia, and five CIS) and in four patients with invasive cancer, as well as in three patients with normal cervical epithelium. Samples used for diagnosis and study were collected at the same patient visit. Patients were diagnosed according to cytological and histological criteria by the appropriate services within the Pathology Departments. Bioptical samples were stored in liquid nitrogen; then 4 μm frozen sections were cut in a cryostat at −20°C. Histological diagnosis was performed with hematoxylin-eosin staining using routine methods.

RESULTS
Specificity of H17 Antibody

These studies were designed to define the protein specificity of mAb H17 by comparing it to mAb 48S, which recognizes virus type-common determinants on the ICP6 protein of HSV_1 [10], and mAb 20αD4, which recognizes the HSV_2-specified glycoprotein gA/B [12]. Extracts of 12 hr HSV_2 (Fig. 1A, lane 1)- or mock (Fig. 1A, lane 2)-infected HEp-2 cells labeled with ^{35}S-methionine [0–12 hrs. postinfection (PI)] were immunoprecipitated with mAbs H17, 48S, and 20αD4 and with antisera to total HSV_2 proteins or to a viral protein (ICP10) encoded by one set of transforming DNA sequences. Preimmune mouse serum and ascites fluid were used as negative controls.

Infected cell extracts contained virtually all the viral proteins (Fig. 1A, lane 1), and these were immunoprecipitated by antiserum to total HSV_2 proteins (Fig. 1C, lane 11). However, mAbs H17 and 48S precipitated only a 144 K protein from the infected cell extract (Fig. 1B, lanes 5,7). They did not recognize any protein in the mock-infected cells (Fig. 1B, lanes 6,8). The 144 K protein was also precipitated from the infected (Fig. 1A, lane 4) but not mock-infected cells (Fig. 1A, lane 3) by antiserum to ICP10 and not by mAb 20αD4 (Fig. 2, lane 2). The preimmune mouse serum (Fig. 1C, lane 10) and the ascitic fluid (Fig. 1B, lane 9) were negative.

Antigenic Relationship Between Antiserum to ICP10 and mAbs H17 and 48S

To determine whether the 144 K proteins precipitated by the three reagents studied in these series (H17, 48S, anti-ICP10) share antigenic determinants, extracts of HEp-2 cells

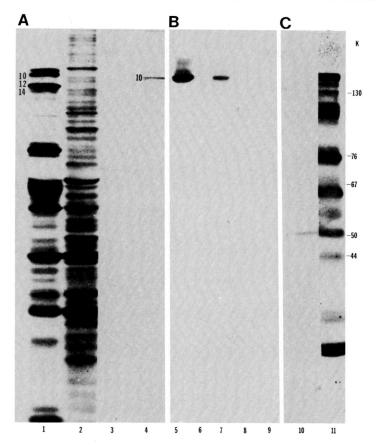

Fig. 1.   Immunoprecipitates resulting from the reaction of extracts of HEp-2 cells infected with HSV$_2$ and labeled with ^{35}S-methionine at 0–12 hr PI (lane 1) and anti-ICP10 serum (lane 4), mAb 48S (lane 5), mAb H17 (lane 7), NS-1 control (lane 9), preimmune serum (lane 10), or antiserum to total HSV$_2$ proteins (lane 11). HEp-2 cells simultaneously mock-infected with PBS and labeled with ^{35}S-methionine (lane 2) were also immunoprecipitated with anti-ICP10 serum (lane 3), mAb 48S (lane 6), and mAb H17 (lane 8). Gels in A–C are not directly comparable in that they were run independently. MW markers (K) are listed on the left. Infected cell protein (ICP) nomenclature is shown on the right.

infected with HSV$_2$ or mock-infected with PBS and labeled with ^{35}S-methionine at 0–12 hr PI, were adsorbed with one of the reagents (48S, H17, or anti-ICP10 serum) and cross-adsorbed with the heterologous ones. The products of the cross-adsorbtion reactions were analyzed by SDS-acrylamide gel electrophoresis. mAb 20αD4 was used as control.

Adsorption with mAb 48S (Fig. 2, lane 4) removed the antigenic determinants recognized by the homologous antibody (Fig. 2, lane 3) as well as those recognized by mAb H17 (Fig. 2, lane 6) and anti-ICP10 serum (Fig. 2, lane 7). Reciprocally, adsorption with mAb H17 (Fig. 2, lane 1) removed the antigenic determinants recognized by mAb 48S (Fig. 2, lane 5; Fig. 3, lane 6) or anti-ICP10 serum (Fig. 3, lane 7). It did not remove the antigenic determinants recognized by mAb 20αD4 (Fig. 2, lane 2). Adsorbtion of the infected cell extracts with anti-ICP10 serum (Fig. 3, lane 2) removed the antigenic determinants recognized by mAb 48S (Fig. 3, lane 3), mAb H17 (Fig. 3, lane 4), and anti-ICP10 serum (Fig. 3, lane 5). We interpret these data to indicate that mAb H17 has an antigenic specificity similar to that of mAb 48S and polyclonal anti-ICP10 serum but not mAb 20αD4.

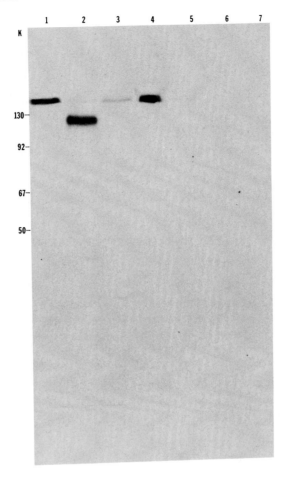

Fig. 2. Cross-reactivity between H17 and 48S mAbs. Extracts (500 μl) of 12 hr-infected cells were incubated with H17 (50 μl) in the presence of protein A-sepharose Cl-4B beads (100 μl) for 2 hr at 4°C with constant mixing. The immunoprecipitates were collected by centrifugation (lane 1) and the super-natants reacted with MAB 20αD4 (lane 2) or mAb 48S (lane 5). Reciprocally, the extracts were adsorbed with 48S antibody (lane 4) and then reacted with the homologous 48S (lane 3) or with the heterologous mAb H17 (lane 6) or anti-ICP10 serum (lane 7). The immunoprecipitates were solubilized and electro-phoresed on 8.5% SDS-acrylamide gels. MW markers (K) are on the left.

Staining of Exfoliated Cervical Cells

Atypical cells from five of nine (55.5%) cases of mild dysplasia and all cases of moderate or marked dysplasia, CIS, or invasive cancer stained with mAb H17 (Tables I–V). The proportion of staining cells increased with the progression of the lesion. Thus, in the five positive mild dysplasia cases, 20–53% (mean 32.6 ± 6.3%) of the atypical cells were H17-positive. In the moderate dysplasia group, the proportion of H17 staining cells ranged between 48% and 76.9% (mean 63.5± 2.7%) in the marked and CIS groups, the percentages were, respectively 33.3%–92.5% (mean 67.9 ± 8.1%) and 52.9–98.2% (mean 81.4 ± 10.12%). In the invasive cancer series, the proportion of H17-positive cells ranged between 75.4% and 96% (mean 85.6 ± 2.0%). The staining was cytoplasmic and/or intranuclear (Figs. 4–6).

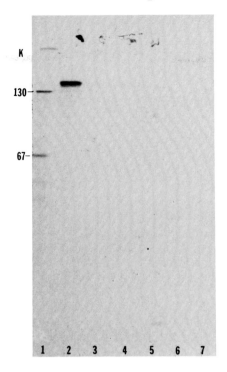

Fig. 3.   Cross-reactivity between anti-ICP10 serum and mAbs 48S and H17. Extracts of 12 hr-infected cells were reacted with anti-ICP10 serum (lane 2) as described in Figure 2 and the supernatants readsorbed with mAb 48S (lane 3), mAb H17 (lane 4), or anti-ICP10 serum (lane 5). The supernatants obtained after adsorbtion of the infected cell antigen with mAb H17 (Fig. 2, lane 1) were reacted with mAb 48S (lane 6) or anti-ICP10 serum (lane 7). ^{125}I-labeled β-galactosidase (130 K) and bovine serum albumin (67 K) were used as MW markers.

TABLE I. Staining of Exfoliated Cells From Patients With Mild Dysplasia

Patient No.	Atypical cells staining with*		
	H17	20αD4	Anti-ICP10
823	6/30 (20)	0/31 (0)	2/35 (5.7)
824	2/10 (20)	0/22 (0)	1/15 (6.7)
829	13/33 (39.3)	0/51 (0)	5/40 (12.5)
831	0/36 (0)	0/34 (0)	3/30 (10)
837	0/31 (0)	0/25 (0)	0/29 (0)
838	8/26 (30.7)	0/38 (0)	2/30 (6.7)
841	27/51 (53.1)	0/65 (0)	6/80 (7.5)
845	0/44 (0)	0/29 (0)	0/50 (0)
846	0/21 (0)	0/15 (0)	0/18 (0)
Mean (positive cases)	11.2/30 (32.6)	0/34 (0)	3.2/38 (8.7)

*All atypical cells on the slide were counted, and the proportion staining with the respective antibody was identified. Parentheses represent percentage of positive cells. Preimmune serum did not stain. Normal squamous cells and koilocytes (No. 829) did not stain with mAbs H17 and 20αD4. Metaplastic cells from patients No. 829 (3%) and No. 837 (6%) stained with anti-ICP10 serum.

TABLE II. Staining of Exfoliated Cells From Patients With Moderate Dysplasia

Patient No.	Atypical cells staining with*		
	H17	20αD4	Anti-ICP10
717	25/52 (48)	0/30 (0)	12/50 (24)
725	80/104 (76.9)	0/77 (0)	29/100 (29)
741	25/37 (67.5)	0/60 (0)	0/51 (0)
754	4/6 (66.6)	0/27 (0)	0/9 (0)
755	43/65 (66.1)	0/69 (0)	6/40 (15)
758	29/41 (70.7)	0/53 (0)	0/71 (0)
783	21/31 (65.6)	0/27 (0)	9/37 (24)
793	21/43 (48.8)	0/65 (0)	20/60 (33.3)
795	20/36 (55.5)	0/33 (0)	0/22 (0)
820	15/22 (68.1)	0/27 (0)	0/23 (0)
826	78/120 (65)	17/209 (8)	20/97 (20.6)
Mean (positive cases)	32.8/50.7 (63.5)		16/64 (25)

*All atypical cells on the slide were counted, and the proportion staining with the respective antibody was identified. Parentheses represent percentage of positive cells. Preimmune serum did not stain. Normal squamous and inflammatory cells did not stain with mAbs H17 and 20αD4. Metaplastic cells from patients No. 758 (7%) and No. 795 (2%) stained with antiserum to ICP10.

TABLE III. Staining of Exfoliated Cells From Patients With Marked Dysplasia

Patient No.	Atypical cells staining with*		
	H17	20αD4	anti-ICP10
764	3/9 (33.3)	0/12 (0)	0/21 (0)
822	37/40 (92.5)	0/72 (0)	10/50 (20)
827	20/24 (83.3)	0/43 (0)	5/35 (14.3)
835	52/76 (68.4)	0/62 (0)	0/88 (0)
842	61/70 (87.1)	3/67 (4.4)	11/109 (10.1)
844	8/15 (53.3)	0/35 (0)	5/27 (18.5)
848	15/26 (57.6)	0/27 (0)	8/41 (19.5)
Mean (positive cases)	28/37.1 (67.9)		7.8/52.4 (14.9)

*All atypical cells on the slide were counted, and the proportion staining with the appropriate antibody was determined. Parentheses represent percentage of positive cells. Preimmune serum did not stain. Normal squamous cells and koilocytes (No. 827) did not stain with mAbs H17 and 20αD4. Metaplastic cells from patient No. 822 (6%) stained with anti-ICP10 serum.

TABLE IV. Staining of Exfoliated Cells From Patients With CIS

Patient No.	Atypical cells staining with*	
	H17	20αD4
825	50/54 (92.6)	0/53 (0)
830	221/225 (98.2)	0/127 (0)
833	9/17 (52.9)	0/25 (0)
836	96/117 (82)	0/81 (0)
Mean (positive cases)	94/103.2 (81.4)	

*All atypical cells on the slide were counted, and the proportion staining with the respective antibody was identified. Parentheses represent the percentage of staining cells. Preimmune serum did not stain. Normal squamous cells did not stain.

**TABLE V. Staining of Exfoliated Cells From Patients
With Invasive Cancer**

Patient	Atypical cells staining with H17*
N.H.	106/127 (83.5)
D.G.	98/130 (75.4)
B.K.	103/115 (89.6)
B.D.	83/97 (85.6)
R.L.	105/121 (86.8)
G.A.	77/93 (82.8)
B.A.	121/150 (80.7)
S.L.	181/194 (93.3)
T.T.	121/132 (91.7)
S.I.	82/107 (76.6)
M.M.	120/125 (96)
Mean (positive cases)	108.8/126.4 (85.6)

*All atypical cells on the slide were counted, and the proportion staining with the H17 antibody was determined. Parentheses represent percentage of staining cells. Preimmune serum did not stain and normal squamous cells were negative.

The percentage of patients with mild dysplasia who had atypical cells reactive with anti-ICP10 serum [six of nine (66.7%)] was essentially similar to that [five of nine (55.5%)] reacting with mAb H17. However, the percentage of patients with ICP10-positive atypical cells was lower in the moderate (25%) and marked (14.9%) dysplasia groups (Tables I–III). Furthermore, anti-ICP10 serum also stained a small proportion (1–3%) of metaplastic cells from four of 27 patients and normal cells from three of 20 normal control women. Cell-by-cell analysis of the staining cells from these latter samples (after Papanicolaou staining) indicated that most of the FA-positive cells (85%) were metaplastic; the others were classified as dyskaryotic.

Only two of the 34 patients studied in these series had atypical cells that stained with mAb 20αD4. One was a case of moderate dysplasia (No. 826) and the other a case of marked dysplasia (No. 842). The proportion of atypical cells that stained with 20αD4 was much lower than that staining with mAb H17. Thus only 8% of the atypical cells from patient No. 826 stained with 20αD4 vs 65% staining with H17 antibody. Duplicate slides from three patients (Nos. 841, 725, and 842) were also stained with mAb 48S. The proportion of atypical cells staining with mAb 48S was similar to that (Tables I–III) recognized by mAb H17.

In all patients, normal squamous cells, metaplastic cells, and, whenever present, koilocytes (Nos. 827, 829) and diskaryoctyes did not stain with any one of the mAbs and antisersa tested in these series. Similarly, these reagents did not stain abnormal cells from patients with condylomatous features only (Nos. 821, 823) or normal squamous cells from the 20 subjects with normal exfoliative cytology. Similarly, in the case of patient No. 842, only 4.4% of the atypical cells stained with 20αD4 vs 87.1% with antibody H17. 20αD4 staining was strictly cytoplasmic.

Staining of the Fresh Tissue Sections

The results with mAb H17 using avidin-biotin staining on fresh tissue sections were essentially similar to those with the FA technique on exfoliated cells. All patients with various degrees of CIN were positive; only one case of invasive cancer did not stain, and all the controls were negative (Table VI).

A large number of epithelial cells, mostly in the basal layer, showed positive staining with various degrees of intensity, indicating a wide but very specific distribution of the antigen recognized by mAb H17. The positivity was often confined to the nucleus, although in the

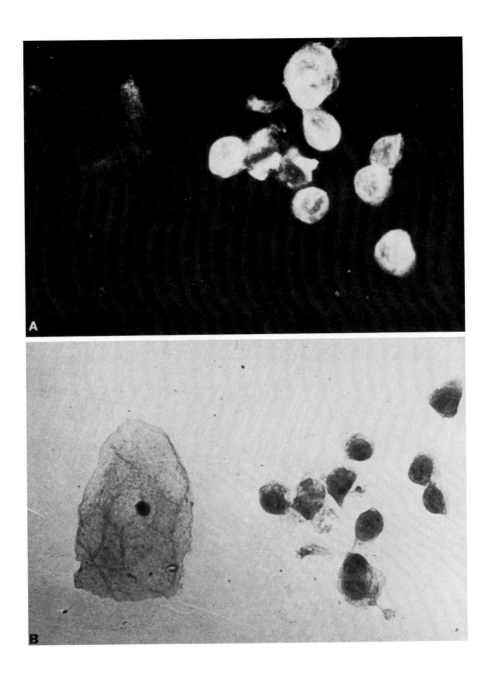

Fig. 4.   A, indirect immunofluorescent staining with H17 of a cluster of atypical cells from a patient with CIS. The normal superficial cell on the left is negative. B, the same group of cells after Papanicolaou staining.

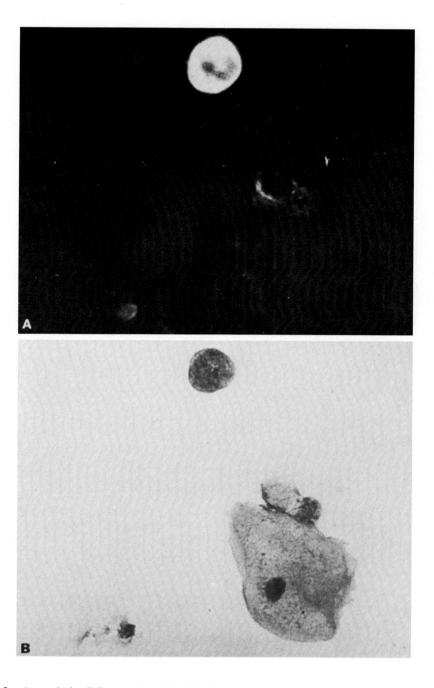

Fig. 5.   A, atypical cell from patient with CIS stained with mAb H17 shows cytoplasmic staining. The normal superficial cell on the bottom is negative. B, same as in A after Papanicolaou staining.

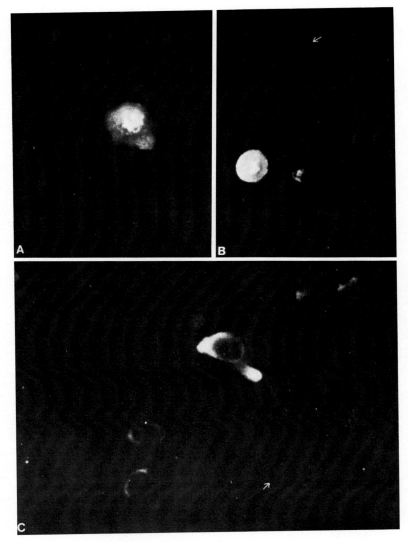

Fig. 6. Different compartmentalization of the H17 staining. A, atypical cells from a patient with marked dysplasia displaying nuclear localization of the staining. Nuclear membrane staining appears as an irregular ring delimiting the chromatin. B, atypical cell from patient with marked dysplasia (No. 827) shows nuclear and cytoplasmic staining. Koilocyte (arrow) and normal cell do not stain. C, cell from CIS patient with cytoplasmic staining only. The intensity of the fluorescence differs in the various atypical cells. Cluster of inflammatory cells (arrow) does not stain.

same cases the cytoplasm of the atypical cells showed a granular positivity (Fig. 7). The stroma cells were negative.

DISCUSSION

The progression of precancerous cervical lesions to invasive cancer is unpredictable and cannot be prognosticated from morphology alone. Although it is believed that 5–20% of mild dysplasias and 40% of severe ones progress to cancer [16], the questions still remain: (1) What proportion of precancerous lesions eventually become invasive? (2) At what rate do cervical

**TABLE VI. Positive PAP Staining of mAb H17 in
the 15 Cases
Examined by Cryostatic Fresh Sections***

Histological diagnosis	No.	No. positive cases
Moderate dysplasia	1	1
Marked dysplasia	5	5
In situ carcinoma	5	5
Invasive cancer	4	3
Normal cervical tissue	3	0

*Fifteen patients with dysplasia and in situ and invasive cancer were tested with mAb H17 on cryostatic fresh sections, by means of peroxidase-antiperoxidase (PAP); 14 of 15 patients showed positive PAP staining. As a control, three patients with normal cervical tissue were negative.

dysplasias progress? and 3) Is there any way of distinguishing between precancerous lesions that are destined to advance (in a high-risk patient) and those that are not?

Answers to these questions are not readily available. The diagnosis of dysplasia or other presumed precursor lesions requires surgical excision that in turn can cure, partly miss, or otherwise modify the biologic behavior. However, it seems reasonable to believe that if a certain precursor lesion is destined to undergo malignant transformation, whereas others are not, the two types may be biochemically, immunologically, or otherwise distinguishable. In theory, the existence of a test capable of differentiating between those cytologically identified precursor lesions with neoplastic or invasive potential and the similarly identified lesions that do not have such potential could have a major impact on the efficacy and yield of cancer screening programs as well as on the precision and validity of clinical diagnosis. Improvement in the diagnostic precision of the initial cytologic smear by the incorporation of immune criteria of neoplastic potential (such as might be revealed by staining with specific mAbs) could, when applied to precancerous lesions, prevent unnecessary procedures and lead to a more rational clinical management.

mAbs H17 and 48S precipitate the 144 K protein previously identified as a component of the viral ribonucleotide reductase [11,17]. Since extracts of 12 hr-infected cells contain virutally all the viral proteins, the data suggest that antigenic determinants recognized by the two mAbs are located only on the 144 K protein. This protein is also precipitated by antiserum to ICP10, a protein independently identified in cervical tumor but not normal cells [18], but not by mAb 20αD4, which recognizes the viral glycoprotein gA/B [11]. Cross-adsorbtion studies indicate that the antigenic specificity of mAb H17 is similar to that of mAb 48S and polyclonal anti-ICP10 serum. However, we cannot exclude the possibility that the two mAbs recognize different epitopes on the 144 K protein that are differentially expressed in atypical cells from various patients.

Two comments seem pertinent with respect to these findings. First, the function relating the logarithm of the MW to the distance of migration is nonlinear for proteins > 100 K, so estimates of their MWs are subject to considerable error. Taking into consideration these limitations, our original studies using bis-acrylamide cross-linked gels estimated that ICP10 has a MW of 160 K ± 10% [8]. In the present series, we used N,N′-diallyltartardiamide cross-linked gels and found that, under these more accurate sizing conditions, the MW of ICP10 is

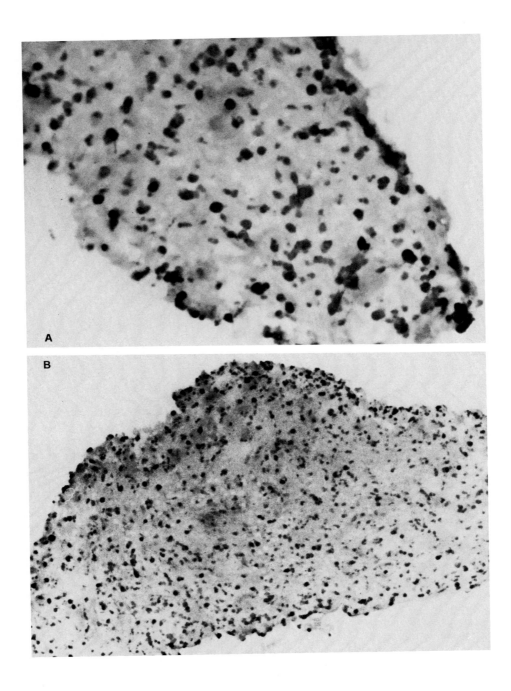

Fig. 7.   Severe dysplasia. All the nuclei are stained with mAb H17. Frozen section, avidin-biotin-peroxidase complex method. Original magnifications: A, ×100; B, ×50.

144 K. This estimate is within the original 10% margin of error and is in line with independent reports of the MW of ICP6, the HSV$_1$ homologue of ICP10 [10,11,15]. Similar findings pertaining to differences in MW estimates obtained on bis-acrylamide as compared to N,N′-diallytartardiamide cross-linked gels were independently reported by Pereira et al [19].

The second comment that seems pertinent with respect to these findings is that ICP10 is associated with neoplastic transformation. It is encoded by transforming sequences within the BglII C fragment of HSV$_2$ DNA and is expressed in the transformed cells [4]. It was independently identified in cervical tumor cells [18]. Derangements in dNTP pools increase the rate of spontaneous mutation [20] and are linked to transformation [21]. Ribonucleotide reductases altered in their regulatory control can confer a mutator phenotype [20].

Significantly, mAb H17 (and, whenever tested, 48S) stains atypical cells from patients with CIN or invasive cervical cancer with a high degree of specificity and sensitivity. Thus 55% of patients with mild dysplasia and those with more advanced lesions have H17-positive atypical cells. The percentage of positive cells increases with the severity of the lesion. It reaches maximal levels in patients with CIS and invasive cancer (mild dysplasia, 32.6%; moderate dysplasia, 63.5%; marked dysplasia, 67.9%; CIS, 81.4%; invasive cancer, 85.6%). This is consistent with the interpretation that H17 might be able to identify CIN cells capable of progressing to a more advanced stage. Also consistent with this interpretation, mAb H17 staining is restricted to the atypical cells. Normal epithelial cells from the same patients and from 20 women with normal cytology and, whenever present, inflammatory cells, koilocytes, and dyskaryocytes do not stain. In this context, it must be stressed that the antigenic specificity of mAb is of little clinical significance. On the other hand, its ability to reproducibly identify CIN cells with a high degree of specificity and sensitivity is of major importance. Indeed, it is possible that proteins others than those studied in these series and that are not encoded by HSV$_2$ will prove to be better immunodiagnostic markers than the 144 K protein recognized by mAbs H17 and 48S. However, antisera and mAbs to the same or other HSV$_2$ proteins cannnot be used indiscriminately to stain cervical atypical cells. Thus we find that mAb 20αD4 stains only a small proportion of atypical cells (4.4–8%) and from only two of the 34 patients studied in this series (Nos. 826 and 842). Similarly, another mAb (6A6) that precipitates the 144 K protein, presumably by recognizing epitopes different from those identified by mAb 48S, does not stain atypical cells from patients with CIN or cervical cancer.

How do we explain the consistent detection of ICP10 in cervical tumor cells when it is generally accepted that viral DNA sequences are not detectable in cervical cancer or, at best, can be identified only in a significantly smaller proportion of cervical tumors than those staining with anti-ICP10 serum [22]? The assumption that HSV$_2$ DNA sequences are not detectable in cervical cancer tissue is misleading. Cervical cancer DNA was not extensively probed with the 4.4 kb BamHI/SacI fragment that codes for ICP10, nor with any other sequences that overlap the ICP10-coding region but that unlike the entire BglII C, are not homologous to normal human DNA [22]. Preliminary studies from our laboratory using the 4.4 kb BamHI/SacI fragment as hybridization probe have identified the presence of homologous DNA sequences in five of seven cervical tumors tissues but not in normal human DNA [23].

From a clinical standpoint, it is most important to remember that not all dysplasias identified cytologically will progress to invasive cancer. Final decisions pertaining to the prognostication of the progression from CIN 1 to invasive cancer depend on a better understanding of the biology of the intraepithelial lesions. Since we find that in our hands only 55.5% of patients with mild dysplasia stain with the H17 antibody, it would be very interesting to verify whether the presence of the viral antigen recognized by this mAb can accurately reflect the risk of progression towards more severe forms of cervical anaplasia. Such studies are presently underway in our laboratories.

ACKNOWLEDGMENTS

We thank Dr. P.K. Gupta for help with the pathological classification of the stained cervical cells and Mrs. Rita Fishelevich for excellent technical assistance. These studies were supported in part by grant CA-39691 from the NCI to Dr. L. Aurelian and in part by the Italian National Research Council (CNR) grant No. 84.000707.44.

REFERENCES

1. Aurelian L. Herpes virus and cervical cancer. In Phillips LA ed. Viruses associated with human cancer. New York, Marcel Dekker Inc., 1983; 79–123.
2. Durst M, Gissman L, Ikenberg H, zur Hausen H. A papillomavirus DNA from cervical carcinomas and its prevalence in cancer biopsy samples from different geographic regions. Proc Natl Acad Sci USA 1983; 80:3812–5.
3. Morin C, Braun L, Casas-Cordero M, Shah KV, Roy M, Fortier M, Meisels A. Confirmation of the papillomavirus etiology of condylomatous cervix lesions by the Peroxidase-Antiperoxidase technique. J Natl Cancer Inst 1981; 66:831–5.
4. Hayashi Y, Iwasaka T, Smith CC, Aurelian L, Lewis GK, Ts'o POP. Multistep transformation by defined fragments of herpes simplex virus type 2 DNA: Oncogenic region and its gene product. Proc Natl Acad Sci USA 1985; 82:8493–7.
5. Aurelian L, Smith CC, Klacsman KT, Gupta PK, Frost JK. Expression and cellular compartmentalization of a herpes simplex virus type 2 protein (ICP 10) in productively infected and cervical tumor cells. Cancer Invest 1983; 1:301–13.
6. Oi V, Herzenberg L. Immunoglobulin producing hybrid cell lines. In Mishell B, Schiigi S, eds: Selected methods in cellular immunology. San Francisco: W.H. Freeman Co. 1980; 351–71.
7. Littlefield JW. Selection of hybrid from mating of fibroblasts in vitro and their presumed recombinants. Science 1964; 145:709.
8. Strnad BC, Aurelian L. Proteins of herpesvirus type 2. III. Isolation and immunologic characterization of a large molecular weight viral protein. Virology 1978; 87:401–15.
9. Smith CC, Aurelian L. Proteins of herpesvirus type 2. V. Isolation and immunologic characterization of two viral proteins in a virus specific antigenic fraction. Virology 1979; 98:255–60.
10. Showalter SD, Zweig M, Hampar B. Monoclonal antibodies to herpes simplex virus type 1 proteins including the immediate early protein ICP 4. Infect Immun 1981; 34:684–93.
11. Bacchetti S, Evelegh MJ, Muirhead B, Sartari CS, Huszar D. Immunological characterization of herpes simplex virus type 1 and 2 polypeptide(s) involved in viral ribonucleotide reductase activity. J Virol 1984; 49:591–3.
12. Balachandran N, Bacchetti S, Rawls W. Protection against lethal challenge of Balb/c mice by passive transfer of monoclonal antibodies to five glycoproteins of herpes simplex virus type 2. Infect Immun 1982; 37:1132–7.
13. Heine JW, Honess RW, Cassai E, Roizman B. Proteins specified by herpes simplex virus. XII. The virion polypeptides of type 1 strains. J Virol 1974; 14:640–51.
14. Hsu SM, Raine L, Fanger H. Use of avidin-biotin-peroxidase complex (ABC) in immunoperoxidase techniques: A comparison between ABC and unlabelled antibody (PAP) procedures. J Histochem Cytochem 1981; 29:577–80.
15. Hsu SM, Raine L, Fanger H. The use of antiavidin antibody and avidin-biotin-peroxidase-complex in immunoperoxidase technics. Am J Clin Pathol 1981; 75:816–21.
16. Koss LG. Concept of genesis and development of carcinoma of the cervix. Obstet Gynecol 1969; 24:850–60.
17. Dutia BM. Ribonucleotide reductase induced by herpes simplex virus has a virus specific constituent. J Gen Virol 1983; 64:513–21.
18. Flanders R, Iyer N, Brokan J, Ricardo M Jr, Kucera L. Reactivity of rabbit polyclonal AG4/ICP10 antibodies with HSV-2 induced ribonucleotide reductase and human cervical carcinoma cells In: Proceedings of the 10th International Herpesvirus Workshop. Ann Arbor, Michigan, 1985; 295.
19. Pereira L, Wolff MH, Fenwick M, Roizman B. Regulation of herpesvirus macromolecular synthesis. V. Properties of polypeptides made in HSV-1 and HSV-2 infected cells. Virology, 1977; 77:733–49.
20. Weinberg G, Velman B, Martin DW Jr. Mutator phenotypes in mammalian cell mutants with distinct biochemical defects and abnormal deoxyribonucleotide triphosphate pools. Proc Natl Acad Sci USA 1981; 78:2447–51.

21. Weber G. Biochemical strategy of cancer cells and the design of chemotherapy: G.H.A. Clowes Memorial Lecture. Cancer Res 1983; 43:3466–92.
22. McDougall JK, Smith P, Tamimi HK, Tolentino E, Galloway DA. Molecular Biology of the relationship between Herpes simplex virus-2 and cervical cancer. In Giraldo G, and Beth E, eds: The role of viruses in human cancer. Amsterdam: Elsevier Science Publishers, 1984; 59–71.
23. Aurelian L. In de Palo G, Zur Hausen H, Rilke F, eds: Herpes and papilloma viruses. Their role in the carcinogenesis of the lower genital tract. New York: Raven Press 1986; 31:63–82.

Human-Human Hybridomas Generated With Lymphocytes From Patients With Colorectal Cancer

Per Borup-Christensen, MD
Karin Erb, CS
Jens Christian Jensenius, PhD
Sven-Erik Svehag, PhD
Bjarne Nielsen, MD

Biomedical Laboratory, Institute of Surgery (P.B.-C.), Institute of Medical Microbiology (K.E., J.C.J., S.-E.S.), and Institute of Pathology (B.N.), University of Odense, Odense, Denmark

ABSTRACT   Human-human hybridoma technology was used to produce human monoclonal antibodies with reactivity to colorectal cancer antigens. Two different B-lymphoma cell lines were fused with lymphocytes obtained from mesenteric lymph nodes from colorectal cancer patients. The fusion frequency was 11% with LICR-LON-HMy-2. Out of 294 growing hybridomas 26 secreted antibodies reacting with epitopes on cultured colon adenocarcinoma cells. Only one (D4213) was established and has now been in culture for 1.5 years. D4213 antibody shows a strong reaction with colon cancer tissue compared with normal colon epithelium. Using W1-L2-729-HF2 the fusion frequency was about 50%. Of 2,487 hybridomas 499 produced immunoglobulin and 44 of these reacted with colon cancer tissues or cultured cancer cells. One of the established hybridomas produces antibody reacting with cancer cell membrane antigens, and on immunoblotting a number of components were stained. The antibody from the other hybridomas reacts with cytoplasmatic antigens, and only one of these showed reactivity in immunoblotting where it bound to a component with M_r of about 60K.

Key words: human monoclonal antibodies, tumor marker

INTRODUCTION

The aim of the present work was to study the humoral immune response in cancer patients and to exploit the possibility of obtaining human monoclonal antibodies that might prove useful in diagnosis and/or treatment of cancer patients. We chose colorectal cancer for the present investigation since it is one of the most frequent cancers, and the prognosis has not improved during the last 20 years in spite of optimal surgical technique. There is significantly no beneficial effect of radiotherapy or chemotherapy.

Address reprint requets to Dr. Per Borup-Christensen, Biomedical Laboratory, J.B. Winsløwsvej 21, DK-5000 Odense C, Denmark.

The production of murine monoclonal antibodies is well established and has facilitated the definition of tumor-associated antigens. Preliminary experiments indicate that such antibodies may be useful not only in immunohistochemically aided diagnosis but also in localization of tumor metastasis by scintigraphy. The more recent availability of suitable fusion partners for the production of human monoclonals has widened this perspective. This has created the possibility of obtaining antibodies against other types of tumor-associated epitopes and may provide some insight into the interplay between the tumor and the humoral immune system of the host.

MATERIALS AND METHODS
Fusion Cell Lines

The human B-lymphoma cell line LICR-LON-HMy-2 (HMy-2) [1] was a gift from Dr. M.J. O'Hara (The Ludwig Institute, London). It produces IgG$_1$ (kappa) and has a doubling time of 20–30 hr. The human B-lymphoma cell line WI-L2-729-HF2 (729-HF2) was obtained from Techniclone International (Santa Ana, CA) [2]. This cell line produces no immunoglobulin. Prior to fusion both cell lines were grown in RPMI-1640 medium (Gibco, Grand Island, NY) supplemented with 10% fetal calf serum (FCS) (Gibco), 100 units penicillin and 100 μg streptomycin per ml, and either 8-azaguanine (Sigma, St. Louis, MO), 4 mM (HMy-2), or 6-thioguanine (Sigma) 0.1 mM (729-HF2).

Human Tissues

Lymphocytes were obtained from the mesenteric lymph nodes draining the tumor region in patients with colorectal cancer. The lymph nodes were minced under sterile conditions. Debris was removed by filtration through cotton wool, and the lymphocytes were separated on Ficoll-Isopaque (Lymphocyte separation medium, Boehringer-Mannheim, Mannheim, FRG). Lymphocytes used for fusion with HMy-2 were suspended in RPMI-1640, 10% FCS, supplemented with pokeweed mitogen (PWM) (Flow Laboratories) at 2.5 μg/ml [3] and cultured for 4–6 days at 37°C in 5% CO$_2$. Lymphocytes used for fusion with 729-HF-2 were used without in vitro stimulation.

Fusion Procedure

Fusions were performed according to the methods described by Köhler [4]. The ratio between HMy-2 or 729-HF-2 and lymphocytes (10^7–10^8) was 1:2, and the cells were plated at 2×10^5 cells in 200 μl per well of 96-well microplates (Costar, Cat. No. 3596, Cambridge, MA). Lymphocytes fused with HMy-2 were seeded on plates with feeder cells. Peritoneal macrophages from one untreated BALB/c mouse were distributed as feeder cells on two microplates. Feeder cells were not necessary when 729-HF-2 was used for fusions.

The cells were maintained in HAT medium for either 6 (HMy-2) or 2 (729-HF-2) weeks. Further culture was done in RPMI-1640, 10% FCS, supplemented with hypoxanthine and thymidine. Growing hybrids appeared 3 to 6 weeks after fusion with HMy-2 and 10 days to 4 weeks after fusion with 729-HF-2. Cloning by limiting dilution was carried out with feeder cells (HMy-2) or without feeder cells (729-HF-2).

ELISA for Antibody Activity

Supernatant from wells containing growing cells was assayed for reactivity toward cell surface antigens by enzyme-linked-immunosorbent assay (ELISA) on the following cells: Colon 137 and Colon 138 (obtained from Dr. P. Ebbesen, The Cancer Research Institute, Århus, Denmark) and COLO 201 (American Type Culture Collection [ATCC], Rockville, MD). These cell lines are derived from human colon adenocarcinomas. COLO 201 was removed from culture bottles by shaking, while Colon 137 and Colon 138 were detached by trypzination and seeded at 5×10^4 cells per well in 100 μl PBS on polystyrene microplates (Cat. No. 269620, Nunc A/S, Kamstrup, Denmark) precoated with 10 μg/ml poly-L-lysine

(Sigma). After centrifugation (200g, 10 min) the cells were fixed with 0.17% glutaraldehyde in PBS [5], quenched with 0.1% bovine serum albumin (BSA, Cohn fraction V, Sigma) in PBS, 100 mM glycine/HCl, pH 7.4, and kept at 20°C with 0.1% BSA in PBS.

The microplates with fixed colon cancer cells were incubated for 2 to 16 hr at room temperature with 100 μl cell culture supernatants per well. The wells were washed three times with PBS, 0.05% Tween-20 (PBS-Tween); (Merck, Darmstadt, FRG), incubated for 1 hr with horseradish peroxidase-coupled rabbit antihuman immunoglobulin (HRP-anti-Ig: antibody against IgG, IgA, IgM, kappa, and lambda; Cat. No. P212, Dakopatts, Copenhagen, Denmark) diluted 1/1,000 in PBS-Tween. After washing the plates three times with PBS-Tween, the substrate (0.015% H_2O_2 in a solution of ortho-phenylendiamine [OPD] at 0.4 mg/ml 0.1 M phosphate, 0.2 M citrate, pH 5.0) was added. After 1 hr at 37°C the plates were read at 450 nm using a multichannel spectrophotometer (Immuno Reader NJ-2000, Inter Med., Tokyo, Japan).

Immunohistochemical Analyses

Supernatants collected 2 to 4 weeks after fusions with 729-HF-2 were screened on formalin-fixed, paraffin-embedded autologous tumor. Tissue sections were deparaffinized and rehydrated through graded alcohols to PBS. The sections were incubated overnight at 4°C in a humidified chamber with 50 μl undiluted supernatant. After incubation the slides were washed for 15 min in PBS followed by incubation for 0.05 hr at 4°C with HRP rabbit antihuman IgM (Cat. No. P215, Dakopatts) or with HRP rabbit antihuman IgG (Cat. No. P214, Dakopatts), both diluted 1:50 in PBS-Tween. The slides were washed and incubated in the chromogenic substrate (0.01% H_2O_2 in PBS, pH 7.4, with diaminobenzidine at 0.6 mg/ml). After washing the sections were counterstained with hematoxylin for 5 min and mounted with Eukitt (O. Kindler, Freiburg, FRG).

Immunoglobulin Assays

Immunoglobulin (Ig) in hybridoma supernatants were quantified, and the classes, sub-classes, and light chain types were determined by ELISA as described previously [6]. In brief, classes and subclasses were determined on plates coated with antihuman IgG (H and L chains), and the binding of hybridoma Ig was detected with alkaline phosphatase (AP)-coupled anti-H chain antibodies, the subclasses with monoclonal murine antibodies and enzyme-labeled anti-mouse Ig.

Light chain type was determined on plates coated with F(ab')$_2$-antikappa or F(ab')$_2$-antilambda antibody and developed with AP-antigamma, AP-anti-my, or AP-antialpha chain antibody.

The distribution of kappa and lambda chains in individual IgM molecules was analyzed for the affinity-purified D4213 IgM and for normal human IgM. The samples were applied to wells coated with F(ab')$_2$-antikappa or antilambda followed by development with beta-galactosidase-coupled antikappa and antilambda antibody.

Immunocytochemical Analysis

Cell smears were prepared from human tumor cell lines and peripheral human blood leukocytes and fixed in buffered formol-acetone [6]. Approximately 50 μl of culture supernatant was placed on the smear and incubated at room temperature in a humidified chamber for 1 hr before rinsing and incubation at room temperature for 0.05 hr with HRP-anti-IgM (Dakopatts) (diluted 1/20 in TBS-Tween). The slides were washed and developed in chromogenic substrata (diaminobenzidine). The smears were lightly counterstained with hematoxylin.

Flow Cytometry

The DNA distribution of nuclear suspensions prepared from hybridoma and parental cultures was analyzed by flow cytometry as previously described [7]. Chicken and trout erythrocytes were added as internal DNA standards.

Colon Cancer Cell Membranes

Solid tumors were surgically removed from colon cancer patients and homogenized on ice in an MSE homogenizer at maximum speed, 3×20 sec. The homogenization was carried out in 10 vol of Tris-buffered saline (TBS: 0.14 M NaCl, 10 mM Tris HCl, 0.1% NaN$_3$, pH 7.4) containing enzyme-inhibitors: iodoacetamid, tranexamic acid (Cyclocapron, KABI, Stockholm, Sweden), ethylene diamine tetraacetic acid (EDTA), and phenylmethylsulfonylfluoride (PMSF), all at 5 mM, and 10 units aprotein (Trasylol, Bayer, Leverkusen, FRG) per ml. After filtration the suspension was further homogenized by five strokes in a Potter Elvhjelm glass homogenator followed by centrifugation (500g, 10 min). The 500g sediment was reextracted, and the combined supernatants were ultracentrifuged (1.5×10^5g, 30 min). The sediment was washed once and resuspended in TBS with enzyme inhibitors to a volume corresponding to the original tumor volume. The protein concentration was estimated to 10–20 mg/ml by E$_{280}$ measurements of membranes solubilized in 1% SDS. The preparation was aliquoted and stored at $-70°$C.

SDS-Polyacrylamide Gel Electrophoresis and Immunoblotting

The colon cancer membrane preparation was diluted in 100 mM Tris/HCl, pH 6.7, with enzyme inhibitors (as above), 1% sodium dodecyl sulfate (SDS), 8.5% glycerol, and 25 ppm pyronine G. Polyacrylamide gel electrophoresis (PAGE) followed by blotting to nitrocellulose sheets was performed as previously described [8].

The nitrocellulose sheets were cut in 2 mm strips. Proteins were stained by colloidal gold [9]. Blots were quenched in TBS, 0.1% Tween-20, pH 6.8, for 10 min and incubated overnight at 4°C with hybridoma supernatant diluted 1/4 in TBS, followed by three washes in TBS, 0.01% Tween. Bound antibody was detected by a 2 hr incubation with AP-rabbit antihuman IgM (Sigma), 1/1,000 in TBS, 0.05% Tween. After incubation with secondary antibody the blots were washed with PBS and fixed by 15 min incubation with 0.2% glutaraldehyde in PBS. The glutaraldehyde was removed by washing with PBS and 0.1 M ethanolamine buffer, pH 9.0. The alkaline phosphatase was visualized with substrate, nitro blue tetrazolium (NBT), 100 μg/ml, and 5-bromo-4-chloroindoxyl phosphate (BCIP) 50 μg/ml of 0.1 m ethanolamine, 4 mM MgCl$_2$, pH 9.0 [10].

RESULTS

Six fusions between HMy-2 and PWM-stimulated B-lymphocytes from patients with colorectal cancer were performed (Table I). There was a great variation in the fusion frequency. Out of 294 hybridomas, 26 produced antibodies that reacted with one or more colon cancer cell lines in ELISA, but only one, D4213, was established and has been kept in culture for 1.05 years. The parental cell line produces IgG$_1$(kappa), while D4213 produces IgM containing both kappa and lambda light chains. D4213 also secretes IgG$_1$(kappa) and a small amount of

TABLE I. Results of Fusion With LICR-LON-HMy 2

Fusion No.	Wells seeded	Wells with hybridoma	Supernatants positive in ELISA with colon cancer cell lines
1	480	6	0
2	480	10	3
3	480	0	0
4	480	153	8
5	480	124	15*
6	288	1	0
Total	2,688	294	26

*One of these was D4213.

IgG$_1$(lambda). The IgM concentration in the supernatant is 1 to 2 μg/ml. Only the IgM reacts with human colon cancer cell lines in ELISA. This reaction was found to be sensitive to variations of pH and ionic strength, with the reactivity disappearing at above pH 8.5 and NaCl concentration above 1 M.

The parental cell line HMy-2 is Epstein-Barr virus (EBV) infected, and flow cytometry was performed to verify if D4213 is an EBV-transformed B lymphocyte or a true hybridoma (Fig. 1). HMy-2 is a diploid cell line showing cells in G$_1$, S, G$_2$, and M phases. D4213 has twice the DNA content of the parental cell line, showing that D4213 is tetraploid.

D4213 antibody has abeen tested on cell smears of different cancer cell lines and normal human leukocytes (Table II). In this analysis the IgM antibody reacts with different colon cancer cell lines and melanoma cell lines but not with other cancer cell lines tested or normal human leukocytes. This suggests that the D4213 antigen is a differentiation antigen. D4213 antibody was further tested by an indirect immunohistochemical technique on both autologous paraffin-embedded, formalin-fixed colon cancer tissue and autologous normal colon epithelium. It appears that D4213 reacts strongly with colon cancer cells, while none or only a slight reaction was seen in normal colon epithelium.

Twenty-eight fusions have been performed between 729-HF-2 and unstimulated lymphocytes from patients with colorectal cancer (Table III). The first 25 fusions gave very poor results. Only one hybridoma produced antibody that reacted with colorectal cancer cells and tissue. The following three fusions gave the same fusion frequency (about 50%), but much higher frequency of hybridomas producing antibodies that reacted with colorectal cancer.

The reactivity against colorectal cancer was estimated in two different analyses (Table IV). All the hybridomas have been frozen for subsequent cloning. Until now 11 of these

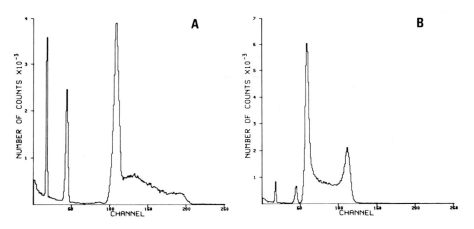

Fig. 1. DNA distribution analyzed by flow cytometry of **A:** D4213 and **B:** HMy-2. The first two peaks represent chicken and trout erythrocytes used as internal DNA standards. Abscissa, fluorescence intensity. Ordinate, number of cells.

TABLE II. Results of Fusion With 729-HF-2

	Fusions 1–25	Fusions 26–28
Wells seeded	4,390	540
Wells with hybridomas	2,214	273
Wells with Ig production	330	169
Wells positive with colorectal cancer	1	43

TABLE III. Reactivity of D4213 Antibody Assayed on Cell Smears

Type of cell	Name	Reaction
Colon adenocarcinoma	Colon 137	+++*
Colon adenocarcinoma	Colon 138	++
Colon adenocarcinoma	COLO 201	++
Mammae carcinoma	MCF-7	−
Duodenum adenocarcinoma	HUTU 80	−
Kidney adenocarcinoma	A 704	−
Burkitt lymphoma	EB-2	−
Melanoma	109 HME	++
Melanoma	HU 373	+
Melanoma	IGR-1	++
Blood leukocytes	PBL	−

*Strong reaction, +++; moderate reaction, ++; weak reaction, +; no reaction, −.

TABLE IV. Reactivity Pattern of Hybridoma Supernatants Obtained by Fusion With 729-HF2

Immunoglobulin	Positive only on colon cancer tissue sections	Positive only in ELISA on cell lines	Positive both in ELISA and on tissue sections	Total
IgM	7	10	13	30
IgG	10	0	4	14
Total	17	10	17	44

hybridomas had been cloned. All of them produce IgM at a concentration in the rage of 300 ng to 2 μg/ml.

The supernatants have been analyzed for reactivity to tumor membrane antigens. Colon cancer cell membranes were treated with SDS and separated on PAGE, followed by blotting onto nitrocellulose sheets. Figure 2 shows some of the results. One hybridoma supernatant (F11348) reacted with several components (lane 2) and another (G4146) with a single component with a molecular weight of about 60K (lane 7), while none of the other hybridoma supernatants showed reaction. F11348 did not react with cytosol similarly separated by SDS-PAGE and blotted onto nitrocellulose, while G4146 gave a strong reaction with a molecule of identical mobility to that seen with membranes.

We have investigated the reactivity of the 11 established hybridomas on colon cancer cell lines by immunocytochemical technique. One of the hybridomas (F11348) produced antibody directed against antigen determinants located on the cell membrane, while the other hybridoma supernatants reacted with cytoplasmic components (Fig. 3).

DISCUSSION

We have produced human monoclonal antibodies using two different human B-lymphoma cell lines, HMy-2 and 729-HF-2. The fusions between HMy-2 and PWM-stimulated lymphocytes obtained from mesenteric lymph nodes resulted in an average fusion frequency of about 11% compared to 50% for fusions between 729-HF-2 and unstimulated lymphocytes. In vitro stimulation was recommended by Warenius et al [3] to increase the fusion frequency but appears superfluous when 729-HF-2 is used as fusion partner (Torben Plesner and Thomas Kellsen, Copenhagen, personal communication).

The fusions have resulted in a number of hybridomas that have been established and that produce antibodies reactive with antigens located in autologous and allogeneic tumor tissue as judged by immunohistochemical analysis on formalin-fixed, paraffin-embedded tissue. The reactivity was also analyzed on colon cancer cell lines by ELISA. A proportion of the monoclonal antibodies reacted only with the tumor tissues, while others reacted only in ELISA,

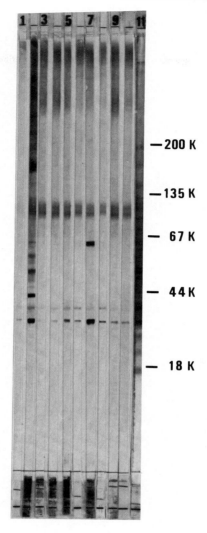

Fig. 2. Immunoblotting of colon cancer cell membranes. Samples were separated by SDS-PAGE, transferred onto nitrocellulose sheets, and incubated with supernatants containing human monoclonal antibodies followed by alkaline phosphatase-conjugated rabbit antihuman IgM (lanes 1–10). Lane 11 was stained for protein with colloidal gold.

and some reacted in both techniques. An explanation of this pattern could be that some of the antigenic determinants are lost in the established cell lines, while other determinants are destroyed in the histochemical procedure. The target antigens of two of the monoclonal antibodies were further characterized by the Western-blot technique. One of the antibodies (F11348) reacts with a number of protein bands on separated cell membranes but not on cytosol. On cell smears this antibody shows surface membrane reactivity. This reactivity pattern would be in concordance with a carbohydrate nature of the target epitope. Preliminary experiments showing sensitivity to periodate oxidation supports this supposition. Only one other monoclonal antibody (G4146) reacted on Western blots, identifying a distinct antigen present in both the crude cell membrane fraction and the cytosol. On cell smears this antibody shows intracellular staining as do the rest of the antibodies. Further analyses of the binding

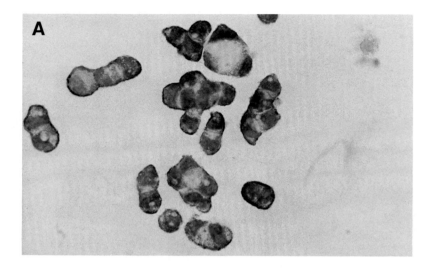

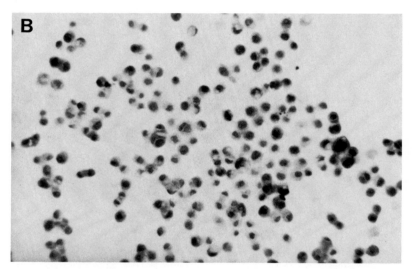

Fig. 3.   Staining of smears of Colon 137 cells with **A:** F11348 (×200; note the membrane staining) and **B:** D4213 (×80; note the cytoplasmatic staining).

patterns of the antibodies and characterization of the antigens will show if some of the human monoclonal antibodies will be useful in tumor localization and therapy or for the detection of circulating tumor-associated antigens. For tumor localization and therapy only antibodies against cell membrane antigens can be expected to be useful. Unfortunately, it appears that only one of the established hybridomas produces antibody with such reactivity. This is similar to observations made by other groups. Cote et al [11] found that only 0.7% of human monoclonal antibodies binding to tumor cells reacted with cell surface antigens, and Imam et al [12] reported that none of 81 human monoclonal antibodies binding to breast cancer reacted with surface antigens. A greater frequency of human monoclonal antibodies directed against epitopes in the cancer cell membrane may possibly be obtained by the use of lymphocytes from cancer patients immunized by the injection of autologous tumor cells [13].

It is established that IgM extravasates more slowly [14] and less extensively [15] than IgG when injected intravenously. On this basis one may assume that for tumor localization IgG will prove more useful than IgM [16]. All our established hybridomas produces IgM. However, it may be possible to Ig class switch [17,18] and thereby obtain antibodies more suitable for in vivo use. Another possibility might be to change the pentameric IgM to monomers by reduction.

ACKNOWLEDGMENTS

This investigation was supported by grants from The Danish Cancer Society, The Danish Medical Research Council, and The Katrine og Vigo Skovgaards Foundation. Kirsten Wedel Riisberg, Maj-Britt Linn Jørgensen, Birgitte Nørrelund, and Jette Bøhrk have provided skilled technical assistance. We also thank Jørgen K. Larsen and Ib Jarle Christensen, The Finsen Laboratory, The Finsen Institute, Copenhagen, for the flow cytometry analysis.

REFERENCES

1. Edwards PAW, Smith CM, Neville AM, O'Hare MJ. A human-human hybridoma system based on a fastgrowing mutant of the ARH-77 plasma cell leukemiaderived line. Eur J Immunol 1982; 12:641–8.

2. Abrams PG, Knost JA, Clarke G, Wilburn S, Oldham RK, Foon KA. Determination of the optimal human cell lines for development of human hybridomas. J Immunol 1983; 131:1201–4.

3. Warenius HM, Taylor JW, Durack BE, Cross PA. The production of human hybridomas from patients with malignant melanoma. The effect of pre-stimulation of lymphocytes with poke-weed mitogen. Eur J Cancer Clin Oncol 1983; 19:347–55.

4. Köhler G. The technique of hybridoma production. In: I. Lefkovitz (ed): Immunological methods, Vol II. New York: Academic Press, Inc., 1981: 285–98.

5. Suter L, Brügger J, Sorg C. Use of an enzyme-linked immunosorbent assay (ELISA) for screening of hybridoma antibodies against cell surface antigens. J Immunol Methods 1980; 39:407–11.

6. Borup-Christensen P, Erb Karin, Jensenius JC, Nielsen B, Svehag S-E. Human-human hybridomas for the study of anti-tumor immune response in patients with colo-rectal cancer. Int J Cancer 1986; 37:83–8.

7. Ralfkiaer E, Wantzin GL, Larsen JK, Christensen IJ, Thomsen K. Single cell DNA measurements in benign cutaneous lymphoid infiltrates and in positive patch tests. Br J Dermatol 1985; 112:253–62.

8. Towbin H, Strehelin T, Gordon J. Electrophoretic transfer of proteins from polyacrylamide gels to nitrocellulose sheets: Procedure and some applications. Proc Natl Acad Sci USA 1979; 76:4350–4.

9. Mocrenans M, Daneels G, DeMey J. Sensitive colloidal metal (gold or silver) staining of protein blots on nitrocellulose membranes. Anal Biochem 1985; 145:315–21.

10. Blake MS, Johnston KH, Russell-Jones GJ, Gotschlich, EC. A rapid, sensitive method for detection of alkaline phosphatase-conjugated anti-antibody on Western blots. Anal Biochem 1984; 136:175–9.

11. Cote RJ, Morrissey DM, Houghton AN, Beattie EJ, Oettgen HF, Old LJ. Generation of human monoclonal antibodies reactive with cellular antigens. Proc Natl Acad Sci USA 1983; 80:2026–30.

12. Imam A, Drushella Mary M, Taylor CR, Tökés ZA. Generation and immunohistological characterization of human monoclonal antibodies to mammary carcinoma cells. Cancer Res 1985; 45:263–71.

13. Haspel MV, McCabe RP, Pomato N, et al. Generation of tumor cell-reactive human monoclonal antibodies using peripheral blood lymphocytes from actively immunized colorectal carcinoma patients. Cancer Res 1985; 45:3951–61.

14. Julien-Vitoux D, Voisin GA. Studies in vascular permeability. II. Comparative extravasation of different immunoglobulin classes in normal guinea pig skin. Eur J Immunol 1973; 3:663–7.

15. Cohen S, Freeman T. Metabolic heterogeneity of human γ-globulin. Biochem J 1960; 76:775–87.

16. Pimm MV, Baldwin RW. Distribution of IgM monoclonal antibody in mice with human tumor xenografts: Lack of tumor localization. Eur J Cancer Clin Oncol 1985; 21:765–8.

17. Müller Christa E, Rajewsky K. Isolation of immunoglobulin class switch variants from hybridoma lines secreting antiidiotape antibodies by sequential sublining. J Immunol 1983; 131:877–81.

18. Steplewski Z, Spira G, Blaszczyk M, et al. Isolation and characterization of anti-monosialoganglioside monoclonal antibody 19-9 class-switch variants. Proc Natl Acad Sci USA 1985; 82(24):8653–7.

Cancer Detection and Prevention Supplement 1:217–223 (1987)

Immunologic Markers for Epstein-Barr Virus in the Control of Nasopharyngeal Carcinoma and Burkitt Lymphoma

Paul H. Levine, MD

Environmental Epidemiology Branch, National Cancer Institute, National Institutes of Health, Bethesda, MD 20892

ABSTRACT Immunologic assays have been instrumental in implicating the Epstein-Barr virus (EBV) as an etiologic factor in nasopharyngeal carcinoma (NPC) and Burkitt lymphoma (BL). In this report, the importance of a variety of specific assays to detect EBV in tumor biopsies and antibodies to EBV antigens in serum from patients with NPC and BL is reviewed. In both NPC and BL, the involvement of EBV appears to differ in various geographic locations. Therefore, it is necessary to be able to interpret the available immunologic laboratory tests to know if a specific patient has "EBV-associated" or "non-EBV-associated" cancer. Such information is not only relevant to etiologic studies in different populations but to identifying individuals at high risk for NPC and BL, to monitoring their response to therapy, and to determining the most appropriate forms of therapy.

Key words: laboratory assays, clinical application, tumor biopsies, EBV antigens

INTRODUCTION

The Epstein-Barr virus (EBV), known to be the cause of infectious mononucleosis [1], has been etiologically implicated in Burkitt lymphoma (BL) and nasopharyngeal carcinoma (NPC) [2]. Although there are many apparent obstacles to proving a viral etiology for any human malignancy, thereby resulting in a modification of the Henle-Koch postulates for EBV-related tumors [3], laboratory assays for detection of the virus and immune reactivity to various EBV antigens have been shown to play an important role in the diagnosis and management of patients with BL and NPC. The applications of these assays, which have had an increasingly significant impact on the clinical approach to EBV-associated malignancies in the past 2 decades, may provide a model for more recently identified human tumor viruses.

DEFINITION OF EBV-ASSOCIATED DISEASE

In considering the application of EBV-related assays to disease control, it is important to define at the outset the group of individuals for which the assays are most appropriate. Disease heterogeneity is a common problem for clinicians as well as epidemiologists, particularly in BL and NPC, where it is important to distinguish between EBV-associated and non-

Address reprint requests to Dr. Paul H. Levine, Environmental Epidemiology Branch, NCI, NIH, Landow Building, Room 3C25, Bethesda, MD 20892.

EBV-associated cases. It must be stressed that "EBV-associated" refers to the detection of the viral genome in tumor cells and not the presence or titer of EBV antibody in the patient's serum. Although the presence of EBV in the tumor cells often correlates with an elevated antibody titer to the viral capsid antigen, the correlation is not 100%, with many EBV-associated cases having minimal rises in antibody and some non-EBV-associated cases having elevated titers. For both BL and NPC, there are apparent differences between EBV-associated and non-EBV-associated disease, particularly in regard to geographic pattern and response to treatment. More cases appear to be EBV-associated in endemic areas (subsaharan Africa for BL and southern China for NPC), and there is indirect evidence that the EBV-associated cases respond better to therapy than the non-EBV-associated cases [4,5]. Whereas these general patterns hold true for both BL and NPC, it should be understood that the characterization of an individual case as EBV-associated or non-EBV-associated is far less difficult in BL, in which the tumor is homogenous and virtually all tumor cells in the patients with EBV-related tumors contain the viral genome, whereas NPCs usually are composed of a mixture of neoplastic and nonneoplastic cells that contain varying proportions of EBV genome-positive cells and are often difficult to classify in the standard WHO classification [6,7], which has a useful but incomplete correlation with EBV association [8,9].

DISEASE SUSCEPTIBILITY

The applicability of EBV serology to disease susceptibility, an important area of investigation relevant to etiology, first became apparent in a prospective study of BL in Africa [10]. In this study, sera were obtained from 42,000 children under age 9, and this population was observed for the subsequent development of lymphoma. Fourteen individuals in this group eventually developed BL 7–54 months after their blood samples had been obtained, and it was observed that the EBV antibody titers to the viral capsid antigen (VCA) in this group of pre-BL sera were significantly higher than those of the general age-matched population as well as specific controls. Because the particular antibody identified in this study was also widespread in the general population and the difference was solely one of titer, it was not possible to apply this finding to the control of BL in Africa readily. In the People's Republic of China, however, a similar effort to identify individuals at risk of developing NPC could be carried out because it was found that a similar antibody, the IgA antibody to the EBV VCA, was closely associated with NPC but was rarely found in a variety of control groups. The relative disease specificity of this antibody [8,9] plus the identification of a lesion that was an apparent precursor of NPC made a significant impact on the detection of individuals at risk for NPC. In a mass screening of 242,000 residents of Zhongshan County by postnasal mirror, Li and his colleagues [11] found 555 to have nasopharyngeal hyperplastic lesions (NPHL). Four of the findings resulting from this study led these investigators to conclude that NPHL was a precursor of NPC: 1) Of the 555 NPHL lesions, occult NPC was detected in 33; 2) of 307 NPHL lesions that were biopsied and classified into simple and heterotypic hyperplasia or metaplasia, the five subsequent NPC lesions that were detected were all in the group with metaplasia; 3) nasopharyngeal smears in another group of 1,650 NPHL patients identified three cases classified cytologically as having malignant cells without overt tumors; 4) EBV titers in the NPHL group were intermediate between the NPC cases and the IgA-positive normal controls. Extensive studies concentrating on the role of EBV assays in detecting individuals at risk for NPC have been implemented by Zeng et al [12–14], who have utilized immunoenzymatic tests for IgA antibody against VCA and EA antigens in saliva as well as serum, the immunoenzymatic tests being more sensitive than the immunofluorescence tests. These investigators continue to apply new assays to detect virus as well as antibody, further defining the profile of individuals at highest risk for developing NPC [14]. Identification of such individuals is of more than academic interest. Not only can this lead to a better understanding of pathogenesis but also a group can be identified that can be targeted for studies of prevention applying the information on etiology that has been obtained in recent years.

EARLY DETECTION

The role of laboratory assays in the early detection of disease is to bring the patient to the therapist while the disease is still curable. For NPC, the success rate of radiotherapy is considerably different between early disease and the more advanced stages [15]. The implementation of mass clinical screening was already observed to have an impact on early detection [11], but additional progress has been made possible by the application of immunoenzymatic assays [12–14]. In a series of hospitalized patients reported by Li et al [11], 32.1% and 18.7% of hospitalized patients had stage III and IV disease present at the time of diagnosis, respectively. Screening by nasopharyngoscope reduced the percentage of stage III and stage IV cases to 10% and 2.5% [11] and seroepidemiologic screening further reduced the percentage of stage III and stage IV cases to 8.5% and 0% [14], respectively.

DIFFERENTIAL DIAGNOSIS

EBV-related assays in differential diagnosis have been particularly useful in patients presenting with a cervical lymph node containing a metastatic carcinoma with no identifiable primary lesion. In areas that are endemic and nonendemic for NPC, the identification of EBV nuclear antigen (EBNA) by immunofluorescence has been virtually diagnostic for NPC and has been successfully used in clinical situations (Ablashi and Prasad, personal communication).

Because of logistic difficulties in having such assays directly available in many hospitals, reference laboratories able to perform the IgA/VCA antibody test have been helpful in a number of circumstances. As a diagnostic tool, this assay not only has been useful in endemic areas [11] but has been particularly helpful in nonendemic areas [8,9]. Transient high titers of IgA antibody to VCA have been noted in acute infectious mononucleosis [16] but this disease is unlikely to be confused with NPC and does not pose a problem in differential diagnosis. Low titers of IgA antibody to VCA can be seen in other head and neck lesions, benign and malignant, as well as in occasional healthy individuals; therefore, this test is not completely specific for NPC, but it has proven to be helpful to ENT surgeons on many occasions. Negative tests for IgA antibody to VCA are not of clinical value in that IgA antibody frequently is not detected in patients with keratinizing squamous cell NPC. However, the diagnostic value of this assay is enhanced by the fact that the undifferentiated NPCs associated with high IgA antibodies to VCA often occur submucosally and are less accessible to direct visualization than those that are not EBV-associated. The latter frequently are mucosal with ulcerations and are more likely to be seen by the ENT surgeon (Weiland, personal communication).

PREVENTION AND THERAPY

Although EBV vaccines for the prevention of EBV-induced lymphoma have been utilized in an experimental model [17], clinical trials have not been initiated, so in this review only applications to treatment of BL and NPC patients will be discussed. The utilization of assays in monitoring disease status and predicting response to therapy is of potentially great value in that it can guide the clinician to selecting patients for more aggressive therapy at the outset, and, in addition, it may be possible to detect relapse at an early subclinical stage. In regard to predicting the response to standard therapy, the test that appears to be most useful at the present time is the antibody-dependent cellular cytoxicity (ADCC) assay. Initially adapted to the EBV system by Pearson and Orr [18], the potential of this assay for identifying patients according to prognosis is suggested by the similar findings for BL and NPC in two separate laboratories [19–22]. Although immunofluorescent assays for antibody to the early antigens [23,24] and IgA antibody to VCA [25] correlate with stage of disease, elevated antibodies indicating a poor prognosis, longitudinal studies have failed to provide a clinically useful marker of practical assistance to the physician. Individual case reports have also suggested that declines in membrane antibody occur prior to relapse in BL [26], but, in a clinical situation, consistency is necessary for such assays to be of practical value. An example of the inconsistency of EBV serologic in a clinical situation is provided by our experience with BL patients treated by the

Burkitt Tumor Project [27]. We were able to select from our serum bank sera from 12 patients who had a clinical relapse more than 1 year after remission induction. Although there is evidence that late relapse is actually tumor reinduction rather than a recurrence of resistant disease [28], these sera provided an important opportunity to evaluate assays that were suggested as monitors of disease status. As is noted in Fig 1, the antibody to EBV early antigen and nuclear antigen were on occasion able to predict clinical relapse but only in a small proportion of patients. Although there has not been a study in which serologic assays have been used successfully by clinicians in adjusting the treatment of patients with BL and NPC, perhaps in part because of the frequent separation of the EBV laboratory from the clinical setting, the development of more sensitive assays and the improvement of methodology in the clinical setting makes future utilization of serology by clinicians quite feasible. One example of a promising assay that has been applied to patients with NPC is the lymphocyte stimulation

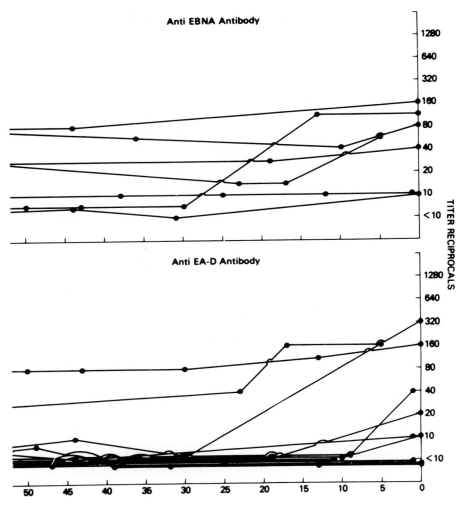

Fig. 1. EBV-specific antibody changes in the year prior to late relapse in African Burkitt lymphoma cases (see reference 27 for details). Although elevations of EBNA and EA-D antibody occurred more than 15 weeks prior to clinical relapse in several patients, changes were not consistent enough to be clinically useful in predicting relapse.

inhibition assay [29], which appears to be a more sensitive monitor of tumor burden than antibody to the early antigen or IgA antibody to VCA. However, although this assay has been applied to patients in Europe, the United States, and Malaysia [30], it is expensive to perform, and, by measuring the ability of serum to block EBV-induced lymphocyte stimulation, it is too complex for many clinical laboratories to perform routinely. Newer serological assays using EBV fragments, such as that recently reported by Halprin et al [31], show greater potential in a clinical setting.

A more direct application of immunologic techniques to therapy has been developed in two clinical trials, one of EBV-specific transfer factor in African BL [32] and one in U.S. patients with NPC (Pearson, personal communication). In the African BL study, 11 patients have thus far been randomized to standard chemotherapy with oral cyclophosphamide and intrathecal methotrexate as compared to the same chemotherapy but with monthly injections of transfer factor. In their initial report, Nkrumah et al [32] showed a significantly greater disease-free interval in the patients treated with transfer factor.

In the pilot study at the Mayo Clinic, four patients were given gammaglobulin with high levels of antibody cytotoxic for EBV. This study was based on the effect of cytotoxic antibody in the mouse sarcoma virus system [33] as well as early reports of regression of BL following serotherapy [34]. This Phase I pilot study demonstrated that serotherapy with cytotoxic EBV antibody is not toxic, and the first patients appeared to show a prolongation of survival. Laboratory assays are being applied to each of these studies (leukocyte migration assay to monitor the effect of transfer factor and the ADCC assay to monitor the effect of serotherapy), but thus far the number of patients and the length of study have been inadequate to determine whether a consistent improvement of laboratory parameters or a consistent therapeutic response can be obtained in these diseases.

In summary, EBV-related assays have been successfully applied to several areas relevant to the control of BL and NPC. This review has been restricted to assays that have already been applied to clinical situations, but there are many new assays that are on the verge of clinical application. The field continues to be a dynamic one, and, as noted at the beginning of this review, it could be useful for virologists outside the EBV field to note the successes as well as the failures in the application of EBV assays to clinical problems as future efforts in viral oncology are contemplated.

REFERENCES

1. Henle W, Henle G. Epstein-Barr virus: The cause of infectious mononucleosis. A review. In: Biggs P, de The G, Payne L, eds. Oncogenesis and herpesviruses. Lyon: IARC, 1972; 269–74.
2. de The G. Role of Epstein-Barr virus in human diseases: Infectious mononucleosis, Burkitt's lymphoma, and nasopharyngeal carcinoma. In: Klein G, ed. Viral oncology. New York: Raven Press, 1980; 769–97.
3. Evans AS. Causation and disease: The Henle-Koch postulates revisited. Yale J Biol Med 1976; 49:175–95.
4. Levine PH, Kamaraju LS, Connelly RR, et al. The American Burkitt lymphoma registry: Eight years' experience. Cancer 1982; 49:1016–22.
5. Levine PH, Connelly RR, Easton JM. Demographic patterns for nasopharyngeal carcinoma in the United States. Int J Cancer 1980; 26:741–48.
6. Shanmugaratnam K, Sobin LH. Histological typing of upper respiratory tract tumours. Geneva: WHO, 1978; 32–3 (International histological typing of tumors; No 19).
7. Prathap K, Prasad U, Ablashi DV. The pathology of nasopharyngeal carcinoma in Malaysians. In: Prasad U, Ablashi DV, Levine PH, Pearson GR, eds. Nasopharyngeal carcinoma: Current concepts. Kuala Lumpur: University of Malaysia Press, 1983; 55–63.
8. Levine PH, Pearson GR, Armstrong M, et al. The reliability of IgA antibody to Epstein-Barr virus (EBV) capsid antigen as a test for diagnosis of nasopharyngeal carcinoma (NPC). Cancer Detect Prevent 1981; 4:307–12.
9. Pearson GR, Weiland LH, Neel HB, et al. Application of Epstein-Barr virus (EBV) serology to the diagnosis of North American nasopharyngeal carcinoma. Cancer 1983; 51:260–8.

10. de The G, Geser A, Day NE, et al. Epidemiological evidence for causal relationship between Epstein-Barr virus and Burkitt's lymphoma from Ugandan prospective study. Nature 1978; 274:756–61.

11. Li ZQ, Chen JJ, Li WJ. Early detection of nasopharyngeal carcinoma (NPC) and nasopharyngeal mucosal hyperplastic lesion (NPHL) with its relationship to carcinomatous change. In: Prasad U, Ablashi DV, Levine PH, Pearson GR, eds. Nasopharyngeal carcinoma: Current concepts. Kuala Lumpur: University of Malaya Press, 1983; 17–23.

12. Zeng Y, Liu UX, Liu C, et al. Application of immunoenzymatic method and immuno-autoradiographic method for the mass survey of nasopharyngeal carcinoma. Intervirology 1980; 13:162–8.

13. Zeng Y, Zhang LG, Li HY, et al. Serological mass survey for early detection of nasopharyngeal carcinoma in Wuzhou City, China. Int J Cancer 1982; 29:139–41.

14. Zeng Y, de The G. Nasopharyngeal carcinoma: Early detection and IgA-related pre-NPC condition. Achievements and perspectives. In: Levine PH, Ablashi DV, Pearson GR, Kottaridis SD, eds. Epstein-Barr virus and associated diseases. Boston: Martinus-Nijhoff 1985; 151–63.

15. Ho HC. An epidemiologic and clinical study of nasopharyngeal carcinoma. Int J Rad Oncol Biol Phys 1978; 4:181–98.

16. Nikoskelainen J, Ablashi DV, Isenberg RA, Neel EU, Miller RG, Stevens DA. Cellular immunity in infectious mononucleosis. II. Specific reactivity to Epstein-Barr virus antigens and correlation with clinical and hematological parameters. J. Immunol 1978; 121:1239–44.

17. Epstein MA. A prototype vaccine to present Epstein-Barr (EB) virus-associated tumors. Proc Soc Lond [Biol] 1984; 221:1–20.

18. Pearson GR, Orr TW. Antibody-dependent lymphocyte cytotoxicity against cells expressing Epstein-Barr virus antigens. JNCI 1976; 56:485–8.

19. Pearson GR, Johansson B, Klein G. Antibody-dependent lymphocyte cytotoxicity against EBV-associated antigens in African patients with nasopharyngeal carcinoma. Int J Cancer 1978; 22:120–5.

20. Chan SH, Levine PH, de The G, et al. A comparison of the prognostic value of antibody-dependent lymphocyte cytotoxicity and other EBV antibody assays in Chinese patients with nasopharyngeal carcinoma. Int J Cancer 1979; 23:181–5.

21. Pearson GR, Qualtiere LF, Klein G, Norin T, Bal IS. Epstein-Barr virus-specific antibody-dependent cellular cytotoxicity in patients with Burkitt's lymphoma. Int J Cancer 1979; 24:402–6.

22. Granlund DJ, Biggar RJ, Levine PH, Fuccillo DA, Nkrumah F. Antibody-dependent cell-mediated cytotoxicity against Epstein-Barr virus membrane antigen in African Burkitt's lymphoma. Int J Cancer 1979; 24:567–71.

23. Henle W, Henle G, Gunven P, Klein G, Clifford P, Singh S. Patterns of antibodies to Epstein-Barr virus-induced early antigens in Burkitt's Lymphoma. Comparison of dying patients with long term survivors. JNCI 1973; 50:1163–73.

24. Henle W, Ho JHC, Henle G, Kwan HC. Antibodies to Epstein-Barr virus-related antigens in nasopharyngeal carcinoma. Comparison of active cases with long term survivors. JNCI 1973; 51:361–9.

25. Henle, W, Ho JHC, Henle G, Chau CW, Kwan HC. Nasopharyngeal carcinoma: Significance of changes in Epstein-Barr virus-related antibody patterns following therapy. Int J Cancer 1977; 20:663–72.

26. Gunven P, Klein G. Circulating antigen-antibody complex associated with Epstein-Barr virus in recurrent Burkitt's Lymphoma. JNCI 1973; 51:1319–21.

27. Biggar RB, Nkrumah FK, Henle W, Levine PH. Very late relapse in patients with Burkitt's Lymphoma: Clinical and serological studies. JNCI 1981; 66:439–44.

28. Ziegler JL, Bluming AZ, Fass L, Morrow R. Relapse patterns in Burkitt's Lymphoma. Cancer Res 1972; 32:1267–72.

29. Kamaraju LS, Levine PH, Sundar SK, et al. Epstein-Barr virus related lymphocyte stimulation inhibitor: A possible prognostic tool for undifferentiated nasopharyngeal carcinoma. JNCI 1983; 70:643–7.

30. Kamaraju LS, Levine PH, Sundar SK, et al. Detection of Epstein-Barr virus-related lymphocyte stimulation inhibitor in Malaysian, European and North American patients with nasopharyngeal carcinoma. In: Prasad U, Ablashi DV, Levine PH, Pearson GR. Kuala Lumpur: University of Malaya Press, 1983;99–102.

31. Halprin J, Scott AL, Jacobson L, et al. Enzyme-linked immunoabsorbent Assays (ELISA) using bacterially synthesized Epstein-Barr virus nuclear and early antigens: Clinical studies of patients with infectious mononucleosis and nasopharyngeal carcinoma. Ann Intern Med 1986; 104:331–7.

32. Nkrumah FK, Pizza G, Viza D, Neequaye J, DeVinci C, Levine PH. EBV-specific transfer factor in the treatment of African Burkitt's Lymphoma: A pilot study. In: Levine PH, Ablashi DV, Pearson GR, Kottaridis SD, eds. Epstein-Barr virus and associated diseases. Boston: Martinus Nijhoff, 1985; 666–72.

33. Pearson GR, Redmon LW, Pearson GW. Serochemotherapy against a Moloney-virus induced leukemia. Cancer Res 1973; 33:1854–7.

34. Ngu VA. Clinical evidence of host defenses in Burkitt tumor. In: Burchenal JH, Burkitt DP, eds. Treatment of Burkitt's tumor. New York: Springer-Verlag, 1967; 204–8.

Cancer Detection and Prevention Supplement 1:225–229 (1987)

Common Acute Lymphoblastic Leukemia Antigen: Partial Characterization by In Vivo Labeling and Isolation of Its Messenger RNA

Susanne Heinsohn
Hartmut Kabisch

*Kinderklinik, Abteilung für Hämatologie und Onkologie,
Universitätskrankenhaus Eppendorf, Hamburg, Federal Republic of Germany*

ABSTRACT   Common acute lymphoblastic leukemia (ALL) antigen (CALLA)-like proteins were detected by in vivo labeling experiments carried out with human lymphoblastoid cell line KM3 and also in cell-free translation, directed by CALLA–specific mRNA prepared from immunoadsorbed KM3 polysomes. The CALLA-like structure found in both systems shows an M_r of 95kDa. Additional CALLA-like proteins could be identified in the in vivo experiments with calculated M_rs of 40kDa in the cells and 85 and 38kDa in the culture medium. In the cell-free translation system, an additional product of M_r 80kDa could be detected.

Key words: common ALL antigen, cell surface marker, lymphoblastic leukemia, in vitro translation

INTRODUCTION

The common acute lymphoblastic leukemia antigen (CALLA) is a cell surface marker expressed on leukemic cells of patients with non-B, non-T acute lumphoblastic leukemia and lymphoid blast crisis. It was also identified on a number of malignancies of the B-cell lineage including Burkitt lymphoma and lymphocytic lymphoma of the nodular, poorly differentiated type and on chronic myelocytic leukemia (CML) cells.

Using immunobiochemical methods, CALLA was originally described by Greaves and colleagues [1] as a glycosylated polypeptide with an M_r of 100kDa. Later, Metzger et al [2] found a 90kDa CALLA-like protein on hematopoetic kidney cells. This poses the question of whether both antigenic structures are expressed by the same gene or part of it, or whether the antigens, coded by different genes, have similar antigenic epitopes. CALLA has also been studied by other investigators using several heteroantisera [3–6]. In agreement with other studies, we found a 95kDa CALLA-like protein in a cell-free translation system directed by mRNA from human lymphoblastoid cell line KM3 using a specific combination of anti-CALLA monoclonal antibodies and heteroantiserum [7].

The significance of CALLA as an immunological marker in classifying acute lympho-blastic leukemias has been shown by several groups [8–10], so it is now a standard in prognosis

---

Address reprint requests to Susanne Heinsohn, UKE-Kinderklinik-Neubau, Abt. f. Hämatologie & Onkologie, Martinistraße 52, D-2000 Hamburg 20, Federal Republic of Germany.

of this disease. However, the mechanisms leading to leukemic transformation are not yet discovered and cannot be answered without studying the CALLA-gene complex. In our studies, we give a partial characterization of CALLA-like proteins using in vivo labeling experiments and cell-free translation of CALLA-specific mRNA leading to the cloning of CALLA-cDNA as a basic step in analyzing the CALLA-gene complex.

MATERIAL AND METHODS
Materials

Monoclonal antibody J5 was purchased from Coulter (Hialeah, FL). Antibody A12 was a gift from Dr. Carrel (Epalinges, Switzerland); antiserum 399 was prepared in our laboratory. Reticulocyte lysate N 90, ^{35}S-methionine, and ^{14}C-protein mixture were purchased from Amersham, protein A-Sepharose CL-4B from Pharmacia (Uppsala, Sweden), oligo-(dT) cellulose type 2 from Collaborative Research, acrylamide and agarose from BRL, components for cell-growth from Gibco (Grand Island, NY), and fetal calf serum (FCS) from Seromed.

Preparation of Antiserum

Antiserum 399 against CALLA, raised in rabbits, was diluted with TBS (20 mM Tris, pH8, 140 mM NaCl, 0.04% NaN, 1 mM EDTA) and applied to a protein A-Sepharose CL-4B column, and purified IgG fraction was eluted with 0.1 M Na-citrat, pH 2.5, and immediately neutralized with Tris.

Growth of Cell Culture

Human lymphoblastoid cell line KM3 of pre-B-cell type (CALLA$^+$) was grown in RPMI 1640 media supplemented with L-glutamine, heat-inactivated FCS (10%), 1 mM sodium pyrophosphate, and 100 U/ml penicillin/streptomycin.

In Vivo Labeling of Cell Culture

For internal labeling experiments, KM3 cells were grown overnight in MEM (Eagle) medium without methionine (Gibco), supplemented with 10 μCi ^{35}S-methionine/ml. Up to 1×10^8 cells were harvested and separated from radioactive media. Cells were washed three times with PBS (140 mM NaCl/2.5 mM KCl/8 mM Na$_2$HPO$_4$/1.5 mM KH$_2$PO$_4$) supplemented with 5 mM methionine and then solubilized with TBS (s.o.) supplemented with 0.4% Triton X-100 for 1 hr at 4°C and finally used for immunoprecipitation of translational products.

Isolation of Specific Polysomes by Immunoadsorption Procedure

Up to 8×10^9 cells were harvested and used for specific polysome isolation. The procedure was carried out as previously described [11].

Isolation of Polyadenylated mRNA

RNA extraction and preparation and purification of polyadenylated mRNA were carried out as described elsewhere [12,13].

In Vitro Translation of Polyadenylated mRNA

The rabbit reticulocyte lysate translation kit was used according to the suppliers instructions: About 1 μg poly-A$^+$ mRNA was translated in a 25 μl translation assay supplemented with 50 μCi ^{35}S-methionine, incubated 1 hr at 30°C, then diluted 1:3 with dilution buffer [10 mM Na$_2$HPO$_4$, 1 mM EDTA, 1% Triton X-100 (w/w), 2% methionine, 1%·Antagosan, (Behringwerke), pH 7.6], and used for immunoprecipitation of translational products.

Immunoprecipitation of In Vitro or In Vivo Translational Products

Thirty to fifty micrograms of protein A-Sepharose (PAS)-bound anti-CALLA antibodies and/or antiserum was added to the translation assay and incubated for 30 min at room temperature and overnight at 4°C. Subsequent washes of PAS followed: twice with buffer TEN 500 (20 mM Tris, pH 7.5, 1 mM EDTA, 0.5% Triton X-100, 500 mM NaCl) and once with buffer TEN 100 (100 mM NaCl instead of 500 mM).

PAGE

NaDodSO$_4$ PAGE was performed as previously described [14]. Gels were fixed with 7% acetic acid, fluorographed using Amplify (Amersham), dried, and exposed to preflashed Fuji RX X-ray films at 80°C. Exposures of 1–3 weeks were necessary to give satisfying results.

RESULTS
CALLA-Like Products Detected With In Vivo Labeling Experiments

Up to 10^8 lymphoblastoid KM3 cells are grown overnight in ^{35}S-methionine-supplemented media. The translation products of cells and media are identified by precipitation with anti-CALLA antibody J5 and anti-CALLA heteroantiserum 399. Both, the monoclonal antibody J5 and the heteroantiserum 399 precipitate a CALLA-like protein of M_r 95kDa, not seen in any control, when mouse IgG$_2$a and rabbit normal serum are used for precipitation. This protein does not appear in the culture media. Heteroantiserum 399 precipitates one additional protein of M_r 40kDa in the cell solubilisate not precipitable with antibody J5. In the culture media, we get specific products only with heteroantiserum 399 with calculated M_rs of 85 and 38kDa (Fig. 1).

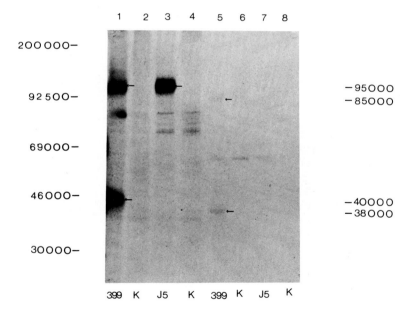

Fig. 1. SDS-PAGE analysis of translational products derived from in vivo ^{35}S-methionine-labeled KM3 cells with human lymphoblastoid phenotype. Lanes 1–4 present the precipitation products of the cell solubilisate, lanes 5–8 the products of the culture media. At the bottom, the anti-CALLA heteroantiserum and antibody used for precipitation are listed. In the controls (lanes 2, 4, 6, 8), a combination of mouse IgG$_2$a and rabbit normal serum are used for precipitation. As protein markers, a ^{14}C-methylated protein mixture was used (listed at left): myosin (200kDa), phosphorylase b (92.5kDa), bovine serum albumin (69kDa), ovalbumin (46kDa), carbonic anhydrase (30kDa). At right, the calculated molecular weights of the precipitable CALLA-like structures are indicated.

Cell-Free Translation Products of mRNA Derived From Polysome Precipitation

The cell-free analysis of mRNA derived from precipitated polysomes shows one antigenic structure of M_r 95kDa appearing with each polysomal mRNA using heteroantiserum 399 or antibody J5 alone for polysomal precipitation. Even when using all combinations of available antibodies and heteroantiserum, only one precipitable CALLA-like protein of M_r 95kDa is obtained as shown by earlier data [7]. Application of only rabbit anti-CALLA heteroantiserum 399 for polysomal precipitation results in two additional cell-free translation products of M_rs 80 and 38kDa (Fig. 2).

DISCUSSION

In this study, we demonstrate that CALLA-like proteins can be identified using in vivo labeling experiments as well as cell-free translation systems directed by mRNA derived from specific immunoprecipitated polysomes. In the cell-free translation system, only a combination of monoclonal antibody and heteroantiserum yields the specific product, whereas the internal labeling experiments use only one, antibody or heteroantiserum, to bring up the very strong CALLA-like product of M_r 95kDa. In further experiments (data not shown), using several combinations of anti-CALLA antibodies and anti-CALLA heteroantiserum for precipitation of translational products from internal labeled KM3 cells, it could be seen that every time heteroantiserum 399 is used the M_r 95kDa Dalton CALLA-like protein is obtained and every time anti-CALLA antibody J5 is used the M_r 40kDa protein is obtained. These two products appear to be the basic CALL antigen structures. As we postulated in earlier experiments [7], it can be suggested that the large CALLA-like antigen of M_r 95kDa is a precursor that will be processed into smaller proteins before or after attachment to the membrane. This thesis is supported by our in vivo labeling experiments in which translation and processing can take

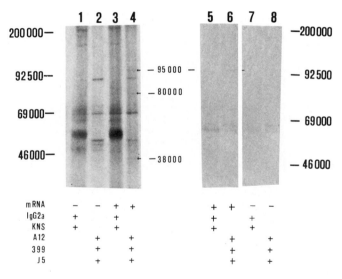

Fig. 2. SDS-PAGE analysis of cell-free translational products directed by mRNA, derived from polysomal immunoprecipitation of KM3 cells. At the bottom, the anti-CALLA antibodies and heteroantiserum used for precipitation are listed. Crosses under each lane indicate the employed antibody(ies)/antiserum. Lanes 1, 2, 7, 8, represent the control minus mRNA. In lanes 3 and 5, representing the control with mRNA, mouse IgG$_2$a and rabbit normal serum (KNS) are used for precipitation. Lanes 1–4 and 5–8 represent different gels. At the left and the right sides, the protein markers (same as in Fig. 1) are indicated. In the middle are the calculated molecular weights of the precipitable CALLA-like products.

place in the presence of natural membranes of the cells, which are necessary for processing and glycosylation. This experiment supports the hypothesis [15,16] that the membrane-derived CALLA has an M_r of 97–100kDa, but with its sugar residues stripped off, a protein of 75–80kDa is defined. The smaller proteins of 38 and 40kDa seem to be further processing products. Several other membrane-bound proteins are known to be processed like the mouse myeloma immunoglobulin L-chain precursor, in which a primary product contains additional amino acids [17]. Our studies are a further step in characterizing the CALL antigen. We isolated specific CALLA mRNA performing the polysomal adsorption procedure and used it for constructing a cDNA library as the first step in isolating the CALLA structural gene.

ACKNOWLEDGMENTS

We thank M.-T. Fichelscher for excellent technical assistance and Ralf Heinsohn for critical reading of the manuscript. A12 antibody was a kind gift from Dr. Carrel (Ludwig Institute of Cancer Research, Lausanne Branch, Epalinges, Switzerland). This work was financially supported by the Deutsche Forschungsgemeinschaft (Bonn), Werner Otto Stiftung (Hamburg), and Förderungsgemeinschaft zur Erforschung und Heilung von Krebskrankheiten bei Kindern e.V. (Hamburg).

REFERENCES

1. Newman RA, Sutherland A, Greaves MF. The biochemical characterization of a cell surface antigen associated with lymphoblastic leukemia and lymphocyte precursors. J Immunol 1981; 126:2024.
2. Metzger RS, Borowitz MJ, Jones NH, Dowell BL. Distribution of common acute lymphoblastic leukemia antigen on haematopoetic tissues. J Exp Med 1981; 154:1249.
3. Billig R, Minowada J, Cline M, Clark B, Lee K. Acute lymphocytic leukemia associated cell membrane antigen. J Natl Cancer Inst 1978; 61:423.
4. Carrel S, de Tribolet N, Gross N. Expression of HLA-DR and common acute lymphoblastic leukemia antigens on glioma cells. Eur J Immunol 1982; 12:354.
5. Kabisch H, Arndt R, Thiele HG, Winkler K, Landbeck G. Partial molecular characterization of an antigenic structure associated to cells of common acute lymphocytic leukemia (ALL). Clin Exp Immunol 1978; 32:399.
6. Rodt H, Netzel B, Thiel E, Laeger G, Huhn D, Hass R, Goetze D, Therfelder S. Classification of leukemic cells with T- and O-ALL specific antisera. Haematol Blood Transf 1977; 20:87.
7. Kabisch H, Fichelscher MTH, Becker WM, Heinsohn S. Isolation of the specific mRNA coding for a CALLA-like protein and partial characterization of its cell-free translational products. Leuk Res 1985; 9:1405.
8. Carrel S, Neuman D, Sekaby RP, Zaech P, Buchegger F, Giradet C. Characterization of a monoclonal antibody (A12) that defines a human acute lymphoblastic leukemia associated differentiation antigen. Hybridoma 1983; 2:11.
9. Chessels JM, Hardesty RM, Rapson NT, Greaves MF. Acute lymphoblastic leukemia in children: Classification and prognosis. Lancet 1977; ii:1307.
10. Thoene I, Kabisch H. Multimarker analysis of childhood lymphoblastic leukemia (ALL): Heterogeneity of cellular phenotypes and clinical relevance of immunological defined subclasses. Blood Transf 1983; 28:100.
11. Kraus PJ, Rosenberg LE. Purification of low-abundance messenger RNAs from rat liver by polysome immuno-adsorption. Proc Natl Acad Sci USA 1982; 79:4015.
12. Aviv H, Leder P. Purification of biologically active mRNA by chromatography on oligothymidylic acid-cellulose. Proc Natl Acad Sci USA 1972; 69:1408.
13. Palmiter RD. Magnesium precipitation of ribonucleoprotein complexes. Expedient technique for the isolation of undegraded polysomes and messenger ribonucleic acid. Biochemistry 1974; 13:3606.
14. Laemmli U. Cleavage of structural proteins during the assembly of the head of bacteriophage T4. Nature 1970; 226:680.
15. Le Baco-Verheyden AM, Ravoet AM, Bazin H, Sutherland DR, Tidman N, Greaves MF. Rat AL2, AL3, AL4 and AL5 monoclonal antibodies bind to common acute lymphoblastic leukemia antigen (CALLA gp 100). Int J Cancer 1983; 32:273.
16. Le Bien TW, Boue DR, Bradley JR, Kersey JH. Antibody affinity may influence antigenic modulation of the common acute lymphoblastic leukemia antigen in vitro. J Immunol 1982; 122:82.
17. Wolf O, Zemell R, Burstein Y, Schlechter J. Partial sequence of immunoglobulin light chain isolated from purified plasma membranes of mouse myeloma cells. Biochem Biophys Res Commun 1977; 78:1383.

Cancer Detection and Prevention Supplement 1:231–234 (1987)

Comparison of CEA Polyclonal Antibodies, CEA Monoclonal Antibodies, Tissue Polypeptide Antigen in the Sera of Supposedly Healthy Individuals

Eric P. Pluygers, MD
Marc P. Beauduin, MD
Paul E. Baldewyns, BSc

*Cancer Detection Unit and Radioimmunology Laboratory, Oncology and
Nuclear Medicine Department, Jolimont Hospital, La Louvière, Belgium*

ABSTRACT   Serum determinations of carcinoembryonic antigen (CEA) using both polyclonal antibodies (PAbs) and monoclonal antibodies (MAbs) were carried out in 348 supposedly healthy screenees. A correlation of the two CEA-detection methods was observed for MAb values higher than 0.5 ng/ml, but not for the lower MAb values that failed to detect CEA. Of 162 such cases (46.5% of the total population that were screened by MAbs), only 39 (11.2%) remained undetected by PAbs, with values as high as 3–4 ng/ml. CEA PAbs thus enabled a more subtle analysis of values in the lower range, a potentially useful factor in screening. In 18 screenees (5.1%) the values were above 2 SD of the mean by MAbs against 13 by PAbs; values above 3 SD were present in three by MAbs and in none by PAbs. In 14 of 18 cases high CEA values were related to smoking and to chronic gastrointestinal disease. The suggested specificity of CEA MAbs for cancer cells thus could not be confirmed because no cancer was detected in this series. Elevated tissue polypeptide antigen values were observed in 14 individuals and were not correlated with either CEA or smoking. Estrogens and estrogen-progestogens were administered to five females whereas four males had gynecomasty, and in three cases leukemia was reported among close relatives.

Key words: screening, cancer tests, tumor immunology, cancer-associated antigens, immunodiagnosis

INTRODUCTION

The value of carcinoembryonic antigen (CEA) determinations using monoclonal antibodies (CEA MAbs) in the staging and monitoring of known cancer cases is now well established and has become a routine procedure in all cases with elevated CEA serum levels. Conversely, CEA determinations for early cancer screening of a supposedly healthy population are generally considered to be of little use. However, we found that individuals having even slightly raised CEA values were at higher risk (up to ten times) of developing an overt cancer [1,2]. It also appears that the population at risk was more readily identified when using a combination of tumor markers.

Address reprint requests to Dr. Eric P. Pluygers, Oncology and Nuclear Medicine Department, Jolimont Hospital, 7161 Haine-Saint-Paul, La Louvière, Belgium.

In this study, which was initiated 8 years ago, CEA assessments, during the first 7 years were carried out using polyclonal antibodies (PAbs). Monoclonal antibodies (MAbs) were used in the most recent year of the study. Other markers were gradually introduced, such as tissue polypeptide antigen (TPA), N.S. enolase, carbohydrate antigen CA 12.5, carbohydrate antigen CA 19.9, and, more recently, carbohydrate antigen CA 15.3. The purpose of this study was the comparison of values obtained from determinations of TPA and CEA by PAbs and by MAbs for the screening of a supposedly healthy population.

MATERIALS AND METHODS
Population Screened

The population under study was made up of 348 supposedly healthy individuals of both sexes who attended a cancer detection center: 266 females (age range 19 to 83 years, mean 46 years) and 82 males (age range 22 to 70 years, mean 45 years). No selections of any kind were made in this group; particularly, no attempt was made to correlate smoking habits with the marker levels except in those cases that revealed abnormal values. Symptomatic individuals, especially those with tumor-related symptoms, were excluded from the study.

Marker Determinations

All individuals attending the screening center had determinations of CEA PAbs, CEA MAbs, and TPA; the determinations were carried out on the same blood sample and in the same laboratory by the same technical staff. Each determination was performed in duplicate, and the mean value of both determinations was recorded using nonautomated equipment. Strict quality control requirements were satisfied, a point of major importance when comparing values in the lower level range. For all assays, commercially available kits were used. CEA PAbs were determined by IRMA technique using a kit produced by Pharmacia Diagnostica A.B., (Uppsala, Sweden). Assays were carried out for CEA MAbs, by IRMA technique (kit produced by Abbott Diagnostics (Abbott Park, Il) and for TPA PAbs by RIA technique (kit produced by Sangtec Medical, Bromma, Sweden). Threshold levels of these markers, at 2 SD from the mean, were set at 7.5 ng/ml for CEA PAbs, at 5 ng/ml for CEA MAbs, and at 100 U/liter for TPA. Values over 5 ng/ml for CEA PAbs and over 3 ng/ml for CEA MAbs were considered "suspicious." A higher threshold that was considered "abnormal" and initiated a more thorough investigation of the case was set at 3 SD from mean for TPA (representing 120 U/liter) and at 15 and 10 ng/ml for CEA PAbs and CEA MAbs, respectively. These latter figures represented the highest values that had been observed in a normal population (N = 283) consisting of blood donors (around 80% of total) and patients attending a thyroid clinic (about 20% of total) in whom any kind of pathology was ruled out.

RESULTS
Comparison Between CEA PAbs and CEA MAbs

Contrary to the good correlation between both techniques that was observed in proven cases of cancer and in follow-up studies, the CEA levels in supposedly healthy screenees revealed marked differences in relation to the technique used (Fig. 1). As could be expected, values obtained by use of MAbs were always lower. In the range of lower values, CEA determined by use of MAbs remained undetected in 162 screenees (46.5% of the total population) while it was undetected by use of PAbs in 39 cases (11.2%). In the range of higher values, 15 screenees had serum levels between 2 SD and "abnormal" threshold when MAbs were used, against ten with the use of PAbs. The values were above the "abnormal" threshold in three screenees by MAbs and in none by PAbs.

Comparison Between CEA PAbs, CEA MAbs, and TPA

In 14 of 348 screenees (4.02%) the values of TPA were above 3 SD, and in 19 cases (5.46%) values ranged between 2 and 3 SD. These 33 cases were evenly distributed between CEA values (Fig. 1).

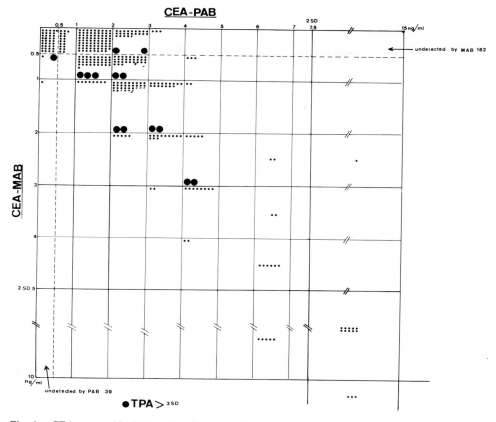

Fig. 1.   CEA assessed by MAbs plotted against CEA assessed by PAbs. Large-sized dots represent TPA values in excess of 3 SD.

DISCUSSION

The presence of a range of lower values in a supposedly healthy population that was screened for cancer requires assessment of minute differences of CEA during yearly follow-up determinations even in cases of the so-called "normal" range of values. We have previously reported [1,2] that in the follow-up of proven cancer cases a steady rise in CEA even below the threshold range points to development of disease. For this reason it is important to assess CEA with great accuracy in the lower level range. In cases in which CEA remains undetected, it loses its usefulness as a possible risk indicator, because a steady rise within the "normal" range may be missed during yearly follow-up determinations. This occurred in 46.5% of the screenees using MAbs against 11.2% with PAbs.

The precise antigen that is determined by CEA immunoassays remains a matter of speculation because of the strong antigenic heterogeneity of the CEA molecule leading to the identification of two molecular forms with a molecular weight difference of 20,000 D [3], several CEA-like substances, the nonspecific cross-reacting antigen NCA [3], and others. It is suggested that careful methodology is essential to obtain valid data [4], and that radioimmunoassays will not be disturbed by cross-reactions as long as competition methods are used, however this is not entirely the case with the actual sandwich techniques in which the use of monoclonal antibodies was hoped to offer a solution to the problem. However, Oehr et al [5] observed that MAb assays did not differ significantly from the former polyclonal CEA assays. According to our observations in a screened population values above 2 SD with MAbs were found in 18 and with PAbs in 10 without any case of cancer detected in a 1 year follow-up. In three individuals, values above 3 SD were found by MAbs, against none by PAbs. In 14 of 18 cases, the elevated CEA level was related to smoking and chronic gastrointestinal tract disease. Hence, the suggested specificity of CEA MAbs (determined by available kits) for cancer cells could not be confirmed. In contrast CEA PAbs were clearly more discriminating in this series.

High TPA values (over 3 SD from mean) were found in 14 screenees and did not correlate in all cases with CEA levels (see figure 1). The precise function of TPA is not yet fully understood, but lead times of 6 months and more were observed on several occasions in cancer patients when compared to other markers. Evaluation of the 14 screenees with high levels of TPA failed to reveal any correlation with smoking; five female screenees were receiving estrogen therapy and four of the five males in this group had gynecomasty. Two screenees had chronic gastrointestinal tract disease, and three of the 14 close relatives (one sister and two brothers) were receiving treatment for leukemia. No explanation is attempted for this surprising observation because TPA is considered to be a marker of epithelial cell proliferation in malignant neoplasms [6].

In the screening of a healthy population, CEA PAbs were found to be more sensitive in the lower range of values only 11.2% were "undetected" against 46.5% of MAbs. It appeared that CEA MAbs were not specific because most values above 2 SD could be explained by smoking and chronic nonneoplastic diseases. For screening purposes, we recommend the use of CEA PAbs because they permit a more sensitive analysis in the lower range of values, and is therefore more favorable for follow-up studies. The addition of TPA determinations in the protocol revealed promising results providing increased sensitivity and therefore decreasing the number of screenees suspected to be at risk of developing overt cancer.

ACKNOWLEDGMENTS

We express our gratitude to Mrs. Danielle Dupont and Mr. Etienne Failly for expert technical assistance and Miss Catherine Leloir for secretarial assistance.

REFERENCES

1. Pluygers E, Beauduin M, Baldewyns P, Burion J. Tumor markers for cancer detection. I. Cancer Detect Prevent 1986; 9:495–504.
2. Pluygers E, Beauduin M, Baldewyns P, Burion J. Tumor markers for cancer detection. II. Cancer Detect Prevent 1986; 9:505–10.
3. von Kleist S. A molecular analysis of the carcino-embryonic antigen (CEA) by monoclonal antibodies. In Anon: Abstracts, 3rd Int Conf Human Tumor Markers, Naples 1986. ALM, Milan, 40–41 (abst).
4. Burtin M, Escribano MJ. The carcinoembryonic antigen and its cross-reacting antigens. In Fishman WH, ed: Oncodevelopmental markers. New York: Academic Press, 1983:315–32.
5. Oehr F, Beesten B, Biersack HJ. The importance of low plasma CEA-values in healthy smokers for the sensitivity of CEA-asssys in tumor patients. In Anon: Abstracts, 3rd Int Conf Human Tumor Markers, Naples 1986. ALM, Milan, 279(abst).
6. Björklund B, Björklund V. The enigma of a human tumor marker: TPA revisited. In Anon: Abstracts, 3rd Int Conf Human Tumor Markers, Naples 1986. ALM, Milan, 24 (abst).

Cancer Detection and Prevention Supplement 1:235–239 (1987)

Screening of Hybridoma Supernatants Raised Against Membrane Fractions From Breast Cancer Using an Immunodot Assay

Ralf Heinsohn
Christiane R. Seitz
Ariel C. Hollinshead
William Hyun
Alois Poschmann

Universitätskrankenhaus Eppendorf Kinderklinik, Abteilung für Klinische Immunpathologie, Hamburg, Federal Republic of Germany (R.H., C.R.S., A.P.); Department of Medicine, The George Washington University Medical Center, Washington, DC (A.C.H., W.H.)

ABSTRACT   Membranes were prepared from mammary tumors and fractionized using gel filtration and gradient polyacrylamide gel electrophoresis. To obtain monoclonal antibodies against tumor-associated antigens, mice were immunized against membrane fraction 2a. After hybridization, we obtained 746 hybridoma cell lines. We performed the immunodot assay for screening. Every supernatant was tested against 15 antigens. Eight antigens were purified fractions from tumor membrane preparation, and five were crude membrane preparations from benign and malignant breast cell lines. Additionally, the Thomsen-Friedenreich antigen of erythrocytes was tested. We selected 83 hybridomas for further characterization.

Key words: tumor-associated antigens, monoclonal antibodies, mammary tumor

INTRODUCTION

Preparation of monoclonal antibodies against tumor-associated antigens requires screening of a great number of hybridoma supernatants. Since there is little knowledge about the nature of tumor-associated antigens, one has to assay against a spectrum of different antigens. Interesting hybridomas are then subject to further characterization. Using conventional screening assays (eg, radioimmunoassay) the consumption of time and materials (supernatants, radioactive reagents) is enormous when a great number of antigens are used. Therefore, we used the immunodot assay, which is easy to perform and rapid to handle.

Membrane fractions used for immunization were originally prepared for skin testing [3]. Two fractions showed skin-reactive antigens when applied to patients with breast carcinomas. Since membrane preparation was done without use of detergents, we did not expect any

---

Address reprint requests to Ralf Heinsohn, UKE Kinderklinik, Abt. f. Klin. Immunpathologie, Martini-straße 52, D-2000 Hamburg 52, Federal Republic of Germany.

denaturation of antigenic epitopes caused by detergents. In this article we present data derived from screening hybridoma supernatants raised against the so-called fraction 2a. This was eluted from gradient polyacrylamide tube gels.

MATERIALS AND METHODS
Immunization and Hybridization

Hybridoma cell lines were established as described previously [1,2].

Preparation of Membrane Fractions

Mammary tumor tissue was pressed through a stainless steel sieve, frozen, and rethawed. After sonification the soluble pool was fractionized using Sephadex G-200 gel filtration and gradient polyacrylamide gel electrophoresis (see Fig. 1). Details of this procedure have been described previously [3].

Immunodot Assay

Antigen solutions were adjusted to 1 mg/ml and 0.5 μl dotted on nitrocellulose sheets using a microliter pipette (Varipette cristal, Eppendorf, Hamburg, FRG) [4]. Nitrocellulose sheets were blocked with 10% sheep serum in 0.1 M phosphate-buffered saline (PBS), pH 7.2. By combining different antigens on a single strip of nitrocellulose it was possible to assay one hybridoma supernatant with 15 antigens simultaneously. Nitrocellulose strips were each incubated with 0.5 ml supernatant for 1 hr and washed twice with 1% sheep serum in 0.1 M PBS. Horseradish peroxidase-linked goat antimouse IgG + IgM (Jackson, Avondale, PA) was used as a second antibody. It was diluted 1:1,000 with 1% sheep serum in 0.1 M PBS; incubation time was 3 hr. After washing (see above) development was performed using 4-chloro-1-

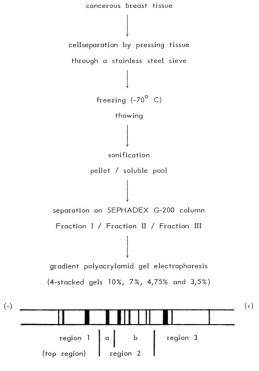

Fig. 1.   Preparation of membrane fractions [3].

naphthol and H_2O_2. Positive spots showed a dark-blue color. Developed nitrocellulose strips were dried, fixed to paper, and stored in the dark without loosing their color for more than 1 year.

Cell Binding Radioimmunoassay

Cell lines were grown to monolayers and trypsinized [5]. Cells were washed, resuspended in medium, and incubated in microtiter plates coated with poly-l-lysine (48 hr, 37°C). Following fixation of cells with 0.25% glutaraldehyde, plates were blocked using 100 mM glycine and 10% bovine serum albumin (BSA) in 0.1 M PBS. Coating of microtiter plates with erythrocytes was also done in this way.

Microtiter plates were then incubated each with 50 μl hybridoma supernatant for 1 hr and washed twice with 1% BSA in 0.1 M PBS, followed by an incubation with rabbit antimouse IgG (Miles). After washing, plates were incubated with ^{125}I protein A (Amersham, Buckinghamshire, England) (1 hr). Then cells were lysed by 0.1 M NaOH, and lysate was absorbed to cotton plugs and transferred to a gamma-counter.

Immunocytological Screening Assay

Cell line MCF-7 was grown and trypsinized, and single cell suspension was adjusted to 6×10^6 cells/ml [6]. Fifty microliters of this suspension were dropped to coated, sterilized slides (Flow No. 60-418-05, Irvine, Scotland). Slides were incubated at 37°C for 24 hr until cells yielded a monolayer. After fixation with acetone/ethanol (1:1, room temperature) and blocking with 10% sheep serum in PBS, slides were incubated with hybridoma supernatants for 1 hr. Slides were then washed three times (1% sheep serum in PBS) and incubated with peroxidase-linked goat antimouse IgG + IgM (Jackson). Binding of second antibody was detected by reaction with aminoethylcarbazol (AEC).

RESULTS

After immunization of mice with membrane fraction region 2a and hybridization of spleen cells with myelomas, we yielded 746 hybridoma cell lines. All of these hybridomas were screened against 15 different antigens using the immunodot assay (Table I).

One antigen was rabbit antimouse IgG + IgM, serving as a catcher assay for production of immunoglobulins. Seven hundred twelve hybridomas produced immunoglobulins. Eight antigens were membrane fractions from mammary tumor tissue (prepared as described above) (see Fig. 1). With antigen fraction "pellet" (after sonification) 55 hybridomas reacted positive; with "soluble pool" (after sonification), 63 hybridomas; with "fraction I" (after gel filtration), 115 hybridomas; with "fraction II" (after gel filtration), 43; with "fraction III" (after gel filtration), 30; with the so-called "top region" (=region 1 in gradient PAGE), 26; with "region 2b$_{4-6}$" (in gradient PAGE), 16; and with "region 2a" (in gradient PAGE), 41 hybridomas gave positive results.

In addition we chose six crude membrane preparations for further screening. One hundred fifty hybridomas reacted positive with membranes from breast cancer liver metastasis. With membrane preparations from normal breast cell line HB-100 and mammary tumor cell lines MCF-7 and SK-BR-3 there was only one positive per cell line. None of the hybridomas reacted with mammary tumor cell line EFM-19 and Thomsen-Friedenreich antigen from erythrocytes.

Since crude membrane preparations from tumor cell lines gave poor results, we decided also to use the cell binding RIA. In this way we hoped to circumvent problems arising from possible denaturing of proteins by binding to nitrocellulose. We tested all hybridomas against erythrocytes (blood group O)-treated nitrocellulose. We tested all hybridomas against erythrocytes (blood group O) treated with neuraminidase from *Vibrio cholerae* (O_{vcn}), against T_n blood (blood group O), and against mammary tumor cell line MCF-7. In the case of O_{vcn}, 95 hybridomas were positive, and in the case of T_n 99 and MCF-7, 48 were positive.

TABLE I. Results from Hybridoma Screening (2a Fusion)

	No.	%	%	%
Total number of supernatants	746	100		
Ig-producing supernatants	712	95	100	
1. Immuno-dot assay				
With positive dot pattern	240	32	34	100
1.1. Membrane fractions				
Pellet (after sonification)	55	7	8	23
Soluble pool (after sonification)	63	8	9	26
Fraction I	115	15	16	48
Fraction II	43	6	6	18
Fraction III	30	4	4	12
Region 1 (top region)	26	3	4	11
Region $2b_{4-6}$	16	2	2	7
Region 2a	41	5	6	17
1.2. Crude membrane preparations				
HB-100	1	0	0	0
MCF-7	1	0	0	0
SK-BR-3	1	0	0	0
EFM-19	0	0	0	0
Breast cancer liver metastasis	150	20	21	62
2. Cell-binding RIA				
(more than 10% binding activity)				
MCF-7	48	6	7	
O_{vcn}	95	13	13	
T_n	99	13	14	
3. Immunocytological assay				
MCF-7	122	16	17	

Unfortunately the reproducibility of cell binding RIA was not very good because of some fluctuation in measuring. So we performed the immunocytological screening assay using cell line MCF-7. In this assay 122 positive hybridomas were found. All of the 48 MCF-7 positives from the cell binding RIA were also positive in the immunocytological assay.

We have assayed all 746 hybridoma supernatants against 19 different antigens and have obtained 14,174 single results (positive or negative). We used a personal computer to evaluate the data. Database software dBASE II (Ashton-Tate) was used for managing and sorting of screening data.

Eighty-three interesting hybridomas were selected. These were rethawed from liquid nitrogen, and 46 of them began to grow. These were reassayed using the immunodot assay. Eighteen hybridoma cell lines were recloned. In recloning we also performed the immunodot assay. The 18 hybridomas are now ready for further characterization.

DISCUSSION

The immunodot assay is a convenient procedure for large-scale screening of hybridoma supernatants. This is especially important in searching for monoclonal antibodies against tumor-associated antigens, where screening with a spectrum of antigens is necessary. Consumption of time and material is very low. We used 12-well reservoir trays (Dynatech No. 002-520-1312, Alexandria, VA) that were staggered on a special shaker (Heidolph, Kehlheim, FRG) and a 12-channel immunowash (Nunc, Roskilde, Denmark) as equipment for the immunodot assay. Staggering the trays made 0.5 ml supernatant sufficient for incubating a nitrocellulose strip dotted with 15 antigens. The immunowash apparatus allowed rapid change of solutions or washing and incubating. This enabled us to assay about 100 to 200 supernatants per day.

The large amount of data resulting from a screening assay with many different antigens require computerized data handling. A personal computer and commercially available database software (dBASE II) have been successfully used for that purpose. We are now developing individual menu-driven computer programs for evaluation of hybridoma screening. Software for interfacing a reflectance densitometer to a computer integrator has been written for automatic densitometric quantification of immunodot assays [7]. Using such equipment offers the possibility of automatic hybridoma screening and interpretation.

The greatest disadvantage of the immunodot assay is the risk of proteins being denatured by absorption to nitrocellulose. In our case dot assays with crude membrane preparations of tumor cell lines gave only poor results. When using other screening assays (cell binding RIA, immunocytological assay) we were able to detect noteworthy amounts of positives. Since we do not know how far other antigens are fully or partly denatured too, some uncertainty remains.

To overcome this uncertainty other techniques are required. The newly developed titerplane and fragmentation technique [8, 9] allows immunohistological screening using frozen sections of tissues fixed on chemically activated glass fragments. It allows histological screening of large numbers of hybridoma supernatants in a short time with less consumption of material, and it has been successfully applied to hybridoma screening [10].

ACKNOWLEDGMENTS

We thank G. Dubberke and K. Lüdemann for excellent technical assistance and the Deutsche Krebshilfe e.V. for financial support.

REFERENCES

1. Köhler G, Milstein C. Continuous cultures of fused cells secreting antibody of predefined specificity. Nature 1975; 256:495–7.
2. Stähli C, Staehelin T, Miggiano V, Schmidt J, Häring P. High frequencies of antigen-specific hybridomas: dependence on immunization parameters and prediction by spleen cell analysis. J Immunol Methods 1980; 32:297–304.
3. Hollinshead AC, Jaffurs WT, Alpert LK, Harris JE, Herberman RB. Isolation and Identification of Soluble Skin-reactive Membrane Antigens of Malignant and Normal Human Breast Cells. Cancer Res 1974; 34:2961–68.
4. Hawkes R, Niday E, Gordon J. A Dot-Immunobinding Assay for Monoclonal and Other Antibodies. Anal Biochem 1982; 119:142–47.
5. Colcher D, Hand PH, Nuti M, Schlom J. A spectrum of monoclonal antibodies reactive with human mammary tumor cells. Proc Natl Acad Sci USA 1981; 78:3199–203.
6. Uhlig H, Rutter G, Dernick R. Self-reactive B lymphocytes detected in young adults, children and newborns after in vitro infection with Epstein-Barr virus. Clin Exp Immunol 1985; 62:75–84.
7. Towbin H, Gordon J. Immunoblotting and Dot Immunobinding — Current Status and Outlook. J Immunol Methods 1984; 72:313–340.
8. Stöcker W. Rationelle Histochemie mit einer neuen Mikroanalysemethode. Acta Histochem (Suppl) 1985; 31:269–81.
9. Stöcker K, Stöcker W, Rittner-Frank Y, Scriba PC. Chemisch aktivierte Glasobjektträger für Gefrierschnitte und ihre Anwendung in der Autoantikörper-Diagnostik. Acta Histochem (Suppl) 1985; 31:283–94.
10. Poschmann A, Seitz Chr, Bein G, Böcker W, Geusendam G, Stöcker W. Rapid histochemical screening of monoclonal antibodies against tumor associated and other antigens using the "titerplane-technique". Immunobiology 1985; 170:1.

Cancer Detection and Prevention Supplement 1:241–247 (1987)

Strategies for the Development of Monoclonal Antibodies for In Vivo Imaging: Their Use in the Imaging of Ovarian Carcinoma

Joy Burchell, PhD
Joyce Taylor-Papadimitriou, PhD
Andrew B. Griffiths, MB, FRCS

Imperial Cancer Research Fund, London, England

ABSTRACT   There are a number of strategies that have been used for the development of monoclonal antibodies which recognise tumour associated antigens. These include the use of whole tumour cells or membrane components as the immunogen, and the use of differentiation antigens, for example the human milk fat globule. The monoclonal antibody HMFG-2 was developed using the latter strategy and has been shown to react with a large molecular weight mucin-like molecule which appears to be highly immunogenic in the mouse. The HMFG-2 antibody is proving to be extremely useful in the localisation of ovarian tumours and is being used in a number of clinics. This antibody and its antigen have a number of characteristics which have contributed to its success in imaging ovarian carcinomas, including the repetitive nature of the antigenic epitope and the antibody's affinity.

Key words: monoclonal antibodies, tumour associated antigens, in vivo imaging, ovarian carcinoma

INTRODUCTION

Although a considerable amount of work has been published on the in vivo imaging of tumours using polyclonal antisera [1–4], the introduction of monoclonal antibodies has given new impetus to this field of cancer research and cancer treatment. Successful in vivo imaging of tumours using radiolabelled antibodies relies on a number of factors including the isotope used for labelling, the type and location of the tumour, and, of course, the antibody and the properties of the molecules carrying the antigenic determinants. This article will describe some of the strategies that have been employed for the production of monoclonal antibodies and then discuss some properties of the HMFG-2 monoclonal antibody that have contributed to its success in imaging ovarian carcinomas.

STRATEGIES FOR THE PRODUCTION OF MONOCLONAL ANTIBODIES
"Shotgun" Approach

In this approach, whole tumour cells are used to immunize the animal and differential screens are performed to select for antibodies recognizing tumour-associated antigens. A

Address reprint requests to Joy Burchell, Imperial Cancer Research Fund, PO Box 123, Lincoln's Inn Fields, London WC2A 3PX, England.

number of monoclonal antibodies have been produced using this immunization method, normally with cells obtained from tumour cell lines [for review, see 5], including the 19.9 and 17.1A antibodies. These antibodies have been extensively used for in vivo imaging [6] and were isolated from a mouse that had been immunized with a colorectal carcinoma cell line [7].

We have used whole, metastatic breast carcinoma cells, isolated from pleural effusion fluid, as an immunogen and fused the spleen cells of the mouse with the myeloma cell line NS1 [8]. The hybridoma supernatants were screened against a variety of cell lines using a live cell binding assay [5], and a number of monoclonal antibodies with varying degrees of tumour specificity have been isolated (see Table I). One antibody, 15.20, looks particularly interesting in that it does not react with normal breast tissue or cell strains derived from normal tissue (see Table I) but does react with all breast carcinomas (10/10) tested. However, this antibody has two disadvantages; 1) It is of the IgM class and so is a large molecule often forming aggregates, and 2) the antibody reacts with an antigen that is destroyed by all forms of fixation. Attempts have been made to isolate mutant clones secreting immunoglobulin of the IgG type, but as yet this has proved unsuccessful. The inability of the antigen to resist any form of fixation makes the widespread characterisation of this antibody difficult; working with unfixed sections is tedious and the availability of normal tissue limited. Antibodies to antigens that are extremely sensitive to fixation might be useful for in vivo imaging, but the difficulties encountered in characterising such antibodies have so far excluded their use in the clinic.

Use of Membrane Components as Antigens

Extracts of the extranuclear cell membranes have been used effectively to produce antibodies to tumour-associated antigens [9–11]. Many of these monoclonal antibodies and antibodies raised against whole cells have been shown to react with carbohydrate determinants [10,12], and indeed a number of the antibodies most widely used for in vivo imaging are directed to antigens that may be wholly or partially carbohydrate [13,14]. The predominance of antibodies with this kind of specificity could be a reflection merely of the highly immunogenic nature of some oligosaccharides in the mouse. However, it has been known for some time that changes in carbohydrate moieties are associated with the malignant change [15–17]. Immunogens can be enriched for oligosaccharide determinants by passing membrane prepara-

TABLE I. Reactivity of Hybridoma S Supernatents With Various Cell Lines

Cell line tested	Antibody						
	8.12	9.11	9.16	11.21	12.10	14.6	15.20
HumE*	+	+	+ +	−	±	−	−
BT20†	±	±	+	−	±	−	+
SKBr3†	−	−	+	−	±	−	+
MB157†	+	+ + +	±	+	+	+ + +	+ + +
734B†	±	+	±	−	−	±	+
CamaI†	+	+ +	+ +	+	±	−	+ +
T47D†	+	+ +	+ +	+	−	+	+ +
Du4475†	±	+	±	+	+	+	+ +
Hs578T‡	−	+	+ + +	±	−	+ + +	+ +
HumF§	±	±	±	−	−	±	±
HEL-F‖	−	−	±	−	−	−	−
Bris8¶	−	−	−	−	−	−	−

*Normal human breast epithelial cells isolated from human milk.
†Cell lines derived from breast carcinomas.
‡Cell line derived from a breast carcinosarcoma.
§Normal human breast fibroblasts.
‖Human embryo lung fibroblasts.
¶Lymphoblastoid cell line.

tions of tumour cells through lectin affinity columns, and this was the technique employed in the isolation of the Ca1 antibody [18]. Because some oligosaccharides have been shown to be especially immunogenic in the mouse [19], a new spectrum of antibodies could perhaps be obtained if these antigens were removed from the membrane preparation (by affinity chromatography using existing antibodies) before immunization.

Production of Antibodies to Differentiation Antigens, eg, the Human Milk Fat Globule

The human milk fat globule (HMFG) membrane, which can be extracted by churning or by solvent extraction of the cream fraction of milk, provides a ready source of membrane representative of a functionally differentiated breast epithelial cell. Polyclonal antisera have been prepared to the HMFG membranes [20,21] and have been used to identify metastatic carcinoma deposits in liver, bone, and serous effusions [22]. More recently, at least three groups have prepared monoclonals to HMFG [23–25]. Of all the components present in the HMFG (15–20 polypeptides on a polyacrylamide gel), a large-molecular-weight glycoprotein appears to be the most immunogenic; the MAM6 series of antibodies [25], M8 and M18 [24], and HMFG-1 and HMFG-2 [23] all seem to be directed to epitopes carried on this molecule. This protein has been shown to be a mucin molecule containing 50% carbohydrate, which is O-linked to serine and threonine residues [26]. HMFG-1, HMFG-2, and M8 have all been used for in vivo imaging [27–29].

HMFG-2 Monoclonal Antibody

The epitope recognised by HMFG-2 is epithelial-specific and is strongly expressed by a variety of carcinomas [30]. It is proving to be extremely useful in the localisation of ovarian tumours and is being used in a number of clinics [28,29]. In one study, 60 patients with a known history of ovarian carcinoma were scanned after the administration of ^{123}I-HMFG-2 and the results obtained from imaging compared with the surgical findings. It was shown that in 94% of cases the imaging results agreed with the surgical findings (N. Pasteisky, personal communication), and this type of success rate has also been reported by other authors [29]. HMFG-2 is now also being used to deliver therapeutic doses of radiation via direct administration into the pleural or peritoneal cavities [31]. This antibody and its antigen have a number of characteristics that have contributed to its success in imaging ovarian carcinomas.

Properties of the HMFG-2 Antigen

The exact nature of the HMFG-2 antigen has yet to be elucidated, but there is some evidence that the epitope is, at least in part, carbohydrate [14]. In the milk fat globule membranes, this epitope is carried on the mucin molecule, which has a molecular weight of greater than 400 Kd, but in tumours and in cultured cells the antigen can be carried on a variety of molecular weight components ranging from 80 to >300 Kd [14]. The epitope is found in the membrane of tumour cells (a necessary prerequisite for in vivo localisation) but has also been observed in the cytoplasm (J. Burchell, R. Tilly, and J. Taylor-Papadimitriou, unpublished observations). This component seems to have a relatively low turnover within the cell, and the HMFG-2 epitope has the advantage of being a repetitive antigen within the same molecule [32]. This allows a number of antibody molecules to bind to a single molecule bearing the antigen and so to deliver a louder radioactive signal when imaging in vivo.

It could be assumed that circulating levels of antigen would be a disadvantage when using antibodies for imaging, although in practice this does not seem to be the case. Anti-CEA antibodies are being used to image carcinomas of the colon [1,33], although elevated levels of CEA have been shown to be present in the serum of carcinoma patients [34]. The HMFG-2 antigen has been demonstrated in the serum of patients with ovarian carcinoma [32], but still the antibody is very successful in imaging ovarian tumours. This might be due to the circulating antigen having a lower affinity for the antibody than membrane-bound antigen and/or the concentration of antigen in the blood stream being much lower than that found within the tumour.

Antibody Specificity

As the catalogue of monoclonal antibodies reactive with tumours increases, the existence of a truly tumour-specific antigen becomes less and less likely. Thus, for the present, in vivo imaging must proceed using antibodies to tumour-associated rather than tumour-specific markers.

As well as being highly expressed by many carcinomas, the HMFG-2 antigen is also found on some normal tissue, especially secretory organs [30], and has been reported to be expressed by normal ovaries. This spectrum of reactivity established using tissue sections is not, however, observed when imaging; normal tissues do not concentrate antibody [29]. Thus, from experience obtained with the HMFG-2 antibody and other antibodies used for in vivo imaging, the spectrum of reactivity seen with normal cells in vitro is not necessarily observed in vivo. This might be due to a number of factors. In normal organs antigens may not be exposed to the blood stream, and only in the malignant change, when the normal architecture of the organ is disrupted, might the antigen be exposed to circulating antibody. Another factor that may restrict access of antibodies to normal tissue is that epithelial cells commonly secrete mucins, which form a barrier over the cells preventing an antibody access to the cell membrane. In addition, there may well be quantitative differences between the level of expression of the antigen by normal tissues and the level of expression by tumours. This is in fact observed in the ovary, where the expression of the HMFG-2 antigen is extremely weak in normal tissue when compared with ovarian tumours (B. Ward, personal communication).

One problem that has been encountered using HMFG-2 is that this antibody localises in benign as well as malignant ovarian tumours (29). This excludes the use of HMFG-2 for the initial diagnosis of ovarian carcinoma and restricts its use to identifying metastatic deposits and estimating the spread of the disease. However, this is still an extremely useful function in that the antibody may alleviate the requirement for a second-look operation.

Antibody Affinity

To obtain efficient tumour imaging, it is important to use an antibody that shows high-affinity binding to its antigen, and the kinetics involved in the association and dissociation of an antibody with its antigen.

It has been shown that differences in an antibody's avidity are due mainly to differences in the rate at which it dissociates from the antigen [35,36]. Thus, by measuring the rates of dissociation, an idea of the antibody's relative affinity for different tumours can be found. Figure 1 shows the curves obtained when the rate of dissociation of HMFG-2 from breast cell lines and strains was measured. It can be observed that, although HMFG-2 bound with relatively high affinity to normal breast epithelial cells, it showed differing affinities in its binding to the cell lines derived from breast tumours. The curves obtained were not straight lines, and this departure from first-order kinetics indicates that there is antigenic heterogeneity within a cell line as well as among different cells [36]. The differences in affinities may result from the antigenic determinants being carried on a number of different molecular weight components [14], which would affect the microenvironment of the epitope. Alternatively, the antibody may show some cross-reaction with determinants that are slightly different from the high-affinity binding site of the antibody. The fact that HMFG-2 binds to different tumours with different avidities may well be important in deciding on the time for imaging patients; the period of time that the antibody will remain bound to a tumour may differ with the individual.

The affinity of an antibody might also play a role in deciding whether subtraction techniques should be employed in imaging. The advantage of labelling the antibody with ^{131}I is that it has a half-life of 8 days, so scanning may be carried out a few days after the administration of the antibody, by which time nonspecific radioactivity should have cleared

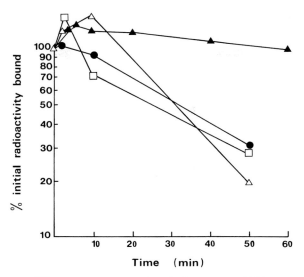

Figure 1:   Dissociation of ^{125}I-labelled HMFG-2 after binding to MCF-7 (□), ZR75-1 (△) T47D (●), all breast cancer cell lines, normal breast epithelial cells from human milk (▲). Cells were incubated for 40 min with ^{125}I-labelled antibody, then a 1,000 times excess of cold antibody was added and radioactivity associated with the cells measured at the times indicated.

from the blood pool. This requires a high-affinity antibody that remains bound to the antigen for a number of days.

CONCLUSIONS

Although in vivo imaging of ovarian cancer using HMFG-2 has been relatively success-ful, there is scope for improvement, especially in the specificity of the antibody. The compo-nent carrying the HMFG-2 determinant has recently been purified from the membranes of the breast cacinoma cell line T47D [37] and used to generate a second series of monoclonal antibodies. It is hoped that by this strategy antibodies will be generated that show many of the characteristics of HMFG-2 but have an increased specificity for tumour cells.

REFERENCES

1. Goldenberg DM, Kim EE, DeLane FH, Bennett S, Primus J. Radioimmunodection of cancer with radioactive antibodies to carcinoembryonic antigen. Cancer Res 1980; 40:2984–92.
2. Mach J-P, Carrel S, Forni M, Ritschard J, Dorath A, Alberto P. Tumour localisation of radiolabelled antibodies against carcinoembryonic antigen in patients with carcinoma. Engl J Med 1980; 303:5–10.
3. Kim EE, DeLand FM, Nelson MD, Bennett S, Simmons G, Alport E, Goldenberg DM Radioim-munodection of cancer with radiolabelled antibodies to -fetoproteins. Cancer Res 1980; 40:3008–12.
4. Goldenberg DM, Kim EE, DeLand FM. Human chorionic gonadotropin radioantibodies in the radioimmunodection of cancer and for disclosure of occult metastases. Proc Natl Acad Sci USA 1981; 78:7754–8.
5. Taylor-Papadimitriou J, Griffiths AB. Development of monoclonal antibodies with specificity for human epithelial cells. Gregoriadis G, Poste G, Senior J, Trouet A, eds: In *Receptor mediated targeting of drugs*. New York: Plenum Publishing, 1985; 201–34
6. Chatal JF, Saccavivi JC, Fumoleau P, Douillard JY, Curtet C, Kremer M, Le Meuel B, Koprowski H. Immunoscintigraphy of colon carcinoma. J Nuclear Med 1984; 25:307–14.
7. Koprowski H, Steplewski Z, Mitchell K, Herlyn M, Herlyn D, Fuhrer P. Colorectal carcinoma antigens, detection by hybridoma antibodies. Somatic Cell Genet 1979; 5:957–61.

8. Kohler G, Milstein C. Derivation of specific antibody producing tissue culture and tumour cell lines by cell fusion. Eur J Immunol 1976; 6:511.

9. Colcher D, Horan Hand P, Nuti M, Schlom J. A spectrum of monoclonal antibodies reactive with human mammary tumour cells. Proc Natl Acad Sci USA 1981; 78:3199–203.

10. Brown A, Feizi T, Gooi MC, Embleton MJ, Picard JK, Baldwin RW. A monoclonal antibody against human colonic adenoma recognises difucosylated type-2-blood-group chains. Biosci Rep 1983; 3:163–70.

11. Inez-Colnaghi M. Antibodies to ovarian cancer. In, Monoclonal antibodies and cancer. Dulbecco R, Langman R, eds: New York; Academic Press, 1983; 239–49,

12. Canevari S, Fossat G, Balsari A, Sonnio S, Colnaghi M. Immunochemical analysis of the determinant recognised by a monoclonal antibody (MBr1) which specifically binds to human mammary epithelial cells. Cancer Res 1983; 43:301–5.

13. Magnani JL, Nilsson-Brockhaus M, Zopf D, Steplewski Z, Koprowski H, Ginsberg V. A monoclonal antibody-defined antigen associated with gastrointestinal cancer is a ganglioside containing sialylated Lacto-H-fucopentaose II. J Biol Chem 1982; 257:14365–9.

14. Burchell J, Durbin H, Taylor-Papadimitriou J. Complexity of expression of antigenic determinants, recognised by monoclonal antibodies HMFG-1 and HMFG-2, in normal and malignant human mammary epithelial cells. J Immunol 1983; 131:508–13.

15. Javadpour N. Immunocytochemical localisation of various markers in cancer cells and tumours. Urology 1983; LI:7.

16. Feizi T. Carbohydrate differentiation antigens. TIBS 1981; 6:333–5.

17. Hounsell EF, Feizi T. Gastrointestinal mucins—Structures and antigenicities of their carbohydrate chains in health and disease. Med Biol 1982; 60:227–36.

18. Ashall F, Bramwell ME, Harrid M. A new marker for human cancer cell. The Ca antigen and the Cal antibody. Lancet 1982; ii:1–6.

19. Brockhaus M, Magnani J, Herlyn M, Blaszcyk M, Steplewski Z, Koprowski M, Ginsberg V. Monoclonal antibodies directed against the sugar sequence of lacto-N-fucopentaose III are obtained from mice immunized with human tumours. Arch Biochem Biophys 1982; 217:647–51.

20. Ceriani RL, Thompson KE, Peterson JA, Abraham S. Surface differentiation antigens on human mammary epithelial cells carried on the human milk fat globule. Proc Natl Acad Sci USA 1977; 74:582–6.

21. Heyderman E, Stule K, Ormerod MG. A new antigen on the epithelial membrane: Its immunoperoxidase localisation in normal and neoplastic tissue. J Clin Pathol 1979; 32:35–44.

22. Dearnaley DP, Sloane JP, Ormerod MG, Steele K, et al. Increased detection of mammary carcinoma cells in marrow using antisera to epithelial membrane antigens. Br J Cancer 1981; 44:85–90.

23. Taylor-Papadimitriou J, Peterson J, Arklie JA, Burchell J, Ceriani RL, Bodmer WF. Monoclonal antibodies to epithelium-specific components of the human milk fat globule membrane: Production and reaction with cells in culture. Int J Cancer 1981; 28:17–21.

24. Foster CS, Edwards PAW, Dinsdale EA, Neville AM. Monoclonal antibodies to the human mammary gland. 1. Distribution of determinants in non-neoplastic mammary and extra mammary tissues. Virchows Arch Pathol Anat Physiol Kin Med 1982; 39:279–82.

25. Hilkens J, Buijs F, Hilgers J, Hageman P, Calafact J, Sonnerberg A, Van-der-Valk M. Monoclonal antibodies against human milk fat globule membranes detecting differentiation antigens of the mammary gland and its tumours. Int J Cancer 1984; 34:197–206.

26. Shimizu M, Yamauchi K. Isolation and characterisation of mucin-like glycoprotein in human milk fat globule membrane. J Biochem 1982; 91:515–21.

27. Rainsbury RM, Westwood JM, Coombes RC, Neville AM, et al. Location of metastatic breast carcinoma by a monoclonal antibody chelate labelled with Indium-111. Lancet 1983; ii:934–8.

28. Epenetos AA, Britton KE, Mather S, Shepherd J, Granowska M, Taylor-Papadimitriou J, Nimmon CC, Durbin H, Hawkins LR, Malpas JS, Bodmer WF. Targeting of iodine-123-labelled tumour-associated monoclonal antibodies to ovarian, breast and gastrointestinal tumours. Lancet 1982; ii:999–1005.

29. Granowska M, Shepherd J, Britton K, Ward B, et al. Ovarian Cancer: Diagnosis using ^{123}I monoclonal antibody in comparison with surgical findings. Nuclear Med Commun 1984; 5:485–99.

30. Arklie J, Taylor-Papadimitriou J, Bodmer W, Egan M, Millis R. Differentiation antigens expressed by epithelial cells in the lactating breast are also detectable in breast cancers. Int J Cancer 1981; 28:23–9.

31. Epenetos AA, Courtenay-Luck N, Halnan K, Hooker G, et al. Antibody guided irradiation of malignant lesions. Three cases illustrating a new method of treatment. Lancet 1984; ii:441–3.

32. Burchell, JM, Wang D, Taylor-Papadimitriou J. Detection of the tumour-associated antigens recognized by the monoclonal antibodies HMFG-1 and 2 in serum from patients with breast cancer. Int J Cancer 1984; 34:763–8.

33. Mach J-P, Buchegger, F , Farni M, Ritschard J, Berche C, Lunbroso J -D, Schreyer M, Girandet C, Accolla RS, Carrel S. Use of radiolabelled monoclonal anti-CEA antibodies for the detection of human carcinomas by external photoscanning and tomoscintigraphy. Immunol Today 1981; 2:239–249.

34. Shively J, Spayth V, Chamg F-F, Metter G, et al. Serum levels of carcinoembryonic antigen and a tumor-extracted carcinoembryonic antigen-related antigen in cancer patients. Cancer Res 1982; 42:2506–13.

35. Froese, A. Kinetic arid equilibrium studies on 2,4-diniterophenyl hapten antibody systems. Immunochemistry 1968; 5:253–64.

36. Mason D, Williams AF. The kinetics of antibody binding to membrane antigens in solution and at the cell surface. Biochem J 1980; 187–20.

37. Griffiths AB, Burchell J, Taylor-Papadimitriou J, Gendler S, Lewis A, Blight K, Tilly R. Immunological analysis of mucin molecules expressed by normal and malignant mammary epithelial cells. Int J Cancer (submitted).

Cancer Detection and Prevention Supplement 1:249–262 (1987)

Imaging of Primary and Metastatic Colorectal Carcinoma With Monoclonal Antibody 791T/36 and the Therapeutic Potential of Antibody-Drug Conjugates

M.V. Pimm, PhD
N.C. Armitage, FRCS
K. Ballantyne, FRCS
R.W. Baldwin, PhD

A.C. Perkins, PhD
L.G. Durrant, PhD
M.C. Garnett, PhD
J.D. Hardcastle, FRCS

Cancer Research Campaign Laboratories, University of Nottingham (M.V.P., L.G.D., M.C.G., R.W.B.) and Departments of Medical Physics, (A.C.P.) and Surgery (N.C.A., K.B., J.D.H.), Queens's Medical Centre, Nottingham, England

ABSTRACT   Monoclonal antibody 791T/36, prepared against a tumour-associated 72,000 dalton glycoprotein, reacted with cells from primary and metastatic colorectal carcinomas. I-131 or In-111-labelled antibody localized in xenografts of colorectal carcinomas established from in vitro clonogenic populations. Clinically, with I-131-labelled antibody, 8/11 colonic tumours imaged positively. Imaging was negative in four patients with benign colon disease. 5/11 rectal tumours were positively imaged, but excreted I-131 in the bladder obscured tumours in several studies. In-111-labelled antibody gave superior images and positively imaged primary and metastatic sites in 13/14 patients. Prospectively in the detection of recurrent disease, I-131 or In-111-antibody detected 29/33 separate sites in 24 patients. Seven negative patients remain disease free. There were 3 false positives; overall sensitivity was 88%, with 70% specificity. Specific localization of radiolabel was confirmed immunochemically and by counting radioactivity in resected specimens. Antibody conjugates with methotrexate, vindesine and daunomycin retained drug activity and antibody function, including xenograft localization and conjugates were therapeutically effective against xenografts. 791T/36 antibody has potential for immunodetection of primary and recurrent colorectal carcinoma and for targeting of therapeutic agents.

Key words: drug targeting, immunodetection, tumors

INTRODUCTION

Colorectal carcinoma is one of the major malignant neoplasms of the Western world, yet, in spite of significant advances in surgical techniques, the survival rate has not improved over the past two decades [1]. The major reasons are the advanced stage of majority of

Address reprint requests to Dr. M.V. Pimm, Cancer Research Campaign Laboratories, University of Nottingham, Nottingham, England NG7 2RD.

colorectal carcinomas at presentation and that anticancer drugs have proven largely ineffective against the disseminated disease [2].

Monoclonal antibodies recognising antigens expressed selectively on human tumours offer new approaches for detection of recurrent and metastatic disease if these antibodies, carrying an appropriate radiolabel, localise sufficiently in tumour sites for visualisation of tumour deposits by external imaging techniques. Moreover, these antibodies potentially offer an approach for selective tumour targeting of antitumour agents. This may improve the drugs' therapeutic indices either by improving the localisation of the agent in the tumour or in metastatses and/or by minimising toxicity to normal tissues.

Antibodies that have been shown clinically to localise in colorectal carcinomas include predominantly those to CEA [3] and other tumour-associated antigens such as those identified by the 19.9 and 17-1A antibodies [4,5]. The monoclonal antibody 791T/36 was raised against a cultured cell line of human osteogenic sarcoma [6], but the antigen it identifies, a 72,000 dalton glycoprotein, was also shown to be expressed in a variety of human malignancies, including colorectal carcinoma [6,7]. This antibody was initially shown to localise in a primary human osteogenic sarcoma by γ camera imaging of the distribution of ^{131}I-labeled antibody [8]. Its reaction with cells of more common malignancies, including colorectal cancer, prompted clinical imaging trials in this disease [9–12]. The studies in colorectal carcinoma will be reviewed here, together with those on the development of drug antibody conjugates with clinical therapeutic potential in this disease.

Reaction of 791T/36 Antibody With Cells of Colorectal Carcinomas

Early studies with 791T/36 antibody showed its reactivity with some long-term culture lines of colorectal carcinoma [6]. More appropriately, before clinical imaging trials with radiolabeled 791T/36 antibody, the expression of 791T/36-defined antigen on cells of primary colon carcinomas and their metastases was assessed. Here cells from tumour, lymph node, and hepatic metastases, brought into suspension by collagenase, were reacted with 791T/36 antibody [13]. Cell-bound antibody was then detected with fluorescein isothiocyanate-labeled rabbit antimouse IgG and analysed by flow cytofluorimetry, using appropriate gating procedures to select tumour cell populations.

Of 31 primary colorectal carcinomas tested 67% showed reaction with 791T/36 antibody significantly greater than that with normal mouse imunoglobulin (Table I). When fluorescence was quantitated in terms of the mean linear fluorescence, the majority (45%) of tumours yielded cells showing "weak" reactivity (MLF < 100), 22% of tumours showed more intense reactivity (MLF > 100), and overall cells from 33% of tumours were considered unreactive. In comparative studies with an anti-CEA antibody, a higher proportion of tumours (97%) yielded reactive cells, but, although these too showed a range of fluorescent staining intensities, reactions were generally greater than those with 791T/36 antibody.

When metastatic as well as primary tumours were available for analysis cells from these metastases reacted at least as well with 791T/36 antibody as those from primary tumour (Fig. 1).

TABLE I. Reactivity of Cells From Primary Colorectal Carcinomas With 791T/36 and Anti-CEA Monoclonal Antibodies

Anitbody	No. of Tumours examined	% of tumours showing reaction of mean linear flourescence			
		> 1,000	100–1,000	< 100	Negative
791T/36	31	3	19	45	33
Anti-CEA*	47	19	62	11	8

*Anti-CEA antibody C24/1/39/11 [13,14].

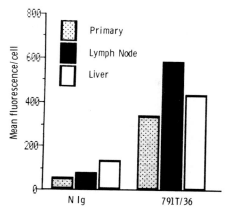

Fig. 1. Binding of 791T/36 monoclonal antibody to primary and metastatic colon carcinoma cells (analysed by flow cytofluorimetry).

TABLE II. Biological Characteristics of Cells of Colorectal Carcinoma Grown In Athymic Mice

| | In vitro doubling time/hr* | | Reaction with 791T/36† | |
	Xenograft-derived cells	Cultured cells	Xenograft-derived cells	Cultured cells
Tumour designated				
C146	21 ± 1	16 ± 1	157 ± 30	80 ± 9
C168	23 ± 2	25 ± 2	62 ± 20	109 ± 9
C170	27 ± 1	26 ± 0.5	111 ± 6	92 ± 29

*Cells were injected into mice at passage 30 and analysed following two passages in mice or 32 passages in culture.
†Determined by indirect immunofluorescence assay (see text). Figures are mean linear fluorescence values obtained by flow cytometry.

ESTABLISHMENT OF COLORECTAL CARCINOMA XENOGRAFTS FOR TUMOUR LOCALISATION STUDIES WITH RADIOLABELED 791T/36

In vitro-cultured cell lines were established from primary colorectal carcinomas. In these studies cells from enzymically disaggregated tumours were initially plated onto 0.3% agar to establish colonies from clonogenic populations, and cells from these were subsequently passaged in conventional monolayer culture [14]. Xenograft lines of three of these colorectal carcinomas (C146, C168, and C170) were established in nude athymic mice or mice immunodeprived by thymectomy and whole body irradiation with cytosine arabinoside protection [15]. In addition, the LS174T colon tissue culture carcinoma cell line [16] was similarly used to establish a xenograft line. When xenografted tumours were resected and disaggregated and their cells analysed for expression of the 791T/36-defined antigen using the fluorescent antibody technique outlined above, levels of expression similar to those in the corresponding cells maintained in culture were seen (Table II). Slightly higher doubling times were observed for all the xenograft-derived cells when they were originally reestablished in culture, but after several passages they were indistinguishable from their continuous culture counterparts (Table II). These observations indicate that these colorectal carcinoma xenografts are appropriate models in which to assess in vivo localisation of 791T/36 antibody since they retain the 791T/36 antigen expression of their corresponding primary tumours.

For these xenograft localisation tests 791T/36 antibody was radiolabeled with ^{125}I and normal mouse immunoglobulin of the same isotype (IgG2b) with ^{131}I to specific activities of approximately 1 mCi; (37MBq)/mg. Groups of mice with established tumour xenografts were injected intraperitoneally with 3 μg of each preparation. Their drinking water was supplemented with 0.1% NaI, and they were killed after 4 days and blood, tumour, and visceral organs and remaining carcass counted for radioactivity. There was preferential accumulation of ^{125}I-791T/36 in all four xenograft lines (Fig. 2). The tissue to blood ratio of ^{125}I in the tumours for the three xenografts derived from C146, C168, and C170 were 1.45:1, 1.01:1, and 1.96:1 compared to a maximum of 0.37:1, 0.36:1, and 0.45:1, respectively, for any of the normal organs. ^{125}I normal IgG2b levels in the tumour tissue were comparable to normal organs. A localisation index calculated as the ratio of the tumour:blood ratio of ^{125}I antibody to the tumour:blood ratio of ^{131}I normal IgG2b was 3.0 $\pm$ 0.2:1, 2.2 $\pm$ 0.5:1, and 3.3 $\pm$ 0.7:1 for lines 146, 168, and 170, respectively.

For imaging of xenografts, 791T/36 antibody was labeled with ^{111}In to a specific activity of 1 mCi; (37MBq)/mg by chelation to DTPA-conjugated antibody [17]. Mice were injected intraperitoneally with 40–80 μCi; (2-4MBq) of ^{111}In-antibody and were imaged 2 to 5 days later with a 40 cm-field of view γ camera fitted with a pin hole collimator. Mice were anaesthetised and placed prone beneath the collimator to give a posterior view. Images were recorded using a dual 20% window centred at the 245 and 171 keV photo peaks. Images containing counts were stored by computer in a 128 × 128 matrix. Regions of interest were drawn on the images around the whole body, the xenograft site, and a contralateral position and count rates from each region used to calculate a tumour to normal tissue (T:NT) ratio and the percentage of whole body activity within the tumour.

Images of mice with both xenograft types examined (C170 and LS174T) showed clear localisation of radioactivity in tumours (eg, Fig. 3). Tumour to nontumour ratios of radioactivity of up to 4.6:1 were achieved, the counts in the tumour region being up to 18% of those in the whole mouse.

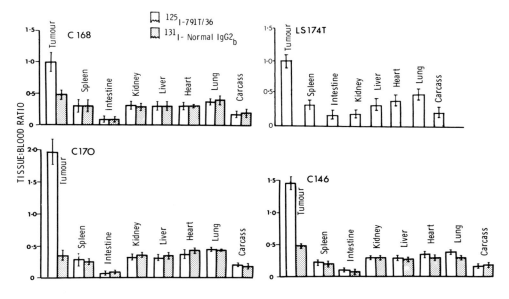

Fig. 2.   Distribution of radiolabeled 791T/36 monoclonal antibody in nude mice with colorectal carcinoma xenografts. Groups of three to four mice with established xenograft were injected intraperitoneally with a mixture of ^{125}I-791T/36 and ^{131}I-normal mouse serum IgG2b and killed after 4 days. The tissue:blood ratio of each isotope in the organs is expressed as (cpm/gm tissue)/(cpm/gm blood).

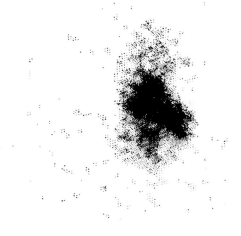

C170 XENOGRAFT

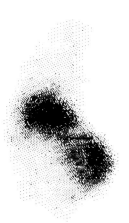

LS174 XENOGRAFT

^{111}In-791T/36

Fig. 3.   Examples of γ camera images of the localisation of ^{111}In-791T/36 monoclonal antibody in mice with xenografts of C170 and LS174T colon carcinomas. Images acquired 2 days after intraperitoneal injection of 40 μCi and 80 μCi of ^{111}In-791T/36, respectively. Tumour to nontumour ratios of ^{111}In counts in these images were 1.5:1 and 2.7:1

CLINICAL IMAGING STUDIES WITH ^{131}I- and ^{111}In-LABELED 791T/36 ANTIBODY IN PRIMARY AND RECURRENT DISEASE

The successful localisation of radiolabeled 791T/36 antibody in xenografts of colorectal carcinomas subsequently formed the basis of clinical imagining trials in patients with primary, recurrent, or metastatic colorectal carcinoma [9–11]. Patients were imaged 48 to 72 h after the administration of ^{131}I- or ^{111}-In labeled 791T/36 antibody (200μg to 1 mg of antibody, 70MBq

[131]I or ^{111}In). Images were acquired with a γ camera including anterior and posterior views of the abdomen and pelvis, a "sitting view" for pelvic lesions, and, if appropriate, a thoracic view. With [131]I- labeled antibody, image enhancement by blood pool subtraction was carried out using ^{99m}Tc labeling of patient red bood cells or [113m]In labeling of transferrin [18]. In patients from whom tumours were resected after imaging resected tissue was also imaged and tumour:nontumour (T:NT) tissue ratios of radioactivity calculated from these images. In addition, samples of tumour and adjacent normal tissue were counted for radioactivity and results expressed as tumour:nontumour radioactivity per gram of tissue. Figures 4 and 5 show examples of patient images with ^{131}I-and [111]In- labeled 791T/36 antibody. With primary malignancy [131]I-791T/36 detected eight of 11 colonic tumours and five of 12 rectal tumours (Table III). The low detection rate in rectal tumours was due primarily to ^{131}I in the urinary bladder masking tumour sites, as examination of resected tumours showed T:NT ratios virtually identical to those with colonic tumours. All of seven benign conditions gave negative images and T:NT ratios of 1:1 of resected specimens. In secondary disease ^{131}I antibody successfully imaged all but two of 19 sites.

The use of ^{111}In as a radiolabel for immunoscintigraphs has several advantages over ^{131}I, particularly lower energy of γ emission, shorter physical half-life, and little urinary excretion, although high liver uptake of ^{111}In causes problems in imaging hepatic and upper abdominal tumours [19,20]. In a small series of imaging studies with [111]In-791T/36, primary tumours were imaged in three of four patients and metastatic sites in eight of ten (Table IV). The mean T:NT ratios of primary resected specimens was 3.3:1 (N = 3).

In a prospective trial to determine the clinical value of antibody imaging compared to conventional imaging modalities, 35 patients with suspected colorectal cancer have been studied using either ^{131}I or [111]In- labeled antibody. Overall, 25 of these patients were subsequently found to have recurrent disease in a total of 37 sites. Antibody imaging detected 30 sites in 21 of these patients [21].

PREPARATION AND THERAPEUTIC EFFICACY OF 791T/36-DRUG CONJUGATES

Since 791T/36 antibody reacts with colorectal carcinoma cells and localises in vivo in colorectal tumours, it is a good candidate antibody for selective tumour targeting of therapeutic agent, and methods of conjugation of 791T/36 antibody to methotrexate [22] and daunomycin [23] have been described previously.

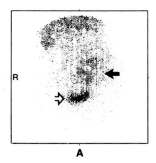 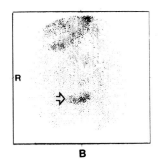 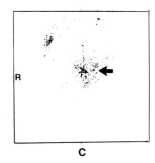

A   B   C

Fig. 4. An example of the imaging of ^{131}I-labeled 791T/36 localisation in colorectal carcinoma. Anterior images of the pelvic region of a patient with recurrent carcinoma of the colon. **A:**[131]I-labelled 791T/36 antibody image recorded 48 hr after administration. **B:**[99m]Tc-labeled human serum albumin and pertechnetate. **C:**Subtracted image. Solid arrows show tumour; open arrows show tracer in the urinary bladder. R, patient's right.

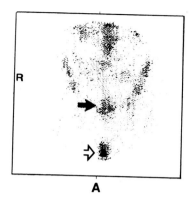

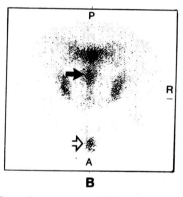

Fig. 5. Images of a patient with a primary tumour of the rectum recorded 72 hr following injection of ^{111}In-labeled 791T/36 antibody. **A:** Anterior view of the pelvic region. **B:** Sitting view. Solid arrows point to the tumour. Uptake of tracer can also be seen throughout the skeleton and in the testes (open arrows), a common feature with ^{111}In-labeled antibodies [19,30]. A, anterior; P, posterior; R, right.

Methotrexate

Initially, methotrexate (MTX)-791T/36 conjugates were prepared by a direct conjugation procedure using the N-hydroxysuccinimide ester of MTX. Assessment of these conjugates for antibody reactivity was carried out by a competitive binding assay in which binding of FITC 791T/36 antibody to tumour target cells was assessed by flow cytometry (Table V). With three separate conjugates with MTX: antibody molar ratios of 1.9:1–2.7:1, the retained antibody activity was 36–75% (Table V) indicating that conjugates can be prepared in this way that retain significant antibody activity. The in vitro cytotoxicity of MTX-791T/36 conjugates was measured by incubating target tumour cells with a range of concentrations of conjugate and measuring cell survival by postincubation labeling with ^{75}Se-selenomethionine [22]. The reactivity of drug or conjugates is conveniently expressed as an IC_{50}, this being the concentration of drug, free or as conjugate, required to produce a 50% inhibition of tumour cell survival. Cells of the colon carcinoma lines C146, C168, and C170 were relatively resistant to free MTX, with an IC_{50} over 1,000 ng/ml. In contrast, the IC_{50} of MTX conjugated to 791T/36 antibody was ten to 20 times lower (Table VI), indicating that cell surface binding of MTX via antibody recognition of antigen facilitated cell killing. Most significantly, this enhanced cell killing with conjugate was also seen with cells prepared directly from xenograft growths.

TABLE III. Localisation of ^{131}I-791T/36 in Gastrointestinal Malignancy

| Disease | Site | Total No. cases | No. positive images | Resected specimen examination | | |
| | | | | No. | Mean tumour:nontumour ratio assessed by | |
					Imaging	Counting
Malignant primaries	Colonic	13	8/11	13	2.3:1	2.6:1
	Rectal	16	5/12	15	2.2:1	2.5:1
Malignant secondaries	Liver	9	8/9	—	—	
	Abdomen	2	2/2	—	—	—
	Pelvis/perineum	6	5/6	—	—	—
	Pulmonary	1	1/1	—	—	—
	Brain	1	1/1	—	—	—
Benign	Diverticular stricture	2	0/2	1	1:1	
	Villous adenoma	3	0/3	2	1.2:1	0.9:1
	Polyposis	1	0/1	1	1.0:1	1.0:1
	Adenoma	1	0/1	—	—	—

TABLE IV. Imaging of Primary and Recurrent Colorectal Carcinoma With ^{111}In-791T/36

| Patient No. | Primary carcinoma | | Metastatic/recurrent carcinoma | |
	Site	Image result	Site	Image result
1	Recto sigmond	Positive	Liver	Positive
2	Sigmond	Positive	–	–
3	Sigmond	Negative	Liver	Negative
	Caecum	Negative		
4	Recto sigmond	Positive	Liver	Negative
5	–	–	Pelvis	Positive
6	–	–	Pelvis	Positive
7	–	–	R. upper abdomen	Positive
8	–	–	L. upper abdomen	Positive
9	–	–	Pelvis	Positive
10	–	–	Pelvis	Positive
11	–	–	Pelvis	Positive

Since these MTX-791T/36 antibody conjugates are highly cytotoxic to colorectal carcinoma cells expressing the 791T/36 antigen, they may be expected to show therapeutic advantages over the free drug if the conjugates can survive in vivo and localise sufficiently in tumours. In vivo distribution studies in mice, including those with colorectal carcinoma xenografts, have been carried out following radioiodine labeling of the antibody component of these conjugates. Blood distribution and clearance rates were virtually identical to those of unconjugated antibody (Fig. 6). Moreover, significant tumour localisation, visualised by γ camera imaging, occurred into C170 colon carcinoma xenografts (Fig. 7). Similar preliminary studies in colorectal carcinoma patients showed blood clearance and tumour imaging virtually identical to that seen with unconjugated antibody (Ballantyne et al, unpublished observations).

In addition to directly linked MTX-791T/36 conjugates, bridged conjugates with human serum albumin (HSA) as a carrier for MTX are also available [22]. These have the advantage of molar substitution ratios at least ten times higher than is feasible with direct linkage, albeit with a somewhat lower retention of antibody binding activity (Table V). The availability of

TABLE V. Characteristics of Methotrexate-791T/36 Monoclonal Antibody Conjugates

Preparation and lot No.	Molar ratio of MTX substitution (MTX:791T/36)	Antibody reactivity (%)*
MTX-791T/36		
MDC26	2.5:1	36
MDC29	1.9:1	68
MDC31	2.7:1	75
MTX-HSA-791T/36		
MT1	32:1	28
MT7	27:1	36
MT11	23:1	32
MT17	38:1	32

*Determined by competition binding assay in which binding of FITC-labeled 791T/36 antibody to tumour cell is measured by flow cytometry.

TABLE VI. Cytotoxicity of 791T/36-Methotrexate Conjugate for Colorectal Carcinoma Cells

	Target cells	IC_{50} (ng/ml) of	
Designation	Derived from	MTX	MTX-791T/36*
C146	In vitro culture	1,000	50
C168	In vitro culture	3,000	300
C170	In vitro culture	2,000	100
C170	Xenograft†	2,000	150

*Lot No. MDC31. See Table V.
†Cells prepared by collagenase digestion of tumour growing as a xenograft in nude mice.

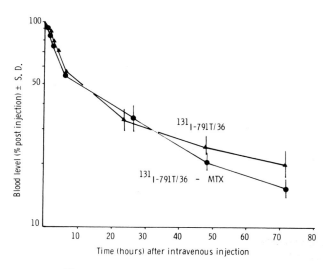

Fig. 6. Blood clearance of ^{131}I-labeled 791T/36 antibody and 791T/36-MTX conjugates in mice. Groups of four mice were injected intravenously with ^{131}I-791T/36 or ^{131}I-791T/36-MTX and 10 μl blood sample obtained periodically from the tail vein.

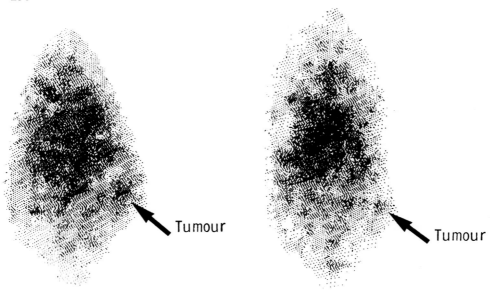

Fig. 7. γ Camera images of the localisation of [131]I-791T/36 methotrexate in xenografts of colorectal carcinoma C170. Two mice with C170 xenografts were injected intraperitoneally with 100 μC: of [131]I-791T/36 methotrexate conjugate and imaged after 3 days. No blood pool subtraction was used.

these conjugates with higher substitution ratios expands the possiblity of conjugate therapy of tumour, since a limiting factor here is the amount of drug potentially deposited in tumour tissue by localising antibody. The validity of this approach is shown by significant retardation of growth of xenografts of the colon carcinoma C170 (Fig. 8). In these studies mice were implanted with tumour tissue and subsequently treated by intraperitoneal injection of free or conjugated MTX. Free drug exerted no therapeutic response, as might be expected from its cells' relative resistance to MTX assessed in vitro (Table IV). In contrast, conjugated drug significantly retarded tumour growth, as evidenced by retarded growth rate and reduced final tumour weights (Fig. 8).

Daunomycin

Daunomycin has been conjugated to 791T/36 antibody using four different linkages [23], but that involving direct linkage by reaction of 14-Bromo daunomycin with the antibody's amino group is technically the most simple and yields a product retaining significant drug and antibody reactivity [23]. The potential in vivo killing of colorectal carcinoma cells with these conjugates has been assessed initially using an in vivo isotopic release assay. Cells of the colon carcinoma line LS174T were labeled with ^{125}I-Iodo-deoxyuridine (^{125}I-UdR) by incubation of cultured cells in ^{125}I-UdR–containing medium. Cells were harvested, washed, and injected intraperitoneally into groups of athymic (nude) mice. Twenty-four hours after cell injection ^{125}I in individual mice was counted in a γ- scintillation well crystal detector. Therapy was initiated by intraperitoneal injection of free daunomycin or daunomycin antibody conjugate and mice counted for ^{125}I at daily intervals (Fig. 9). [125]I cell label was lost with a half-life of 3.5 days from untreated mice. A total of 6 mg/kg of free daunomycin shortened this half-life to 2.2 days, indicating an acceleration of tumour cell death. The same dose of daunomycin conjugated to 791T/36 antibody had a more pronounced effect, the in vivo half-life of radiolabel being only 1.5 days, virtually identical to that from labeled tumour cells damaged by heating (80°C, 5 min) before injection. Daunomycin conjugated to normal IgG had a less

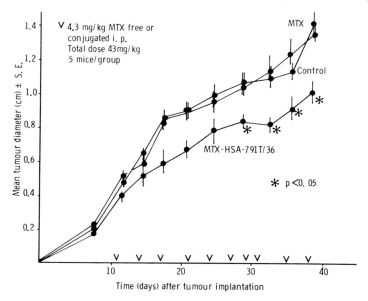

Fig. 8. Therapeutic effect of 791T/36-methotrexate conjugate against xenografts of colorectal carcinoma C170. A group of nude mice implanted subcutaneously with C170 tissue were given twice weekly injections of free or 791T/36-conjugated methotrexate as shown. Only the conjugated drug produced significant retardation of tumour growth as assessed by the Student t test from tumour diameters.

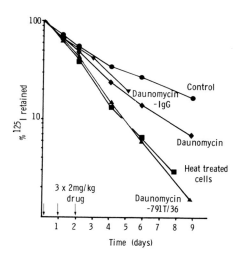

Fig. 9. In vivo killing of tumour cells by free or conjugated daunomycin monitored by release of ^{125}I from ^{125}I–UdR–labeled cells. Groups of three mice were injected with viable or heat-treated ^{125}I-UdR–labeled LS174T colon carcinoma cells (1×10^6 cells/mouse; $6 \times 10^{-2} \mu$Ci ^{125}I/10^6 cells). Twenty-four hours later and then at daily intervals, mice were counted for radioactivity. Treatment was given intraperitoneally starting 24 hr after radiolabeled cell injection. Total dose of daunomycin, either free or in conjugated form, was 6 mg/kg body weight.

pronounced effect, the rate of radiolabel excretion being similar to that seen only with free drug. These findings indicate that daunomycin-antibody conjugates can exert in vivo cytotoxicity against tumour cells and the effect can be greater than that achieved with the free drug. The lack of accelerated cell death following administration of daunomycin conjugated to normal immunoglobulin indicates that the effect with antibody conjugate is associated with tumour target cell expression of 791T/36- defined antigen.

In addition to improved in vivo killing of tumour cells by daunomycin following conjugation to 791T/36 monoclonal antibody, in vivo toxicity tests have demonstrated that conjugated drug is significantly less toxic than the free material. Thus, the LD_{50} of free drug for mice given twice weekly injections is 14 mg/kg, while drug conjugated to 791T/36 antibody showed no toxicity at up to 30 mg/kg (Fig. 10). Tests with daunomycin similarly conjugated to normal IgG have demonstrated no toxicity with total doses up to 80 mg/kg of drug in conjugated form. These findings indicate that treatment schedules with conjugated drug can be designed to contain far more drug that can be tolerated in free form, and, as with methotrexate conjugates, we are now planning to compare free and 791T/36-conjugated daunomycin on the basis of their therapeutic indices against human tumours developing as xenografts in immuno-deprived mice.

DISCUSSION

These and related studies [7,14,24] have shown that the antigen identified by the 791T/36 monoclonal antibody is expressed in colorectal carcinomas. Consequently, radiolabeled antibody, but not normal IgG2b, shows localisation in primary and metastatic tumour deposits [9–11,24]. The ultimate value of this as a diagnostic tool, particularly in recurrent and metastatic disease, cannot yet be evaluated since these trials are still in progress. It can be envisaged, however, that further refinements, including the use of 791T/36 antibody fragments such as Fab [25] the further use of ^{111}In rather than ^{131}I, and other radiolabels with more suitable physical characteristics, such as [99m]Tc [26], will further improve imaging quality and reliability.

These studies also show that conjugates of 791T/36 with the antitumour agents methotrexate and daunomycin are cytotoxic for colorectal tumour cells both in vivo and in vitro. Clearly, full analysis of the therapeutic efficacy of these conjugates requires dose response and toxicity tests to establish the therapeutic indices of the conjugates in relation to those of the free drugs. However, therapeutic advantages are already emerging from, for example, the finding that colorectal carcinomas, relatively insensitive to methotrexate, are suppressed in vitro and, even more importantly, in vivo by MTX-791T/36 conjugates. Similarly with daunomycin, enhanced cell killing in vivo has been achieved with the drug following conjuga-

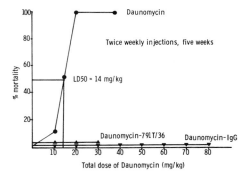

Fig. 10.   Toxicity of daunomycin and daunomycin-conjugates in mice. Groups of ten mice were given twice-weekly intraperitoneal injections for 5 weeks of daunomycin or daunomycin conjugated to 791T/36 monoclonal antibody or to normal human IgG. Numbers of mice surviving or dying during and up to 2 weeks after the injection were assessed.

tion to 791T/36 antibody. In addition, it has been demonstrated that these conjugates are markedly less toxic than free drug, and these two findings indicate that conjugated drug could have a therapeutic advantage.

In addition to methotrexate and daunomycin, 791T/36 has also been conjugated to immunological agents such as interferon [27] and to the A chain of the plant toxin richin [28]. Thus, a wide range of conjugates is becoming available for therapeutic assessment, initially in mice with colorectal carcinoma xenografts and then, potentially, for clinical assessment. However, 791T/36 is only one of a number of monoclonal antibodies [3–5] shown to localise in primary and recurrent colorectal carcinoma. Clearly further development of this approach may rest on the use not of single antibodies but of cocktails of antibodies each to different tumour-associated antigens. Thus, it has already been shown that 791T/36 antibody and the C/24 anti-CEA antibody can localise simultaneously in xenografts of the LS174T colon carcinoma [29], and clinically improved imaging detection rates have been obtained with mixtures of the 17-1A and 19.9 antibodies [4]. Therapeutically this approach might enable simultaneous localisation of more than one agent, higher total drug levels in tumour, and partly overcome the problem of possible heterogeneity of expression of antigens within tumours and their metastases.

ACKNOWLEDGMENTS

This work was supported by grants from the Cancer Research Campaign, UK. We thank Dr. J. Gallego for making antibody-daunomycin conjugates available.

REFERENCES

1. Stower MJ, Hardcastle JD. The results of 1115 patients with colorectal cancer treated over an 8 year period in a single hospital. Eur J Surg Oncol 1985; 11:119–23.
2. Moertel CG. Cancer of the large bowel. In Frei E, Holland JF, eds: Cancer medicine. Philadelphia: Lea and Febiger 1973: 1597–621.
3. Mach JP, Buchegger F, Forni M, et al. Use of radiolabelled monoclonal anti-CEA antibodies for the detection of human carcinomas by external photoscanning and tomoscintigraphy. Immunol Today 1981; 2:239–49.
4. Chatal JF, Saccavini JC, Fumoleau P, et al. Immunoscintigraphy of colon carcinoma. J Nucl Med 1984; 25:307–14.
5. Mach JP, Chatal JF, Lumbroso JD, et al. Tumour localization in patients by radiolabelled monoclonal antibodies against colon carcinoma. Cancer Res 1983; 43:5593–600.
6. Embleton MJ, Gunn B, Byers VS, Baldwin RW. Antitumour reactions of monoclonal antibody against a human osteogenic sarcoma cell line. Br J Cancer 1981; 43:582–7.
7. Campbell DG, Price MR, Baldwin RW. Analysis of a human osteogenic sarcoma antigen and its expression on various human tumour cell lines. Int J Cancer 1984; 34:31–7.
8. Farrands PA, Perkins A, Sully L, et al. Localization of human osteosarcoma by antitumour monoclonal antibody. J Bone Joint Surg 1983; 65B:638–40.
9. Farrands PA, Perkins AC, Pimm MV Hardy JG, Baldwin RW, Hardcastle JD. Radioimmunodetection of human colorectal cancers using an anti-tumour monoclonal antibody. Lancet 1982; 2:387–400.
10. Armitage NC, Perkins AC, Pimm MV, Farrands PA, Baldwin RW, Hardcastle JD. The localization of an antitumour monoclonal antibody (79IT/36) in gastrointestinal tumours. Br J Surg 1984; 71:407–12.
11. Armitage NC, Perkins AC, Pimm MV, Wastie MC, Baldwin RW, Hardcastle JD. Imaging of primary and metastatic colorectal cancer using an ^{111}In-labelled antitumour monoclonal antibody (791T/36). Nucl Med Commun 1985; 6:623–31.
12. Pimm MV, Baldwin RW. Immunoscintigraphy of tumours: Experience with the monoclonal antibody 791T/36. Clin Immunol Newsl 1984;5:150–2.
13. Durrant LG, Robins RA, Armitage NC, Brown A, Baldwin RW, Hardcastle JD. Association of antigen expression and DNA ploidy in colorectal tumours. Cancer Res 1986; 46:3543–9.
14. Durrant LG, Robins RA, Pimm MV et al. Antigenicity of newly established colorectal cell lines. Br J Cancer 1986; 53:37–45.

15. Pimm, MV, Embleton MJ, Perkins AC, et al. In vivo localization of anti-osteogenic sarcoma 791T monoclonal antibody in osteogenic sarcoma xenografts. Int J Cancer 1982; 30:75–85.
16. Tom BH, Rutzky LP, Oyasu R, Tomita JT, Goldenberg DM, Kahan BD. Human colon adenocarcinoma cells. II. Tumorigenic and organoid expression in vivo and in vitro. JNCI 1977; 58:1507–12.
17. Perkins AC, Pimm MV, Birch MK. The preparation and characterization of ^{111}In-labelled 791T/36 monoclonal antibody for tumour immunoscintigraphy. Eur J Nucl Med 1985; 10:296–301.
18. Perkins AC, Whalley DR, Hardy JG. Physical approach for the reduction of dual radionuclide image subtraction artefacts in immunoscintigraphy. Nucl Med Commun 1984;5:501–12.
19. Perkins AC, Pimm MV. Differences in tumour and normal tissue concentrations of iodine and indium labelled monoclonal antibody. I. The effect of image contrast in clinical studies. Eur J Nucl Med 1985; 11:295–9.
20. Pimm MV, Perkins AC, Baldwin RW. Differences in tumour and normal tissue concentrations of iodine and indium labelled monoclonal antibody. II. Biodistrbution studies in mice with human tumour xenografts. Eur J Nucl Med 1985; 11:300–4.
21. Ballantyne KC, Armitage NC, Perkins AC, et al. Monoclonal antibody 791T/36 imaging in the detection of recurrent colorectal cancer. Eur J Surg Oncol 1985; 11:313.
22. Garnett MC, Embleton MJ, Jacobs E, Baldwin RW. Preparation and properties of a drug-carrier-antibody conjugate showing selective antibody-directed cytotoxicity in vitro. Int J Cancer 1983; 31:661–70.
23. Gallego J, Price MR, Baldwin RW. Preparation of four daunomycin-monoclonal antibody 791T/36 conjugates with anti-tumour activity. Int J Cancer 1984; 33:737–44.
24. Price MR, Pimm MV, Page CM, Armitage NC, Hardcastle JD, Baldwin RW. Immunolocalization of the murine monoclonal antibody 791T/36 within primary human colorectal carcinomas and identification of the target antigen. Br J Cancer 1984; 49:809–12.
25. Pimm MV, Baldwin RW. Localization of an anti-tumour monoclonal antibody in human tomour xenografts: Kinetic and qualitative studies with the 791T/36 antibody. In Monoclonal antibodies for tumour detection and drug targeting. New York: Academic Press, 1985.
26. Childs RL, Hnatowich DJ. Optimum conditions for labeling of DTPA-coupled antibodies with technetium-99m. J Nucl Med 1985; 26:293–9.
27. Pelham JM, Gray JD, Flannery GR, Pimm MV, Baldwin RW. Interferon α conjugation to human osteogenic sarcoma monoclonal antibody 791T/36. Cancer Immunol Immunother 1983;15:210–6.
28. Embleton MJ, Byers, VS, Garnett MC, Baldwin RW. In vitro comparisons between monoclonal antibody-targeted drug and toxin conjugates. Br J Cancer 1985;52:432.
29. Pimm MV, Perkins AC, Baldwin RW. Simultaneous localization of two monoclonal antibodies in a human colon carcinoma xenograft. IRCS Med Sci 1985; 13:499–500.
30. Epenetos AA, Snook D, Hooker G, Lavender JP, Halnan KE. Tumour imaging using an improved method of DTPA-coupled monoclonal antibodies radiolabelled with metallic radionuclides. Lancet 1984; 2:169.

Cancer Detection and Prevention Supplement 1:263–268 (1987)

Monoclonal Islet Antibody Hisl-19 as a Tool in the Diagnosis of Neuroendocrine Carcinomas of the Skin

Peter Buxbaum, MD
Gabriele Horvat
Christian Gamper, MD
Klaus Krisch, MD

Department of Pathology, University of Vienna, Medical School, Vienna, Austria

ABSTRACT   The monoclonal islet cell antibody HISL-19 generated after immunization of BALB/c mice with human pancreatic islet cell preparations, demonstrated specific immunoreactivity for neuroendocrine (Merkel) cells of the skin as shown by successive and simultaneous localization of neuron-specific enolase and the antigen detected by mab HISL-19 in the same cells of the bovine epidermis. Following these observations, we tested nine neuroendocrine carcinomas of the skin that were believed to be of Merkel cell origin for their immunoreactivity with mab HISL-19 using an indirect immunoperoxidase technique on formalin-fixed and paraplast-embedded tissues. In contrast to malignant lymphomas, poorly differentiated squamous cell carcinomas, and malignant melanomas, all nine neuroendocrine carcinomas reacted strongly with mab HISL-19, indicating its potential as a useful immunohistochemical probe for the distinction of neuroendocrine carcinomas of the skin from other cutaneous neoplasms with similar histological appearance.

Key words: Merkel cells, immunohistochemical marker, neuron-specific enolase

INTRODUCTION

Neuroendocrine carcinomas of the skin (Merkel cell tumors) represent a group of skin neoplasms with features of neuroendocrine differentiation such as their content of typical neurosecretory granules ranging in size from 80 to 350 nm, immunocytochemically demonstrable expression of peptide hormones, and constant neuron-specific enolase (NSE) immunoreactivity [for review, see 1]. The latter has been reported to be the most reliabale immunocytochemical marker for the delineation of neuroendocrine skin carcinomas and for distinguishing them from other skin tumors with similar light microscopic appearance such as malignant melanomas, malignant lymphomas, and poorly differentiated squamous cell carcinomas that (with the exception of some malignant melanomas) do not express NSE [2].

In this article we describe the immunocytochemical identification of another neuroendocrine-specific antigen detected by a monoclonal antibody (mab) HISL-19 [3,4] in normal

---

Address reprint requests to Dr. Klaus Krisch, Institut für Pathologische Anatomie der Universität Wien, Spitalgasse 4, A-1090 Wien, Austria.

Merkel cells of the skin and a series of nine Merkel cell tumors using formalin-fixed and paraplast-embedded tissues to investigate its potential as a tool for the identification of these tumors in specimens processed by the routine pathology laboratory.

MATERIALS AND METHODS
Materials

Monoclonal antibody HISL-19 was produced as previously described [3] and kindly supplied by Dr. Srikanta (Joslin Diabetes Center, Boston, MA). Briefly, 4- to 6-week-old female BALB/c mice were immunized with human islet cells isolated from cadaveric human pancreatic specimens by enzymatic digestion and gradient centrifugations [5]. Spleen cells from the immunized mice were fused with the nonsecretor murine myeloma cell line P3×63, 653 using the standard polyethylene glycol technique [6,7]. The resulting hybrids were initially screened for reactivity with human islets, performing the indirect immunofluorescence technique on cryostat sections of human pancreas. Positive colonies were cloned several times, expanded, and monoclonal antibody ascites raised in mice. Rabbit antiserum to bovine NSE was obtained from Dako Immunoglobulins (Guldborgvej, Copenhagen, Denmark) as were the bridge swine antirabbit Ig antibody, the rabbit peroxidase antiperoxidase (PAP) complex, the peroxidase-conjugated rabbit antimouse Ig and swine antirabbit Ig antibodies, and the alkaline phosphatase monoclonal antialkaline phosphatase (APAAP) complex.

Immunohistochemistry

Formalin-fixed (10%), routinely processed, and paraplast-embedded specimens from nine neuroendocrine carcinomas of the skin, eight malignant melanomas, seven malignant lymphomas, and five poorly differentiated squamos cell carcinomas (grade 3–4) were retrieved from the surgical pathology files of the Institute of Pathological Anatomy, University of Vienna, School of Medicine. The immunoreactivity of mab HISL-19 was evaluated using an indirect immunoperoxidase technique. The sections were incubated with mab HISL-19 (dilution 1/4,000 of ascites fluid) and subsequently incubated with peroxidase-conjugated rabbit antimouse Ig antibody (dilution 1/100) followed by a peroxidase-conjugated swine antirabbit Ig antibody (dilution 1/100). For the demonstration of the antigen detected by mab HISL-19 in malignant melanomas, the APAAP technique was used essentially as described by Cordell et al [8] to avoid problems in the distinction of specific immunostaining and melanin. Immunostaining for NSE was done with the well-established peroxidase antiperoxidase (PAP) method [9] using a 1/3,000 dilution of the rabbit antibovine NSE antibody. Peroxidase activity was detected by the 3,3'-diaminobenzidine tetrahydrochloride (DAB) or the 4-chloro-1-naphtol reaction, and the sections were counterstained with hematoxylin. Controls included replacement of each of the first antibodies with normal mouse or rabbit serum, respectively.

For the successive and simultaneous localization of the antigen detected by mab HISL-19 and NSE in Merkel cells, fresh specimens of normal skin were taken from the noses of calfs obtained from the local slaughterhouse. After formalin fixation (10%) and paraplast embedding, sections were immunostained with mab HISL-19 using the indirect peroxidase method as described above, the site of specific immunoreactivity was made visible by the DAB procedure, and the sections were then photographed. The antibodies were eluted by immersion in glycine HC1 buffer (pH 2.0) for 2 hr and the sections were reimmersed in TBS and then reacted for NSE with DAB and again photographed.

RESULTS
Immunostaining of Normal Merkel Cells by mab HISL-19

Immunostaining for the antigen detected by mab HISL-19 revealed positive reactivity in few cells of the bovine epidermis. These cells were found above the basement membrane in the basal layer of the epidermis lying singly or in small groups (Fig. 1A). They were typically oriented with their main axis parallel to that of the epidermis. The pattern of HISL-19

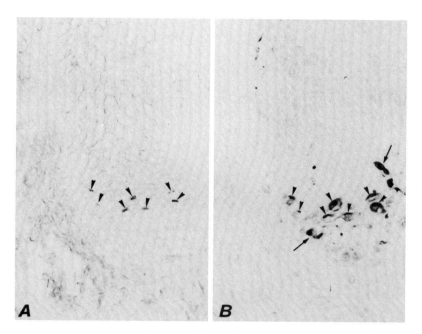

Fig. 1. Normal bovine skin stained by the immunoperoxidase technique using DAB substrate. The section was reached first for the antigen detected by mab HISL-19 (**A**), yielding a dot-like immunoreaction product (arrowheads) in some cells lying above the basement membrane of the epidermis. After elution of the antibodies with glycine HC1 buffer the same section was reacted for NSE (**B**). Note the characteristic ringlike appearance of the NSE immunoreaction in Merkel cells, which is in contrast to the still visible mab HISL-19 binding sites (arrowheads). Some NSE-positive nerve fibers (arrows) are also present. No counterstain. ×500.

immunoreactivity was restricted to an irregular, dot-like cytoplasmic structure while the rest of the cell body was unstained. No nerve fibers of the skin were stained by mab HISL-19.

To assess the nature of the mab HISL-19 immunoreactive cells, subsequent NSE immunostaining of the same section was performed after elution of the antibodies used for the detection of the HISL-19-antigen. In this way, all HISL-19 immunoreactive cells also were strongly stained by NSE antibody (Fig. 1B). The NSE immunoreaction was diffuse, distributed in the cytoplasm, but sometimes appeared particularly concentrated at the cell periphery, giving the cell a ring-like appearance. The differences in the immunoreactive pattern of the antigen detected by mab HISL-19 and NSE allowed the identification of both antigens within the same cell. Therefore, removal of the reaction product produced by the first antibody (HISL-19) before NSE immunostaining was not necessary. The coexpression of the HISL-19 antigen and NSE indicates that the HISL-19 immunoreactive cells are indeed Merkel cells.

Immunostaining of Cutaneous Neoplasms by mab HISL-19 and NSE Antibody

According to the classification suggested by Gould et al [1], seven neuroendocrine carcinomas in this series were of the intermediate cell type and two of the trabecular type. All cases strongly reacted with mab HISL-19 (Fig. 2A) as well as with NSE antibody (data not shown). In contrast to the diffuse NSE immunostaining in the tumor cells, the cytoplasmic distribution of the HISL-19 antigen was similar as described above for the normal Merkel cells exhibiting solitary or multiple irregular-shaped cytoplasmic clots of specific reaction product.

Among the eight malignant melanomas, four did not show any immunoreactivity for the HISL-19 antigen. In the remaining four cases the HISL-19 antigen was present only in a few

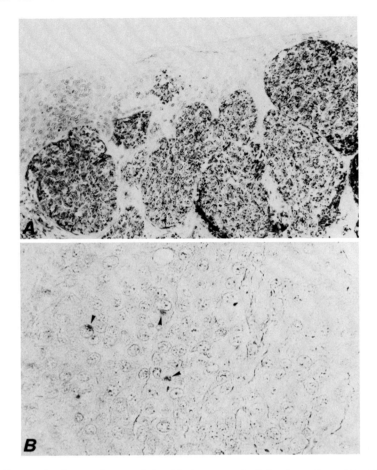

Fig. 2. **A:** Neuroendocrine carcinoma of the skin immunostained for the antigen detected by mab HISL-19. All tumor cells are strongly stained. Indirect peroxidase technique using DAB substrate, hematoxylin counterstain. ×220. **B:** Malignant melanoma exhibits only a few mab HISL-19 immuno-reactive cells (arrowheads). APAAP method using fast red as substrate, hematoxylin counterstain. ×500.

scattered isolated cells, while the large majority of the tumor cells remained unstained (Fig. 2B). Positive NSE immunostaining was observed in three cases of malignant melanomas represented by moderate to strong uniform cytoplasmic reactivity. Malignant lymphomas and squamous cell carcinomas, grade 3–4, contained no detectable amount of HISL-19 antigen or NSE. The results are summarized in Table I.

DISCUSSION

The monoclonal islet antibody HISL-19 was raised in mice using human islet cell preparations as immunogen [3]. Using immunocytochemical methods, the antigen detected by mab HISL-19 was identified not only in pancreatic islet cells but also in central and peripheral neurons as well as in a large number of cells of the diffuse neuroendocrine system such as neuroendocrine cells of the gut, C cells of the thyroid, anterior pituitary cells, and adrenal medulla [4]. As determined by the "Western" immunoblotting technique, mab HISL-19 recognizes a novel group of neuroendocrine cell proteins that are not related to NSE [3,4]. In

TABLE I. Immunoreactive* for the Antigen Detected by Mab HISL-19 and NSE in 29 Malignant Cutaneous Neoplasms

Histologic type	HISL-19 Antigen			NSE	
	+	±	−	+	−
Neuroendocrine skin carcinomas (N = 9)	9	0	0	9	0
Malignant melanomas (N = 8)	0	4	4	3	5
Squamous cell carcinomas (N = 5)	0	0	5	0	5
Malignant lymphomas (N = 7)	0	0	7	0	7

*Staining: +, positive; ±, few immunoreactive cells; −, negative.

this study we have shown that normal Merkel cells, which represent the neuroendocrine cell of the skin [10] and are the only nonkeratinocytes that express NSE [11], also express the neuroendocrine antigen detected by mab HISL-19. The cells in the skin immunoreactive for mab HISL-19 were identified as Merkel cells by their typical location above the basement membrane of the squamous epithelium and by their content of NSE as demonstrated by successive and simultaneous NSE immunostaining of the same tissue section.

Mainly on the bases of ultrastructural features neuroendocrine carcinomas of the skin are believed to arise from the Merkel cell [12,13]. This suggestion is supported by the capability of normal Merkel cells as well as of cells of neuroendocrine skin tumors to express various neuropeptides such as ACTH, bombesin, vasoactive intestinal polypeptide, and leu-enkephalin [1], in addition to NSE. The well-known variability in the light microscopic appearance of these tumors may lead to considerable difficulties in distinguishing them from other skin neoplasms such as malignant melanomas, malignant lymphomas, or poorly differentiated squamous carcinomas [1,2]. So far, NSE has been reported to be the most reliable marker for the delineation of neuroendocrine skin carcinomas in surgical pathology [2]. However, NSE immunoreactivity was not exclusively found in neuroendocrine carcinomas of the skin but also in some malignant melanomas [1,2,14]. In addition, positive NSE immunostaining has since also been rarely identified in lymphomas [15]. Furthermore, NSE immunostaining is influenced by formalin fixation, which sometimes leads to interpretation problems of immunostaining results [16,17].

In a previous study we reported the presence of the neuroendocrine antigen detected by mab HISL-19, which is not significantly altered by routine fixation procedures, in various tumors of the diffuse neuroendocrine system such as insulomas, carcinoids, paraganglimas, and pheochromocytomas, implicating its usefulness as marker for tumors of neuroendocrine differentiation in surgical pathology [4]. In this study we investigated a series of skin neoplasms including neuroendocrine skin carcinomas, malignant melanomas, malignant lymphomas, and poorly differentiated squamous cell carcinomas for their expression of the antigen detected by mab HISL-19 (using an indirect peroxidase technique on formalin-fixed and paraffin-embedded specimens). Mab HISL-19 strongly reacted with all neuroendocrine skin carcinomas tested, but not at all with malignant lymphomas and undifferentiated carcinomas. Malignant melanomas were also negatiave or exhibited only very few positive cells scattered throughout the tumor. These findings may have practical application in the distinction between neuroendocrine skin carcinomas and other skin neoplasms with similar light microscopic appearance.

As suggested by Gould et al [1] neuroendocrine carcinomas of the skin may be divided into at least three histologically distinct types, the trabecular type, the intermediate cell type, which represents the most frequent variant, and the small cell type. According to this classification, seven of our nine cases were of the intermediate cell type and two of the trabecular type. No case of the small cell type could be investigated for the expression of the HISL-19 antigen. Since this variant is morphologically indistinguishable from small cell carcinomas from other sites [1] such as from the lung, which were reported not to express the HISL-19 antigen [4], it seems to be very likely that neuroendocrine skin carcinomas of small cell type also may not be detected by mab HISL-19. Further studies have to be performed to prove this possible limitation of mab HISL-19 as an immunocytochemical probe for the diagnosis of neuroendocrine skin carcinomas.

REFERENCES

1. Gould VE, Moll R, Moll I, Lee I, Franke WW. Biology of disease. Neuroendocrine (Merkel) cells of the skin: Hyperplasias, dysplasias, and neoplasms. Lab Invest 1985; 52:334–53.
2. Gu J, Polak JM, Van Noorden S, Pearse AGE, Marangos PJ, Azzopardi JG. Immunostaining of neuron-specific enolase a a diagnostic tool for Merkel cell tumors. Cancer 1983; 52:1039–43.
3. Srikanta S, Krisch K, Eisenbarth GS. Novel islet proteins defined by monoclonal islet cell antibody HISL-19: identification and characterization. Diabetes 1986; 35:300–5.
4. Krisch K, Buxbaum P, Horvat G, et al. Monoclonal antibody HISL-19 as an immunocytochemical probe for neuroendocrine differentiation. Its application in diagnostic pathology. Am J Pathol 1986; 123:100–8.
5. Kortz WJ, Reiman TH, Bollinger RR, Eisenbarth GS. Identification and isolation of rat and human islet cells using monoclonal antibodies. Surg Forum 1982; 33:354–6.
6. Scearce RM, Eisenbarth GS. Production of monoclonal antibodies reacting with the cytoplasm and surface of differentiated cells. Methods enzymol 1983; 103:459–69.
7. Srikanta, S, Eisenbarth GS. Anti-islet cell monoclonal antibodies. In Larner J, Pohl SL, eds: Methods in diabetic research. I. Laboratory methods, part C. New York: John Wiley and Sons, Inc. 1984: 195–208.
8. Cordell JL, Falini B, Erber WN, et al. Immunoenzymatic labeling of monoclonal antibodies using immune complexes of alkaline phosphatase and monoclonal anti-alkaline phosphatase (APAAP complexes). J Histochem Cytochem 1984; 32:219–29.
9. Sternberger LA. Immunocytochemistry. 2nd ed. New York: John Wiley and Sons, Inc., 1979.
10. Pearse AGE. The neuroendocrine (APUD) cells of the skin. Am J Dermatopathol 1980; 2:121–3.
11. Gu J, Polak M, Tapia FJ, Marangos PJ, Pearse AGE. Neuron-specific enolase in the Merkel cells of mammalian skin. The use of specific antibody as a simple and reliable histologic marker. Am J Pathol 1981; 104:63–8.
12. Tang CK, Toker C. Trabecular carcinoma of the skin. An ultrastructural study. Cancer 1978; 42:2311–21.
13. Sibley RK, Rosai J, Foucar E, Dehner LP, Bosl G. Neuroendocrine (Merkel cell) carcinoma of the skin. A histologic and ultra-structural study of two cases. Am J Pathol 1980; 4:211–21.
14. Dhillon AP, Rhode J. Patterns of staining for neuron specific enolase in benign and malignant melanocytic lesions of the skin. Diagn Histopathol 1982; 5:169.
15. Wick MR Scheithauer BW, Kovacs K. Neuron-specific enolase in neuroendocrine tumors of the thymus, brochus, and skin. Am J Clin Pathol 1983; 79:703–7.
16. Haimoto H, Takahaski Y, Koshikawa T, Nagura H, Kato K. Immunohistochemical localization of gamma-enolase in normal human tissues other than nervous and neuroendocrine tissues. Lab Invest 1985; 52:257–3.
17. Siegal GP, Groben P, Hyman BD, Roberson JB, Reddick RL, Askin FG. Neuron-specific enolase immunoreactivity in small-cell carcinoma of the uterine cervix. Arch Pathol Lab Med 1985; 109: 5–6.

Cancer Detection and Prevention Supplement 1:269–277 (1987)

Monoclonal Antibodies Detecting Plasminogen Activators on the Membrane of Leukemic Lymphoid Cells of T-Cell Origin

Klaus G. Stünkel, PhD
Eckhard Thiel, MD
Hans G. Opitz, PhD
H.D. Schlumberger, MD

Uta Opitz, PhD
Daniel Catovsky, MD, MRC Path
Volker Klimetzek, PhD

Bayer AG, Wuppertal (K.G.S., U.O., H.G.O., V.K., H.D.S.) and Hematology, GSF, Munich (E.T.), Federal Republic of Germany, Royal Postgraduate Medical School, Hammersmith Hospital, London, England (D.C.)

ABSTRACT The specificities of six monoclonal antibodies produced against plasminogen activator of the human Bowes melanoma cell line are described. They have been used to detect membrane-bound plasminogen activator on cultured human lymphoid cell lines and on neoplastic human lymphocytic and myeloid cells of leukemic patients. These studies indicate that only certain phenotypic subsets of the T-cell lineage derived from patients with chronic lymphocytic leukemia or with Szezary syndrome express plasminogen activator on their surface membrane.

Key words: lyphoblastoid cell lines, fibrinolysis, immunofluorescence

INTRODUCTION

Plasminogen activators (PA) are serine proteases that catalyze the conversion of plasminogen to plasmin and are involved in the regulation of various vital physiological processes such as fibrinolysis, degradation of extracellular matrix, cell migration, tissue remodelling, and embryogenesis [1]. At least two types of PA exist in the human organism [2–4]. One is the urokinase type of activator (u-PA), the other the tissue type activator (t-PA).

A variety of tumor cells of solid tumors and of leukemia are known to secrete both types of PA [5–7]. Recently it was reported that in acute myeloid leukemia (AML) the molecular species secreted by these cells might have prognostic significance. Patients with AML whose cells release only t-PA do not respond to combination chemotherapy [8].

In this article we report on the production and characterization of six selected monoclonal antibodies (Moab) with specificity against t-PA and on the studies to detect membrane-associated PA on cultured human lymphoid cell lines and on neoplastic human lymphocytic and myeloid cells of leukemic patients. Our results indicate that only certain phenotypic subsets of leukemic cells of the T-cell lineage derived from patients with chronic lymphocytic leukemia or with Sezary syndrome express t-PA on their surface membrane.

Address reprint requests to Dr. Klaus G. Stünkel, Bayer AG, D-5600 Wuppertal 1, FRG.

MATERIALS AND METHODS
Chemicals

Dulbecco's modified Eagle's medium (D-MEM), RPMI 1640, Hank's balanced salt solution (HBSS), L-glutamine, fetal calf serum (FCS), and newborn calf serum (NCS) were purchased from Gibco (Karlsruhe, FRG). Pentex bovine fibrinogen (lot 23 A, free of plasminogen), rabbit antimouse IgM, IgG1, IgG2a, Ig2b, and IgG3 sera were from Miles (Frankfurt, FRG). Fluorescein isothiocyanate (FITC)-labeled goat antimouse serum was from Tago (Burlingame, CA). Pristane was from Roth (Karlsruhe, FRG). Human plasminogen and plasmin and S-2251 (H-D-valyl-L-leucyl-L-lysine-p-nitroanilide dihydrochloride) were from Kabi (Stockholm, Sweden). ^{125}Iodine was from NEN (Dreieich, FRG). Iodination of fibrinogen and antibodies was done according to Helmkamp et al [9]. Low molecular weight (33,000) urokinase (Abbokinase) was from Abbot (Delkenheim, FRG); high molecular weight (54,000) urikinase (Ukidan) was from Serono (Freiburg, FRG).

Mice

Balb/c and NMRI mice were purchased from Bomholtgaard (Rye, Denmark).

Cell Cultures

The established human Bowes melanoma cell line (kindly donated by D. Collen, University of Leuven, Belgium) was maintained in D-MEM supplemented with 10% FCS. Serum-free t-PA–containing cell supernatants were prepared from confluent monolayer cultures. The human lymphoblastoid cell lines and the cell line K-562 were cultured in RPMI 1640 supplemented with 10% FCS and 1% L-glutamine.

Cell Samples of Leukemic Patients

All cell samples were derived from leukemia cell preparations, which had been recently classified according to standard hematological and immunological criteria [10,11], which includes conventional surface markers [10] and surface markers characterized by monoclonal antibodies [13]. The remaining cells were suspended in RPMI 1640 containing 10% dimethylsulfoxide and 10% FCS and then frozen in a Controlled Rate Freezer (Union Carbide Cryogenics, Duisburg, FRG) with a cooling rate of 1°C/min. The samples were then stored in liquid nitrogen. Only those cell samples were used in this study that contained less than 10% dead (trypan blue positive) cells after thawing and washing.

Immunofluorescence

For indirect immunoflourescence, 1.2×10^6 cells, suspended in HBSS containing 0.3% BSA, were incubated with monoclonal antibodies in appropriate dilutions for 30 min at 4°C. After two washes, 25 μl of affinity-purified FITC-labeled goat antimouse serum (diluted 1:10) was added. After further incubation at 4°C for 30 min and washing twice, the percentage of positive cells was determined using a Leitz microscope with epiillumination. Before use, the reagents were ultracentrifuged and checked for unspecific binding using the K-562 cell line. Control incubations were performed with Balb/c mouse ascites.

Production and Characterization of Monoclonal Antibodies

The antibodies were derived from hybrid cell lines produced by the polyethylene glycol-mediated fusion of spleen cells with the myeloma cell line X63AG, 8653. In brief, spleens of Balb/c mice immunized with purified t-PA (see below) were removed, single cell suspensions were prepared, and cell fusions was carried out according to the procedure described by Köhler and Milstein [14]. Subsequently, growing cells were selected in HAT medium, composed of D-MEM supplemented with 1×10^{-4} M hypoxanthine, 4×10^{-7} M aminopterin, and 1.6×10^{-5} M thymidine.

Supernatants from hybridoma cells were tested for reactivity using a solid phase radioimmunoassay (see below). Hybrids producing anti-t-PA antibodies were cloned by limiting dilution.

For antibody production, $2-4 \times 10^6$ hybridoma cells were injected into Balb/c mice pretreated with 0.5 ml Pristane.

Isotyping of Monoclonal Antibodies

The isotype of monoclonal antibodies was determined by immunoelectrophoresis in agarose using rabbit antimouse IgM, IgG1, IgG2a, Ig2b, and IgG3 sera.

Purification of t-PA

Convential purification. t-PA was purified according to the procedure described by Rijken and Collen [4]. The purification procedure consisted of chromatography on zinc chelate-agarose, concanavalin A-agarose, and Sephadex G-150 in the presence of 0.01% Tween 80.

Affinity chromatography. Monoclonal anti- t-PA IgG antibodies were coupled to cyanogen bromide-activated Sepharose according to the procedure of March et al [15]. The columns were eliquibrated with 0.1 M Tris-HCl (pH 7.4) containing 0.3 M KCl and 0.05% Tween 80. Cell supernatants containing t-PA were then added at a flow rate of 3 ml/min. The unspecific adsorbed proteins were removed by washing with the equilibrating buffer. t-PA was eluted with 2 M MgBr2 (pH 7.4).

Plasminogen Activator Assays

Cell-associated PA activity was assayed by using ^{125}I-labeled fibrinogen-coated microtiter plates [16]. These plates were washed once with PBS and used immediately for the PA assay without prior conversion of the fibrinogen to fibrin [17]. Cells ($0.5-8 \times 10^5$ cells/ml) were added in quantities of 140 μl together with 20 μl of plasminogen (4 CU/ml). PBS served as control. After an incubation of 4 hr at 37°C, the radioactivity released into the supernatant was counted. The amount of total digestible ^{125}I-labeled fibrinogen was determined by a 4 hr incubation with 160 μl of plasmin (4 CU/ml).

The PA activity of cell supernatants was determined by the esterolysis of the chromogenic substrate S-2251 [18]. PA-containing supernatants (140 μl) and 20 μl 0.5 M Tris-HCl (pH 7.4) were added in triplicate to wells of a flat-bottomed microtiter plate (#655 101, Greiner, Nürtingen, FRG). The microtiter plates were then incubated for 15 min on a warm plate (37°C). After the addition of 20 μl S-2251 (6.0 mM) and 20 μl plasminogen (4 CU/ml) to each well, the release of p-nitroaniline was measured at 405μm with a Microelisa Auto Reader (MR 580, Dynatech, Plochingen, FRG). The controls contained PA-free medium, S-2251, and plasminogen. The activity of the samples was calculated by plotting the increase of extinction against the square of time, as described by Drapier et al [19]. Affinity-purified t-PA served as standard.

Solid Phase Radioimmunoassay

Remova wells (Flow M 17451) were coated with t-PA, u-PA, or control antigen in 0.05 M Tris-HCl (pH 9.5) at 4°C overnight. Wells were washed three times with PBS containing 3% BSA and then incubated with the same buffer for 2 hr at room temperature. The wells were washed again three times with PBS alone. One hundred microliters of antibody-containing culture supernatants was incubated for 2 hr at room temperature and the cells were then washed three times with PBS. One hundred microliters of ^{125}I-labeled antimouse IgG antibodies was added and incubated for 2 hr at room temperature. After five washings with PBS, the wells were counted in a γ counter.

RESULTS
Characterization of Anti-t-PA Monoclonal Antibodies

Fifty-five different hybridoma cell lines secreting anti-t-PA antibodies were established. Most of these clones secreted antibodies that showed cross-reaction with high and/or low molecular weight urokinase (u-PA). Only very few clones secreted antibodies that reacted exclusively with t-PA. For the present study six monoclonal antibodies (Moab) were selected: Moab 131, 206, and 282, reacting exclusively with t-PA, and Moab 7, 33, and 280, cross-reacting with high and low molecular weight u-PA (Table I). None of the six Moab bind to the catalytically active site of the two proteases. Binding studies with proteolytically degraded fragments of u-PA and t-PA, as well as activity measurements in the presence of the antibodies, revealed that the three t-PA–specific Moab (131, 206, and 282) bind to the fibrin binding site specific for t-PA. Furthermore, competition studies showed that the t-PA–specific Moab recognize different epitopes within the fibrin binding sites. The isotypes of the six Moab as determined by immunoelectrophoresis are show in Table I.

Binding Properties of Anti-PA Antibodies to Cultured Lymphoid Cell Lines

Several T- and B-lymphoid cell lines of different maturation stages and the multipotential stem cell K-562 were studied for the binding of the six Moab by indirect immunofluorescence. As seen in Table II, cell lines of B-cell origin, a cell line expressing the common ALL antigen, and the multipotential stem cell K 562 bound none of the six antibodies. The two T-cell lines HSB-2 and Molt-4, on the other hand, showed positive immunofluorescence. In the case of

TABLE I. Isotype and Specificity of Moab Established Against Tissue Type Plasminogen Activator (t-PA)*

Moab code	Isotype	Tissue type (t-PA)	Urokinase Type (u-PA)	
			HMW	LMW
131	G_1	+	−	−
206	G_1	+	−	−
282	G_1	+	−	−
7	G_2	+	+	+
33	M	+	+	+
280	M	+	+	+

*Cross-reactivity of Moab with u-PA was tested using high molecular weight urokinase (HMW) and low molecular weight urokinase (LMW).

TABLE II. Reactivity of Moab With Permanent Cell Lines*

Cell line	Phenotype	PA-antigen expression	Monoclonal antibody code					
			131	206	282	7	33	280
Molt 4	T-BL III	+	NT†	NT	NT	< 10	NT	NT
Jurkat	T-BL III	−						
HSB-2	T-BL IV	+	> 90	0	0	> 90	> 90	0
HUT-78	T-BL V	−						
Raji	B-BL I	−						
PDe-B1‡	B	−						
Wichmann‡	B	−						
MH-3	cALL	−						
K-562	Multipotential stem cell	−						

*All antibodies were tested by indirect immunofluorescence. The results are expressed as percent positive cells. The classification of the different cell lines was done according Minowada et al [11] and Drexler et al [12].
†Not tested.
‡Epstein Barr virus-transformed.

Molt-4, which were tested only with Moab 7, less than 10% of the cells were positively stained. HSB-2, which reacted with Moab 131, 7, and 33, contained >90% of positively stained cells. These cells displayed a very bright and intensive fluorescence, whereas cells of Molt-4 exhibited only a faint staining pattern. This suggests differences in antigen density or the insertion of PA in the cell membrane. It is of interest to note that HSB-2 bound the t-PA–specific Moab 131 but did not bind the two other t-PA–specific antibodies 282 and 206. This indicates that the two epitopes of the fibrin binding site recognized by these two antibodies are possibly buried in the membrane and, therefore, not accessible for the two antibodies.

Plasminogen-Dependent Proteolytic Activities of Lymphoid Cell Lines

After having shown by immunological methods the presence of surface-associated t-PA on only two of the tested cell lines, it was of interest to see whether the selective distribution of t-PA could also be demonstrated by measuring the plasminogen-dependent and -independent proteolytic activity of these cell lines. To determine the cell-associated proteolytic activities, cells of the different cell lines were plated with or without plasminogen in ^{125}I-fibrinogen-coated wells and tested for their ability to degrade the fibrinogen. As shown in Table III none of the cell lines possessed significant plasminogen-independent proteolytic activity. Only at very high cell densities was some plasminogen-independent proteolytic fibrinolysis observed with the HSB-2 cell line. High levels of plasminogen-dependent fibrinolysis were found for the HSB-2 and the K-562 cell lines. The other five cell lines, including Molt-4, were devoid of any plasminogen-dependent proteolytic activity.

Since the proteolytic activities of the two positive cell lines could be due to membrane-bound proteases or to extracellular released proteases, it was tested whether the plasminogen-dependent proteolytic activities could also be detected in cell-free supernatants. As shown in Table IV K-562 possessed high extracellular proteolytic activity, whereas HSB-2 was devoid of significant activities.

TABLE III. Plasminogen-Dependent and -Independent Fibrinolytical Activities of Different Cell Lines*

Cell lines	Plasminogen	No. of cells/cm^2 × 10^6				
		8	6	4	2	1
HSB-2	+	100	87	81	57	33
	−	11	6	2	2	1
Molt-4	+	2	2	3	2	2
	−	3	2	2	1	2
Jurkat	+	3	3	2	2	1
	−	2	3	2	2	2
HUT-78	+	3	2	1	2	2
	−	2	2	3	2	1
Wichmann	+	4	2	2	2	2
	−	2	1	3	2	1
MH3	+	5	3	3	2	1
	−	4	3	2	2	2
K 562	+	100	86	78	50	29
	−	5	3	2	2	2

*Cells were plated at different cell densities in microtiter wells coated with ^{125}-I-fibrinogen in the presence (+) or absence (−) of plasminogen (0.4 caseinolytical units (CU/ml)). After 4 hr the amount of solubilized fibrinogen was determined. The total digestible fibrinogen, set to 100%, was determined by adding plasmin (0.4 CU/ml). The zero control contained plasminogen alone and induced an unspecific proteolysis of 2 ± 1%. Each value is the mean of three wells.

**TABLE IV. Plasminogen-Dependent Esterolytic
Activities of HSB -2- and K-562–derived
Cell-Free Supernatants***

Cell lines	Cell density ($\times 10^6$/ml)	CU/ml
HSB-2	1.0	0.78 ± 0.2
	1.5	0.97 ± 0.2
K 562	1.0	13.9 ± 1.5
	1.5	21.5 ± 2.3

*The two cell lines were seeded at two different cell
densities in serum-free D-MEM and cultivated for 48
hr. The esterolytic activity of these supernatants was
quantified by the plasminogen-dependent esterolysis of
S-2251. CU, caseinolytic units.

TABLE V. Analysis of Different Subtypes of Leukemia for the Presence of Membrane-Bound PA*

Differential diagnosis of leukemias	Monoclonal antibody code					
	131	206	282	7	33	280
AML	0/5	0/5	0/5	0/5	0/5	0/5
AMML	0/5	0/5	0/5	0/5	0/5	0/5
A MoL	0/3	0/3	0/3	0/3	0/3	0/3
cALL	0/5	0/5	0/5	0/5	0/5	0/5
T-ALL	0/3	0/3	0/3	0/5	0/3	0/3
B-PLL	0/3	0/3	0/3	0/3	0/3	0/3
T-PLL	0/4	0/4	0/4	0/4	0/4	0/4
B-CLL	0/3	0/3	0/3	0/3	0/3	0/3
T-CLL	3/8	1/7	1/7	4/8	3/6	1/7
Sezary syndrome	2/2	2/2	0/2	1/2	1/2	1/2

*Cell samples containing $\geqslant 20\%$ of positively stained cells were scored as positive. AML, acute myeloid
leukemia; AMML, acute myelomonocytic leukemia; A MoL, acute monocytic leukemia; cALL, acute
lymphoblastic leukemia of common type; T-ALL, acute lymphoblastic leukemia of T-cell type; B-PLL,
T-PLL, prolymphocytic leukemia of B- or T-cell type; B-CLL, T-CLL, chronic lymphocytic leukemia
of B- or T-cell type.

These data show that a good correlation exists between the immunological and enzymological data. All lymphoid cell lines of B-cell origin were negative in both tests. HSB-2, which
showed a high percentage of immunologically positive cells, was also high in plasminogen-
dependent fibrinolysis. Molt-4, which possessed only a low percentage of faintly stained cells,
had no proteolytic activity. K-562, however, which showed no immunological evidence for
the presence of t-PA, secreted high amounts of a plasminogen-splitting enzyme. Affinity
chromatography and radioimmunoassays performed with the extracellular enzyme, indicated,
however, that this enzyme is not related to t-PA (data not shown).

Reaction Pattern of Anti-t-PA Moab With Leukemia Cells

After having established that t-PA is only expressed on certain lymphoid cell lines, it
was investigated as to whether a similar pattern could be found with leukemic cells of patients.
Different types and subtypes of prescreened acute and chronic lymphoid and myelomonocytic
leukemias classified according to cytological and immunological criteria (Table V) were
screened for immunofluorescence-positive cells. As shown in Table V, none of the leukemic
cells of the myelomonocytic lineage expressed detectable amounts of t-PA on their surface
membrane. The same was true for leukemic cells of B-cell origin. Interestingly, only cells of

patients with a chronic lymphocytic leukemia of T-cell type (T-CLL) and those with Sezary syndrome bound PA-specific Moab.

The individual T-cell marker profiles and the binding properties of the different Moab are summarized for all cases of T-CLL and of Sezary syndrome in Table VI. The leukemic cells of patients with T-CLL could be classified in three phenotypically different groups: Subtype 1, (two patients) displaying the T4-helper phenotype, was t-PA and u-PA negative. Subtype 2, displaying the T8-suppressor/cytotoxic phenotype, expressed membrane-bound PA in two out of four patients. Cells of patient Do. stained for u-PA, while cells from patient Ge. stained specifically for t-PA. Subtype 3 cells, displaying a mixed phenotype of T8-suppressor/cytotoxic cells and the M1 antigen of the myelomonocytic cells, were found to be t-PA positive in both cases. The leukemic cells of the two patients with Sezary syndrome showed a T-helper phenotype and expressed membrane-bound plasminogen activator of tissue type in both cases.

DISCUSSION

The existence of two types of plasminogen activator, urokinase-type (u-PA) and tissue-type (t-PA) has now been definitely established. They are two separate gene products and show differences in immunological reactivity, molecular weight, and amino acid sequence [1,5].

Human tumor cells are known to release both types [5–7]. Recently it was reported that the determination of the type of PA might serve as a useful aid for prognosis in leukemic patients [7,8]. Rapid detection of plasminogen activators on cells and tissues by immunocyto-chemical methods, however, has been hampered by the lack of sufficiently strong and specific antibodies. In this article we described six monoclonal antibodies that could be used to detect t-PA and u-PA by immunofluorescence. The corresponding hybridomas were established from spleen cells of a mouse immunized with purified t-PA from the human Bowes melanoma cell line [4]. Three Moab (131, 206, and 282) react selectively with t-PA, whereas the other three recognize t-PA as well as u-PA. They show no cross-reactivity with other serine proteases, such as kallikrein, trypsin, or chymotrypsin. None of the six Moab alone or a cocktail of six inhibit the catalytic activity of t-PA or u-PA. The t-PA–specific Moab (131, 206, and 282) recognizing different epitopes of the fibrin binding site, however, inhibit the binding of t-PA to fibrin.

When different lymphoid cell lines and a multipotential stem cell line were tested with these Moab, suprisingly only the T-cell line HSB-2 showed strong positive immunofluores-

TABLE VI. Reactivity of Anti-PA Moab With Lymphocytes of Chronic Lymphocytic Leukemia of T-Cell Origin (T-CLL) and Szezary Syndrome*

Patients	Phenotype	Monoclonal antibody code						Evaluation
		131	206	282	7	33	280	
T-CLL								
Kl.	E, T3, T4, T 11	3	0	3	4	3	9	Negative
Wi.	E, T3, T4, T10, T11	0	0	0	2	2	1	Negative
Su.	E, T3, T8, T11	7	0	1	8	14	6	Negative
Mk.	E, T3, T8, T11	0	0	0	2	1	0	Negative
Do.	E, T3, T8, T11	0	0	0	86	72	0	7, 33
Ge.	E, T3, T8, T11	65	35	0	61	49	6	131, 206, 7, 33
Si.	E, T3, T8, T10, T11, M1	21	NT†	NT	20	NT	13	131, 7
Ma.	E, T3, T8, T11, M1	71	0	55	64	69	74	131, 282, 7, 33, 280
Sezary syndrome								
Ste.	T3, T4	74	19	0	9	0	0	131
Ho.	T3, T4	48	62	4	59	41	28	131, 206, 7, 33, 280

*The data are given as percentages of immunofluorescence-positive cells. All cell samples contained less than 10% of dead cells. In the case of patient Si., the sample used contained about 55% viable cells.
†Not tested.

cence staining of their cell membrane with the t-PA–specific Moab. The presence of plasminogen activator on the membrane of this cell line and not on other lymphoid cell lines could also be demonstrated by enzymological tests. During this investigation it was found that K-562, a multipotential stem cell line, secrete a plasminogen-splitting enzyme, which is obviously not related to t-PA or u-PA.

When the expression of PA on leukemic cells of different lineages and maturation stages was investigated, no PA could be detected on the surface of leukemic cells of myelomonocytic origin, which are known to secrete both types of PA [8]. These data suggest that the PA of these cells is stored in cytoplasmic vacuoles and is therefore not detected by immunocytological methods on the cell surface membrane.

The results of the cell line study indicated that certain T-leukemias would be recognized by the Moab specific for t-PA. As expected, only certain subsets of T-cell leukemia bound anti-PA Moab. Cells from T-ALL patients were found to be negative as well as those cases classified as prolymphocytic leukemia of T-cell lineage. Cells from patients with chronic lymphocytic T-cell leukemia (four of eight cases) and cells from patients with Szezary syndrome (two of two cases), both being malignancies involving mature T cells [20,21], were positively stained by the anti-PA Moab. The T-CLL leukemia can be divided into two groups, one having an antigenic profile of suppressor T lymphocytes (T4$^-$/T8$^+$) and the other displaying a mixed phenotype of T4$^-$/T8$^+$ and of M1, a myelomonocytic antigen. The latter phenotype is also observed on cells expressing natural cytotoxic activity [22]. Cells derived from the two Sezary syndrome patients expressing a helper/inducer phenotype (T4$^+$/T8$^-$) were PA positive, whereas T-CLL (two cases) belonging also to the helper/inducer phenotype were negative.

This study indicates that membrane-bound PA might be a useful marker for the characterization of further subsets within the T-suppressor/cytotoxic and the T-inducer/helper population.

REFERENCES

1. Saksela O. Plasminogen activation and regulation of pericellular proteolysis. Biochim Biophys Acta 1985; 823:35–65.
2. Wilson EL, Becker MLB, Hoal EG, Dowdle EB. Molecular species of plasminogen activators secreted by normal and neoplastic human cells. Cancer Res 1980; 40:933–8.
3. Astedt B, Wallen P, Assted B. Occurrence of both urokinase and tissue plasminogen activator in human seminal plasma. Thrombos Res 1979; 16:463–72.
4. Rijken DC, Collen D. Purification and characterization of multiple molecular weight forms of human cell plasminogen activators. J Biol Chem 1981; 256:7035–41.
5. Dano K, Andreasen PA, Grondahl-Hansen J, Kristensen P, Nielsen LS, Skriver L. Plasminogen activators, tissue degradation, and cancer. Adv Cancer Res 1985; 44:139–266.
6. Quigley JP. Proetolytic enzymes. In Hynes RO, ed: Surfaces of normal and malignant cells. Sussex: John Wiley and Sons, Inc. 1979; 247–285.
7. Wilson EL, Jacobs P, Dowdle EB. The secretion of plasminogen activators by human myeloid leukemic cells in vitro. Blood 1983; 61:568–74.
8. Wilson EL, Jacobs P, Oliver L. Plasminogen activator as a prognostic factor in hematological malignancies. In Neth R, Gallo RC, Greaves MF, Janka G, eds: Modern trends in human leukemia. Berlin: Springer, 1985; 4:197–9.
9. Helmkamp RW, Goodland RL, Bale WF, Spar IL, Mutschler LE. High specific activity Iodination of gamma-globulin with Iodine-131 monochloride. Cancer Res 1960; 20:1495–500.
10. Thiel E, Rodt H, Huhn D, et al. Multimarker classfication of acute lymphoblastic leukemia: evidence for further T subgroups and evaluation of their clinical significance. Blood 1980; 56:759–72.
11. Minowada J, Drexler HG, Menon M, et al. A model scheme of hemopetic cell differentiation based on multiple marker analysis of leukemia-lymphomas: T-cell lineage. In Neth R, Gallo RC, Greaves MF, Janka G, eds: Modern trends in human leukemia. Berlin: Springer, 1985; 4:426–9.

12. Drexler HG, Otsuka K, Martin PJ, Gaedicke G, Minowada J. Changes in isoenzyme patterns expressed by the erythroleukemia cell lines K-562 and HEL after induction of differentiation. In Neth R, Gallo RC, Greaves MF, Janka G, eds: Modern trends in human leukemia. Berlin: Springer 1985; 4:430–2.

13. Thiel E, Kummer U, Rodt H, et al. Comparison of currently available monoclonal antibodies with conventional markers for phenotyping opf one hundred acute leukemias. Blut 1982; 44:95–100.

14. Köhler G, Milstein C. Continuous cultures of fused cells secreting antibody of predefined specificity. Nature 1975; 256:495–8.

15. March SC, Parikh J, Cuatrecasas P. A simplified method for cyanogene bromide activation of agarose for affinity chromatography. Anal Biochem 1974; 60:149–55.

16. Klimetzek V, Sorg C. Lymphokine-induced secretion of plasminogen activator by murine macrophages. Eur J Immunol 1977; 7:185–7.

17. Klimetzek V, Sorg C. The production of fibrinolysis inhibitors as a parameter of the activation state in murine macrophages. Eur J Immunol 1979; 9:613–9.

18. Klimetzek V, Schlumberger HD. Functional heterogeneity of macrophages in age-dependent modulation of oxidative metabolism and secretion of proteases. Agent Actions 1984; 15:41–2.

19. Drapier JC, Tenu JP, Lemaire G, Petit JR. Regulation of plasminogen activator secretion in mouse peritoneal macrophages. Biochimie 1979; 61:463–9.

20. Greaves MF, Rao J, Hariri G et al. Phenotypic heterogeneity and cellular origins of T cell malignancies. Leuk Res 1981; 5:281–99.

21. Broder S, Edelson RL, Lutzner MA, et al. The Sezary syndrome: a malignant proliferation of helper T cells. J Clin Invest 1976; 58:1297–306.

22. Thiel E, Schlimok G, Stünkel K, Rieber EP, Huhn D, Feucht H. Chronic lymphocytic leukemia of T-gamma-type with NK and ADCC activity: Demonstration of T-lymphocytic and monocytic antigens. In Resch K, Kirchner H, eds: Mechanisms of lymphocyte activation. Amsterdam: Elsevier, 1981; 294–8.

Cancer Detection and Prevention Supplement 1:279–290 (1987)

Passive, Adoptive, and Active Immunotherapy:
A Review of Clinical Trials in Cancer

Georges Mathé, MD

*Service des Maladies Sanguines et Tumorales and ICIG (Univ. Paris—Sud,
CNRS UA 04-1163; Assoc. Claude Bernard and ARC), Hôpital Paul-Brousse,
Villejuif, France*

ABSTRACT The results today of passive immunotherapy with monoclonal antibodies (MAb) are still very limited, even via its indirect methods (in vitro tumor cell clearance of bone marrow before autologous retransplantation, transport of cytostatic chemicals, and radiation). Tumor cell heterogeneity requires the use of several MAb. Adoptive immunotherapy in the form of the graft vs leukemia (GVL) reaction associated with the graft vs host (GVH) reaction, after an allogeneic bone marrow transplantation, first demonstrated in animals in 1962, has been confirmed in man. The material and operational development of tumor immunology, immunopharmacology, and clinical trial methodology should improve active immunotherapy results and help to convert into a cure what is often a significant but only marginal increase: 1) of disease-free survival or 2) of survival or 3) of survival after relapse. The general ineffective management and use of adjuvant chemotherapy for all tumors except breast carcinoma before menopause will, on the other hand, contribute to necessary new concepts of how to manage the postremission, residual, minimal disease.

Key words: monoclonal antibodies, GVH and GVL reactions, immunopharmacology

INTRODUCTION

Cancer immunotherapy has been divided into three forms: passive, adoptive, and active.

PASSIVE IMMUNOTHERAPY

The passive forms, using mainly heterologous sera [1–7] have given remarkable results in many experimental systems. In 1958, we even successfully applied the carrier property of antibodies to transport a cytostatic drug, methotrexate [8]. Even before the discovery of monoclonal antibodies (MAb) [9], clinical passive immunotherapy had been applied with the help of heterologous antisera [10–12], especially of antithymocyte serum for Sezary's disease [13]. It is the availability of MAb, however, that has induced the present interest in passive immunotherapy in man.

After Bernstein et al [14] had shown the effect of MAb in mouse lymphoma, Ritz et al [15] injected J5 antibody into CALLA$^+$ acute lymphoid leukemia (ALL) patients with spectac-

---

Address reprint requests to Dr. Georges Mathé, Service des Maladies Sanguines et Tumorales and ICIG, Hôpital Paul-Brousse, 12-16 av. Paul-Vaillant-Couturier, 94804-Villejuif, Cédex, France.

ular but transitory effects, Miller and Levy [16] administered a murine antihuman T-cell differentiation antigen to T-cell leukemias and lymphomas with the same effect, and Miller et al [17] used antiidiotypic antibodies against B-lymphoid neoplasias. Other clinical researchers have used MAb to clear the bone marrow from neoplastic cells before it is retransplanted and while the patient is subjected to very intensive chemotherapy [18,19].

We use, in our protocol [20], several MAb, because J5 and VILAI do not react against exactly the same human ALL cells (Table I) [21], and several monoclonals are necessary to cure leukemic mice because of tumor heterogeneity [22]. These antibodies can either kill the neoplastic cells with complement [18,19] or serve as carriers of metals [23] that render tumor cells sensitive to a magnetic field [24].

The possible future of these two forms of passive immunotherapy remains to be determined. It does not seem realistic to expect much from the in vivo effects of MAb against bulky disease. In the treatment of residual disease for which no immediate, visible effect may be expected, a comparative study is necessary. Moreover, passive immunotherapy with hetero-specific G2a immunoglobulin (Ig) MAb could be used in human cancer because macrophages of tumor-bearing patients express Pc receptors that cross-react strongly with murine Ig of the G2a subclass to kill tumor cells [25].

The action of neoplastic cell destruction by complement lysis or opsonization depends on several factors such as antibody specificity, properties of target cell antigens, and especially antigenic modulation. The latter generally depends on bivalent antibody binding, hence the interest in trying monovalent MAb [26]. The results of the Hammersmith Oncology Group [27] in the treatment of malignant effusions with antibody-guided irradiation suggest that passive local immunotherapy may be effective.

ADOPTIVE IMMUNOTHERAPY

We proposed the adoptive form of immunotherapy in 1962 (Fig. 1) [28,29] after several experiments showing reduction of neoplastic cells by the graft versus leukemia (GVL) reaction (Table II) [29] and the reduction of a leukemogenic virus (Table III) [30]. Bortin's group [31] confirmed the effect of the GVL effect in their analysis of the different immunogenetic conditions and of the possibility of enhancing GVL without augmenting GVH.

In 1959, we obtained in man the first partial [32–35] and total human chimera with a complete remission without relapse [36,37] in an ALL patient. He died 2 years later of encephalitis. Weiden et al [38] repeated such results in Seattle and were able to show statistically that the long-term survival (Fig. 2) after bone marrow graft is better when it is complicated by GVH than when it is not. We also obtained an antileukemic effect with white cell transfusions [39].

What is the future of allogeneic bone marrow transplantation? Its use in acute myeloid leukemia (AML) patients in first remission renders results inferior to those that we obtained with cytostatic treatment [40]. Therefore, in both AML and ALL, we only use allogeneic bone marrow grafts in second or later remissions [20]. In chronic myeloid leukemia (CML), it is presently the best treatment [41]. Before allogeneic transplants are used, their results should be compared to those of other treatment modalities. The sequelae of immunosuppression and the harmful effects on fertility and endocrine function, especially in children, should be seriously considered [42].

Transfusions of in vitro tuftsin-activated white cells should be tried to see if tuftsin activation of polymorphs and monocytes and the indirect effect on lymphocytes [43–45] are able to enhance the effects of these cells against tumor cells.

ACTIVE IMMUNOTHERAPY

We proposed active immunotherapy in 1968 after observing that immunostimulation, when applied after tumor take, was equally effective in murine leukemia [46,47] as when

TABLE I. Differences Between Monoclonal Antibodies (J_5 and Vil-A_1) Produced by Two Different Hybridomas

	No. of studies	J_5 (Mean ± SD percent of pos. cells)	Vil-A_1 (Mean ± SD percent of pos. cells)	Mean difference J_5 minus Vil-A_1 ± SE	Level of significance between mean differences (P)	Significance between mean difference in different groups (P)
1. Nonmalignant, inflamed childhood and adult tonsils	16	18.62 ± 9.42	9.25 ± 6.86	9.38 ± 1.99	≈0.00001	
2. B-cell lymphoma (non-Hodgkin lymphoma lymph nodes and chronic lymphatic leukemia peripheral blood)	10 3	18.69 ± 26.22	6.69 ± 12.43	12.00 ± 4.65	≈0.05	
1 + 2	29	18.65 ± 18.50	5.10 ± 9.64	10.55 ± 2.32	≈0.00001	
3. Pre-B lymphatic tumors (ALL marrows at diagnosis or in remission, or peripheral blood at diagnosis)	19	13.89 ± 23.83	11.39 ± 19.38	2.29 ± 3.70	>0.5	=0.0006*

*Wilcoxon rank test.
Adapted from Canon et al [21] with permission of the publisher.

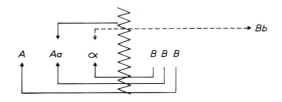

Fig. 1.   Our 1962 concept of adoptive immunotherapy [29,30].

TABLE II. Adoptive Immunotherapy of Leukemia DBA$_2$ In F$_1$ (DBA/2 × C57Bl/6)

	Survival (median)	Cure
Control	11	0
850 rads + isogeneic bone marrow graft*	14.4	0
850 rads + C57Bl/6 bone marrow graft	22.6	1

*Isogeneic bone marrow graft after irradiation is not very efficient. The survival is better after allogeneic bone marrow graft.
Adapted from Mathé et al [29] with permission of the publisher.

applied before tumor take [48]. We also observed an absolute condition for the effect of immunotherapy that depended on the presence of a small number of residual tumor cells, less than 10^5 in mice [47]. We were able to demonstrate that a bulky tumor, reduced by surgery [49], chemotherapy [50], and even radiotherapy [51], could be cured by adjuvant immunotherapy.

In a clinical, comparative, phase II trial of active immunotherapy in ALL in remission, seven patients of 20 were cured with a 16 year follow-up [52]. This result is based on the comparative "fixed response rate" method [53], highly significant because there were no cures of ALL prior to 1968. Moreover, immunotherapy has, in this trial, resulted in a genetic selection. The cured patients belong to two HLA groups (A33 and B17) with a significantly higher frequency than the long-term survivors after chemotherapy and the normal population (Table IV) [54,55]. Although the effect of active immunotherapy as adjuvant treatment of minimal residual disease is still very controversial [56], a critical review of the literature of most clinical trials may reveal the reasons for many "negative" results.

In many trials, a comparative evaluation is made of the effect of *chemoimmunotherapy* and *chemotherapy* [57]. However, in the experimental systems [58], and in the OncoFrance phase III trial on melanoma [59], and in the Edsmyr et al trial on prostatic carcinoma [60], chemoimmunotherapy was less effective than immunotherapy alone, because of the possible immunosuppressive effects of most cytostatics. Comparative trials with randomized controls seemed to produce a high incidence of negative results, not only in cases of adjuvant immunotherapy but also in cases of adjuvant chemotherapy of all tumors except breast carcinoma before the menopause [57,61].

Although immunotherapy does not spectacularly cure many patients, several trials suggest that, similar to adjuvant therapy of minimal residual disease, positive results may be obtained [46,47,49–51]. Examples are the prolonged survival of patients with *ALL* not only in our original trial [52] but also in one trial with controls [62] (Fig. 3) and in two randomized studies [63,64]. Binet and colleagues [65] recently reported significant results after treatment of CLL with levamisole. Salmon et al [66] found good response with the same drug in *myeloma*.

For non-Hodgkin large cell lymphoma, Hoerni et al [67] and Jones and colleagues [68,69] found significant benefits from BCG treatment even after 4–7 years. For *AML,* Reizenstein et al [70] observed significant results from BCG treatment as long as the fourth

TABLE III. Antiviral Effect of Adoptive Immunotherapy*

Treatment of donors	Number of recipients	Animals without leukemia after more than 100 days
First experiment (0.2 ml blood)		
Controls inoculated and not treated	33	0
950 rads	26	0
950 rads + isogeneic marrow	31	0
950 rads + allogeneic marrow	21	7

Treatment of donors	Recipients dying before 57th day	Recipients dying between 58th and 100th days	Recipients without leukemia on 200th day
Second experiment (0.2 ml serum)			
I. Controls inoculated and not treated	45	0	0
II. 950 rads	40	5	0
III. 950 rads + isogeneic marrow	38	7	0
IV. 950 rads + allogeneic marrow	31	13	1
V. 950 rads + allogeneic marrow from vaccinated donors	31	7	7

*(DBA/2 × CBA) F_1 mice inoculated with living Charlotte Friend virus were irradiated with 950 rads and received 10^7 bone marrow cells, isogeneic or allogeneic, from donors vaccinated with formalized virus. Blood or serum from these recipients was subsequently injected into normal isogeneic mice. Comparison of the percentage survival up to the 58th day in group IV or V and group II: $\chi^2 = 5.40$ for 1df, $P < 0.05$. Comparison of the percentage of animals cured in groups IV and V: $\chi^2 = 4.94$ for 1 df, $P < 0.05$.
Adapted from Mathé and Amiel [30] with permission of the publisher.

year, Bekesi and Holland [71] obtained favorable results with neuraminidase-treated neoplastic cells, and Ota [72] reported significant effects with bestatin, all three in randomized trials. Considering all AML active immunotherapy trials (except Ota's study), Foon et al [73] found a significant effect on survival. For *CML*, treatment with BCG and irradiated blastic crisis cells led to highly significant results for survival [74].

In the case of *melanoma*, a very significant response was reported by Eilber et al [75]. The same authors later observed, in a randomized, controlled study, a moderate benefit for disease-free survival (DFS) and overall survival and a very significant effect on survival after relapse [76].

In our OncoFrance trial, therapy with BCG only led to better results than the combination of chemo- and immuno (BCG)-therapy for DFS and overall survival and very significantly for survival after relapse [59]. Spitler et al [77] obtained with levamisole a moderate effect on DFS in melanoma stage I patients and Oka [78] a significant effect with bestatin on DFS and overall survival after relapse of this disease.

In the case of *osteosarcoma*, Strander et al [79] reported significant results with interferon. Regrettably there have been no immunotherapy trials for glioma, a solid tumor known

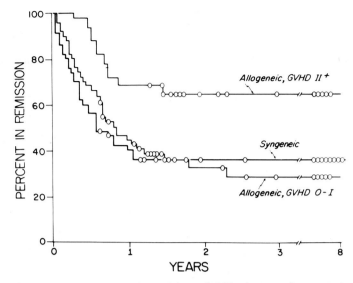

Fig. 2. Kaplan-Meier product limit estimate of the probability (expressed as percent of remaining in remission from acute lymphoblastic or nonlymphoblastic leukemia as a function of time after transplantation. Data are shown for 46 syngeneic marrow recipients, 117 allogeneic marrow recipients with no or grade I GVHD, and 79 allogeneic marrow recipients with grades II–IV or chronic GVHD. Each open symbol represents one patient who is now alive in remission [38].

**TABLE IV. HLA Antigen Frequencies in 14 BCG-Treated Long-Term Survivors
With Acute Lymphatic Leukemia Compared to 14 Chemotherapy Long-Term Survivors
and to 591 Healthy Controls [54,55]**

No.		Percent	Percent	P
14 BCG	HLA-B17	42.8	7.3	<0.01
14 Chemotherapy	HLA-A33	35.7	1.2	<0.01
591 Controls	HLA-B17 or A33	71.4	8.1	<0.001

to be accompanied initially by the most severe immunologic insufficiency [80]. For *bronchial carcinoma*, significant results were obtained by Maver et al [81] with intrapleural BCG, by Stewart et al [82] with a solubilized tumor-associated antigen (TAA) preparation, and by Focan et al [83] with levamisole. For *gastric cancer*, Ochiai [84] had significant results with BCG. Similar to our ALL trials [54,55], this treatment seemed to be influenced by genetic factors. For *colon cancer*, Robinson [85] obtained good results with MER, however, only in patients with low-grade disease. In *bladder cancer*, local immunotherapy has been effective in several phase II trials [86]. For *ovarian cancer*, Alberts et al [87] reported favorable results in residual disease. For uterine *cervix carcinoma*, Okamura [88] obtained significant results with a glucan derivative. Use of polyA-polyU in a randomized study led to significant results in *breast carcinoma* up to the fifth year [89]. In *prostate carcinoma*, Edsmyr et al [60] reported significant results with bestatin.

NEGATIVE TRIALS

Negative results may be explained by an insufficient number of patients or in some cases by use of chemotherapy or immunotherapy following insufficient debulking [57]. The reported results from active immunotherapy need comparison with those from adjuvant chemotherapy with beneficial result in only half of the patients. A good response of breast carcinoma before

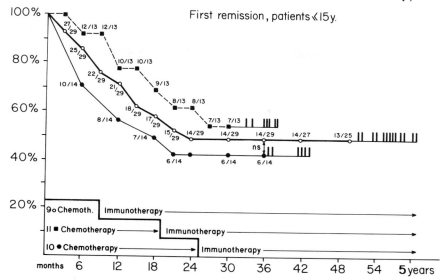

Fig. 3. Cumulative curves of the duration of first remissions in 1976 (established by the "direct" method) for the children submitted to three protocols (9, 10, and 11). Protocol 9 had a short induction and protocol 10 a long induction and maintenance chemotherapy. The result shows either that maintenance chemotherapy was of no use or that active immunotherapy was as effective as chemotherapy [62].

menopause occurred in two of three trials on DFS [90–92] but not on overall survival [91,92]. All other recent trials, including those on breast carcinoma after menopause [90–92] led to negative results [57]. This failure of cytostatics may be explained on the grounds that the residual cells responsible for recurrence were in G0 phase. However, this resting state of cells is a necessary condition for their sensitivity to active immunotherapy [93].

A problem that led to the controversial aspect of immunotherapy arose because Hewitt et al [94] failed to find tumor-associated antigens (TAA) in spontaneous tumors in contrast to induced animal tumors [95,96]. The availability of MAb may change these results [97]. Moreover, based on the discovery of natural immunity, TAA are not required for active immunotherapeutic action and for the immunobiologic control of cancer. NK cells [98], autoreactive cells [99], macrophages, and NK-like cells seem to play an antigen-independent role in tumor surveillance.

TAA, possibly an expression of oncogenes [100] that may be "paranoid" normal growth regulation genes, are probably normal antigens with inappropriate expression [101,102]. The complexity of abnormally expressed or modified normal antigens does not prevent them from being effective in some autoimmune conditions or in tumor surveillance [103]. Occasionally, however, TAA may also be true neoantigens, which, for example, may be associated with chemotherapy resistance [104] or the tendency for metastasis (Olsson, personal communication).

The future of active immunotherapy will be influenced by the availability of new immunodifiers that are used more easily than BCG with scientific pharmacologic methods and with improved purity of substances such as the thymic peptides [105], tuftsin [106–108], bestatin [106,109], and zinc [110]. With improved dosage and application [46], the risk of obtaining immunonsuppressive effects [111] may be reduced.

The future of immunotherapy may be influenced also by the possibilities to measure the effect of immunologic interventions by such parameters as the numbers of inducer-helper and cytotoxic-suppressor T lymphocytes and NK cells [112] bearing in mind the difficulty of interpretating the data especially because of chronobiologic variations [113]. It is hoped that clinical immunopharmacology may develop into a sufficiently precise tool to permit active, efficient immunotherapy.

ACKNOWLEDGMENTS

The author thanks Nicole Vriz and Elisabeth Couvé for efficient editorial assistance.

REFERENCES

1. Moller G. Effect on tumor growth in syngeneic recipients of antibodies against tumor-specific antigens in methyl-cholanthrene-induced mouse sarcomas. Nature 1965;204:846–52.
2. Collins JJ, Sanfilippo F, Tsong-Chou L, Ishizaki T, Metzgar RS. Immunotherapy of murine leukemia. I. Protection against Friend leukemia virus induced disease by passive serum therapy. Int J Cancer 1978;21:51–60.
3. Drake WP, Ungaro PC, Mardiney Mr Jr. Passive administration of antiserum and complement in producing anti-EL4 cytotoxic activity in the serum of C57Bl/6. JNCI 1973;50:909–12.
4. Hu C, Linna TJ. Serotherapy of avian reticulo-endotheliosis virus-induced tumors. Ann NY Acad Sci 1976;277:634–8.
5. Old LJ, Stockert E, Boyse EA, Geering G. A study of passive immunization against a transplanted G$^+$ leukemia with specific antiserum. Proc Soc Exp Biol Med 1967;124:63–7.
6. Pearson GR, Redmon LW, Bass LR. Protective effect of immune sera against transplantable Moloney virus-induced sarcoma and lymphoma. Cancer Res 1979;33:171–4.
7. Wright PW, Bernstein ID. Serotherapy of malignant disease. Prog Exp Tumor Res 1980;25:140–8.
8. Mathé G, Tran Ba Loc, Bernard J. Effet sur la leucémie L1210 d'une combinaison par diazotation d'améthoptérine et de gammaglobulines de hamsters porteurs de cette leucémie par hétérogreffe. CR Acad Sci [III] 1958;246:1626–8.
9. Kohler G, Milstein C. Continuous cultures of fused cells secreting antibody of predefined. Nature 1975;256:495–8.
10. Fefer A. Immunotherapy and chemotherapy of Moloney sarcoma virus-induced tumors in mice. Cancer Res 1969;29:2177–82.
11. Herberman RB, Rogentine GN, Oren ME. Bioassay of anti-tumor effects of human alloantisera. Clin Res 1969;17:328–31.
12. Wright PW, Hellstrom KE, Bernstein ID. Serotherapy of malignant disease. Med Clin North Am 1976;60:607–12.
13. Fisher RI, Kubota TT, Mandel GL, Broder S, Young RC. Regression of a T-cell lymphoma after administration of antithymocyte globulin. Ann Intern Med 1978;88:799–804.
14. Bernstein ID, Tam MR, Nowinski RC. Mouse leukemia: Therapy with monoclonal antibodies against a thymus differentiation antigen. Science 1980;207:68–71.
15. Ritz J, Pesando JM, Sallan SE, et al. Serotherapy of acute lymphoblastic leukemia with monoclonal antibody. Blood 1981;58:141–5.
16. Miller RA, Levy R. In vivo effect of murine hybridoma monoclonal antibody on human T-cell neoplasm. In: Rosenberg SA, Kaplan HS, eds. Malignant lymphoma. New York: Academic Press, 1982;1:553–8.
17. Miller RA, Maloney DG, Warnke R. Treatment of a B-cell lymphoma with monoclonal anti-idiotype antibody. N Engl J Med 1982;306:517–22.
18. Ritz J, Schlossman SF. Utilization of monoclonal antibodies in the treatment of leukemia and lymphoma. Blood 1982;59:1–9.
19. Ritz J, Sallan SE, Bast RC Jr, et al. Autologous bone marrow transplantation in calla-positive acute lymphoblastic leukaemia after in vitro treatment with J5 monoclonal antibody and complement. Lancet 1982;ii:60–8.
20. Mathé G, Misset JL, Machover D, et al. Protocoles des traitements des leucémies et des lymphomes: Vers l'escalade ou vers la réduction de l'intensité. Biomed Pharmacother 1984;38:13–32.
21. Canon C, Eichler-Reiss F, Reizenstein P, Mathé G. Difference between monoclonal antibodies against the common acute leukemia antigen from two different hybridomas. Anticancer Res 1983;3:407–8.
22. Olsson L, Mathé G. Antigenic heterogeneity of leukemia. Blood Cells 1981;7:281–6.

23. Balercia G, Canon C, Cinti S, Marabello G, Dantchev D, Mathé G. Immunoelectron microscopy with immunogold staining method and monoclonal antibodies. A promising tool in ultrastructural study of lymphatic subpopulations. Biomed Pharmacother 1984;38:114–6.

24. Treleaven JG, Gibson FM, Ugelstad J, et al. Removal of neuroblastoma cells from bone marrow with monoclonal antibodies conjugated to magnetic microspheres. Lancet 1984; i:70–2.

25. Steplewski Z, Lubeck MD, Koprowski H. Human macrophages armed with murine immunoglobulin G2a antibodies to tumors destroy human cancer cells. Science 1983;221:865–8.

26. Cobbolt SP, Waldmann H. Therapeutic potential of monovalent monoclonal antibodies. Nature 1984;308:460–2.

27. Anon. Report from the Hammersmith Oncology Group and the Imperial Cancer Research Fund: Antibody-guided irradiation of malignant lesions: Three cases illustrating a new method of treatment. Lancet 1984; i:1441–3.

28. Mathé G, Amiel JL, Schwarzenberg L. Bone marrow transplantation and leucocyte transfusions. Springfield, IL:Charles C. Thomas, 1971.

29. Mathé G, Amiel JL, Niemetz J. Greffe de moelle osseuse après irradiation totale chez des souris leucémiques, suivie de l'administration d'un antimitotique pour réduire la fréquence du syndrome secondaire et ajouter á l'effet antileucémique. CR Acad Sci [III] 1962; 254:3602–5.

30. Mathé G, Amiel JL. Réduction de la concentration plasmatique du virus leucémigène de Charlotte Friend par immunothérapie adoptive (greffe de moelle oseuse allogénique). CR Acad Sci [III] 1964;259:4408–10.

31. Tempelis L, Wasik MR, Bortin MM: Adoptive immunotherapy of disseminated malignancies. La Ricerca Clin Lab 1983;13:163–6.

32. Mathé G, Jammet H, Pendic B, et al. Transfusions et greffes de moelle osseuse homologue chez des humains irradiés à haute dose accidentellement. Rev Franç Etud Clin Biol 1959;4:226–38.

33. Mathé G, Jammet H, Playfair J, Amiel JL: Irradiation totale et greffe de moelle osseuse chez l'homme. In CR 8th Congr Soc Europ Hematol Basel: Karger, 1962:67–75.

34. Mathé G, Bernard J, Schwarzenberg L, et al. Essai de traitement de sujets atteints de leucémie aigue par irradiation suivie de transfusion de moelle oseuse homologue. Rev Franç Etud Clin Biol 1959;4:675–704.

35. Mathé G, Bernard J, Vries MJ de, et al. Nouveaux essais de greffe de moelle osseuse homologue après irradiation totale chez des enfants atteints de leucémie aigue en rémission. Le problèmes du syndrome secondaire chez l'homme. Rev Hematol 1960;15:115–61.

36. Mathé G, Amiel JL, Schwarzenberg L, Cattan A, Schneider M: Haematopoietic chimera in man after allogenic (homologous) bone marrow transplantation. Control of the secondary syndrome. Specific tolerance due to the chimerism. Br Med J 1963;5373:1633–5.

37. Mathé G, Amiel JL, Schwarzenberg L, et al. Successful allogenic bone marrow transplantation in man. Chimerism induced specific tolerance and possible antileukemic effects. Blood 1965;25:179–96.

38. Weiden PL, Flournoy N, Thomas ED, et al. Antileukemic effect of graft-versus-host disease in human recipients of allogeneic-marrow grafts. N Engl J Med 1979;300:1068–71.

39. Schwarzenberg L, Mathé G, Schneider M, Amiel JL, Cattan A, Schlumberger JR. Attempted adoptive immunotherapy of acute leukemia by leucocyte transfusions. Lancet 1966;ii:365–8.

40. Machover D, Rappaport H, Schwarzenberg L, et al. Treatment of acute myeloid leukemia with a combination of intensive induction chemotherapy. Early consolidation, splenectomy and long-term maintenance chemotherapy. Cancer 1984;53:1644–50.

41. Speck B, Bortin MM, Champlin R, et al. Allogeneic bone marrow transplantation for chronic myelogenous leukaemia. Lancet 1984; i:665–8.

42. Sklar CA, Kim TH, Ramsay NKC. Testicular function following bone marrow transplantation performed during or after puberty. Cancer 1984;53:1498–501.

43. Florentin I, Martinez J, Maral J, et al. Immunopharmacological properties of tuftsin and of some analogs In: Najjar VA, Fridkin M, eds. Antineoplastic immunogenic and other effects of the tetrapeptide tuftsin: A natural macrophage activator. New York: New York Acad Sci, 1983:177–91.

44. Bruley-Rosset M, Hercend T, Rappaport H, Mathé G: Immunorestorative capacity of tuftsin after long-term administration to aging mice. In: Najjar VA, Fridkin M, eds. Antineoplastic immunogenic and other effects of the tetrapeptide tuftsin: A natural macrophage activator. New York: New York Acad Sci, 1983:242–50.

45. Mathé G, Florentin I, Bruley-Rosset M, Martinez J, Winternitz F. Modifiers of normal immune status and restorators or immunodepressed animals. Paper presented at the Conference on Clinical and Biological Evaluation of the Immunomodifiers, San Rocco, Italia, Oct. 1–4, 1983.

46. Mathé G. Cancer active immunotherapy, immunoprophylaxis and immunorestoration. An introduction. New York: Springer Verlag, 1976.

47. Mathé G. Immunothérapie active de la leucémie L1210 appliquée après la greffe tumorale. Rev Franç Clin Biol, 1968;13:881–3.

48. Glynn JP, Humphreys SR, Trivers G, Biancao AR, Goldin A. Studies on immunity to leukaemia L1210 in mice. Cancer Res 1963;23:1008–10.

49. Thompson RB, Alberola V, Mathé G. Evaluation of surgery, chemotherapy and immunotherapy on Lewis lung tumor. Eur J Clin Biol Res 1972;17:900–2.

50. Mathé G. Active immunotherapy. Adv Cancer Res 1971;14:1–36.

51. Martin M, Bourut C, Halle-Pannenko O, Mathé G. BCG immunotherapy of Lewis tumor residual disease left after local radiotherapy. Biomedecine 1975;23:337–8.

52. Mathé G, Amiel JL, Schwarzenberg L, et al. Active immunotherapy for acute lymphoblastic leukaemia. Lancet 1969;i:697–9.

53. Lee YJ, Wesley RA. Statistical contributions to phase II trials in cancer: Interpretation, analysis and design. Semin Oncol 1981;8:403–10.

54. Tursz T, Hors J, Lipinski M, Amiel JL, Mathé G. Comparison of HLA phenotypes in long-term survivors with acute lymphoblastic leukemia treated with immunotherapy versus chemotherapy. In: Mathé G, Bonadonna G, Salmon S, eds. Adjuvant therapies of cancer. New York: Springer Verlag, 1982:26–8.

55. Tursz T. Heterogeneity of results correlated to genetics (HLA-DR). Personal Communication.

56. Terry W. Cancer immunotherapy. Paper presented at the Paris Anti-Cancer Congress, 1978.

57. Mathé G, Reizenstein P, Eriguchi M. Cancer residual disease, its chemotherapy and immunotherapy. In press.

58. Mathé G, Halle-Pannenko O, Bourut C. Comparison of various possible chemo-immunotherapy sequences (cyclophosphamide-BCG; BCG-cyclophosphamide interspersion) in the treatment of L1210 leukemia. In: Fourth Annual Conference, International Society for Experimental Hematology, Yugoslavia, Sept 21–24, 1975. Abstract 138, p 61.

59. Mathé G, Misset JL, Serrou B, et al. Immunotherapy versus chemo-immunotherapy as adjuvant treatment of malignant melanoma. In: Torisu M, Yoshida LT, eds. Basic mechanisms and clinical treatment of tumor metastasis. New York: Academic Press, 1985;617–22.

60. Edsmyr F, Esposti PL, Andersson L, Naslund I, Blomgren H. Clinical study on bestatin and peplomycin in treatment of prostatic carcinoma. In: Carter SK, Ultmann J, eds. Peplomycin. 13th Int Congress on Chemotherapy, Vienna, Aug 28–Sept 2, 1983.

61. Mathé G. Lessons from cancer adjuvant therapy comparative trials with randomized controls. Personal Communication.

62. Mathé G, De Vassal F, Schwarzenberg L, et al. Preliminary results of three protocols for the treatment of acute lymphoid leukaemia in children: Distinction of two groups of patients according to predictable prognosis. Med Pediatr Oncol 1978;4:17–27.

63. Stryckmans PA, Otten J, Delbeke MJ, et al. for the EORTC Hemopathies Working Party. Comparison of chemotherapy with immunotherapy for maintenance of acute lymphoblastic leukemia in children and adults. Blood 1983;62:606–10.

64. Pavlovsky S, Sackmann Muriel F, Garay G, et al. Chemoimmunotherapy with levamisole in acute lymphoblastic leukemia. Cancer 1981;48:1500–5.

65. Travade P, Chastang C, Auquier A, et al. Resultats préliminaires du protocole LLC 76. In: Bernard A, Boumsell L, Demeocq F, eds. Biologie des leucémies et hémtosarcomes. Paris: G. Lachurié, 1983:229–35.

66. Salmon SE, Alexanian R, Dixon D. Chemoimmunotherapy for multiple myeloma. Effect of levamisole during maintenance. In: Terry WD, Rosenberg SA, eds. Immunotherapy of human cancer. New York: Excerpta Medica, 1982:61–4.

67. Hoerni B, Durand M, Eghbali H, Hoerni-Simon G, Lagarde C. Adjuvant BCG-therapy of non-Hodgkin's malignant lymphomas. In: Salmon SE, Jones SE, eds. Adjuvant therapy of cancer III. New York: Grune & Stratton, 1981:99–104.

68. Jones SE. Chemoimmunotherapy of malignant lymphoma. In: Terry WD, Rosenberg SA, eds. Immunotherapy of human cancer. New York: Excerpta Medica, 1982:55–8.

69. Jones SE, Salmon SE, Fisher R. Adjuvant immunotherapy with BCG in non-Hodgkin's lymphoma: A Southwest Oncology Group controlled clinical trial. In: Jones SE, Salmon SE, eds. Adjuvant therapy of cancer II. New York: Grune & Stratton, 1979:163–6.

70. Reizenstein P, Andersson B, Bjorkholm M, et al. BCG plus leukemic cell therapy in patients with acute nonlymphoblastic leukemia: Effect in groups with high and low remission rates. In Terry WD, Rosenberg SA, eds. Immunotherapy of human cancer. New York: Excerpta Medica, 1982:17–26.

71. Bekesi JG, Holland JF. Therapeutic effectiveness of neuraminidase-treated allogeneic myeloblasts as immunogen in acute myelocytic leukemia. In: Mathé G, Bonadonna G, Salmon S, eds. Adjuvant therapies of cancer. New York: Springer Verlag, 1982:42–5.

72. Ota K. A phase III study of bestatine as adjuvant immunotherapy of acute myeloid leukemia. Personal Communication.

73. Foon KA, Smaley RV, Riggs CW, Gale RP. The role of immunotherapy in acute myelogenous leukemia. Arch Intern Med 1983;143:1726–30.

74. Mathé G, Schwarzenberg L, Misset JL, et al. The present state of "curability" of leukaemias including polycythaemia vera. In: Tanner E, Hefti ML, eds. Annals of life insurance. New York:Springer Verlag, 1980;6:112–33.

75. Eilber FR, Morton DL, Holmes EC, Sparks FC, Ramming KP. Adjuvant immunotherapy with BCG in treatment of regional lymph node metastases from malignant melanoma. N Engl J Med 1976;294:237–40.

76. Morton DL, Carmack Holmes E, Eilber FR, Ramming KP. Adjuvant immunotherapy of malignant melanoma: Results of a randomized trial in patients with lymph node metastases. In: Terry WD, Rosenberg SA, eds. New York: Excerpta Medica, 1982:245–8.

77. Spitler LE, Sagebiel R. A randomized trial of levamisole versus placebo as adjuvant therapy in malignant melanoma. N Engl J Med 1980;303:1143–6.

78. Oka T. Bestatin as melanoma adjuvant therapy. Personal Communication.

79. Strander H, Aparisi T, Blomgren H, et al. Adjuvant interferon treatment of human osteosarcoma. In: Mathé G, Bonadonna G, Salmon S, eds. Adjuvant therapies of cancer. New York:Springer Verlag, 1982: 103–10.

80. Gerosa MA, Olivi A, Rosenblum ML, Semenzato GP, Pezzutto A. Impaired immunocompetence in patients with malignant gliomas: The possible role of Tg-lymphocyte subpopulations. Neurosurgery 1982;10:571–4.

81. Maver C, Kausel H, Lininger G, McKneally M. Intrapleural BCG immunotherapy of lung cancer patients. In: Mathé G, Bonadonna G, Salmon S, eds. Adjuvant therapies of cancer. New York:Springer Verlag, 1982:227–30.

82. Stewart THM, Hollinshead AC, Harris JE, Raman S. Specific active immunotherapy in lung cancer: The induction of long-lasting cellular responses to tumour associated antigens. In: Mathé G, Bonadonna G, Salmon S, eds. New York: Springer Verlag, 1982:232–5.

83. Focan C, Focan-Henrard D, Schyns-Mosen J, Frere MH, Halen M, Lehung S. Levamisole (L) versus placebo (O) for prolongation of remission and survival in human solid tumors. A double-blind randomized trial. Paper presented at the 10th Congress of the European Society for Medical Oncology, Nice, Dec 7–9, 1984.

84. Ochiai T, Sato H, Okuyama K, Asano T. Immunotherapy of gastric cancer with special reference to Japanese randomized trials. In: Mathé G, Reizenstein P, Di Cato M, eds. Clinical trials in oncology: ethics, errors, methods and results. Geneva: Bioscience Ediprint, Inc, 1985., 87–95.

85. Robinson E, Haim N, Bartal A, Mohilever J, Mekori T. Adjuvant radio chemoimmunotherapy in colorectal cancer: results of a randomized study and review of literature. In: Mathé G, Reizenstein P, Di Cato M, eds. Clinical trials in oncology: ethics, errors, methods and results. Geneva: Bioscience Ediprint, Inc, 1985., 23–9.

86. Camacho F, Pinsky C, Kerr D, Whitmore W, Oettgen H. Treatment of superficial bladder cancer with intra-vesical BCG. In: Proc Int Conf Immunother Cancer, Bethesda, April 28–30, 1980.

87. Alberts D, Moonn T, O'Toole R, Neff J, Tate Thigpen J, Blessing J. BCG as an adjuvant to adriamycin-cyclophosphamide in the treatment of advanced ovarian carcinoma: Ongoing analysis of a Southwest Oncology Study Group. In: Jones SE, Salmon S, eds. Adjuvant therapy of cancer II. New York: Grune & Stratton, 1979:1653–60.

88. Okamura K, Yajima A. Cervical cancer: chemotherapy and immunotherapy. In: Mathé G, Reizenstein P, Di Cato M, eds. Clinical trials in oncology: ethics, errors, methods and results. Geneva: Bioscience Ediprint, Inc, 1985., 101–7.

89. Lacour J, Lacour F, Spira A, et al. Adjuvant treatment with polyadenylic-polyuridylic acid (polyA-polyU) in operable breast cancer. Lancet 1980;ii:161–2.

90. Tancini G, Bajetta E, Marchini S, Valagussa P, Bonadonna G, Veronesi U. Preliminary 3-year results of 12 vs 6 cycles of surgical adjuvant CMF in premenopausal breast cancer. Cancer Clin Trials 1979;2:285–9.

91. Mathé G, Misset JL, Plague R, et al. Superiority of AVCF (ADM, VCR, CPM and 5-FU) over CMF (CPM, MTX and 5-Fu) as adjuvant chemotherapy for breast cancer. A phase III trial of Association Oncofrance. In: Torisu M, Yoshida T, eds. Basic mechanisms and clinical treatment of tumor metastasis. New York: Academic Press, 1985; 477–84.

92. Olsson L, Mathé G. A cytokinetic analysis of bacillus Calmette-Guérin induced growth control of murine leukemia. Cancer Res 1977;37:1743–9.

93. Hewitt HB, Blake ER, Walder AS. A critique of the evidence of host defense against cancer based on personal studies of 27 murine tumors of spontaneous origin. Br J Cancer 1976;33:241–3.

94. Foley EJ. Antigenic properties of methylcholanthrene-induced tumors in moce of the strain of origin. Cancer Res 1953;13:835–8.

95. Prehn RT. Tumor specific immunity to transplanted dibenz(a,h)anthracene induced sarcomas. Cancer Res 1960;20:1614–6.

96. Hellstrom KE, Hellstrom I, Brown JP. Diagnostic and therapeutic use of monoclonal antibodies to human tumor antigens. Med Oncol Tumor Pharmacother 1984;1:143–5.

97. Talmadge JE, Meyers LM, Prieur DJ, Starkey JR. Role of natural killer cells in tumor growth and metastasis: C57Bl/6 normal and beige mice. JNCI 1980;65:929–33.

98. Olsson L, Kiger N, Mathé G. Autoreactive cells in cancer active immunotherapy: Their cytotoxic potential and genetic restriction. Transplant Proc 1980;12:167–71.

99. Kuzumaki N, Minakawa H, Matsuo T, Haraguchi S, Yoshida T. Correlation between tumor-specific surface antigens and *src* gene expression in Rous sarcoma virus-induced rat tumors. Eur J Cancer Clin Oncol 1983;19:401–4.

100. Schatten S, Drebin JA, Granstein RD, Greene MI. Differential antigen presentation in tumor immunity. Fed Proc 1984;43:2460–3.

101. Parmiani G, Carbone G, Invernizzi G, Meschini A, Della Porta G. Expression of genetically inappropriate histocompatibility antigens on the cell surface of experimental tumors and their relationship to tumor-associated transplantation antigens. In: Spreafico F, Arnon R, eds. Tumor-associated antigens and their specific immune response. London: Academic Press, 1979:31–8.

102. Rogers MJ. Tumor-associated transplantation antigens of chemically-induced tumors: New complexities. Immunol Today 1984;5:167–70.

103. O'Hara CJ, Price GB. A monoclonal antibody demonstrating specificity for drug-resistant cells. Immunol Lett 1982;5:15–8.

104. Chretien P, Lipson SD, Makuch R, Benady DE, Cohen MH, Minna JD. Thymosin in cancer patients: in vitro effects and correlations with clinical response to tymosin immunotherapy. Cancer Ther Rep 1978;62:1787–9.

105. Florentin I, Mathé G, Bruley-Rosset M. Do tuftsin and bestatin constitute a biopharmacologic immunoregulatory system? In: Mathé G, Umezawa H, eds. Antibiotics in cancer treatment. Trends Antibiotics Res 1985:1:in press.

106. Timus M, Kim Triana, Mathé G. Biological response modifiers: tuftsin. Personal Communication.

107. Catane R, Sulkes A, Uziely B, Yez E, Isacson R, Treves AJ, Fridkin M. Initial clinical studies with tuftsin. In: Mathé G, Reizenstein P, Di Cato M, eds. Clinical trials in oncology: ethics, errors, methods and results. Geneva: Bioscience Ediprint, Inc, 1985., 81–5.

108. Serrou B, Cupissol D, Flad H, et al. Phase I evaluation of bestatin in patients bearing advanced solid tumors. In: Terry WD, Rosenberg SA, eds. Immunotherapy of human cancer. New York: Excerpta Medica, 1982:454–8.

109. Blazsek I, Mathé G. Zinc and immunity. Biomed Pharmacother 1984;38:187–93.

110. Scott MT. Tumour-induced specific suppression: a limitation to immunotherapy. Immunol Today 1982;3:8–11.

111. Canon C, Mathé G, Reizenstein P. The necessary clinical monitoring of immunopharmacology study and immunotherapeutic trials and its result interpretation. Biomed Pharmacother (in press).

112. Lévi F, Canon C, Blum JP, Reinberg A, Mathé G. Large-amplitude circadian rhythm in helper-suppressor ratio of peripheral blood lymphocytes. Lancet 1983;ii:462–3.

Cancer Detection and Prevention Supplement 1:291–299 (1987)

Metastasis Models for Human Tumors in Athymic Mice:
Useful Models for Drug Development

Donald L. Fine, PhD
Robert Shoemaker, PhD
Adi Gazdar, MD
Joseph G. Mayo, DVM

Oystein Fodstad, MD, PhD
Michael R. Boyd, MD, PhD
Betty J. Abbott, MS
Patricia A. Donovan

Program Resources, Inc. (D.L.F., P.A.D.) and Developmental Therapeutics Program (R.S., J.G.M., B.J.A.), National Cancer Institute/Frederick Cancer Research Facility (NCI-FCRF), Frederick, MD; NCI-Naval Medical Oncology Branch (A.G.) and Developmental Therapeutics Program (M.R.B.), Bethesda, MD; Norsk Hydros Institute for Cancer Research, Oslo, Norway (O.F.)

ABSTRACT Although human tumor xenografts have been extensively used for preclinical evaluation of antitumor agents, most of this work has utilized subcutaneous or subrenal capsule assays based on change in tumor size. To obtain experimental models more reflective of the human clinical situations, we have developed several metastatic models that are based on and complement a panel of cell strains used in large-scale in vitro drug screening. One melanoma and four lung tumors produced metastatic lesions in the lung within 60 days following subcutaneous, intraperitoneal, or intrasplenic inoculation of BALB/C athymic nude mice. Several tumors also produced liver lesions, and one lung tumor strain showed metastasis to the brain. The metastatic lesions histologically resembled the tumors that grew at the inoculation site. In vitro and in vivo cell strains were rederived from the metastatic lesions. These systems may provide practical models for experimental drug and immunotherapeutic trials.

Key words: in vitro drug screening, lung cancer, melanoma, chemotherapy, xenografts

INTRODUCTION

Athymic (nude) mice have provided useful systems for in vivo propagation of xenografted tumors for the testing of chemicals for potential antineoplastic activity. The ability to propagate human tumors in nude mice makes possible the testing of such compounds against specific classes of human tumors [1–3]. Most transplants of human malignant tumors result in localized growth in a rather "benign" pattern, in that the tumor develops as a well circum-

Address reprint requests to Dr. Donald L. Fine, NCI/FCRF, Frederick, MD 21701.

scribed nodule at the site of inoculation [4]. Only a small number of human tumor xenografts have the capability of invading and metastasizing [5,6]. A number of investigators have concluded that various factors influence the ability of a tumor to metastasize; animal age [7], source and health status [8,9], route and site of inoculation [6,10], and inherent tumor properties [11,12] are important in determining the observed metastatic phenotype.

We have been interested in developing metastatic models of human tumors that would be more reflective of human clinical disease and complement a panel of cell lines to be used for in vitro drug screening. Described here are five human tumor cell strains that metastasize in nude mice and some that result in lethal disease and reproducible death patterns. The metastatic lesions morphologically resemble the original tumor. The capacity of these cell strains to be expanded in vitro, cryopreserved, and shipped to different laboratories makes them particularly useful tools for in vivo preclinical evaluation of candidate chemotherapeutic agents.

MATERIALS AND METHODS
Animals

Specific pathogen-free 4–6-week-old athymic female NCr-nu mice were used in all experiments as indicated. The mice were obtained from Animal Production, Harlan Sprague Dawley, Inc., at the NCI-FCRF (Frederick, MD), and were maintained in strict isolation in filter-top cages and fed a diet of autoclavable NIH open formula 31 rodent chow. All food, water, bedding, and cage materials were presterilized.

Tumor Cell Cultures

All tumor cell strains were maintained as monolayer cultures in RPMI-1640 medium supplemented with 10% heat-inactivated fetal bovine serum (FBS). All cells used in these experiments were tested and found to be free of mycoplasma contamination and infection by seven murine adventitious agents including reovirus type 3, pneumonia virus of mice, mouse adenovirus, murine hepatitus virus, lymphocytic choriomeningitis virus, ectromelia virus, and lactic dehydrogenase virus.

Tumor cells were collected from monolayer culture using trypsin-EDTA in Hanks balanced salt solution, washed, and suspended in sterile, normal saline for injection at a concentration of 5×10^7 viable cells/ml. All cell preparations were > 95% viable by trypan blue exclusion staining. Large volume production consisted of growth in roller bottles using the above-mentioned culture medium. Stock ampules of the cell cultures were frozen in RPMI-1640 medium containing 10% heat-inactivated FBS and 10% DMSO at a concentration of 1×10^7 cells/ml.

Mouse Inoculations

Fresh surgical resections were received on wet ice in RPMI-1640 medium containing 10% FBS. Solid tumor specimens were minced into approximately 2 mm^3 fragments devoid of necrotic material. Fragments were implanted into 5 mice SC via a 13-gauge trocar.

Pleural effusions were received as 5 ml cell suspensions in RPMI-1640 medium containing 10% FBS. Two groups of five mice each were injected with 0.2 ml SC or 0.3 ml IP.

Cell strains were implanted into ten mice SC, IP, or intrasplenically (IS) at 1×10^7 cells/animal. All mice were monitored daily for tumor growth. Solid tumors were calipered weekly. Serial passaging was performed on tumors that showed progressive growth. At designated intervals or when moribund, the mice were sacrificed by cervical dislocation and necropsied. Lymph nodes, lungs, liver, spleen, heart, kidneys, small intestine, pancreas, brain, muscle, and skin were fixed in buffered 10% formalin and processed for histological examination.

Histology

Fixed tissues were embedded in paraffin, cut into 5 μm sections, and stained with hematoxylin and eosin.

RESULTS
Development of Metastatic Models

In these studies, a total of 36 fresh tumor resections and 15 established tumor cell strains were inoculated by either SC or IP routes. Growth at the SC inoculation site occurred in 21 of 36 (58%) fresh tumor resections attempted. Of these, 62% were serially transplanted for three or more passages. Growth of tumors in mice inoculated IP with fresh tumor material occurred in only two of 13 (17%) inoculations. Each of these was successfully grown in serial transplants. For those tumors that grew at the SC site, the average appearance of tumor was seen 54 days postinoculation. Growth at the SC inoculation site occurred in 15 of 15 (100%) of the established cell strains tested. For these, appearance of palpable tumors at the site of inoculation averaged 15.8 days postinoculation.

Histological examination of tumor-bearing mice revealed that most of the SC xenografts exhibited noninvasive behavior; however, three nonsmall-cell lung carcinomas (non-SCLC) A549, H460, and H125; one lung adenocarcinoma, H969; and one amelanotic melanoma, LOX, were found to invade and destroy adjacent muscle and metastasize to other soft tissues. Table I summarizes the relevant features and invasive characteristics of these tumors and cell strains.

Four of the five tumors that produced metastatic lesions were from established tumor cell strains. The fifth, H969, was from a pleural effusion of a patient with a lung adenocarcinoma. Although each of the five had distinguishing characteristics, all five metastasized to the lung. Lung lesions were observed within 5 weeks in mice inoculated IP with the four established cell strains (A549, H460, H125, LOX), whereas lung metastasis was seen in the H969 IP-inoculated animals after 22 weeks. In one set of experiments, development of lung

TABLE I. Characteristics of Metastatic Models

Designation cell line/tumor	Original tumor histology	Inoculation routes	In vivo growth*	Characteristics
A549 (cell line)	Bronchioloalveolar carcinoma (adenocarcinoma)	IS IP SC	Liver, lung, spleen, lymph node, metastasis	Alveolar trucking, intrahepatic vessel growth, lymphatic, duct filled
NCI-H125 (cell line)	Adenosquamous carcinoma	SC	Heart, kidney, lung, pancreas, liver, adrenal, spleen, and muscle invasion	Intrahepatic blood vessel invasion, alveolar trucking
NCI-H460 (cell line)	Large-cell carcinoma	IS IP SC	Lung, liver, spleen, gall bladder, kidney metastasis	Poorly differentiated and rapid IP growth
NCI-H969 (malignant effusion)	Adenocarcinoma (pleural effusion)	IP SC	Lung, liver, brain metastasis; ascites	Intrahepatic blood vessel invasion
LOX (cell line)	Amelanotic melanoma	IS IP SC	Heart, lung, pancreas metastasis	Intracapillary transport

*Lung metastases were present after all three routes of inoculation; metastases to and invasion of other organs were present only after IP inoculation.

metastases in A549-inoculated mice appeared to take much longer in SC-inoculated (15 weeks) than in IP-inoculated (3 weeks) animals.

SC Inoculations

For H460, A549, and H125 cell strains, growth at the inoculation site was characterized by invasion of the subcutaneous tissues and body wall. Histologically, each tumor resembled the tumors from which they were originally derived.

IP Inoculations

Each of the cell strains forms solid tumors after IP inoculation. These tumors metastasized to liver (Fig. 1A) and regional lymph nodes (Fig. 1B) and in some cases destroyed the pancreas (Fig. 1C). Each metastatic line invaded abdominal as well as cardiac muscle. IP like SC tumors metastasized to the lung as solid (Fig. 1D) or intravascular (Fig. 1E) lesions. Intrahepatic and lymphatic duct infiltrations were common findings.

Intrasplenic Inoculations

Intrasplenic inoculation of A549, H460, and LOX cell strains yielded results identical to those with IP inoculation. This can be explained in part by leakage of tumor cells back through the inoculation site from the splenic capsule into the peritoneal space.

IP Titrations of Tumor Strains

Titration studies were performed with several of the established tumor strains to determine a usable number of cells, which when inoculated IP would give consistent death patterns within reasonable periods of time for in vivo drug testing (eg, 30–60 days). A linear relationship was seen between survival and the number of cells inoculated for each of the three lines tested (LOX, A549, H460). For example, with H460 cells at a dose of 10^7 cells, nine of ten mice died by day 22; at a dose of 10^6 cells, ten of ten mice died by day 33; at a dose of 10^5, ten of ten mice died by day 78; and at 10^4 cells, eight of ten mice died by day 86. The median survival time for mice inoculated IP with 10^7 H460 cells was 23.1 days. For mice inoculated with 10^7 A549 cells or 10^7 LOX cells, the median survival times were 35.5 and 18.5 days, respectively.

Large-Scale Cell Culture Production

Because these strains grow aggressively in athymic mice, they can be used in survival studies. The ability to grow these cells in vitro in large quantities makes it possible to use cryopreserved tumor cells for direct implantation into experimental animals. Each of these was propagated in roller culture, concentrated, and frozen at $-180°C$. Both A549 and H460 lines produced lethal disease and reproducible death patterns when individual vials containing 1×10^7 cells were shipped frozen to remote screening laboratories, quickly thawed, and inoculated IP into athymic mice (Fig. 2A,B). Histopathological examination of the mice revealed lesions consistent with earlier findings (Table I).

In Vivo Drug Testing

Aggressive growth and reproducible death pattern demonstrated by several of these tumor strains provide suitable models for in vivo drug testing. IP or IV administration of established antitumor drugs, such as melphalan, on days 1, 5, and 9 after IP implantation of 10^6 LOX tumor cells resulted in substantial increases in life span in the group administered melphalan by the IP route, in contrast to administration of the drug by the IV route, which showed prolonged life span only at the 9 mg/kg dose (Fig. 3A,B).

DISCUSSION

Our findings on the incidence of tumor growth and metastasis in nude mice of xenografted fresh human tumors and inoculated human tumor cell strains are similar to previously published findings. In these studies, 58% of the fresh tumor resections or pleural effusions and 100% of establised tumor cell strains grew in the nude mouse host. Sharkey and Fogh [13] reported successful transplantation of human malignant tumors in approximately 50% of all tumors derived from soft tissues, including lung. In their experiments, cultured human tumor cell lines had a successful take rate, approximately twice that observed for tumors derived from surgical specimens. In our studies, one of 36 (2.7%) fresh tumors and four of 15 (27%) of the established tumor cell strains metastasized. In the studies of Sharkey and Fogh [12], growth was observed in 106 tumors implanted in 1,045 mice. However, metastasis was observed in only 14 (1.3%) instances involving 11 different tumor lines. In studying 534 mice grafted with 66 different tumors, Sordat et al [6] found metastasis in only 5.6% of the animals.

Of the surgical specimens that we grew subcutaneously, 13 of 21 (62%) could be passaged sequentially. This was substantially higher than that reported by Fogh et al [14], who accomplished continuous passage of tumors in one-third of the primary transplants. Our higher success rate for growth of fresh tumors and subsequent passage of the primary tumor might be attributable to the relatively young age (4–6 weeks old) and state of health (specific pathogen-free) of the mice used in these studies.

From histological examination of tumor-bearing animals that had been inoculated with the established tumor strains by both IP and SC routes, it was readily apparent that metastasis occurred to a greater extent in the IP-inoculated animals. Similar findings were reported by Kyriazis et al [15]. In their studies, SC-injected tumors developed rapidly at the inoculation site, but the tumor focus was surrounded by a thick fibrous capsule, whereas following IP transplantation tumors spread widely in the peritoneal cavity invading intraabdominal organs and metastasizing to regional lymph nodes and lungs.

In general, the metastatic cell strains that we have isolated displayed an invasive pattern at the SC inoculation site. This characteristic was previously noted [12] as being a marker of more aggressive tumors and can be viewed as an inherent property of the tumor cells of gaining access to blood and/or lymphatic vessels as the first step in the metastatic process [16]. We are now using this marker as a prescreen for tumors and cell lines having metastatic potential.

Over the past 2 years, the National Cancer Institute has switched the emphasis of its drug screening program from a compound-oriented to a disease-oriented approach. The overall strategy in this approach is to provide primary drug screening using panels of human tumor cell strains in vitro. The aim of this screening is to identify compounds that exert selective cytotoxicity and it is hoped selective cytotoxicity toward particular tumor types. As a secondary stage in this testing, it would be highly desirable to perform in vivo testing using one or more of the in vitro-sensitive cell strains. Several of the cell strains described in this report seem to be very well suited to this application and can be manipulated in various ways for in vivo testing. The suitability of some of these for routine assays using a survival end point represents an important advance in drug testing. These assays allow use of an objective end point and require a successful treatment of metastasis in order to produce long-term survivors.

ACKNOWLEDGMENTS

This research was supported through the National Cancer Institute, DHHS, under contract No. N01-23910 with Program Resources, Inc.

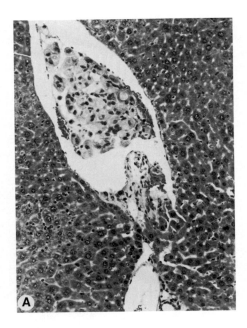

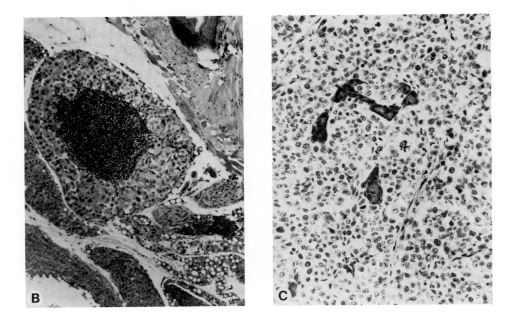

Fig. 1.   IP inoculations of athymic mice with cell strains H460, A549, and H125. Tumor metastases to liver (A), regional lymph nodes (B), and pancreas (C). Tumors metastasized to lung as solid (D) or intravascular (E) lesions. Hematoxylin and eosin stain.

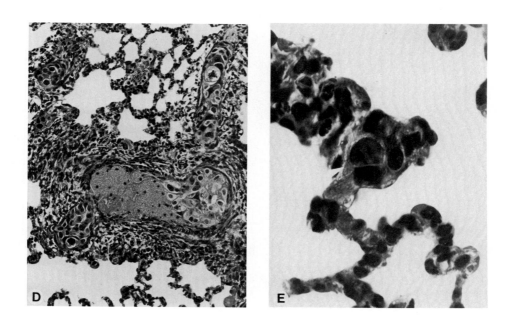

Fig. 1. Continued.

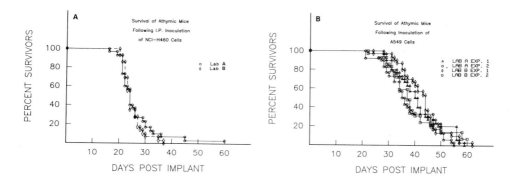

Fig. 2.   Survival experiments.

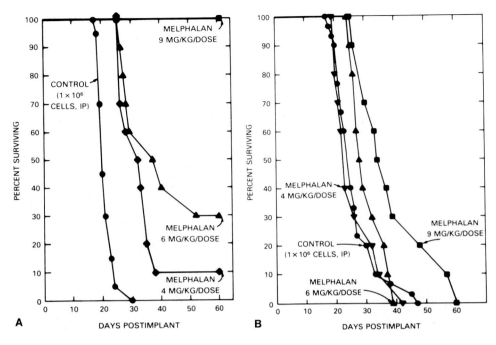

Fig. 3. Response of LOX amelanotic melanoma to IP (A) and IV (B) treatment [Q4d × 3(1)] with melphalan.

REFERENCES

1. Ovejera AA, Houchens DP. Human tumor xenografts in athymic nude mice as a preclinical screen for anticancer agents. Semin Oncol 1981; 8:386–93.
2. Bogden AE, Houchens DP, Ovejera AA, Cobb WR. Advances in chemotherapy studies with the nude mouse. In Fogh J, Giovanilla BC, eds: The nude mouse in experimental and clinical research. New York, Academic Press, Vol 2, 1982; 367–400.
3. Fodstad O, Aamdal S, Pihl A, Boyd M. Activity of mitozolomide (NSC 353451), a new imidazotetrazine, against xenografts from human melanomas, sarcomas, and lung and colon carcinomas. Cancer Res 1985; 45:1778–86.
4. Rygaard J. Mouse models and tumor metastases with special reference to the athymic nude mouse. In Mirand EA, Hutchinson WB, Mihich E, eds: 13th International Cancer Congress, Part C. Biology of cancer (2), New York: Alan R. Liss, Inc, 1983; 37–44.
5. Hanna N. Role of natural killer cells in control of cancer metastasis. Cancer Mestasis Rev 1982; 1:45–65.
6. Sordat BCM, Ueyama Y, Fogh J. Metastasis of tumor xenografts in the nude mouse. In Fogh J, Giovanella BC, eds: The nude mouse in experimental and clinical research. New York: Academic Press, Vol 2, 1982; 95.
7. Hanna N, Fidler IJ. Expression of metastatic potential of allogeneic and xenogeneic neoplasms in young nude mice. Cancer Res 1981; 41:438–44.
8. Sordat B, Bogenmann E. Metastatic behavior of human colon carcinoma in nude mice. In Sparrow S, ed: Immunodeficient animals for cancer research. New York: Macmillian, 1980; 145.
9. Kyriazis AP, DiPersio L, Michael JG, Pesce AJ. Influence of the mouse hepatitis virus (MHV) infection on the growth of human tumors in the athymic mouse. Int J Cancer 1979; 23:402–9.
10. Kyriazis AA, Kyriazis AP. Preferential sites of growth of human tumors in nude mice following subcutaneous transplantation. Cancer Res 1980; 40:4509–11.
11. Ware JL, Lieberman AP, Webb KS, Vollmer RT. Factors influencing phenotypic diversity of human prostate carcinoma cells metastasizing in athymic nude mice. Exp Cell Biol 1985; 53:163–9.

12. Sharkey FE, Fogh J. Metastasis of human tumors in athymic nude mice. Int J Cancer 1979; 24:733–8.
13. Sharkey FE, Fogh J. Considerations in the use of nude mice for cancer research. Cancer Metastasis Rev 1984; 3:341–60.
14. Fogh J, Tiso J, Orfeo T, Sharkey FE, Daniels WP, Fogh JM. Thirty-four lines of six human tumor categories established in nude mice. J Natl Cancer Inst 1980; 64:745–51.
15. Kyriazis AP, DiPersio L, Michael GT, Pesce AJ, Stinnett JD. Growth patterns and metastatic behavior of human tumors growing in athymic mice. Cancer Res 1978; 38:3186–90.
16. Fidler IJ, Gersten DM, Hart IR. The biology of cancer invasion and metastasis. Adv Cancer Res 1978; 28:149–250.

Cancer Detection and Prevention Supplement 1:301–309 (1987)

Effect of Red Ginseng on Natural Killer Cell Activity in Mice With Lung Adenoma Induced by Urethan and Benzo(a)pyrene

Yeon S. Yun, PhD
Hae S. Moon, BS
Yeong R. Oh, BS

Sung K. Jo, BS
Young J. Kim, BS
Taik K. Yun, MD, PhD

Laboratory of Immunology (Y.S.Y., S.K.J., H.S.M.) and Laboratory of Cancer Pathology (Y.J.K., Y.R.O., T.K.Y.), Korea Cancer Center Hospital, Korea Advanced Energy Research Institute, Seoul, Korea

ABSTRACT   It was previously reported that red ginseng extract inhibited carcinogenesis by urethan, DMBA, and aflatoxin B_1 [Yun et al: Cancer Detect Prevent 1983; 6:515–25]. In an attempt to investigate the mechanism of the anticarcinogenic effect of ginseng, the natural killer (NK) activity and the incidence of lung adenoma were followed over a period of 48 weeks postinjection with urethan or benzo(a)pyrene.

The NK activity was markedly depressed from 4 weeks to 24 weeks after injection of carcinogens. This decreased NK activity was returned to the level of controls by administration of ginseng. At the same time, a lower incidence of lung adenoma was noted following administration of ginseng to urethan-injected mice. However, the lung adenoma induced by benzo(a)pyrene began to occur at 48 weeks in which NK activity had naturally declined to a level too low to be affected by ginseng, and administration of ginseng did not decrease the incidence. In conclusion, these results suggest that the anticarcinogenic effect of ginseng may be related to the augmentation of NK activity.

Key words: anticarcinogen, immunomodulator, newborn mice

INTRODUCTION

Ginseng is one of the most popular natural tonics used in oriental countries. Its diverse pharmacological effects on the human body have been the targets of research for many years, and a number of investigators continue to study these effects from various angles. It was suggested that the effect of ginseng might be due to its capacity to increase nonspecific resistance of the organism [1].

The immune system may play an important role in the host-related aspect of resistance to carcinogenesis. In general, there have been numerous indications of increased oncogenesis in immunosuppressed experimental animals and patients. However, there have also been a

---

Address reprint requests to Dr. Yeon S. Yun, Laboratory of Immunology, Korea Cancer Center Hospital, Korea Advanced Energy Research Institute, 215-4, Gongneung-Dong, Dobong-Ku, Seoul, Korea.

number of objections raised against the theory of immune surveillance [2,3]. Most of the apparent contradictions to this theory actually have been related to the postulated central role of T cells in the antitumor defense system [4]. Therefore, increasing attention has been directed toward alternative host defense mechanims, particularly natural antitumor resistance by lymphocytes and macrophages [5–7]. Natural killer (NK) activity appears to be associated with a subpopulation of normal lymphocytes capable of spontaneously lysing certain tumor and normal cell targets [8]. There is now considerable evidence supporting the role of NK cells in in vivo resistance to tumor growth in mice [9–13], and it has been hypothesized that NK activity is a primary mechanism of immune surveillance [8–14]. Although NK activity has been studied extensively in humans and other animals, its regulation is poorly understood. Interferon and substances capable of inducing interferon enhance NK activity [15–17], while a variety of other immunopharmacological agents inhibit NK activity [18–21].

We previously reported that ginseng had anticarcinogenic effects on lung tumors induced by DMBA, urethan, and aflatoxin B_1 [22]. Ginseng extract inhibited the incidence and the proliferation of tumors induced by carcinogens when orally administered in vivo [22]. In addition, urethan and DMBA have been found to depress NK activity strongly during the latent period before tumor development [23,24]. In this regard, it was of interest to determine whether the anticarcinogenic effect of ginseng might be accompanied by resistance to the ability of the agent to depress NK activity. The study reported herein examines the relationship between the effect of ginseng on NK activity and anticarcinogenic resistance.

MATERIALS AND METHODS
Experimental Animals

Noninbred Swiss Webster mice were obtained from NCI (National Cancer Institute [NIH]) and bred at random inter se. All mice were housed in a controlled room with food and water ad libitum. Food was given as solid pellets prescribed by the NIH-7 open formula [25].

Ginseng Extract

Korean red ginseng extract powder, spray-dried, was obtained from the Office of Monopoly (Seoul, Republic of Korea). It was dissolved in tap water at a concentration of 1 mg/ml and administered to mice ad libitum as drinking water from weaning to sacrifice.

Chemical Carcinogens

Newborn mice, less than 24 hr old, were injected subcutaneously in the subscapular region with 0.02 ml of the suspension, containing 1 mg of urethan (Fisher Scientific Co., Fair Lawn, NJ) in 1% aqueous gelatin [26,27]. In the case of benzo(a)pyrene (Sigma Chemical Co., St. Louis, MO), mice were given a single injection with 40 μg in 0.02 ml of 1% aqueous gelatin via the same route as for urethan [28]. The suspension of benzo(a)pyrene was prepared [26] and promptly used after preparation. The weaning rates of mice injected with urethan and benzo(a)pyrene are summarized in Table I. The weaning rates of all experimental groups were above 75% and almost equal.

TABLE I. Weaning Rate in Swiss Webster Mice Treated With Urethan and Benzo(a)pyrene

Treatment of mice	Dose and route	Vehicle	No. of mice	No. of survivors at weaning	%Survivors at weaning
Untreated	—	—	1,880	1,509	80
% Gelatin	0.02 ml × 1, SC	H_2O	889	743	84
Urethan	1 mg/0.02 ml × 1, SC	1% Gelatin	1,883	1,412	75
B(a)P	40 μg/0.02 ml × 1, SC	1% Gelatin	1,757	1,463	83

Controls

There were three controls in this experiment as follows: 1) Untreated control mice were given solid pellets and tap water ad libitum. 2) Ginseng control mice were given solid pellets and the solution of ginseng extract ad libitum as drinking water. 3) Vehicle control mice were injected with 0.02 ml of 1% aqueous gelatin (Difco Lab., Detroit, MI) in the subscapular region within 24 hr after birth.

Naked Eye and Microscopical Examination

Experimental mice were sacrificed at 4, 6, 12, 24, and 48 weeks after birth. Their various organs were examined: lung, heart, salivary gland, liver, thymus, pancreas, spleen, kidney, brain, pituitary gland, testis, and ovary. The organs and tumors were stained by hematoxylin and eosin for microscopical observation. Spleen was used for assay of NK activity.

Preparation of Effector Cells

At different times following carcinogen treatment, 30 mice from every experimental group were sacrificed, and ten spleens were pooled in each petri dish containing 20 ml cold Hank's balanced salt solution (HBSS), obtained from Grand Island Biological Co. (Grand Island, NY) After being washed twice with HBSS, spleen cell suspensions were prepared in cold HBSS by gentle teasing of the organ with forceps and aspirating it through a 10 ml pipette. After allowing the tissue debris to sediment for 5 min at ice-bath, the cell suspensions in HBSS were layered on Ficoll-Hypaque solution (specific gravity 1.078) and centrifuged at 400g for 30 min at 18–20°C. The mononuclear cell band was harvested and washed three times with HBSS. All cells were resuspended to the desired concentration in complete medium: RPMI 1640 medium (Grand Island Biological Co.) supplemented with 10% heat-inactivated fetal bovine serum (Grand Island Biological Co.), 100 units of penicillin, 100 μg of streptomycin, and 2 mM of fresh glutamine [29–31].

Preparation of Target Cells

YAC-1 cell line, a cell line of Moloney virus-induced lymphoma of A/Sn orign, was used for target cells [32]. This cell line was obtained from the Albert Einstein Hospital, and maintained in complete medium. The target cells were labeled by incubating 1×10^7 cells in 1 ml of medium with 100 μCi of $Na_2{}^{51}CrO_4$ (specific activity 283.58 mCi/mg, 1 mCi/ml; New England Nuclear, Boston, MA) in 37°C bath water for 1 hr with occasional shaking. The labeled cells were washed three times with HBSS supplemented with 5% fetal bovine serum (5% FBS-HBSS) and adjusted to the desired concentration (2×10^5 cells/ml).

Assay for Natural Killer (NK) Activity

A 12 hr ^{51}Cr-release assay method was used for NK activity, as described by Nunn and Herberman [33]. The desired concentrations of effector cells were mixed with labeled target cells in 1 ml per culture tube (Falcon, 2058) in triplicate and incubated for 12 hr at 37°C. Most experiments were performed with E:T ratios of 100:1, 50:1, and 25:1. The tubes were centrifuged for 10 min at 500g at 4°C, and 500 μl of the supernatants was collected. Their radioactivities were measured in a well-type γ-counter (Aloka Universal Scaler, Japan).

Calculation of Natural Killer Activity

Spontaneous release (SR) was defined as the counts per minute (cpm) released from targets incubated with medium alone, and maximum release (MR) was determined as the cpm in the supernatants after lysis of the target with 1% Triton X-100. The formula used to calculate the percentage of specific ^{51}Cr-release was

$$\% \text{ specific release} = \frac{\text{cpm experimental} - \text{cpm SR}}{\text{cpm MR} - \text{cpm SR}} \times 100.$$

Throughout the experiments, MR were higher than 95% of total isotope uptake, and SR were less than 10%.

Statistical analysis of each experiment was done with the use of the χ^2 test and the t test for lung adenoma incidence and NK activity, respectively.

RESULTS

Natural killer (NK) activity in the mice was highest at 6 weeks and completely depressed at 48 weeks of age. Its kinetics were similar in all control and experimental groups (Figs. 1, 2). The incidence of tumors occurring in the mice has been carefully followed in controls during the time span of this experiment. Lung adenomas have been found in about 10% of control mice of more than 12 weeks of age but have not been seen prior to this time.

Enhancement of NK activity by ginseng and its correlation with lung adenoma incidence in mice injected with urethan is presented in Table II. Examinations of NK activity of spleen cells of mice in each group at designated time periods following urethan treatment revealed profound and sustained suppression of NK activity in mice treated with urethan only. At 12 weeks following its treatment, NK activity was decreased by half compared to untreated controls. Administration of ginseng to urethan-treated mice resulted in enhancement of NK activity from 4 to 24 weeks. NK activity showed an increase of 18% at 4 weeks, 20% (P < 0.05) at 6 weeks, 29% (P < 0.05) at 12 weeks, and 13% at 24 weeks compared to urethan treatment alone.

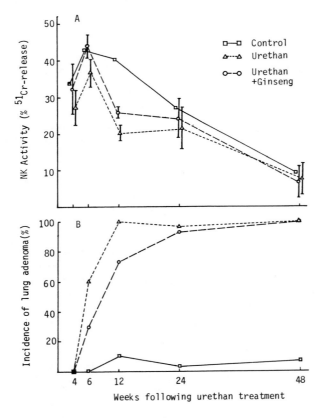

Fig. 1. Enhancement of NK activity by ginseng and its correlation with lung adenoma incidence in mice injected with urethan. Effects of ginseng on NK activity of spleen cells (**A**) and incidence of lung adenoma (**B**) in mice injected with urethan, respectively.

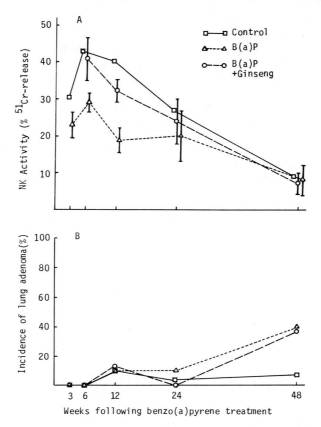

Fig. 2.   Time course of the effect of ginseng on NK activity and lung adenoma incidence in mice injected with benzo(a)pyrene. Effects of ginseng on NK activity of spleen cells (**A**) and incidence of lung adenoma (**B**) in mice injected with benzo(a)pyrene.

TABLE II. Effect of Ginseng on the NK Activity of Spleen Cells in Mice Treated With Urethan

Treatment of mice	No. of mice	NK activity* following weeks of treatment				
		4	6	12	24	48
Untreated	30	33.6 ± 3.8	42.6 ± 0.8	40.1 ± 3.0	27.0 ± 5.7	9.1 ± 5.0
1% Gelatin	30	Not tested	40.1 ± 1.0	35.7 ± 5.5	26.9 ± 8.3	7.8 ± 5.0
Ginseng	30	Not tested	44.5 ± 0.2	41.3 ± 4.6	28.4 ± 6.7	11.2 ± 7.8
Urethan	30	27.3 ± 5.0	36.6 ± 4.0	20.1 ± 2.1†	21.6 ± 5.8	7.5 ± 4.5
Urethan + ginseng	30	32.1 ± 7.2	43.9 ± 3.1‡	25.8 ± 1.3‡	24.3 ± 5.9	6.8 ± 5.0

*Mean ± SD of three pools. Ten spleens of mice were pooled and tested three times. E:T ratio = 25:1. Similar results were obtained with other effector cell:target cell ratios.
†Significantly different (P < 0.05, t test) from untreated group.
‡Significantly different (P < 0.05, t test) from urethan-treated group.

The incidence of lung adenoma was also examined at the same time periods following urethan treatment (Table III). In the urethan-treated group, the lung adenoma was induced in all mice at 12 weeks following urethan treatment. In contrast, it was not until 24 weeks following urethan treatment that lung adenoma was induced in almost all the mice in the combined ginseng and urethan-treated group. The incidence of lung adenoma in the combined ginseng and urethan-treated group showed a significant decrease of 50% (P < 0.05) and 27% (P < 0.05) at 6 and 12 weeks, respectively, following urethan treatment compared to that of the urethan alone-treated group. Thus it appeared that administration of ginseng delayed the occurrence of lung adenoma in urethan-treated mice.

The effects of ginseng on NK activity and lung adenoma incidence in mice treated with benzo(a)pyrene are summarized in Tables IV and V. This experiment was performed to investigate the effects of ginseng on NK activity and the incidence of lung adenoma in mice previously treated with benzo(a)pyrene. The NK activity and incidence of lung adenoma in each group were monitored at designated time intervals following benzo(a)pyrene treatment.

There was a marked reduction of NK activity in benzo(a)pyrene-treated mice as compared to that of untreated mice from 3 to 24 weeks following treatment. Administration of ginseng to benzo(a)pyrene-treated mice resulted in an increase of NK activity by 39% (P < 0.05) at 6 weeks, 69% (P < 0.05) at 12 weeks, and 20% at 24 weeks compared to benzo(a)pyrene treatment alone.

The lung adenoma incidence was less than 10% both in benzo(a)pyrene and combined ginseng with benzo(a)pyrene groups of 24 weeks following benzo(a)pyrene treatment, and the incidence was similar to the spontaneous adenomas in control mice. The lung adenoma induced by benzo(a)pyrene began to occur at 48 weeks at which time NK activity in all experimental mice had naturally declined to a very low level. The incidence of lung adenoma at 48 weeks was 40% in benzo(a)pyrene and 37% in the combined ginseng with benzo(a)pyrene group.

TABLE III. Effect of Ginseng on the Incidence of Lung Adenoma in Mice Treated With Urethan

Treatment of mice	No. of mice	Lung adenoma incidence following weeks of treatment (%)				
		4	6	12	24	48
Untreated	30	0/30 (0)	0/30 (0)	3/30 (10)	1/30 (3)	2/30 (7)
1% Gelatin	30	Not tested	0/30 (0)	3/30 (10)	0/30 (0)	1/30 (3)
Ginseng	30	Not tested	0/30 (0)	1/30 (3)	0/30 (0)	3/30 (10)
Urethan	30	0/30 (0)	18/30 (60)	30/30 (100)	29/30 (97)	30/30 (100)
Urethan + ginseng	30	0/30 (0)	9/30 (30)*	22/30 (73)*	28/30 (93)	30/30 (100)

*Significantly different (P < 0.05, χ^2 test) from urethan-treated group.

TABLE IV. Effect of Ginseng on the NK Activity of Spleen Cells in Mice Treated With Benzo(a)pyrene

Treatment of mice	No. of mice	NK activity* following weeks of treatment				
		3	6	12	24	48
Untreated	30	30.4 ± 10.5	42.6 ± 0.8	40.1 ± 3.0	27.0 ± 5.7	9.1 ± 5.0
1% Gelatin	30	32.9 ± 6.0	40.1 ± 1.0	35.7 ± 5.5	26.9 ± 8.3	7.8 ± 5.0
Ginseng	30	Not tested	44.5 ± 0.2	41.3 ± 4.6	28.4 ± 6.7	11.2 ± 7.8
B(a)P	30	23.2 ± 3.4	29.3 ± 2.4[†]	19.1 ± 3.4[†]	20.3 ± 6.9	8.3 ± 4.3
B(a)P + ginseng	30	Not tested	40.9 ± 5.8[‡]	32.4 ± 3.0[‡]	24.2 ± 6.1	7.4 ± 3.0

*Mean ± SD of three pools. Ten spleens of mice were pooled and tested three times. E:T ratio 25:1. Similar results were obtained with other effector cell:target cell ratios.
†Significantly different (P < 0.05, t test) from untreated group.
‡Significantly different (P < 0.05, t test) from B(a)P-treated group.

TABLE V. Effect of Ginseng on the Incidence of Lung Adenoma in Mice Treated
With Benzo(a)pyrene

Treatment of mice	No. of mice	Lung adenoma incidence following weeks of treatment (%)				
		3	6	12	24	48
Untreated	30	0/30 (0)	0/30 (0)	3/30 (10)	1/30 (3)	2/30 (7)
1% Gelatin	30	0/30 (0)	0/30 (0)	3/30 (10)	0/30 (0)	1/30 (3)
Ginseng	30	Not Tested	0/30 (0)	1/30 (3)	0/30 (0)	3/30 (10)
B(a)P	30	0/30 (0)	0/30 (0)	3/30 (10)	3/30 (10)	12/30 (40)*
B(a)P + ginseng	30	Not tested	0/30 (0)	4/30 (13)	0/30 (0)	11/30 (37)

*Significantly different (P < 0.05, χ^2 test) from untreated group.

DISCUSSION

The results of the present study indicate for the first time that the long-term oral administration of red ginseng extract augments NK activity and, furthermore, that the augmentation correlates with its anticarcinogenic effect in urethan-treated mice. In keeping with reports by others [34] suppression of NK activity by urethan was also detected in the mice (Fig. 1). At 4 weeks following urethan treatment, NK activity decreased by 18% and returned to the level of the untreated control group after red ginseng oral administration prior to appearance of lung adenomas. Administration of ginseng to urethan-treated mice resulted in a significant increase of NK activity as well as in a significant inhibition of the incidence of lung adenomas at 6 and 12 weeks following urethan treatment (Tables II and III). These results indicate a positive correlation between augmentation of NK activity and inhibition of urethan-induced lung carcinogenesis by ginseng and support the hypothesis that NK cells play a role in resistance to urethan-induced lung carcinogenesis [34].

On the other hand, the experimental finding that the administration of ginseng augmented NK activity but did not decrease the incidence of lung adenoma in benzo(a)pyrene-treated mice might be due to the long latent period of carcinogenesis by benzo(a)pyrene. Benzo(a)pyrene significantly decreased NK activity from 6 to 24 weeks following its treatment compared to the untreated groups (Fig. 2). The decreased NK activity was almost recovered by ginseng administration. The NK activity in the mice was highest from 6 to 12 weeks after birth, and, furthermore, the administration of ginseng markedly enhanced the NK activity at that time in benzo(a)pyrene-treated mice. However, the lung adenoma induced by benzo(a)pyrene began to occur at 48 weeks after birth when the NK activity had naturally declined in all experimental mice to a level too low to be affected by ginseng. Benzo(a)pyrene is found in tobacco smoke and the urban atmosphere [35,36]. The increasing sociological impact of environmental carcinogens is most clearly revealed in international epidemiological studies. It appears that the majority of cancers are initiated by external agents. Therefore, the enhancing effect of ginseng on the benzo(a)pyrene-suppressed NK activity might be of some practical benefit for the prevention of carcinogenesis by other agents.

In conclusion, the results support the idea that the anticarcinogenic effect of ginseng in mice treated with urethan may be related, at least in part, to its ability to enhance the NK activity of the host.

REFERENCES

1. Brekhman II, Dardymov IV. New substance of plant origin which increase non-specific resistance. Annu Rev Pharmacol 1969; 9:419–26.
2. Prehn RT. Immunosurveillance, regeneration and oncogenesis. Progr Exp Tumor Res 1971; 14:1–24.
3. Stutman O. Immunodepression and malignancy. Adv Cancer Res 1975;22:261–422.
4. Burnet FM. The concept of immunological surveillance. Progr Exp Tumor Res 1970; 13:1–27.

5. Herberman RB, Holden HT. Natural cell-mediated immunity. Adv Cancer Res 1978; 27:305–77.
6. Kiessling R, Wigzell H. An analysis of the murine NK cell as to structure, function and biological relevance. Immunol Rev 1979; 44:165–208.
7. Keller R. Regulatory capacities of mononuclear phagocytes with particular reference to natural immunity against tumors. In Herberman RB, ed: Natural cell-mediated immunity against tumors. New York: Academic Press, 1980:1219–69.
8. Herberman RB. Natural killer (NK) cells. Progr Clin Biol Res 1981; 58:33–43.
9. Hanna N, Burton RC. Definitive evidence that natural killer (NK) cells inhibit experimental tumor metastasis in vivo. J Immunol 1981; 127:1754–8.
10. Pollack SB, Hallenbeck LA. In vivo reduction of NK activity with anti-NK 1 serum: Direct evaluation of NK cells in tumor clearance. Int J Cancer 1982; 29:203–7.
11. Riesenfeld I, Örn A, Gidlund M, Axberg I, Alm GV, Wigzell H. Positive correlation between in vitro NK activity and in vivo resistance toward AKR lymphoma cells. Int J Cancer 1980; 25:399–403.
12. Talmadge JE, Meyers KM, Prieur DJ, Starkey JR. Role of natural killer cells in tumor growth and metastasis: C57BL/6 normal and beige mice. JNCI 1980; 65:929–35.
13. Talmadge JE, Meyers KM, Prieur DJ, Starkey JR. Role of NK cells in tumor growth and metastasis in beige mice. Nature (Lond) 1980; 284:622–4.
14. Herberman RB, Ortaldo JR. Natural killer cells: Their role in defenses against disease. Science 1981; 214:24–30.
15. Gidlund M, Örn A, Wigzell H, Senik A, Gresser I. Enhanced NK cell activity in mice injected with interferon and interferon inducers. Nature 1978; 273:759–61.
16. Lee, SH, Kelley S, Chiu H, Stebbing N. Stimulation of natural killer activity and inhibition of proliferation of various leukemic cells by purified human leukocyte interferon subtypes. Cancer Res 1982; 42:1312–6.
17. Timonen T, Ortaldo JR, Herberman RB. Analysis by a single cell cytotoxicity assay of natural killer (NK) cell frequencies among human large granular lymphocytes and of the effects of interferon on their activity. J Immunol 1982; 82:2514–21.
18. Djeu JY, Heinbaugh JA, Vieira WD, Holden HT, Herberman RB. The effect of immunopharmacological agents on mouse natural cell-mediated cytoxocity and on its augmentation by poly I.C. Immunopharmacology 1979; 1:231–44.
19. Hochman PS, Cudkowicz G. Suppression of natural cytotoxicity by spleen cells of hydrocortison-treated mice. J Immunol 1979; 123:968–76.
20. Introna M, Allavena P, Spreafico F, Mantovani A. Inhibition of human natural killer activity by cyclosporin A. Transplantation (Baltimore) 1981; 31:113–6.
21. Oehler JR, Herberman RB. Natural cell-mediated cytotoxicity in rats. III. Effects of immunopharmacologic treatments on natural reactivity and on reactivity augmented by polyinosinic-polycytidylic acid. Int J Cancer 1978; 21:221–9.
22. Yun TK, Yun YS, Han IW. Anticarcinogenic effect of long-term oral administration of red ginseng on newborn mice exposed to various chemical carcinogens. Cancer Detect Prevent 1983; 6:515–25.
23. Ehrlich R, Efrati M, Bar-Eyal A, et al. Natural cellular reactivities mediated by splenocytes from mice bearing three types of primary tumor. Int J Cancer 1980; 26:315–23.
24. Gorelik E, Herberman RB. Inhibition of the activity of mouse natural killer cells by urethan. JNCI 1981; 66:543–7.
25. Anonymous. Report of the American Institute of Nutrition Ad Hoc Committee on Standards for Nutritional Studies. J Nutr 1977; 107:1340–8.
26. Pietra G, Spencer K, Shubik P. Response of newly born mice to chemical carcinogen. Nature 1959; 183:1689.
27. Brenblum I, Haran GN. The initiating action of ethyl carbamate (urethan) on mouse skin. Br J Cancer 1965; 9:453–6.
28. Pietra G, Rappaport H, Shubik P. The effect of carcinogenic chemicals in newborn mice. Cancer 1961; 14:308–17.
29. Böyum A. Isolation of mononuclear cells and granulocytes from human blood. Scand J Clin Lab Invest 1968; 21(Suppl 97):77–89.
30. Dutton RW. Further studies of the stimulation of DNA synthesis in cultures of spleen cell suspension by homologous cells in inbred strains of mice and rats. J Exp Med 1965; 122:759–63.
31. Heumer RP, Keller LS, Lee KD. Thymidine incorporation in mixed cultures in spleen cells from mice of differing H-2 types. Transplantation 1968; 6:706–10.

32. Kiessling R, Klein E, Wigzell H. Natural killer cells in mouse. I. Cytotoxic cells with specificity for mouse Molony leukemia cells. Specificity and distribution according to genotype. Eur J Immunol 1975; 5:112–7.

33. Nunn ME, Herberman RB. Natural cytotoxicity of mouse, rat, and human lymphocytes against heterologous target cells. JNCI 1979; 62:765–71.

34. Gorelik E, Herberman RB. Susceptibility of various strains of mice to urethan-induced lung tumors and depressed natural killer cell activity. JNCI 1981; 67:1317–22.

35. Harris CC. Cause and prevention of lung cancer. Semin Oncol 1974; 1:163–6.

36. Menck HR, Casagrande JT, Henderson BE. Industrial air pollution: Possible effect on lung cancer. Science 1974; 183:210–2.

Cancer Detection and Prevention Supplement 1:311–316 (1987)

DNA Methylating Activity in Murine Lymphoma Cells Treated With Xenogenizing Chemicals

P. Puccetti, MD, PhD L. Romani, MD, PhD
M. Allegrucci, PhD P. Dominici, PhD
C. Borri Voltattorni, PhD M.C. Fioretti, PhD

*Institutes of Pharmacology (P.P., L.R., M.A., M.C.F.) and Biochemistry
(P.D., C.B.V.), University of Perugia, Perugia, Italy*

ABSTRACT We investigated whether epigenetic rather than mutational events might be involved in the induction of immunogenicity by the triazene derivative 1-(p-chlorophenyl)-3,3-dimethyltriazene (DM-Cl). To this purpose, we assessed the DNA methylation pattern of murine lymphoma cells xenogenized by DM-Cl and compared it with the changes induced by the DNA hypomethylating agent 5-azacytidine (5-Aza), which is also capable of affecting tumor cell immunogenicity. Both agents were found to increase the immunogenic potential of the treated tumor but according to different modalities. In particular, the novel immunogenicity conferred by 5-Aza treatment correlated well with the extent of hypomethylation induced, as opposed to what was observed for tumor xenogenization by DM-Cl.

Key words: DNA methylation, murine lymphomas, chemical xenogenization

INTRODUCTION

Immunogenic variants of animal tumor have been successfully employed in experimental models of tumor immunotherapy; they often possess the ability to induce strong immunity against the original poorly immunogenic neoplasms. Such nontumorigenic variants, which grow and regress in immunologically intact hosts, may either preexist in the parental tumor—and thus be selected by cloning [1]—or appear at very high frequencies following treatment of tumor cells by mutagens [2,3]. This latter phenomenon is generally referred to as *chemical xenogenization* [4].

Two major classes of mutagenic compounds have been used in the past to effect xenogenization of tumor cells, namely, triazene and nitrosoguanidine derivatives [5]. Recently, immunogenic variants of tumors were also reported to occur following treatment of tumor cells with the DNA hypomethylating agent and gene activator 5-azacytidine (5-Aza) [6]. Based on the observation that 5-Aza is a very strong hypomethylating agent but lacks mutagenic activity in eukaryotic cells, it has been hypothesized that DNA hypomethylation is a common

Address reprint requests to P. Puccetti, Institute of Pharmacology, University of Perugia, Via del Giochetto, I-06100 Perugia, Italy.

mechanism through which xenogenizing compounds affect the immunogenic potential of tumor cells [6,7].

In the present study, we comparatively analyzed the induction of tumor immunogenicity by 5-Aza and a triazene derivative as we assessed the DNA methylation patterns of the tumor cells undergoing xenogenization. Although both the induction and reversion of a weak immunogenicity by 5-Aza correlated well with the levels of DNA methylation, the appearance of a stable, highly immunogenic phenotype in the cells treated with the triazene derivative was found to be independent of DNA methylating activity.

MATERIALS AND METHODS
Mice

Hybrid (BALB/c Cr $\times$ DBA/2 Cr)F1 (CD2F1) male mice (H-2^d/H-2^d) were obtained from the Mammalian Genetics and Animal Production Section, Division of Cancer Treatment, National Cancer Institute (NCI), National Institutes of Health (NIH) (Bethesda, MD).

Drugs

5-Aza was purchased from Sigma Chemical Co. (St. Louis, MO). 1-(p-Chlorophenyl)-3,3-dimethyltriazene (DM-Cl) was obtained according to a previously described procedure [8]. N,N-bis(2-chloroethyl)-N-nitroso-urea (BCNU) was obtained from the Drug Synthesis and Chemistry Branch, Divison of Cancer Treatment, NCI, NIH.

Tumor

In vivo L1210Ha, an ascitic leukemia of DBA/2 origin, was maintained in histocompatible CD2F1 mice by serial IP transplantation of neoplastic cells suspended in 0.2 ml medium 199.

Treatment of Cells With 5-Aza and Establishment of an L1210Ha/5-Aza Line

L1210Ha cells ex vivo (TG 0) were treated in vitro for 24 hr at 37°C in a 5% CO_2 atmosphere with 3 μM 5-Aza at a concentration of 1 $\times$ 10^6/ml RPMI medium containing 10% fetal calf serum. At the end of the incubation, the cells were extensively washed and injected IP into mice (10^5/mouse; TG 1). This procedure was repeated up to TG 10.

Treatment of Cells With DM-Cl and Establishment of an L1210Ha/DM-Cl Line

The experimental procedure for obtaining an L1210Ha/DM-Cl line was similar to that described for the 5-Aza-treated tumor, with the major exception that the incubation of tumor cells with DM-Cl was carried out for 1 hr and required the presence of a mouse liver preparation for metabolic activation of the drug. The entire procedure for obtaining in vitro xenogenization of leukemic cells by triazene derivatives has been previously described [9].

Immunogenicity Test

According to this procedure [10], tumor cells to be assayed for immunogenicity were injected (IP, 10^5/mouse) in four groups of histocompatible mice as follows: 1) intact recipients; 2) intact recipients further treated with BCNU, 10 mg/kg, IP, 3 days after tumor challenge; 3) immunodepressed recipients (400 R, 1 hr before tumor inoculation); and 4) immunodepressed recipients treated with BCNU. The degree of immunogenicity was quantitated by analyzing the mortality parameters of intact vs immunodepressed hosts treated or not with chemotherapy.

Evaluation of DNA 5-Methylcytosine Content by High-Performance Liquid Chromatography (HPLC)

The HPLC method used to quantitate 5-methylcytosine was based on that described by Flateau et al [11]. Cells were labeled with (6-^{3}H)-uridine by incubating 2 $\times$ 10^5 cells/ml with

2 μCi/ml uridine. A Beckman HPLC system with an Altex Ultrasil-CX column was used with isocratic elution using 0.035 M KH_2PO_4, pH 2.5, containing 5% vol/vol MeOH at a flow rate of 2.5 ml/min. The elution of the bases was measured using known standards. The fractions containing the cytosine (C) and 5-methylcytosine (MC) were assayed for radioactivity by scintillation counting. Percentage MC was calculated as follows: %MC = cpm(MC)/cpm(C) + cpm(MC) $\times$ 100%.

RESULTS

In a first series of experiments, we investigated whether exposure of L1210 tumor cells to 5-Aza would result in immunogenic changes that could be detected in the "immunogenicity test" routinely used in our laboratory to monitor the changes induced by triazene derivatives. To this purpose, the leukemic cells were treated in vitro with 5-Aza over the course of ten transplant generations (TG) according to the scheme illustrated in Materials and Methods. At each TG, the degree of immunogenicity was tested by recovering the leukemic cells from the tumor-bearing hosts and injecting them into intact or immunodepressed animals treated or not with cytoreductive chemotherapy (for details, see Immunogenicity Test). Figure 1 shows the results. It is apparent that treatment of tumor cells with 5-Aza failed to result in immunogenic changes that could per se modify the mortality parameters of tumor-bearing mice not subject to chemotherapy. However, if BCNU was administered to intact hosts challenged with the 5-Aza-treated tumor, there was an increase in MST proportial to the number of tumor treatments with 5-Aza. In particular, at TG 7, the synergistic effects of chemotherapy and host immune responses resulted in survival of the challenged mice, the MST exceeding the 60 day observation period. No such effects were observed in tumor-bearing mice treated with BCNU but previously immunodepressed by radiation.

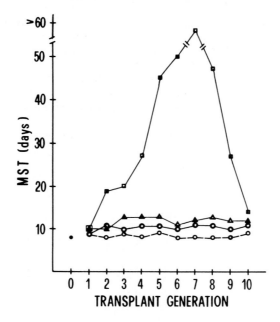

Fig. 1. Median survival time of CD2F1 mice inoculated with L1210Ha/5-Aza cells at different TGs. Cells to be assayed for immunogenicity were recovered 7–8 days after in vitro treatment with 5-Aza and transplantation. Recipient mice were as follows: ○—○, intact; ○---○, irradiated; □—□, intact treated with BCNU; △—△, irradiated treated with BCNU. ●, Control mice receiving nonxenogenized tumor cells.

At each TG, a portion of the cells recovered to be assayed for immunogenicity as analyzed for their content of 5-methylcytosine. Table I illustrates the results. It appears that the development of a 5-Aza-treated tumor subline was accompanied by a progressive decrease in DNA methylating activity, with a negative peak at TG 7 (85.3% of control). However, starting from this TG, a reversion of the pattern was observed so that, at TG 10, the 5-methylcytosine content was 96.9% of control.

An experimental design similar to the one described for 5-Aza was used to evaluate the effects of the triazene derivative DM-Cl. L1210Ha leukemic cells were treated with DM-Cl for ten TG, each in vitro drug exposure preceding the serial transplantation of the tumor. Figure 2 shows that, as early as TG 2, the increase in immunogenicity was so marked as to result, by itself, in survival of the tumor-challenged mice with no need for the synergistic effects of cytoreductive chemotherapy. Once again, the beneficial effects of xenogenization were lost in irradiated mice. When the analysis of 5-methylcytosine pattern was extended to the cells undergoing treatment with DM-Cl, no evidence could be found for any impairment of DNA methylating activity (Table II).

DISCUSSION

The availability of strongly immunogenic variants of feebly immunogenic tumors has opened up new perspectives in experimental studies of tumor immunotherapy [12], and particularly encouraging results have been obtained with chemical xenogenization of murine lymphoma cells [4,5]. Most xenogenizing chemicals are endowed with potent mutagenic activity, which makes it conceivable that the mechanism(s) of action of these compounds involves somatic mutation of tumor cells [5,13]. Frost et al [6] have reported the occurrence of highly immunogenic tumor variants following treatment of mouse cell lines with the poorly mutagenic cytidine analog 5-azacytidine, a strong DNA hypomethylating agent. This finding has led to the proposal that a common mechanism of induction of immunogenicity might be transcriptional activation of previously "silent" genes due to DNA hypomethylation. Such a proposed mechanism, epigenetic in nature, has recently found additional support in studies by other groups [7,14]. In the present investigation, we addressed the problem of the methylation pattern in murine lymphoma cells xenogenized by DM-Cl according to a repeated mutagenesis protocol that has long been used in our laboratory to study the effects of most triazene derivatives. At the same time, we evaluated the impact of repeated exposure of tumor cells to 5-Aza on both tumor immunogenicity and DNA methylation. We thus developed two L1210Ha

TABLE I. Quantitation of DNA 5-Methylcytosine Content by HPLC in L1210Ha/5-Aza Cells*

L1210Ha (TG)	5-Methylcytosine (%)	Percent of control
0	4.22 ± 0.05	—
1	4.24 ± 0.16	100.4
2	3.89 ± 0.15	92.7
3	3.86 ± 0.02	91.4
4	3.93 ± 0.01	93.1
5	3.90 ± 0.01	92.4
6	3.66 ± 0.03	86.7
7	3.60 ± 0.07	85.3
8	3.72 ± 0.15	88.7
9	3.82 ± 0.17	90.5
10	4.09 ± 0.08	96.9

*At each transplant generation, cells were recovered to be labeled with (6-^{3}H)-uridine 7–8 days after in vitro treatment with 5-Aza and transplantation. Results are ± SE from three to five separate determinations.

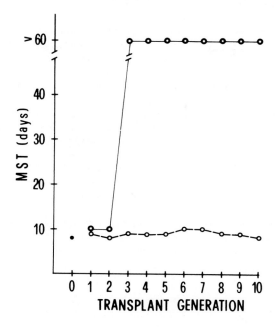

Fig. 2.   Median survival time of CD2F1 mice inoculated with L1210Ha/DM-Cl cells at different TGs. Cells to be assayed for immunogenicity were recovered 7–8 days after in vitro treatment with DM-Cl and transplantation. Recipient mice were as follows: ○—○, intact; ○- - -○, irradiated. ●, Control mice receiving nonxenogenized tumor cells.

TABLE II. Quantitation of DNA 5-Methylcytosine Content by HPLC in L1210Ha/DM-Cl Cells*

L1210Ha (TG)	5-Methylcytosine (%)	Percent of control
0	4.22 ± 0.05	—
1	4.49 ± 0.17	106.3
2	4.45 ± 0.12	105.4
3	4.41 ± 0.11	104.5
4	4.32 ± 0.01	102.3
5	4.32 ± 0.05	102.3
6	4.24 ± 0.05	100.4
7	4.37 ± 0.12	103.5
8	4.35 ± 0.04	103.8
9	4.32 ± 0.05	102.3
10	4.37 ± 0.01	103.5

*At each transplant generation, cells were recovered to be labeled with $(6-^3H)$-uridine 7–8 days after in vitro treatment with DM-Cl and transplantation. Results are ± SE from three to five separate determinations.

tumor sublines, namely L1210Ha/5-Aza and L1210Ha/DM-Cl. The two sublines showed different characteristics with respect to both induction of immunogenicity and DNA methylation pattern. In the L1210Ha/5-Aza tumor, the newly acquired immunogenic strength never reached the levels typical of the DM-Cl line, and the appearance of the immunogenic phenotype was soon followed by reversal of the phenomenon. Interestingly, there was a close correlation between the degree of immunogenicity and the extent of hypomethylation induced by treatment with 5-Aza. Thus, in particular, at TG 7—a time when the 5-methylcytosine value was 85.3% of control—the combined effects of host antitumor response and cytoreductive chemotherapy resulted in survival of the animals challenged with the L1210Ha/5-Aza tumor cells. In contrast, treatment of leukemic cells with DM-Cl was accompanied by early appearance of high levels of immunogenicity so that L1210Ha/DM-Cl TG2 cells were rejected by intact recipient mice even in the absence of BCNU chemotherapy. Furthermore, the DM-Cl line remained immunogenic over the course of the subsequent transplant generations. When the cells were assayed for 5-methylcytosine content, no evidence could be found for a decreased DNA methylating activity. In fact, a limited but consistent hypermethylation was disclosed for the tumor cells at all tested TGs. In conclusion, the studies summarized in the present report show that DNA hypomethylation is not associated with xenogenization of tumor cells by the triazene derivative DM-Cl, as opposed to that observed with the immunogenic changes induced by 5-Aza. Further studies will be needed to elucidate better the nature of the mechanism(s) involved in xenogenization of tumor cells.

ACKNOWLEDGMENTS

This study was supported by CNR-Rome, Italy, Grant No. 84.00577.44 of Special Project "Oncology."

REFERENCES

1. Kreider JW, Bartlett GL. Increased immunogenicity of a spontaneous variant clone of the 13762A rat mammary adenocarcinoma. JNCI 1985; 75:141–6.
2. Bonmassar E, Bonmassar A, Vadlamudi S, Goldin A. Changes of L1210 leukemia in mice treated with 5-(3-3'-dimethyl-1-triazeno) imidazole-4-carboxamide. Cancer Res 1972; 32:1446–50.
3. Boon T, Kellerman O. Rejection by syngeneic mice of cell variants obtained by mutagenesis of a malignant teratocarcinoma line. Proc Natl Acad Sci USA 1977; 74:272–5.
4. Puccetti P, Romani L, Fioretti MC. Chemical xenogenization of tumor cells. Trends Pharmacol Sci 1985; 6:485–7.
5. Boon T. Antigenic tumor cell variants obtained with mutagens. Adv Cancer Res 1983; 39:121–51.
6. Frost P, Liteplo RG, Donaghue TP, Kerbel RS. Selection of strongly immunogenic "tum⁻" variants from tumors at high frequency using 5-Azacytidine. J Exp Med 1984; 159:1491–501.
7. Altevogt P, von Hoegen P, Leidig S, Schirrmacher V. Effects of mutagens on the immunogenicity of murine tumor cells: immunological and biochemical evidence for altered cell surface antigens. Cancer Res 1985; 45:4270–7.
8. Johnson AW. Synthesis of 2-arylfurans. J Chem Soc 1946; 895.
9. Nardelli B, Contessa AR, Romani L, Sava G, Nisi C, Fioretti MC. Immunogenic changes of murine lymphoma cells following in vitro treatment with aryl-triazene derivatives. Cancer Immunol Immunother 1984; 16:157–61.
10. Riccardi C, Bartocci A, Puccetti P, Spreafico F, Bonmassar E, Goldin A. Combined effects of antineoplastic agents and anti-lymphoma allograft reactions. Eur J Cancer 1979; 16:23–33.
11. Flateau E, Bogenmann E, Jones PA. Variable 5-methylcytosine levels in human tumor cell lines and fresh pediatric tumor explants. Cancer Res 1983; 43:4901–5.
12. Giampietri A, Bonmassar A, Puccetti P, Circolo A, Goldin A, Bonmassar E. Drug-mediated increase of tumor immunogenicity in vivo for a new approach to experimental cancer immunotherapy. Cancer Res 1981; 41:681–7.
13. Giampietri A, Fioretti MC, Goldin A, Bonmassar E. Drug-mediated antigenic changes in murine leukemia cells: Antagonistic effects of Quinacrine, an antimutagenic compounds. J Natl Cancer Inst 1980; 64:297–301.
14. Carlow DA, Kerbel RS, Feltis JT, Elliot BE. Enchanced expression of class I major histocompatibility complex gene (D^k) products on immunogenic variants of a spontaneous murine carcinoma. JNCI 1985; 75:291–301.

Cancer Detection and Prevention Supplement 1:317–328 (1987)

Cell Regulatory and Immunorestorative Activity of Picibanil (OK432)

Michael A. Chirigos, PhD, DSc
Tohru Saito, MD
James E. Talmadge, PhD
Wladyslaw Budzynski, MD
Eilene Gruys, BS

Immunopharmacology Section, Biological Therapeutics Branch, Biological Response Modifiers Program, Division of Cancer Treatment (M.A.C.,T.S., E.G., W.B.) and Preclinical Screening Laboratory, Program Resources, Inc. (J.E.T.), National Cancer Institute, NIH, Frederick Cancer Research Facility, Frederick, MD

ABSTRACT   Picibanil (OK432), a pharmaceutical preparation of a low virulent Su strain of *Streptococcus pyogenes*, possesses cell regulatory activity particularly in its ability to augment natural killer (NK) cell activity and to activate macrophages to exert a tumoricidal effect both in vitro and in vivo. It is effective in retarding and/or inhibiting the growth of three different tumors: MBL-2 lymphoma, M109 alveolar adenocarcinoma, and B16 melanoma. The antitumor effect is mediated through regulation of NK cells and macrophages, possibly by its ability to stimulate the production and secretion of interferon and interleukin 1 and 2. It is a very effective adjuvant for tumor cell vaccines that elicit cytotoxic T-cell responses. Following cytoreductive chemotherapy (Cytoxan) Picibanil treatment leads to an earlier reconstitution of both bone marrow cellularity and differentiation to granulocyte-macrophage colonies.

Key words: antitumor, NK augmentation, macrophage, bone marrow, GM-CFU-C

INTRODUCTION

Picibanil (OK432), a pharmaceutical preparation of a low virulent Su strain of *Streptococcus pyogenes* developed in Japan [1], has been reported to possess immunomodulatory activity in preclinical [2,3] and clinical [4] studies. We examined Picibanil in several in vitro and in vivo assays to test its effect on cellular effector cells (natural killer cells [NK] and

Dr. Michael A. Chirigos is now at USAMRIID, Fort Detrick, Frederick, MD 21701. Address reprint requests there.

macrophages [Mϕ]) against various tumor target cells and its capacity to increase bone marrow cellularity and granulocyte-monocyte-colony–forming units (GM-CFU-C). In addition, we evaluated its antitumor activity against three different tumors.

MATERIALS AND METHODS
Mice

Male BALB/c and female C57BL/6 mice were obtained from the Mammalian Genetics and Animal Production Section, Division of Cancer Treatment, National Cancer Institute—Frederick Cancer Research Facility, NIH (Frederick, MD). The animals were 6 to 8 weeks of age when used for experiments.

Biological Response Modifiers

Polyinosinic-polycytidylic acid poly-L-lysine (poly ICLC) was supplied by Dr. Hilton B. Levy (National Institute of Allergy and Infectious Diseases, National Institutes of Health, Bethesda, MD). Cyclophosphamide (Cytoxan [CY]) was obtained from the Division of Cancer Treatment, NCI (Bethesda, MD). Picibanil (OK432) was a generous gift of Dr. H. Nakano, Chugai Pharmaceuticals (Tokyo, Japan). Granulocyte macrophage–colony-stimulating factor (GM-CSF) preparations used were generated by injecting BALB/c mice with 5 μg/mouse of lipopolysaccharide (LPS). Sera and lung conditioned media from these mice were then subjected to concentration and ultrafiltration using Diaflo ultrafilters [5]. The molecular weight of the GM-CSF preparations used ranged between 15 and 35 Kd. Lipopolysaccharide from *Salmonella typhimurium* (LPS) was purchased from Difco Laboratories (Detroit, MI). The media and biological response modifier (BRM) preparations were tested for endotoxin contamination with the Limulus lysate assay and found to contain less than 0.125 ng/ml.

Tumor Cells

The tissue culture cell line of YAC-1, a Moloney virus-induced lymphoma of A/Sn origin, was used as the target for NK activity. MBL-2, a lymphoblastic leukemia cell line derived from C57BL/6, was used as the target for macrophage cytotoxic activity. Cell lines were maintained in tissue culture in RPMI 1640 supplemented with L-glutamine (Grand Island Biological Co., Grand Island, NY), 125 μg/ml of gentamycin (Microbiological Associates, Bethesda, MD), and 10% fetal bovine serum (Associated Biomedic Systems, Buffalo, NY).

Assays

Macrophage-mediated cytotoxicity. The assay for measuring the ability of BRMs to induce macrophage-mediated cytotoxicity against the MBL-2 cell line has been described previously [6].

Natural killer cells. A conventional ^{51}Cr-release assay was employed as previously described [7].

Bone marrow cells. Sterile single cell suspensions from femoral bone marrow were prepared as previously described [8]. The total number of viable nucleated cells per femur was counted for each mouse by hemocytometer. Morphological characterization of the bone marrow cells was done by Giemsa and esterase staining. To determine the number of granulo-cyte-Mϕ–committed stem cells (GM-CFU-C), a previously described in vitro soft agar culture technique was used [9]. Briefly, 10^5 unfractionated bone marrow cells were suspended in 2 ml of 0.3% agar, supplemented with 15% horse serum (Gibco), 15% fetal calf serum (Gibco), 292 μg/ml L-glutamine (Gibco), and 100 μg/ml of gentamycin/ml (Sigma, St. Louis, MD), and were plated in 35 mm Petri dishes (Falcon, Oxnard, CA). As CSF source, 0.2 ml of the described preparation was used. The cultures were incubated at 37°C in a fully humidified atmosphere of 70% CO_2 in air. Colonies (>40 cells) were scored and classified on the basis of their morphology at days 7 and 10 of the culture period.

Other in vitro T-cell functions and tumor assays employed have been adequately described [10,11].

RESULTS

Various concentrations of Picibanil were tested for their in vitro capacity to augment splenic NK cell cytotoxicity (Fig. 1). Significant augmentation of NK cytotoxicity occurred with 0.001 μg/ml, with peak activity occurring with 1 μg/ml and declining with higher concentrations. The response to 1 μg/ml approached that achieved with γIFN or poly I:C. Picibanil was tested for its capacity to activate Mϕ directly in vitro to exert tumoricidal activity on P815 radiolabeled target cells (Fig. 2). Levels of Picibanil beginning with 1 μg/ml directly activated Mϕ. Peak activation was attained with 50 μg/ml and was similar to the Mϕ activation achieved by two other known Mϕ activators, poly ICLC and lipopolysaccharide (LPS).

Different responses in augmentation of NK cells and Mϕ activity were seen depending on the route by which Picibanil was administered (Table I). A significant increase in NK cell and Mϕ activity occurred only in the peritoneal exudate cells (PEC) when the intraperitoneal (ip) route was used. This increased activity correlated with the increased number of peritoneal cells and percentage of Mϕ contained. Following intravenous (iv) injection augmented NK activity in the spleen and peritoneal blood correlated with an increase in the number of splenic monocytes. A significant increase in Mϕ activity was also achieved, with correlated with an increased number of PEC and percentage of Mϕ. Treatment by the intramuscular (im) or oral route did not lead to any response of NK cell or Mϕ activity or any increase in numbers of splenic monocytes or PEC.

We further examined the duration of time that NK cell activity and Mϕ activity remained elevated following one ip injection of Picibanil (Table II). As previously observed, ip inoculation of Picibanil did not lead to any significant splenic NK activity or increase in splenic monocytes. NK cell activity of PEC, however, was significantly elevated within 24 hr and remained elevated for the 8 day observation period, reaching the peak of activity on the third day following treatment. The number of PEC and the percentage of Mϕ within the PEC also were significantly increased and remained elevated during the 8 day period. Mϕ from the PEC exhibited significant tumoricidal activity within 24 hr, reaching maximum activity by day 3.

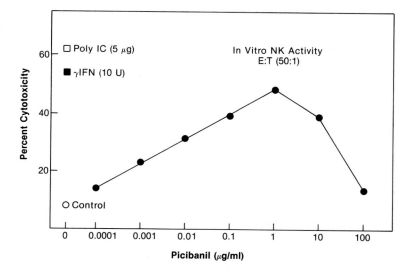

Fig. 1. NK cell activity after various doses of Picibanil in vitro. Spleens from normal C3H mice were titrated and prepared as a single cell suspension and incubated in the presence of increasing concentrations of Picibanil or polyinosinic-polycytidylic acid (poly IC) or murine γ-interferon (γIFN) for 20 hr at 37°C in a humidified 5% CO_2-in-air incubator. The cells were washed free of drugs and an effector (spleen cells) to target cell (YAC) ratio of 50:1 incubated after 4 hr was used to measure cytotoxicity.

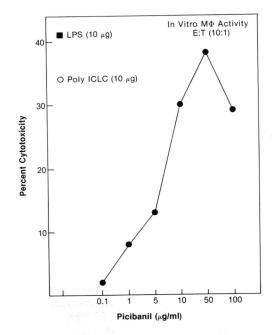

Fig. 2. Macrophage activity after various doses of Picibanil in vitro. Thioglycolate-elicited macrophages from C57BL/6 mice were collected by peritoneum lavage, washed, and allowed to adhere for 4 hr. The effector (Mϕ) to target (^{111}In-labeled P815 tumor cells) ratio of 10:1 was used. Poly ICLC and lipopolysaccharide (LPS) were employed as internal controls. The 72-hr assay was used to measure cytotoxicity.

TABLE I. NK Cell Response to Picibanil Via Various Routes of Injection

Route*	Spleen† 100:1	50:1	25:1	Spleen count ($\times 10^{-7}$)	Blood† 25:1	12:1	6:1	PEC† 12:1	PEC (per ml $\times 10^{-6}$)	Mϕ (per ml $\times 10^{-6}$)	Tumor‡ inhibition (%)
ip	16	9	7	6.4	8	6	3	56	22.0	13.6	67
iv	35	22	18	15.3	25	19	11	7	10.2	7.3	24
im	16	11	8	4.8	2	1	1	4	4.8	3.5	6
Oral	13	8	6	3.6	1	0.5	0.5	3	6.4	4.4	0
Placebo	11	7	5	3.4	3	1	0.5	2	4.4	2.6	0

*Mice sacrificed at 3 days following injection with 4 mg/kg.
†Percentage of cytotoxicity at the indicated effector to target cell ratios.
‡In vitro inhibition of MBL-2 target cells at a 10:1 ratio and 48 hr incubation.

Similar to the NK activity, Mϕ tumoricidal activity also remained elevated for the 8 day observation period.

We examined the extent of Mϕ tumoricidal activity exerted in vivo by separating Mϕ from the peritoneal ascites fluid and incubating them with MBL-2 cells in vitro to assess their ability to inhibit MBL-2 replication (Fig. 3). The results demonstrate that Mϕ from treated mice were capable of a 30 to 70% inhibition of MBL-2 tumor cells, indicating that the tumoricidal activity observed in vitro was also occurring in vivo. This observation was further supported by the significant decrease of viable tumor cells in the ascites fluid. The decrease in tumor cell burden was reflected by an increase in survival time.

Because of the observation that both peritoneal NK cells and Mϕ tumoricidal activity are significantly elevated by Picibanil, we examined whether these two effector cells would

TABLE II. Duration of Picibanil Effect on NK and Macrophage

Picibanil* treatment (day)	Spleen NK† 100:1	50:1	Spleen count ($\times 10^{-7}$)	PEC NK† 50:1	25:1	12:1	PEC (per ml $\times 10^{-6}$)	Mϕ‡ (per ml $\times 10^{-6}$)	Tumor inhibition (%)
Placebo	10	6	10	1	0.3	0.1	5.4	1.8	3
1	7	4	11	14	6	3	17.8	4.5	47
2	11	5	11	33	24	17	26.2	9.8	64
3	15	6	10	56	42	30	28.2	11.0	93
4	13	5	7	44	33	26	24.0	7.8	95
6	20	12	7	45	34	25	27.2	9.5	97
8	11	7	10	32	23	16	22.4	6.1	65

*Mice sacrificed on the indicated day following Picibanil treatment (4 mg/kg ip).
†Percentage of cytotoxicity at the effector to target cell (E:T) ratio indicated.
‡In vitro inhibition of MBL-2 target cells at an E:T cell ratio of 10:1 and 48 hr incubation.

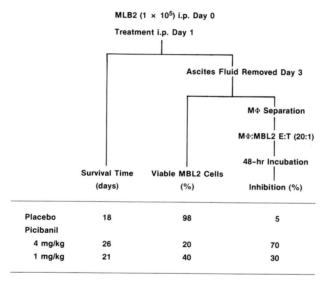

Fig. 3. Separation of Mϕ versus NK cell tumor cell cytotoxicity. Flow chart shows the method for separating Mϕ from the peritoneal ascites fluid for in vitro testing of tumoricidal activity. Percentage of dead versus viable tumor cells in the ascites fluid was determined by trypan blue dye exclusion. Additional mice were observed for survival time.

result in a therapeutic effect in mice with various tumor burdens (Fig. 4). Treatment resulted in a significant extension of survival time, which also led to a substantial number of long-term survivors in mice inoculated with 10^3 to 10^5 tumor cells. The most therapeutic effect was attained in mice inoculated with 10^3 cells.

Figure 5 shows the ability of Picibanil treatment to inhibit establishment of lung tumor colonies. The doses tested were capable of decreasing significantly the establishment of lung tumor colonies when they were administered 1 or 3 days following tumor cell inoculation. When treatment was delayed until day 6, only the 4 mg/kg dose resulted in significant protection. The 4 mg/kg dose was consistently the most effective dose and was well tolerated. Doses greater than 4 mg/kg (5 to 7 mg/kg) were also effective; however, they lead to cachexia and body weight loss.

B16 melanoma cells, similar to the M109 tumor, when inoculated iv, lodge in the lung and grow out into macroscopic colonies of tumor. Proliferation is progressive, and the number

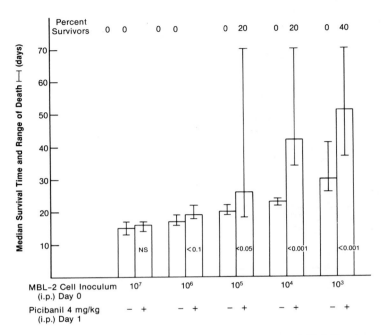

Fig. 4. Therapeutic effect of Picibanil vs different tumor cell inoculums. C57BL/6 male mice received various inoculums of MBL-2 lymphoma cells. One day following tumor cell inoculation, Picibanil or placebo was injected ip. Mice were observed for mortality over a 70 day observation period. Numbers above each column are the percentage of survivors at 70 days. These results represent the average of three experiments.

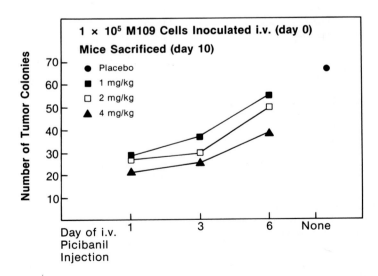

Fig. 5. Effect of Picibanil treatment on the establishment of lung tumor colonies. The alveolar adenocarcinoma M109 was inoculated iv on day 0 and Picibanil was administered iv on either days 1, 3, or 6 following M109 inoculation. Mice were sacrificed 10 days following tumor cell inoculation, and the lungs were scored for the number of tumor colonies formed.

of countable tumor colonies increases with time and they pervade the liver, leading to the eventual death of the animal. In this study, we also examined the role of NK cells in preventing the formation of tumor colonies in the lung and liver by pretreating mice with asialo-GM_1 (as GM_1) antibody, which selectively neutralizes NK cells (Table III).

Pretreating mice with Picibanil 3 days prior to B16 melanoma cell inoculation (at a time when NK cell activity was at its peak on day 3 [see Table I]) led to a significant decrease in tumor colonies in both the lung and liver. Pretreatment with anti-asGM_1 antibody, leading to a suppression of NK cell activity, resulted in an increase in lung tumor colonies particularly in the liver. These results indicate that NK cells were involved in decreasing the establishment of both lung and liver tumor colonies. Picibanil treatment was capable of overcoming the NK cell suppression exerted by anti-asGM_1 antibody. These results indicate that NK cells are responsible, in part, for suppressing B16 metastases. However, the observation that Picibanil also strongly enhances Mϕ tumoricidal activity would indicate that alveolar Mϕ may have also been responsible for the therapeutic effect attained in mice that were treated with both agents.

We tested the prophylactic effect of Picibanil in the B16 melanoma system to assess whether NK cells and/or Mϕ in the lung would prevent establishment of B16 tumor colonies (Table IV). Treatment with 0.5 or 5.0 mg/kg 3 days prior to challenge with B16 melanoma tumor cells resulted in significant protection.

Picibanils, capacity to stimulate cytotoxic T-lymphocyte response in an allogeneic tumor system was also examined using techniques previously reported [12,13]. The results in Table V show that Picibanil admixed with the allogeneic tumor cells significantly augmented the cytotoxic T-lymphocyte response to the tumor antigen. A similar adjuvant effect was observed when Picibanil was mixed with UV2237 fibrosarcoma tumor vaccine and syngeneic mice challenged with viable tumor cells (Table VI). Significant protection was attained when Picibanil was mixed with the irradiated tumor cells. At the 20 and 2 μg doses, significant protection occurred against the syngeneic tumor challenge in both parameters: the percentage of animals that did not develop tumors and the rate of growth of the tumor in animals that developed tumors. These results are in keeping with a T-lymphocyte response and are

TABLE III. Antitumor Activity of Picibanil Against B16 Melanoma in Immunosuppressed Mice

B16 (1×10^5 iv)	Anti-asGM_1 (iv)	BRM*	Day 10 Lung	Day 10 Liver	Day 17 Lung	Day 17 Liver
Day 0	—	—	33 (32–70)	1 (0–4)	182 (34–300)	8 (0–16)
Day 0	—	Picibanil	14 (18–56)	1 (0–2)	33 (12–142)	1 (0–10)
Day 0	Day 3	—	50 (20–76)	46 (32–68)	191 (33–300)	80 (36–111)
Day 0	Day 3	Picibanil	29 (3–141)	17 (1–43)	65 (60–112)	25 (0–75)

Header note: Median No. (range) of metastases spans the four Lung/Liver columns.

*Picibanil 4 mg/kg iv on day −3.

TABLE IV. Antitumor Prophylactic Effect of Picibanil

Drug	Dose (mg/kg)	Lung lesions (median)
HBSS	Placebo	245
Picibanil	5	18
Picibanil	0.5	118
Picibanil	0.05	195
Picibanil	0.005	232

Mice treated with drug iv at 3 days prior to B16 melanoma inoculation (5×10^4 iv). Mice sacrificed 3 weeks after tumor cell injection.

TABLE V. Picibanil Adjuvant Effect on Cytotoxic T-Lymphocyte Response

Picibanil total dose* (μg)	Tumor vaccine†	% Cytotoxicity‡		
		200:1	100:1	50:1
Placebo (HBSS)	−	15	13	12
Placebo (HBSS)	+	13	15	11
100	−	13	11	11
10	−	13	10	8
1	−	12	9	8
100	+	42	31	19
10	+	28	20	13
1	+	19	13	10

*Picibanil mixed with irradiated (10,000 R) tumor cell vaccine at time of intradermal injection (id).
†Irradiated tumor cells (fibrosarcoma UV2237) injected on day 0 (5×10^6 cells, primary) and day 10 (2×10^6 cells, secondary).
‡On day 15, nonadherent spleen cells were incubated with the radiolabeled (^{75}Se-selenium methionine) clone 46 subline (clonal subline of fibrosarcoma UV2237) at the spleen cell to tumor cell target ratios shown.

TABLE VI. Picibanil Adjuvant Effect With Tumor Cell Vaccine

Picibanil total dose* (μg)	Tumor vaccine†	% With Tumor (average size cm^3)‡	
		Day 18	Day 35
Placebo	−	100 (0.15)	100 (1.90)
Placebo	+	80 (0.21)	80 (1.17)
20	−	100 (0.15)	100 (1.73)
2	−	100 (0.12)	100 (1.71)
0.2	−	100 (0.12)	100 (1.96)
20	+	40 (0.05)	60 (0.33)
2	+	40 (0.10)	40 (1.20)
0.2	+	100 (0.10)	100 (2.1)

*Picibanil mixed with irradiated (10,000 R) 10^6 UV2237 tumor cell vaccine at time of intradermal injection (id).
†Tumor cell vaccine injected id on day −10 and viable UV2237 (2×10^5) injected id on day 0.
‡Average size of tumor of animals with tumor.

indicative of the capacity of Picibanil to stimulate the T-cell compartment of the immune system.

Results shown in Table VII demonstrate the increased therapeutic response when cytoreductive chemotherapy (Cytoxan) was combined with Picibanil treatment. An additive therapeutic response was achieved when the combination was employed in both decreasing the number of lung tumors as well as in increasing the survival time. Cytoxan alone was effective (group 2 vs 1), although delaying treatment until 7 days after tumor inoculation was not as effective (group 3 vs 2). Picibanil alone when administered 4 days following tumor inoculation was significantly effective (group 6 vs 1). Delaying treatment with Picibanil until day 7 (group 7) was not markedly effective probably because a greater tumor burden was present by that time. Combined treatment (groups 4 and 5 vs 2 and 4) lead to the most effective therapeutic response.

We have reported that two chemically defined immunoregulatory agents are capable of stimulating bone marrow replication and differentiation to granulocyte-macrophage–committed stem cells (GM-CFU-C) [14]. In addition, these agents were shown to cause earlier reconstitution of bone marrow in mice that received a therapeutic dose of the antitumor agent

TABLE VII. Response of M109 Alveolar Carcinoma to Combined Cytoxan and Picibanil Treatment

Group*	Cytoxan (200 mg/kg ip)	Picibanil (4 mg/kg iv)	Lung foci†	MST (days)^P
1			65	21
2	D4		21‡	32, <0.01
3	D7		52§	27, <0.05
4	D4	D7	10‡·‖	40, <0.001
5	D7	D10	35‡·¶	32, <0.01
6		D4	38§	29, <0.05
7		D7	60	23, <NS

*Mice inoculated iv with 2×10^5 M109 tumor cells.
†Number of lung tumor colonies observed at 12 days following tumor inoculation.
‡P < 0.01.
§P < 0.05 compared to control (group 1).
‖P < 0.05 compared to group 2.
¶P < 0.05 compared to group 3.
^{P}Median survival time and statistical analysis P value (Student's t test) compared to control (group 1).

TABLE VIII. Bone Marrow Reconstitution by Picibanil Following CYP Treatment

Treatment	Effector cell	Control		CYP ± Picibanil treatment* (day of observation)				
		Placebo	Picibanil	4	7	10	13	16
PBS	BM†	9.5	12.3					
	GM-CFU-C‡	100	135					
CYP+PBS	BM			3.5	7.3	10.1	9.8	9.6
	GM-CFU-C			28	62	98	90	92
CYP+	BM			4.5	11.1§	12.4§	13.0§	10.1
Picibanil	GM-CFU-C			42	110§	130§	127§	105

*BALB/c mice received a single ip injection of cyclophosphamide (CYP) 150 mg/kg on various days between day −16 to day −4, which was followed by a single ip injection of PBS or Picibanil (4 mg/kg) on day −3. All mice were sacrificed on day 0 for effector cell assay.
†Bone marrow cells/femur ($\times 10^6$).
‡GM-CFU-C/femur (% of placebo control).
§Statistical analysis (P < 0.01) between CYP+PBS and CYP and Picibanil.

cyclophosphamide (CYP). Picibanil was examined to determine whether it possessed similar properties (Table VIII). Picibanil treatment alone significantly increased bone marrow cellularity as well as the number of GM-CFU-C. CYP treatment resulted in a decease in the number of nucleated bone marrow cells and GM-CFU-C for a period of 10 days at which time they returned to normal values as shown in the placebo-treated controls. Administration of Picibanil to animals pretreated with CYP caused an earlier reconstitution of bone marrow cells and GM-CFU-C, including a pronounced rebound effect with bone marrow cell counts and GM-CFU-C above control values in a much shorter period of time.

DISCUSSION

Table IX summarizes the various cell regulatory and immunomodulating activities of Picibanil. This agent has been shown to possess therapeutic value when administered either alone or in combination with other cancer treatment modalities [4,15–18]. A persistent observation has been the excellent NK cell response achieved in peripheral blood and particularly

TABLE IX. Summary of Cell Regulatory and Immunomodulatory Activity of Picibanil (OK432)

1. Picibanil significantly increases NK cell and macrophage effector cell responses in vitro and in vivo
2. The most efficacious routes of treatment are iv or ip
3. Single treatment leads to elevated NK cell and macrophages for 7 to 10 days
4. Parallel with increased macrophage cytotoxicity is the increased expression of Ia antigen
5. Picibanil treatment is effective in retarding intracavitary tumor cell growth (MBL-2, M109, B16)
6. Combined treatment with Cytoxan and Picibanil leads to an increased therapeutic response through that achieved by single treatment alone
7. Picibanil treatment following cytoreductive drug treatment leads to an earlier myelopoiesis, specifically for bone marrow and GM-CFU-C differentiation probably mediated through colony-stimulating factor production
8. Cytokines that have been reported to be induced by Picibanil are IL-1 , IL-2, colony-stimulating factor, IFNβ, and natural killer activating factor

its capacity to augment NK cells in patients with carcinomatosis pleural effusions after intrapleural injections of Picibanil [19–22].

The current studies show that Picibanil possesses multifaceted immunomodulatory activity. NK cell activity is preferentially augmented in spleen and peripheral blood when Picibanil is administered by the iv route, whereas peritoneal NK cells and Mϕ activity are increased when it is administered by the ip route. NK and Mϕ activation appears to be maintained over a long period following only one treatment. The therapeutic activity appears to be mediated through its ability to increase the tumoricidal activity of NK cells and Mϕ, as well as increasing their numbers. The ability of Picibanil treatment to retard intracavitary tumors (intraperitoneal growth of MBL-2) (Figs. 3, 4), M109 lung tumor colony metastases (Fig. 5), and B16 melanoma (Table IV) would indicate the involvement of both NK cell and Mϕ tumor cell killing.

The role of the NK cell in inhibiting B16 melanoma cell metastases to lung and formation of lung colonies was established with the use of the NK cell neutralizing antibody anti-asGM$_1$. The ability of Picibanil to exert a therapeutic response despite the depletion of NK cells in mice treated with the neutralizing antibody would indicate that Mϕ also played a significant role in inhibiting lung tumor colony formation. Others have reported a similar therapeutic role of NK cells and macrophages in human and animal tumor studies [23–25].

Results of the current studies indicate that Picibanil mediates its effect through its ability to increase NK cell and macrophage tumoricidal activity. Its effect, however, is limited when a large tumor burden is present (Figs. 3–5). It is still effective when tumor burden is reduced by cytoreductive chemotherapy (Table VII).

The observations support the hypothesis that if the ratio of effector (NK cells and macrophages) to tumor target cells is adequate, a sufficient number of tumor cells will be eliminated, resulting in an extended survival.

Picibanil also appears to be an effective vaccine adjuvant capable of eliciting cytotoxic T lymphocytes (Table V) and rejecting a syngeneic tumor cell challenge (Table VI).

Of particular interest is the effect of Picibanil on myelopoiesis. The ability of Picibanil to increase bone marrow cellularity and GM-CFU-C differentiation especially in mice treated with the myelosuppressive drug CYP could be advantageous especially to the tumor-bearing host undergoing cytoreductive chemotherapy. Such treatment has led to infections secondary to depressed monocyte functions and granulocytopenia in cancer patients. In addition to the Picibanil's effect on myelopoiesis, it also activates other limbs of the immune system, including Mϕ and NK cell cytotoxic functions. Further, Picibanil may have therapeutic value through its ability to cause the production and secretion of cellular regulators such as IL-1 and IL-2 [26], as well as tumor necrosis factor.

Picibanil is one of the few agents that have been studied in such detail and found to exert such multifaceted immunomodulatory and cellular regulatory functions. This agent would be of considerable therapeutic value in a combined modality treatment protocol for various human tumors.

ACKNOWLEDGMENTS

W.B. Budzynski is a guest researcher from the Institute of Immunology and Experimental Therapy, Wroclaw, Poland.

This project was supported in part by federal funds from the Department of Health and Human Services, under contract number NO1-CO-23910 with Program Resources, Inc.

REFERENCES

1. Okamoto H, Shain S, Koshimura S. Streptolysin S-forming and antitumor activities of group A streptococci. In Jeljaszewicz J, Wadström T, eds: Bacterial toxins and cell membranes. London: Academic Press, 1979; 254.
2. Ishii Y, Yamaoka H, Toh K, Kikuchi K. Inhibition of tumor growth in vivo and in vitro by machrophages from rats treated with OK432. Gann 1976; 1:115.
3. Chirigos MA, Saito T, Talmadge JE. The immunomodulatory activity of Picibanil (OK432). In Hoshino T, Uchida A, eds: Clinical and experimental studies in immunotherapy. Princeton: Excerpta Medica, 1985; 20.
4. Micksche M, Kokran O, Uchida A. Clinical and immunopharmacological studies with OK432, a streptococcal preparation. In Serrou B, Rosenfeld C, Daniels JC, Saunders JP, eds: Current concepts in human immunology and cancer immunomodulation. Amsterdam: Elsevier Biomedical Press, 1982; 639.
5. Stanley ER, Guilbert LJ. Methods for the purification, assay, characterization, and target cell binding of a colony stimulating factor (CSF). J Immunol Methods 1981; 42:253.
6. Bartocci A, Papadiemtriou V, Chirigos MA. Enhanced macrophage and natural killer cell antitumor activity by various molecular weight maleic anhydride divinyl ethers. J Immunopharmacol 1980; 2:149–58.
7. Herberman RB, Nunn ME, Lavrin DH. Natural cytotoxic reactivity of mouse lymphoid cells against syngeneic and allogeneic tumors. I. Distribution of reactivity and specificity. Int J Cancer 1975; 16:216.
8. Schlick E, Friedberg KD. Bone marrow cells under the influence of low lead doses. Arch Toxicol 1982; 49:227.
9. Schlick E, Bartocci A, Chirigos MA. Effect of azimexone on the bone marrow of normal and γ-irradiated mice. J Biol Resp Modif 1982; 1:179.
10. Fidler IJ, Berendt M, Oldham RK. The rationale for and design of a screening procedure for the assessment of biological response modifiers for cancer treatment. J Biol Resp Modif 1982; 1:15.
11. Talmadge JE, Oldham RK, Fidler IJ. Practical consideration for the establishment of a screening procedure for the assessment of biological response modifiers. J Biol resp Modif 1984; 3:88.
12. Brunner KT, Mauel J, Cerottïni J, Chaperis B. Qualitative assay of the lytic action of immune lymphoid cells on ^{51}Cr labeled allogeneic target cells in vitro. Immunology 1968; 14:181.
13. Henney CS. Quantitation of the cell-mediated immune response. J Immunol 1971; 107:1558.
14. Chirigos MA, Saito T, Schlick E, Ruffmann R. Cellular regulation by immunomodifiers MVE-2 and Poly ICLC and their theraperutic application. Cancer Treat Symp 1985; 1:11.
15. Uchida A, Hoshino T. Clinical studies on cell-mediated immunity in patients with malignant disease. Cancer 1980; 45:476.
16. Wakasugi H, Oshimi K, Miyata M, Morioba Y. Augmentation of natural killer cell activity by a streptococcal preparation, OK432, in patients with malignant tumors. Clin Immunol 1981; 1:154.
17. Yamagota S, Koh T, Oride H, Hattori T. Antitumor effects of levamisole in combination with anaerobic corynebacterium, OK432 (streptococcal preparation) and chemotherapy in mice. Cancer Immunol Immunother 1980; 7:217.
18. Mashiba H, Matsunaga K, Gojobori M. Effect of immunochemotherapy with OK432 and yeast cell wall on the activities of peritoneal macrophages of mice. Gann 1979; 70:687.
19. Watanobe Y, Iwa T. Clinical value of immunotherapy for lung cancer by the Streptococcal preparation OK432. Cancer 1980; 53:248.
20. Uchida A, Hoshino T. Clinical studies on cell mediated immunity in patients with malignant disease. Cancer Immunol Immunother 1980; 9:153.

21. Uchida A, Micksche M. Lysis of fresh human tumor cells by autologous peripheral blood lymphocytes and pleural effusion lymphocytes activated by OK432. JNCI 1983; 71:673.
22. Uchida A, Micksche M, Hoshino T. Intrapleural administration of OK432 in cancer patients: Augmentation of autologous tumor cell killing activity of tumor-associated large granular lymphocytes. Cancer Immunol Immunother 1984; 18:5.
23. Colotta F, Rambaldi A, Colombo N, Tobacchi L, Introna I, Mantovani A. Effect of streptococcal preparation (OK432) on natural killer activity of tumor-associated lymphoid cells in human ovarian carcinoma and on lysis of fresh ovarian tumor cells. Br J Cancer 1983; 48:515.
24. Colotta F, Bersani L, Polentarutti N, Peri G, Mantovani A. Effect of inactivated streptococci (OK432) on macrophage functions in mice. J Immunopharmacol 1985; 7:437.
25. Saito M, Nanjo M, Aonuma E, et al. Activated macrophages are responsible for the tumor-inhibitory effect in mice receiving intravenous injection of OK432. Int J Cancer 33:271, 1984.
26. Ichimura O, Suzuki S, Sugawara Y, Osawa T. Lymphokines inducation by streptococcal preparation OK432 (picibanil) in mice: Characterization of interleukin 1 (IL-1), interleukin 2 (IL-2) and natural killer cell activating factor (NKAF). In Hoshino T, Uchida A, eds: Clinical and experimental studies in immunotherapy. Princeton: Exerpta Medica, 1985; 48.

Cancer Detection and Prevention Supplement 1:329–331 (1987)

Imunovir in the Treatment of Immunodepression of Diverse Etiology

B.B. O'Neill, PhD
A.J. Glasky, PhD

Newport Pharmaceuticals Int. Inc., Newport Beach, CA

ABSTRACT Immunodepression associated with a variety of situations such as cancer or any of its major modalities of treatment (surgery, irradiation, or chemotherapy) has been effectively alleviated with Imunovir (inosine pranobex-BAN), and this has been associated with demonstrable clinical benefit to these patients. One hundred and six immunodepressed patients with solid tumors undergoing radiotherapy were treated with either Imunovir or placebo; 64% of Imunovir-treated patients were immunorestored after 3 months compared to 23% in the placebo group. Imunovir was also effectively used in 75 patients with malignant hematological disorders both as an immunorestorative agent given prophylactically to prevent infection and as a therapeutic agent to treat infections in these immunodepressed patients. In different studies involving surgical patients treated with either Imunovir or placebo, 70–81% of hypoergic or anergic patients in the Imunovir group became normoergic by day 14 of treatment compared to 5–17% of the placebo group, and this enhanced immunorestoration was associated with lower incidence of local sepsis ($P < 0.05$), systemic sepsis ($P < 0.025$), and postoperative mortality ($P < 0.05$).

Key words: immunodepression, management, cancer, surgical patients

INTRODUCTION

Secondary nonspecific immunodeficiency states are linked to a variety of clinical situations such as cancer or any of its major modalities of treatment (surgery, irradiation, or chemotherapy). Irrespective of etiology, the resulting immunodeficiency favors the appearance of viral, bacterial, or parasitic infections, which as well as being more serious and atypical than in a noncompromised host also tend to become more frequent or chronic and resistant to current standard therapy.

It would appear, therefore, that there is certainly a place for a safe and effective immunostimulating drug in such conditions. Imunovir (inosine pranobex-BAN) is one such drug. It is composed of one molecule of inosine and three molecules of the para-acetamidobenzoic acid salt of N,N-dimethylamino-2-propanol. The preclinical in vitro and in vivo immunostimulating properties of the drug are well documented [1]. An abundance of human safety data has also been accumulated sometimes in patients to whom the drug has been given

Address reprint requests to B.B. O'Neill, Newport Pharmaceuticals Int. Inc., Newport Beach, CA 92663.

in relatively high doses (3–4 g/day) continuously for periods of several years [2] and in combination with a wide variety of other drugs (J.S. Meyer, unpublished report).

CLINICAL USAGE IN IMMUNODEFICIENCY STATES

Association of immunorestorative and clinical effects has been established in a series of studies in cancer patients [3–6]. De Simone et al [3] used Imunovir (4 g/day for 28 days) in 20 patients with nonresectable gastric cancer 2 weeks after surgery and compared their clinical immune responses to those of ten similar patients treated with placebo in the same way. A significant improvement in immune status indicated by increased PHA response, E-active rosettes, and delayed type hypersensitivity was evident 14 days after Imunovir therapy, and this was maintained throughout treatment up to 42 days postsurgery. Thus in the period between the surgical act and commencement of either radiotherapy or chemotherapy in patients with nonresectable gastric cancer, it is possible to restore or enhance the cell mediated immunity and enhance the prognosis in this population.

The immunostimulating potential of Imunovir in patients with solid tumors was also examined [4]. One hundred and six patients with solid tumors (46 with breast cancer, 31 with cancer of head and neck, and 29 with uterine cancer) and immunodepression after radiotherapy were randomized and treated daily with either 3 g/day Imunovir or matching placebo for 1 month and then 4 days each week for a further 4 months. On examination, 1, 3, and 5 months after initiation of drug therapy, it was evident that Imunovir-treated patients were more quickly immunorestored, with 23% of placebo patients immunorestored after 3 months compared to 64% of those on active drug (Fig. 1).

The clinical significance of such an immunorestoration in patients immunodepressed whether by the cancer per se or by the treatment of such a disease is illustrated by the studies of Schaison et al [5] and Ochoka et al [6]. Schaison et al [5] investigated both the therapeutic and prophylactic effects of Imunovir on viral infections in patients with malignant hematologic disease, patients in whom these viral infections are common and often much more severe than in the noncompromised host. Twenty-five patients with herpes simplex virus (HSV), cytomegalovirus, varicella zoster virus (VZV), or measles were treated with Imunovir at a dose of 50 mg/kg/day for 10–15 days, and in 19 of these patients an excellent response was observed. A second group of 25 similar patients without infection but at high risk for these infections were treated prophylactically with 50 mg/kg/day in combination with trimethoprim-sulfamethoxazole. No viral or parasitic infections occurred during the period of treatment, and interestingly a prolonged period of remission of hematological disease was also observed.

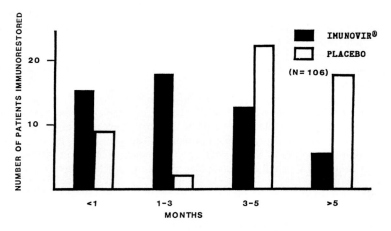

Fig. 1. Immunorestoration of Imunovir in cancer patients.

TABLE I. Effects of Imunovir on Incidence of Complications in Surgical Patients

Treatment	DTH normoergic (%)		Local infection (%)	Generalized infection (%)	Mortality (%)
	Day 0	Day 14			
Imunovir	54.2	87.5	14.6	6.25	2.08
Placebo	58.4	60.5	25.0	18.70	12.50

Similarly, Ochoka et al [6] treated HSV and VZV infections in 15 patients with leukemia or malignant lymphoma. Using a dose of 50 mg/kg/day Imunovir for 10 days, Ochoka et al reported an alleviation of pain and swelling with an acceleration of healing and no further appearance of new lesions. A further ten patients exposed to and at high risk of VZV infection were treated prophylactically with 50 mg/kg/day for 15 days, and in this group only one patient in ten developed VZV infection.

Similar immunorestorative and clinical effects of Imunovir have been seen in immuno-depressed patients undergoing surgery. Gui et al [7], Cirulli and Amico Roxas [8], and Ronconi et al [9] evaluated the immunorestorative effects of Imunovir by performing skin tests on patients prior to surgery and treating those found to be anergic or hypoergic with either Imunovir or matching placebo (4 g/day for either 11 or 14 days and last dose within 3 days of surgery). Gui et al found that 81% of Imunovir-treated patients experienced an increased skin test response posttreatment compared to only 16% of the placebo-treated patients (P < 0.005). Cirulli and Amico Roxas also evaluated the incidence of postoperative complications and found that patients treated with Imunovir experienced a significantly lower incidence of local sepsis (P < 0.05), systemic sepsis (P < 0.25), and postoperative mortality (P < 0.01) which correlated directly with the significant increase in the number of Imunovir-treated patients who became normoergic (Table I).

In conclusion, the potential of Imunovir to modulate the host immune response has important clinical implications that are illustrated in the trials discussed above. In each of these studies, a clinical response has paralleled an effect on the immune response and establishes a link between enhancement of immunological status and clinical improvement in conditions of diverse etiology.

REFERENCES

1. O'Neill BB, Ginsberg T. In: "Proceedings of 13th International Congress of Chemotherapy (Vienna)." 1983; Vol 265; pp 11–24.
2. Jones CJ, Dyken PR, Huttenlocher PR, Jabbour JT, Maxwell KW. Lancet 1982; ii:1034–7.
3. De Simone C, Meli D, Midini G, Ricca D, Di Paola M. Paper presented at the XVIth International Congress of Therapeutics, 1981.
4. Fridman H, Calle R, Morin A. Int J Immunopharmacol 1980; 2:194.
5. Schaison G, Gluckman E, Souillet JF, Ture JM. Paper presented at the 4th International Congress of Immunology, 1980.
6. Ochoka M, Chmielewska D, Matysiak M. Fol Haematol 1984; 3:343–9.
7. Gui D, Borgognone A, Pittiruti M, Ronconi P. Clin Europea XXI, 1982; 2:3–8.
8. Cirulli G, Amico Roxas M. Riv Gen Ital Chir 1980; 31:553–64.
9. Ronconi P, Bellantone R, Pittiruiti M. Chir Patol Sper 1981; 24:20–33.

Cancer Detection and Prevention Supplement 1:333–349 (1987)

Clinical Efficacy of Lentinan on Patients With Stomach Cancer: End Point Results of a Four-Year Follow-Up Survey

T. Taguchi, MD

Department of Oncologic Surgery, Research Institute for Microbiol Diseases, Osaka University, Osaka, Japan

ABSTRACT   End-point results of a 4-yr followup survey and a randomized control trial of lentinan (LNT) on patients with advanced or recurrent stomach cancer have been investigated in order to evaluate the clinical efficacy of LNT in combination with chemotherapeutic agent tegafur (FT). Eligible (68) patients in control groups were administered with FT consecutively at doses of 600 mg/day, and eligible (96) patients in the treated group were administered LNT in combination with FT. LNT was injected intravenously 2 mg weekly. Remarkable lifespan prolongation effects of LNT have been observed both at the end of the control trial and at the end of the followup survey (p < 0.01) using Kaplan-Meier's method and the generalized Wilcoxian test. Remarkable survival at 1, 2 and 3 years has been observed in the treated group using lifetable analysis. Side effects of LNT have been transitional and not serious. Thus, LNT should be effective in combination with FT for patients with stomach cancer.

Key words: cancer treatment, immunomodulation, polysaccharides

INTRODUCTION

Lentinan is a purified polysaccharide extracted from *Lentinus edodes*, which is an edible Japanese mushroom, Shiitake. Lentinan is composed of only glucose, a β-1,3-glucan, with an average molecular weight of 500,000 daltons, and composed of β-1,3-glucopyranoside linkage as a main chain with β-1,6-glucopyranoside–linked branches [1,2]. Lentinan has antitumor activities against allogeneic, syngeneic, and autochthonous tumors in mice or rats. Its mode of action has been extensively studied from an immunological and biological point of view and was found to exert antitumor activities not through a direct cytocidal effect against tumor, but through stimulation of the host-defense mechanisms, such as activation of macrophage differentiation and helper T lymphocyte functions and/or alternative pathways of complements [3–11]. Based on the striking antitumor effect in animal models with analyses of its mode of actions and based on acute, subacute, and chronic toxicological studies in mice, rats, and monkeys, the use of lentinan was considered for the treatment of human cancer. In phase I and

Address reprint requests to T. Taguchi, Department of Oncologic Surgery, Research Institute for Microbiol Diseases, Osaka University, Suita Osaka, 565 Japan.

phase II clinical studies, the optimal dosage range and administration method was determined from the knowledge of its antitumor effect and host immune responses [12–14]. Lentinan was administered to patients with gastrointestinal cancer at doses of 0.5–5.0 mg/person once or twice a week in combination with chemotherapeutic agents such as tegafur (FT) or mitomycin C (MMC) plus 5-fluorouracil (5-FU). Based on these results, the phase III study in a randomized controlled trial with the envelope method was conducted on patients with advanced and recurrent stomach cancers for evaluation of the clinical efficacy of lentinan.

PATIENTS AND METHODS
Administration Schedule

As a basic chemotherapeutic agent, FT was used in the control group at doses of 600 mg/person/day, which varied according to the condition of patients, and was given either orally, intravenously, or by suppository. FT should be administered continuously as long as possible. In the treated group, lentinan was administered in combination with FT at a dose of 2 mg once weekly or 1 mg twice weekly by intravenous injection with either one injection or drip infusion and was continued as long as possible (Fig. 1).

Eligibility of Patients

Eligible conditions for patient selection were cases with either advanced or recurrent histologically proven cancer, in individuals less than 80 years old free of serious complications and without multiple cancer and severe impairment of liver, kidney, and bone marrow. Patients who had prior therapy were given a rest period to eliminate the influence of the prior treatment. Patients were treated according to the protocol of the administration method and were randomized by the envelope method.

Classifications of Patients

Patients were classified as eligible cases, ineligible cases, exclusions, and withdrawals. "Exclusions" consisted of protocol failure, and "withdrawals" included early death, loss to follow-up, and an insufficient observation period of less than 4 weeks and an insufficient administration period of either FT or lentinan for less than 3 weeks.

Evaluation of Clinical Efficacy of Lentinan

Efficacy of lentinan in cancer treatment was determined from the antitumor effect and from prolongation of life span.

Antitumor Effect

Antitumor effect was evaluated using Koyama-Saito's criteria [15].

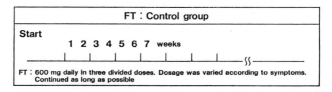

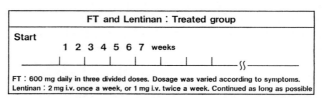

Fig. 1.   Protocols used during the randomized controlled study.

Response Rate

Response rate was calculated as follows: Numerator: effective case, greater than partial response (PR) in evaluated lesion; denominator: evaluated case. "PR" denotes 50% or more decrease in total tumor size of the bidimensionally measurable lesion, which was measured to determine the effect of therapy by two observations not less than 4 weeks apart without appearance of new lesions or progression of any lesion or 30% or more estimated decrease in total tumor size of the unidimensionally measurable lesion, which was measured to determine the effect of therapy by two observations not less than 4 weeks apart without appearance of new lesions or progression of any lesion.

Prolongation of Survival

Kaplan-Meier's method and the generalized Wilcoxon's test were used for the evaluation of life-span prolongation effect. Life table analysis was used for the evaluation of survival ratio.

Follow-Up Survey

To evaluate the life-span prolongation effect and increase in survival ratio, the follow-up survey from September 30, 1980, to May 1, 1984, was performed after the completion of a randomized controlled trial.

RESULTS
Classifications of Patients

One hundred four cases in the control group and 114 cases in the treated group were entered into the trial. Sixty-eight cases and 77 cases were eligible in the control and the treated group, respectively (Table I). Twenty-four cases in both groups were ineligible because of 1) violation of the envelope method (23 cases; ten cases in the control group [C], 13 cases in the treated group [L]); 2) receiving postoperative adjuvant chemotherapy (15 cases; ten cases in C, five cases in L); 3) no histological confirmation (one case in L); 4) age older than 81 years (three cases; one case in C, two cases in L); 5) renal failure (one case in L); 6) insufficient period after prior therapy (two cases; one case in C, one case in L); and 7) protocol failure using anticancer drugs other than FT or other immunotherapeutic agents (three cases; two cases in C, one case in L). A total of seven cases were excluded from evaluation because of protocol failure: Four cases in the control group and one case in the treated group had been treated with other immunotherapeutic agents, two cases in the treated group had more than a 2-week interval between the onset of lentinan and FT administration. A total of 15 cases of withdrawal consisted of the following categories: nine cases of early death, loss to follow-up, or of insufficient observation period of less than 4 weeks (seven cases in C, two cases in L), five cases of insufficient dosage of FT (one case in C, four cases in L), and one case of insufficient dosage of lentinan (one case in L). No significant bias was observed in patient classification between the control group and the treated group (P = 0.91).

Background Factors

Background factors such as sex, age, performance status, prior chemotherapy, primary lesion, and tumor sites were comparatively analyzed between the control group and the treated group. The test of significance of each background factor was examined and no significant difference was observed in either background factors (Tables II, III).

Chemotherapeutic Agents in the Follow-Up Period After the Controlled Trial

The selection of the chemotherapeutic agent was left to the doctor's discretion; therefore, the chemotherapeutic agents that were used have been surveyed (Table IV). Fourteen cases in the control group were alive at the end of the controlled trial as of September 30, 1980. Ten

TABLE I. Summary of Eligible, Ineligible, Exclusion, and Withdrawal Cases

Classification	Criteria for Classification	No. of C	No. of L
Eligible		68	77
	Violation of envelop method	10	13
	Curative resection	10	5
	No histological confirmation	0	1
	Age $\geqslant 81$ years	1	2
Ineligible	Severe complication	0	1
	Resting period $\leqslant 4$ weeks	1	1
	MMC alone or MMC + FT	0	1
	Concomitant use of other anticancer drugs or immunotherapeutic agents	2	0
Exclusion	Use of other anticancer drugs or immunotherapeutic agents in the course of the study	4	1
	Inadequate intervals of lentinan administration (22 weeks)	–	2
Withdrawal	Early death or loss to follow up, within 4 weeks	3	1
	Insufficient observation period ($\leqslant 4$ weeks as of end of Sept. 19)	4	1
	FT $\leqslant 3$ weeks	1	4
	Lentinan $\leqslant 5$ mg	–	1

C, control; L, treated.

out of 14 cases had been treated with chemotherapeutic agents such as FT, 5-FU, FT + MMC, or 5-FU + MMC. Treatment during the follow-up survey was discontinued in three cases, and one case was treated with FT + lentinan. Forty-three cases in the treated group were alive as of September 30, 1980. Ten out of 43 cases received FT, 5-FU, MMC, or a combination of these, 18 cases were treated with lentinan + FT, 5-FU, or MMC, and 15 cases received no chemotherapeutic agents.

Administration Intensity of FT

The administration intensities of FT in both the control and treated groups were analyzed and compared. The administration intensity was expressed as a tangent of the graph consisting of Y-axis as the administration amount of FT to X-axis as the administration interval (Figs. 1, 2, 3).

In the control group, the relationship of the administration amount versus the administration interval is shown as $Y = 0.445X + 4.995$, with a correlation coefficient value of 0.7850, and in the treated group as $Y = 0.3450X + 18.166$, with a correlation coefficient value of 0.6435. The administration intensity of FT in the control and treated groups was 0.445 and 0.345, respectively. Therefore, the administration intensity of FT in the treated group was not stronger than that in the control group.

Antitumor Effect (Incidence of PR Cases)

The response rate of antitumor effect ($\geqq$ PR) in the control and treated groups was 2.0% (1/51) and 16.3% (8/48), respectively. The response rate in the treated group was greater than in the control group with a statistical significance ($P < 0.01$).

TABLE II. Background Factors of Stomach Cancer Patients on FT Regimen

	Tegafur	Lentinan + tegafur
Age (years)		
~ 20 yo	0	0
~ 30 yo	1	1
~ 40 yo	6	4
~ 50 yo	5	12
~ 60 yo	10	19
~ 70 yo	23	20
~ 80 yo	23	21
	t = 1.2592	
	p = 0.2079	
Sex		
Male	50	49
Female	18	28
	$\chi^2 = 1.2069$	
	p = 0.2719	
Performance status		
0	4	3
1	11	14
2	20	29
3	30	31
4	3	0
	t = 0.8586	
	p = 0.3905	
Previous chemotherapy		
+	28	32
−	40	45
	$\chi^2 = 0.0150$	
	p = 0.9026	
Primary lesion		
+	40	44
−	28	33
	$\chi^2 = 0.0013$	
	p = 0.9713	

Prolongation of Survival

Prolongation of survival was analyzed at two periods: at the end of the controlled trial on September 30, 1980, and at the end-point of the follow-up survey on May 1, 1984. Survival curves at the two periods revealed that the life-span prolongation effect of lentinan administration had the same significant tendency ($P < 0.01$), (Fig. 4). Furthermore, life table analysis demonstrated that the 1, 2, 3, and 4 year survival ratio of the treated group was significantly high (Table V).

Prolongation of survival was also analyzed according to correlation with performance status, primary lesion, and prior chemotherapy. In every correlation with performance status of 0–1, 2, and 3, the life-span prolongation effect of lentinan was observed with statistical significance ($P < 0.01$) (Figs. 5–7), and the mean survival days of each group corresponded well to the performance status of patients at the commencement of the trial; that is, mean

TABLE III. Tumor Sites Distribution

	Recurrent cases*	
Tumor Sites	No. of	
	C	L
Anastomotic lesion + lymphnode	5	8
Anastomotic lesion + peritonitis carcinomatosa + liver, or Douglas cul-de-sac	3	2
Liver	4	1
Liver + peritonitis carcinomatosa	4	2
Liver + Douglas cul-de-sac	2	0
Peritonitis carcinomatosa + Virchows node, skin, navel, or Douglas cul-de-sac, ovarium	6	8
Virchows node + regional lymphnode + bone	3	6
Pleuritis carcinomatosa + skin	1	2
Intestine + ovarium	0	4
Stomach + lymphnode	7	8
Stomach + liver	7	8
Stomach + liver + peritonitis carcinoma-tosa + bone, or Douglas cul-de-sac	11	7
Stomach + liver + lung, renal, bone, or Douglas cul-de-sac	6	5
Stomach + peritonitis carcinomatosa	3	3
Stomach + peritonitis + small intestine, spleen or Douglas cul-de-sac, ovarium	2	7
Stomach + lung	3	2
Stomach + esophagus + skin, Douglas cul-de-sac	1	4

C, control; L, treated. $^*\chi^2 = 10.64$; $P = 0.22$. $^+\chi^2 = 5.71$; $P = 0.57$.

TABLE IV. Classification of Treatments in Follow-up Survey (September 30, 1980 to May 1, 1984)

Group	Total	Chemotherapy alone	Lentinan + chemotherapy	No treatment
Control	14	10	1	3
Treated	43	10	18	15

Chemotherapeutic agents were FT, 5-FU, or MMC.

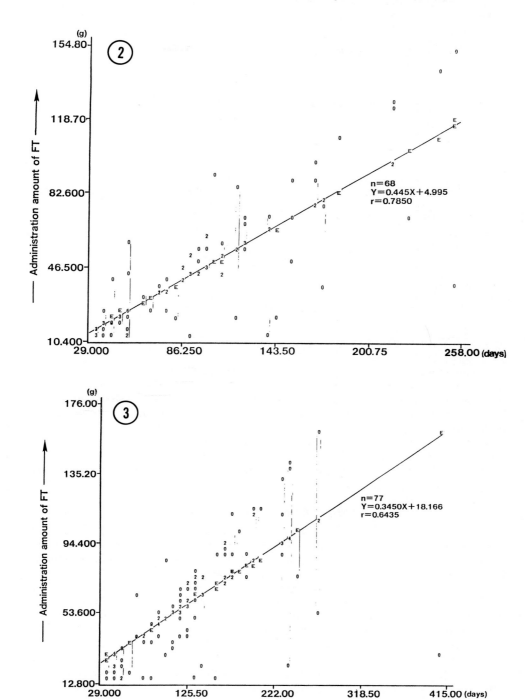

Fig. 2.   Administration amount of FT vs administration duration in control group.

Fig. 3.   Administration amount of FT vs administration duration in treated group.

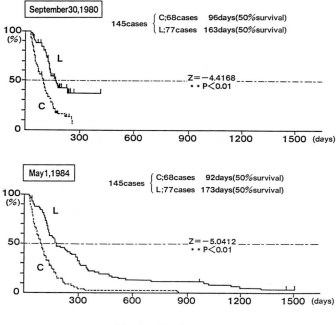

Fig. 4.   Survival curve.

survival days were shorter in cases in which the performance status became worse. In every case of patients with either a primary lesion or recurrence, or of patients with or without prior chemotherapy, the observed life prolongation effect of lentinan was statistically significant at P < 0.01 (Figs. 8–11). Survival curves of patients in the follow-up survey were analyzed in relation to type of treatment such as with either chemotherapy alone or with lentinan plus chemotherapy in the control and treated groups. Comparison of the chemotherapy-treated cases (ten) and patients who were treated with lentinan plus chemotherapy (18) with the untreated group (ten cases) revealed a significant difference in life-span prolongation effect in the treated group (P < 0.05) (Figs. 12, 13).

Survival Curve and Lentinan Dosage

In this randomized controlled study, analysis of lentinan dosage was made in relation to prolongation of life span. Twenty-six cases were treated with a dose of 1 mg/person twice a week, and 51 cases received a dose of 2 mg/person once a week. A significant life-span prolongation effect was observed in both cases of 1 mg and 2 mg of lentinan in comparison to the control group at the end of the controlled trial and at the end of the follow-up survey (Figs. 14–16). Comparing the 2 mg doses (L-2) with the 1 mg dose (L-1) in relation to the survival curve, the survival interval at median survival ratio of L-2 was 227 days, whereas that of L-1 was 132 days at the end of the controlled trial. The same tendency was observed at the end of the follow-up survey. No statistical significance was found between the doses L-1 and L-2 at the end of the controlled trial. Conversely, at the end of the follow-up survey, a significant life-span prolongation effect was observed in cases who had been treated with doses of 2 mg of lentinan (P < 0.05) (Fig. 16).

Side Effects

Subjective and objective side effects of lentinan occurred rarely, and the symptoms were transitional and not serious. The following side effects were noted in six patients (5.4%): a

TABLE V. Analysis of Survival Rates of Stomach Cancer Patients on FT Treatment on the Basis of the Life Table Analysis May 1,1984

Interval (days)	Entered	Dead	Lost	With-drawn	Exposed	Prop. dead	Prop. survived	Cumul. survival	Q/L-d	SE
C										
0–365	68	65	1	0	67.5	0.9630	0.0370	0.0370	0.3852	0.0230
365–730	2	0	0	0	2.0	0.0000	1.0000	0.0370	0.0000	0.0230
730–1,095	2	2	0	0	2.0	1.0000	0.0000	0.0000	0.0000	0.0230
1,095–1,460										
1,460–1,825										
L										
0–365	77	56	6	0	74.0	0.7568	0.2432	0.2432	0.0420	0.0499
365–730	15	7	0	0	15.0	0.4667	0.5333	0.1297	0.0583	0.0411
730–1,095	8	2	1	0	7.5	0.2667	0.7333	0.0951	0.0485	0.0367
1,095–1,460	5	3	0	0	5.0	0.6000	0.4000	0.0381	0.3000	0.0255
1,460–1,825	2	0	0	2	1.0	0.0000	1.0000	0.0381	0.0000	0.0255

Interval (days)	Differ.	SE	Z
0–365	−0.2062	0.0549	−3.75
365–730	−0.0927	0.0471	−1.97
730–1,095	−0.0951	0.0433	−2.20
1,095–1,460			
1,460–1,825			

Generalized Wilcoxon test: $W = 2,480.00000$; $VW = 2,015.54297$; $T = -5.04115$; $P = 0.00000$.

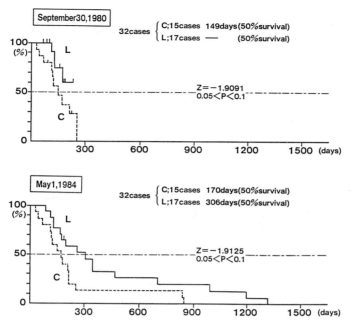

Fig. 5.   Survival curve correlated with performance status of 0–1.

feeling of oppression to the chest in three cases, rash in two cases, heat sensation, sweating, blood pressure rise, and redness in the face in one case, respectively. Lentinan administration was not discontinued as a result of these side effects.

DISCUSSION

Advanced and recurrent stomach cancer is a neoplasm with one of the poorest prognoses. Recent statistics in Japan [16] show that the 2 year survival ratio of patients with advanced stomach cancer is only 0.8% (31/4,020 patients; 1962–1971); from 1962 to 1978 the ratio remained 0.8% (106/13,137 patients). Furthermore, the low 5 year survival ratio was less than 0.1% (6/7,998 patients) in the period from 1962 to 1978. On the other hand, the 2, 3, and 4 year survival ratio of the lentinan-treated group in this study was 13.0, 9.5, and 3.8%, respectively; furthermore, two patients were free from cancer and alive more than 5 years (as of January 31, 1985) from the commencement of the trial. In view of the fact that the life-span prolongation effect of lentinan was significant in the period of controlled trial and follow-up survey and that the survival ratios of 1, 2, 3, and 4 years in the lentinan-treated group were significantly higher than those in the control group, it is suggested that lentinan may be beneficial for patients with advanced and recurrent stomach cancer when administered in combination with FT.

The purpose of cancer therapy is the prolongation of the survival period and possibly to cure the disease, not solely to obtain a transitional regression of tumor size. In spite of the fact that many chemotherapeutic agents have been used for the treatment of stomach cancer, no life-span prolongation effect from these agents was evident from the data of a 14 year survey of survival ratios in Japan. This finding suggests problems in the evaluation of cancer treatment. Chemotherapeutic agents are toxic to the human body, and their effectiveness should not be evaluated on the basis of a transitional regression in tumor size. Assessment of the therapeutic effect of antineoplastic agents should be carried out in a randomized fashion by

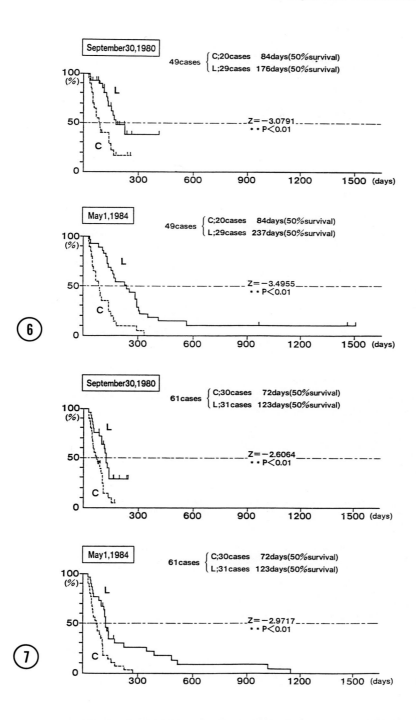

Fig. 6. Survival curve correlated with performance status of 2.

Fig. 7. Survival curve correlated with performance status of 3.

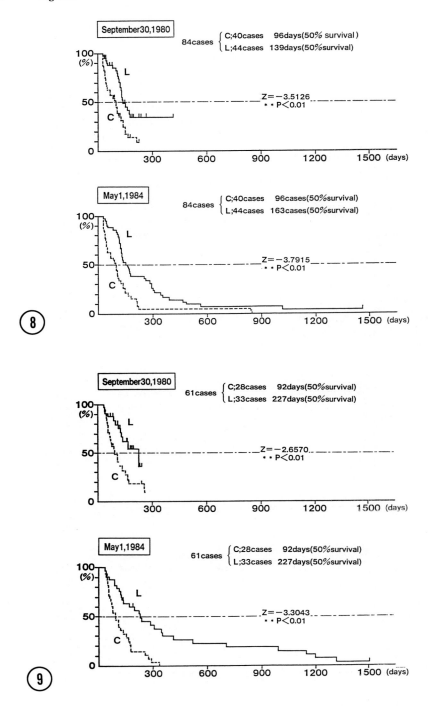

Fig. 8.   Survival curve correlated with primary lesions. Initial occurrence cases of stage IV.

Fig. 9.   Survival curve correlated with absence of primary lesion. Recurrent cases.

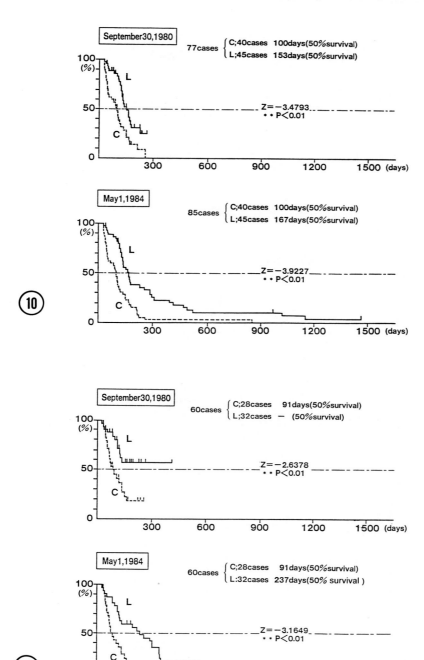

Fig. 10.   Survival curve correlated with absence of prior chemotherapy.

Fig. 11.   Survival curve correlated with prior chemotherapy.

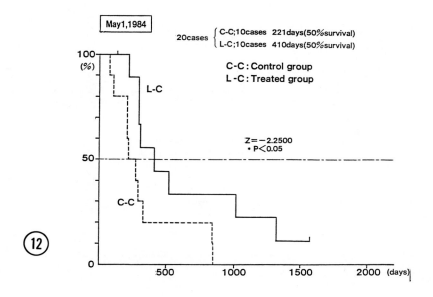

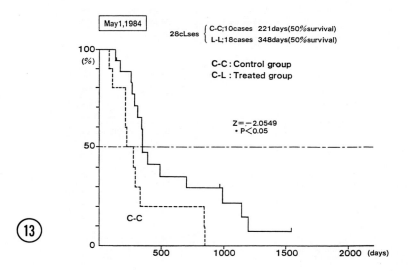

Fig. 12.   Survival curve of cases treated with chemotherapy alone in both control and treated groups in follow-up survey in relation to treatment.

Fig. 13.   Survival curve of cases in the follow-up survey in relation to treatment: chemotherapy alone in the control group vs lentinan plus chemotherapy in the treated group.

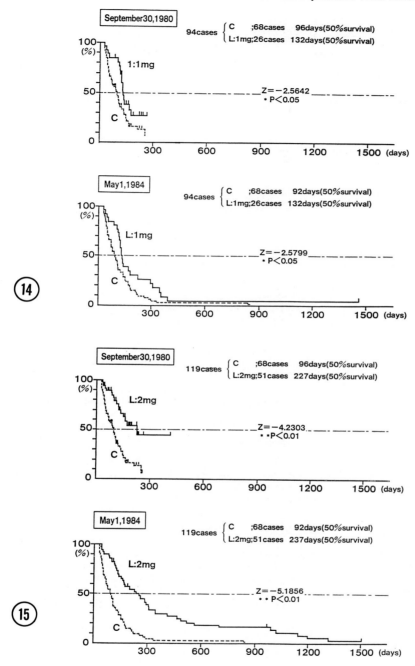

Fig. 14.   Survival curve correlated with doses of lentinan: treated group with 1 mg of lentinan vs control group.

Fig. 15.   Survival curve correlated with doses of lentinan: treated group with 2 mg lentinan vs control group.

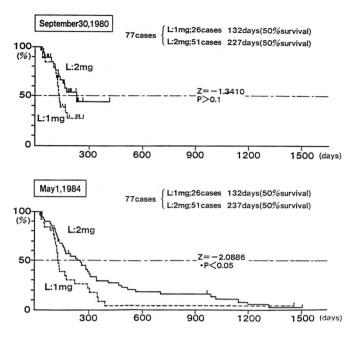

Fig. 16. Survival curve in relation to doses of lentinan: treated group with 2 mg lentinan vs treated group with 1 mg lentinan.

evaluation of the life prolongation effect as an end-point result together with the antitumor effect.

REFERENCES

1. Chihara G, Hamuro J, Maeda YY, Arai Y, Fukuoka F. Fractionation and purification of the polysaccharides with marked antitumor activity, especially lentinan, from *Lentinus edodes* (Berk.) Sing. (an edible mushroom). Cancer Res 1970; 30:2776–81.
2. Saito H, Ohki T, Takauka N, Sasaki T. A ^{13}C-N.M.R.-spectral study of a gel-forming, branched (1-3)-β-D-glucan, (lentinan) from *Lentinus edodes*, and its acid-degraded fractions. Structure, and dependence of conformation on the molecular weight. Carbohydrate Res 1977; 58:293–305.
3. Chihara G, Maeda YY, Hamuro J, Sasaki T, Fukuoka F. Inhibition of mouse sarcoma 180 by polysaccharides from Lentinus edodes, Berk. Sing. Nature 1969; 222:687–8.
4. Maeda YY, Hamuro J, Yamada Y, Ishimura K, Chihara G. The nature of immunepotentiation by the antitumor polysaccharide lentinan and the significance of biogenic amines in its action. Ciba Found Symp 1973; 18:251–86.
5. Dennert G, Tucker D. Antitumor polysaccharide lentinan—A T cell adjuvant. JNCI 1973; 51:1727–9.
6. Maeda YY, Chihara G. The effect of neonatal thymectomy of the antitumor activity of lentinan, carboxymethylpachymaran and zymozan, and their effects on various immune responses. Int J Cancer 1973; 11:153–61.
7. Dresser DW, Phillips JM. The orientation of the adjuvant activities of *Salmonella typhosa* lipopolysaccharide and lentinan. Immunology 1974; 27:895–902.
8. Fachet J, Chihara G. Effect of lentinan on tumor growth in murine allogeneic and syngeneic hosts. Int J Cancer 1980; 25:371–6.
9. Hamuro J, Chihara G. Lentinan: A T-cell-oriented immunopotentiator, its experimental and clinical applications and possible mechanism of immune modulation. In Fenichel RL, Chirigos MA, eds: Immune modulation agents and their mechanisms. Marcel Dekker, NY 1984; 25:409–36.

10. Aoki T. Lentinan. In Fenichel RL, Chirigos MA, eds: Immune modulation agents and their mechanisms. Marcel Dekker, NY 1984; 25:63–77.

11. Herlyn D, Kaneko Y, Powe J, Aoki T, Koprowski H. Monoclonal antibody-dependent murine macrophage-mediated cytotoxicity against human tumors is stimulated by lentinan. Jpn J Cancer Res (Gann) 1985; 76:37–42.

12. Taguchi T, Furue H, Majima H. Phase I study of lentinan. Jpn J Cancer Chemother 1979; 6:619–26.

13. Taguchi T, Furue H, Majima H. Phase II study of lentinan. Jpn J Cancer Chemother 1981; 8:422–34.

14. Furue H, Itoh I, Kimura T et al. Phase III study on lentinan. Jpn J Cancer Chemother 1981; 8:944–66.

15. Koyama Y, Saito T. The criteria of the Japan Society for Cancer Therapy for evaluation of clinical effects of cancer chemotheraphy on solid tumors. In: Reports on activity of cooperative study groups for cancer research by grant-in-aid of the Ministry of Health and Welfare. Tokyo: Ministry of Health and Welfare, 1980.

16. Saito T, Yokoyama M, Nakao I. Results on life prolongation by cancer chemotherapy: Comparison of the results of two surveys carried out seven years apart. Sci. Rep. Res. Inst. Tohoku Univ. Series C (Medicine), The Report of the Research Institute for Tuberculosis and Cancer 1984; 31:42–8.

Cancer Detection and Prevention Supplement 1:351–359 (1987)

Serological Evaluation of Melanoma Patients in a Phase I/II Trial of Vaccinia Melanoma Oncolysate (VMO) Immunotherapy

Marc K. Wallack, MD
Jerry A. Bash, PhD,
Katherine R. McNally, BS
Eleuthere Leftheriotis, DVM

Department of Surgery, Mount Sinai Medical Center, Miami Beach, FL (M.K.W., J.A.B., K.R.M.); Institut Merieux, Lyon, France (E.L.)

ABSTRACT   Vaccinia melanoma oncolysates (VMO) were tested in a Southeastern Cancer Study Group (SECSG)-sponsored phase I/II multiinstitutional trial. Forty-eight patients with stage I or II disease were placed on study at six different dose levels of VMO and two different dose schedules, immediate or delayed. Patients' sera, obtained before treatment and every 3 months following initiation of treatment, were tested for antimelanoma antibodies using a *Staphylococcus* protein A (SpA) assay. Pretreatment sera were negative in 46 of 47 patients, and only two of 19 patients on delayed treatment developed reactivity by 6 months. However, 13 of 23 on immediate treatment developed reactivity, including eight of eight at the higher doses (1.5 and 2.0 mg). Neither anti-HLA antibody tested by a standard microcytotoxicity assay nor circulating immune complexes measured by both Clq and conglutinin bindng assays were produced as a result of the immunization. The demonstration of immunogenicity of VMO at the 2 mg dose and immediate schedule supported the rationale for the use of this dose and schedule for the ongoing second phase Ia/Ib trial and for the future phase III randomized prospective study.

Key words: adjuvant, antibody, vaccine

INTRODUCTION

Specific active immunotherapy of cancer is based on the assumption that tumor-associated antigens are sufficiently immunogeneic to elicit a response in the patient against his own tumor. Although the existence of melanoma-associated antigens has been well documented, immune responses to autologous tumors have been difficult to elicit [1]. The possibility of increasing antitumor responses through the use of vaccines prepared from modified tumor cells has therefore been a goal for many years [2].

One of the more promising approaches to augmentation of antitumor responses is through virus infection of tumor cells. The potential of virus lysis of tumor cells as a means of

Address reprint requests to Dr. M.K. Wallack, Department of General Surgery, Mount Sinai Medical Center, 4300 Alton Road, Miami Beach, FL 33140.

lines were infected with vaccinia vaccine virus at a multiplicity of infection (MOI) of 10:1. These lines were incubated at 37°C for 20 hr at which time the cells were removed and the suspension was centrifuged. The pellet (pellet 1) was sonicated and centrifuged three times. After the final spin, the remaining pellet was discarded and the supernatant retained (supernatant 2). In the meantime, the original supernatant (supernatant 1) was centrifuged at high speed for 2 hr. The remaining supernatant was discarded, and the pellet (pellet 2) was combined with supernatant 2, to make the oncolysate. The preparation was checked for intact cells, and, when these were present, sonication and homogenization were continued. The final product was assayed by the Lowry method to determine total protein concentration and diluted to produce the six different doses. Viral content was monitored, and the presence of intact melanoma antigens was confirmed using a radioimmunoassay technique [9].

VMO Administration

Forty-eight patients were placed on study at six different dose levels (0.05, 0.10, 0.50, 1.0, 1.5, and 2.0 mg protein) and two different treatment arms. Immediate treatment involved VMO injections once per week for 13 weeks followed by injections every other week for 1 year or until a recurrence. Delayed treatment involved an initial injection of VMO followed by a 6 week interval before resumption of treatment as per immediate treatment. Four patients were sequentially assigned to each dose level and treatment arm. Each 1 ml dose of VMO was given intradermally near sites of regional lymphatics excluding the site of node dissection.

Patient Monitoring

All patients had a complete history and physical examination including performance status, temperature, weight, blood pressure, pulse, CBC, differential, platelet count, urinalysis, alkaline phosphatase, bilirubin, BUN, creatinine, LDH, SGOT, and chest X-ray. Both the physical examination and laboratory studies were repeated every 3 months. Prior to the study, liver, bone, and brain scans were generally performed. All scans were optional at yearly intervals. A smallpox booster was given 1 week prior to the initial injection of VMO.

Toxicity

In previous trials, there was both local and systemic toxicity to the VMO 7,8. Local reactions including erythema, swelling, and tenderness at the injection site. Systemic reactions included headache, malaise, nausea, and fever. Toxicity was monitored in all patients after each injection and graded according to SECSG criteria (see Table I).

Immunologic Studies

Staphylococcus protein A (SpA) assay. Blood was obtained from the patients before treatment and every 3 months during treatment. The serum was harvested and tested in an SpA assay as described by Pfreundschuh et al [10]. Briefly, for this test, cells were plated into wells of microtiter plates. After overnight incubation, the melanoma cells were first exposed to the patients' sera diluted 1/10. The plates were washed and the cells subsequently exposed to SpA convalently bound to Type O human erythrocytes. The wells were washed again and scored for rosette formation. A melanoma cell line, Mel 4, used in the preparation of VMO was used as the target cell line.

HLA antibody screen. A standard microcytotoxicity technique [11] was performed by South Florida Blood Services, Miami, and used to screen patients' sera for anti-HLA antibodies. Pretreatment and treatment sera were tested against a panel of 50 HLA-typed lymphocyte donors. Treatment sera to be tested were selected from samples positive in the SpA assay. Rabbit complement was added to initiate lysis of cells with bound antibody. Eosin stain was used to visualize the lysed cells. The results were then interpreted as 1) no cytotoxic antibodies present, 2) cytotoxic antibodies present, specific for HLA, or 3) cytotoxic antibodies, multiple specificities.

patients were originally stage I, 38 stage II. As of December, 1986, 27 patients have had recurrence, including six stage I and 20 stage II. The mean disease-free interval of these patients was 11 months, ranging from 1 to 30 months. Nine patients had recurrence prior to receiving their initial 13 VMO injections. Eight patients had recurrence prior to completion of therapy but after their initial 13 injections. Ten patients have had recurrence since completion of therapy. A total of 21 patients have died. Twenty-one patients (6 stage I and 15 stage II) remain free of disease with a mean disease-free interval of 46 months, ranging from 27 to 52 months.

Toxicity

Toxicities were graded on a scale of 0–4 as shown in Table I. Tables II–IV indicate the highest grade of toxicity noted in each patient during therapy for each of the eight reactions monitored. After 1,230 injections of VMO in these 48 patients, there were no life-threatening reactions. Of the 384 reactions reported, the majority, 328 of 384 (85%) were either grade 0 or grade 1 (see Table IV). Forty-six of forty-eight patients experienced some degree of erythema with the majority demonstrating a grade 1 reaction. Forty-three of forty-eight experienced swelling, the majority (26/48) showing a grade 1 response. Thirty-four of forty-eight patients felt tenderness at the injection site, again, the majority (29/48) with a grade 1 response. Most patients did not suffer from fever. Of the 17 who did, 14 experienced a grade 1 fever. Only five patients suffered nausea and vomiting and four of these showed a grade 1 response. Twenty-four of forty-eight patients did not demonstrate a change in their performance status. Twenty-three suffered a grade 1 response. Twenty-four of forty-eight patients suffered headaches, but 23 of those reactions were grade 1. Fifteen of forty-eight patients suffered lymphadenopathy, 12 of these grade 1 responses. Only 13 severe or grade 3 reactions were reported, eight involving erythema, three involving swelling, one involving tenderness, and one involving nausea and vomiting. Of these, nine were in patients on delayed treatment and four in patients on immediate treatment. Patients in the delayed treatment arm experiencing these reactions included four at the 0.10 mg dose, three at the 0.50 mg dose and two at the 1.0 mg dose (see Table II). Patients in the immediate treatment arm included three at the 0.10 mg dose and one at the 1.5 mg dose (see Table III).

Staphylococcus Protein A Assay (SpA)

Patients in the delayed treatment arm of the study showed minimal SpA reactivity by 6 months. By 3 months, only one of 19 patients showed reactivity. By six months two of 19 were positive (see Table VI). Patients in the immediate treatment arm showed more reactivity. By 3 months, sera from nine of 19 patients tested were positive, and by 6 months sera from 13 of 23 patients tested were positive (see Table V). All four patients at the 1.5 mg dose were positive by 3 months. Two of the four patients at the 2.0 mg dose were positive at 3 months, and all four were positive by 6 months.

HLA Testing

Pretreatment and treatment serum samples were screened for the presence of cytotoxic HLA antibodies using a standard microcytotoxicity technique. Forty-two of forty-six patients were negative both before and during treatment. Three of forty-six patients were positive both before and during treatment, and one patient was positive before treatment but negative during treatment.

Testing for Circulating Immune Complexes (CIC)

Both the conglutinin (K) and Clq binding assays were used to determine if the level of circulating immune complexes was above normal in 42 patients. Pretreatment and treatment samples were tested on each patient. Only one patient showed evidence of CIC above normal by the K binding assay, but that was in the pretreatment sample only. The treatment sample

TABLE II. Toxicity: Local and Systemic Reactions, Delayed Therapy

	0.05 mg					0.10 mg					0.50 mg					1.0 mg					1.5 mg					2.0 mg				
	0	1	2	3	4	0	1	2	3	4	0	1	2	3	4	0	1	2	3	4	0	1	2	3	4	0	1	2	3	4
Erythema	1*	2	0	0	NA†	0	2	0	2	NA	0	1	1	2	NA	0	2	0	2	NA	0	3	1	0	NA	0	3	1	0	
Swelling	1	2	1	0	NA	0	2	1	1	NA	1	1	1	2	NA	1	2	1	0	NA	0	2	2	0	NA	0	2	2	0	NA
Tenderness	1	3	0	0	NA	1	2	1	0	NA	0	2	2	0	NA	1	3	0	0	NA	1	3	0	0	NA	0	3	1	0	NA
Fever	3	1	0	0	0	2	2	0	0	0	3	1	0	0	0	2	2	0	0	0	2	2	0	0	0	1	3	0	0	0
Nausea	3	1	0	0	0	2	1	0	0	0	4	0	0	0	0	4	0	0	0	0	4	0	0	0	0	4	0	0	0	0
Performance status	3	1	0	0	0	2	2	0	0	0	2	2	0	0	0	2	2	0	0	0	2	1	1	0	0	0	4	0	0	0
Headache	3	1	0	0	NA	2	2	0	0	NA	2	2	0	0	NA	2	2	0	0	NA	2	1	1	0	NA	0	4	0	0	NA
Lymphadeno-pathy	2	2	0	0	NA	2	0	2	0	NA	2	2	0	0	NA	2	1	1	0	NA	4	0	0	0	NA	3	1	0	0	NA

*See Table I for abbreviations.

†NA, not applicable.

TABLE III. Toxicity: Local and Systemic Reactions, Immediate Therapy

	0.05 mg					0.10 mg					0.50 mg					1.0 mg					1.5 mg					2.0 mg				
	0*	1	2	3	4	0	1	2	3	4	0	1	2	3	4	0	1	2	3	4	0	1	2	3	4	0	1	2	3	4
Erythema	2	2	2	0	NA†	1	0	2	1	NA	0	1	3	0	NA	0	3	0	0	NA	1	2	1	0	NA	0	3	1	0	NA
Swelling	0	2	2	0	NA	1	0	2	1	NA	0	3	1	0	NA	0	4	0	0	NA	1	2	1	0	NA	0	4	0	0	NA
Tenderness	3	0	1	0	NA	1	1	1	1	NA	1	3	0	0	NA	0	4	0	0	NA	1	3	0	0	NA	1	2	1	0	NA
Fever	4	0	0	0	0	3	1	0	0	0	1	2	1	0	0	4	0	0	0	0	3	1	0	0	0	3	1	0	0	0
Nausea	3	1	0	0	0	4	0	0	0	0	3	1	0	0	0	4	0	0	0	0	4	0	0	0	0	4	0	0	0	0
Performance status	4	0	0	0	0	3	1	0	0	0	3	1	0	0	0	2	2	0	0	0	1	3	0	0	0	1	3	0	0	0
Headache	4	0	0	0	NA	3	1	0	0	NA	3	1	0	0	NA	2	2	0	0	NA	1	3	0	0	NA	1	3	0	0	NA
Lymphadeno-pathy	3	1	0	0	NA	2	2	0	0	NA	3	1	0	0	NA	4	0	0	0	NA	4	0	0	0	NA	2	2	0	0	NA

*See Table I for abbreviations.
†NA, not applicable.

TABLE IV. Summary of Toxicity at All Doses Tested

	Grade				
	0	1	2	3	4
Erythema	2*	24	14	8	NA†
Swelling	5	26	14	3	NA
Tenderness	11	29	7	1	NA
Fever	31	14	3	0	0
Nausea and vomiting	43	4	0	1	0
Performance status (malaise)	24	23	1	0	0
Headache	24	23	1	0	NA
Lymphadenopathy	33	12	3	0	
Total	173	155	43	13	0

*No. reported.
†NA, not applicable.

TABLE V. SpA Reactivity of Patients in the Immediate Treatment Arm

Dose (mg)	Positive by 3 months	Positive by 6 months
0.05	1/3*	1/4
0.10	0/4	0/4
0.50	2/3	2/4
1.0	0/1	2/3
1.5	4/4	4/4
2.0	2/4	4/4

*No. of patients positive/No. tested.

TABLE VI. SpA Reactivity of Patients in the Delayed Treatment Arm

Dose (mg)	Positive by 3 months	Positive by 6 months
0.05	NA*	0/2
0.10	0/1†	0/4
0.50	0/1	0/4
1.0	0/1	1/3
1.5	1/3	1/3
2.0	0/3	0/3

*Not available.
†No. of patients positive/No. tested.

showed a normal level. Twenty-eight patients showed no evidence of CIC levels above normal by the Clq binding assay. Six patients showed CIC levels above normal in their pretreatment samples only. Five patients showed CIC levels above normal in their treatment samples but not in their pretreatment. These five patients included two on delayed treatment and three on immediate treatment. Of the two patients on delayed treatment, one was on the 0.10 mg dose, the other on the 0.50 mg dose. Of the three patients on immediate treatment, one was on the 0.10 mg dose and two were on the 1.0 mg dose. Three patients had CIC levels above normal both in the pretreatment and treatment samples.

DISCUSSION

This multiinstitutional trial was organized through the SECSG. Participating institutions included Duke University, University of Alabama in Birmingham, Washington University in St. Louis, University of Virginia, and University of Miami. The primary objective of the study was to determine toxicity of the VMO on selected melanoma patients with high-risk stage I or II disease at the six different doses tested and the two different treatment schedules. Differences in immunologic testing of these patients were also observed at the different dose levels and schedules in order to determine an appropriate dose to use in the development of future studies.

Both local and systemic reactions were moderate at all the doses tested. The majority of responses to the VMO injections were mild (grade 1). It is important to note that erythema was experienced by 46 of 48 patients monitored. These local reactions were recorded only 24 hr after injection, indicating some type of immunoresponsiveness to the oncolysate. No life-threatening (grade 4) reactions were observed at any dose. The 13 grade 3 reactions seen were not dose-related. There was, therefore, no contraindication for use of the highest (2.0 mg) dose in future trials.

Although disease-free interval and survival were not an end point of this trial, all patients were followed throughout the treatment phase and are continuing to be followed at 6 month intervals. Twenty-one patients remain free from disease with a disease free interval ranging from 27 to 52 months. Twenty-seven patients have had recurrence, but nine of these were before receiving their initial 13 VMO injections. If these nine are excluded from the total number of patients, because of insufficient VMO therapy, then 18 of 39 patients have had recurrence as opposed to 27 of 48. This gives a recurrence rate of 46% vs one of 56% when all patients are included.

Staphylococcus protein A binds most human IgGs. By incubating the patients' sera with adherent cultured melanoma cells, and then adding indicator cells, we may be demonstrating the presence of antibody specific for melanoma antigens in these VMO-treated patients. Only one of 47 patients' pretreatment sample was positive in the SpA assay, indicating a definitive change in reactivity when, after 3–6 months of therapy, the serum became positive. There was minimal reactivity in patients on the delayed treatment arm at all the doses tested. By 6 months, only two of 19 patients had become positive in the SpA assay. In contrast, in the immediate treatment arm, by 3 months, nine of 19 patients were positive. By six months, 13 of 23 patients showed positive reactivity in the SpA assay. More importantly, eight of eight patients on the 1.5 and 2.0 mg doses were positive. This reactivity seen in the immediate treatment arm at the higher doses suggests that this regimen is optimal for immunostimulation of an antimelanoma antibody response, so the 2 mg dose was chosen for a subsequent phase Ia/Ib study for patient accrual. Thirty-nine patients have been put on study at the 2 mg dose. Of 27 patients tested after 3 months of treatment, 14 have become SpA-positive, and of the seven patients who have reached 6 months of treatment five have become SpA-positive. These results support the use of this dose and treatment regimen for the upcoming radomized prospective study.

The possibility had been mentioned that the reactivity seen in the SpA assay was merely antibody production against HLA antigens on the tumor cells used in the oncolysate. Screening of serum samples for the presence of such antibodies indicated no formation of HLA antibodies secondary to VMO stimulation. Forty-two of forty-six patients were negative both before and during treatment; three of 36 were positive both before and during treatment. One patient was positive before treatment but negative during treatment. None of the patients tested developed reactivity after VMO therapy; ie, they were negative pretreatment. There was no correlation between SpA reactivity and the minimal reactivity seen in the HLA screening. We recently noted the development of anti-HLA-3 antibodies in a patient who had been extensively treated with VMO over a 2 year period. Since two of the melanoma lines used in preparation of VMO express HLA-3, we performed further experiments to exclude the possibility that the antimelanoma reactivity observed in the SpA was due to anti-HLA-3. To summarize these findings: 1) The serum showed equal reactivity against all melanoma lines tested independent of their expression of HLA-3; 2) extensive absorption of the serum with pooled platelets to remove anti-HLA-3 antibody had no effect on the titer of reaction with melanoma targets (unpublished observations). These results seemed to preclude the possibility that the SpA reactivity was related to anti-HLA antibodies.

Since patients with circulating antibodies reactive with melanoma continued to be injected with antigen, the development of antigen-antibody complexes presented a potential problem for interpretation of serological data as well as for possible clinical sequelae. However, on the basis of the two assays performed to determine levels of circulating immune complexes, no meaningful evidence for elevation of immune complexes as a result of VMO stimulation was obtained. None of the treatment samples tested by the conglutinin-binding assay showed levels above the normal range. Although five of 42 patients tested showed elevated levels of complexes in treatment samples by the Clq binding assay, six patients showed elevated levels in their pretreatment samples only. Of the five patients showing elevated Clq binding during treatment, there was no correlation with dose, treatment schedule, or clinical course.

Although these serological studies confirm our previous observations concerning the production of antimelanoma antibodies during VMO treatment [7,8], we have only recently begun to study the development of cell-mediated immunity in similar patients. Our preliminary results with peripheral blood lymphocyte cultures demonstrate T-cell priming during treatment, since a proliferative response to VMO can be elicited in vitro in the presence of IL-2 [14]. Moreover, a significant response to uninfected melanoma cells can be demonstrated with lymphocytes from some patients in mixed lymphocyte-tumor cell cultures. Such stimulated cultures expanded in the presence of IL-2 then show a marked increase in melanoma-restricted cytolytic activity (unpublished observations). The relationship of the development of humoral and cellular responses to clinical course will be studied more extensively in the upcoming phase III randomized prospective trial.

Immunotherapy with VMO as an adjuvant to surgery appears to be a promising direction for future management of malignant melanoma. This SECSG phase I/II trial demonstrates that toxicity is minimal and that VMO especially at the higher doses stimulates immunoreactivity as demonstrated by the SpA assay. This reactivity is not HLA-related, nor is there evidence of immune complex formation. Based on the results of this trial, the 2.0 mg dose, immediate treatment, is being used in an ongoing SECSG phase Ia/Ib trial and will be used in the future phase III randomized prospective study.

ACKNOWLEDGMENTS

This study was supported in part by the Southeastern Cancer Study Group.

REFERENCES

1. Livingston PO, Albino AP, Chung TJC, et al. Serological responses of melanoma patients to vaccines prepared from VSV lysates of autologous and allogeneic cultured melanoma cells. Cancer 1985; 55:713-20.
2. Kobayashi H (ed). Immunological xenogenization of tumor cells (GANN Monograph on Cancer Research, No. 23). Tokyo; Japan Scientific Societies Press, and Baltimore: University Park Press, 1979
3. Sharpless GR, Davies MC, Cox HR. Antagonistic action of certain neurotropic viruses toward a lymphoid tumor in chickens with resulting immunity. Proc Soc Exp Biol Med 1950; 73:270-5.
4. Koprowski H, Love R, Koprowski I. Enhancement of susceptibility to viruses in neoplastic tissues. Texas Rep Biol Med 1957; 15:559-76.
5. Lindenmann J, Klein PA. Immunological aspects of viral oncolysis. Rec Results Cancer Res 1967; 9:1-84.
6. Wallack MK, Steplewski Z, Koprowski H, et al. A new approach in specific, active immunotherapy. Cancer 1977; 39:560-4.

7. Wallack MK, Meyer M, Burgoin A, et al. A preliminary trial of vaccinia oncolysates in the treatment of recurrent melanoma with serologic responses to the treatment. J Biol Response Modif 1983; 2:586–96.
8. Wallack MK, Michaelides MC. Serologic response to human melanoma line from patients with melanoma undergoing treatment with vaccinia melanoma oncolysates. Surgery 1984; 96:791–9.
9. Herlyn M, Clark WH, Mastrangelo MJ, et al. Specific immunoreactivity of hybridoma secreted monoclonal anti-melanoma antibodies to cultured cells. Cancer Res 1980; 40:3602–9.
10. Pfreundschuh MG, Ueda R, Rauterberg EW, Dorken BH, Shiku H. Comparison of multiple rosetting assays for detecting antibody reactivity of different immunoglobulin classes against surface antigens of benign and malignant tissue culture cells. J Immunol Meth 1980; 37:71–81.
11. Zachary AA, Braun WE (eds). The AACHT laboratory manual. New York: The American Association for Clinical Histocompatibility Testing, 1981.
12. Zubler RH, Lambert PH. The ^{125}I-Clq binding test for the detection of solid immune complexes. In Bloom BR, David JR, eds: In vitro methods in cell-mediated and tumor immunity. New York: Academic Press, 1976; 565–72.
13. Macanovic M, Lachmann TJ. Conglutinin binding polyethylene glycol precipitation assay for immune complexes. Clin Exp Immunol 1979; 38:274–83.
14. Jacubovich R, Bailly M, Gerlier D, Bourgoin A, Leftheriotis E, Wallack MK. Cellular immune response of melanoma patients to vaccinia oncolysates of allogeneic cultured melanoma cells. Cancer (in press).

Cancer Detection and Prevention Supplement 1:361–371 (1987)

BM 41.440: A New Antineoplastic, Antimetastatic, and Immune-Stimulating Drug

Dieter B.J. Herrmann, MD
Uwe Bicker, MD
Wulf Pahlke, MD

Boehringer Mannheim GmbH, Department of Immunopharmacology and Cancer Research, Mannheim, FRG

ABSTRACT   Alkyllysophospholipids are analogs of the cell membrane component lyso-phosphocholine. The thioether lysophospholipid BM 41.440 (1-hexadecylmercapto-2-methoxymethyl-rac-glycero-3-phosphocholine) is already in use in phase I and II trials in human cancer therapy. A direct antitumor effect of this new compound has been shown in vitro using 35 different cell types of murine and human origin. All normal cells investigated were not affected in the concentration range (1–10 μg/ml) that was cytotoxic for most tumor cells studied. In vivo, antimalignant and antimetastatic actions have been documented in the Meth A sarcoma, L1210 leukemia, B 16 melanoma and the [3]Lewis-lung carcinoma tumor models, respectively. Murine, bone marrow-derived macrophages (Mϕ), preincubated with BM 41.440, showed an increased cytotoxicity in vitro. Addition of syngeneic spleen cells and low doses of BM 41.440 to this system enhanced tumor cell destruction 20- to 100-fold compared to controls dependent on the target cells used (YAC, ABLS-8.1, L1210, and P815). In vivo, Meth A sarcoma growth was dose and time dependently reduced in CB6F$_1$ mice under therapeutic IV application of BM 41.440-activated Mϕ. The mean survival time of DBA mice, treated once IP with BM 41.440 4 days before L1210 challenge, increased from 24 to 38 days.

Key words: alkylglycerophosphatide, ether phospholipid, cytostatics, antimetastatics, macrophages

INTRODUCTION

Alkyllysophospholipids (ALP) are analogs of lysophosphocholine, which is an important intermediate in the continuous exchange and renewal of phospholipids in cellular membranes via a deacylation/reacylation cycle, called Lands pathway [1]. These analogs represent a new family of antitumor drugs [2]. The antineoplastic and antimetastatic effects of ALP, as verified in a variety of tumor models in vitro and in vivo [2–4], have been explained by a direct and

Address reprint requests to Dr. D.B.J. Herrmann, Boehringer Mannheim, GmbH, Department of Immunopharmacology and Cancer Research, Sandhofer Straße 116, 6800 Mannheim 31, FRG.

*When the data are expressed in this form, the figures represent the mean $\pm$ standard deviation, followed by the number of animals in parentheses.

selective cytotoxic activity on malignant cells [2,5] and by the stimulation of specific host-defense mechanisms [6–8].

BM 41.440 is a new thioether lysophospholipid analog. Its chemical structure is shown in Figure 1. The physiological lysophosphocholine molecule has been modified at two different sites: First, the ester bond in the sn-1 position of the glycerol backbone has been replaced by a thioether linkage that cannot be cleaved by phospholipases; second, the hydroxyl group in the sn-2 position has been blocked by a methoxymethyl group thereby preventing acylation of the 1-S-alkyllysophosphocholine via acyltransferases (EC 2.3.1.23) in the Lands pathway [1].

Here we report on the pharmacological in vitro and in vivo effects of BM 41.400. This compound recently entered phase I trials in human cancer therapy in West Germany.

MATERIALS AND METHODS
Chemicals and Media

BM 41.440 was synthesized by Boehringer Mannheim GmbH (Mannheim, FRG). The alkyllysophospholipid analog was supplied as a crystalline powder and stored at 4°C as a stock solution of 100 μg/ml DMEM plus 20% FCS. DMEM, horse serum, and FCS were from Boehringer Mannheim GmbH.

Cells and Continuous Cell Lines

Macrophages (Mϕ) were obtained from bone marrow cells of 8- to 12-week-old (BALB/c $\times$ C57BL/6)F$_1$ (CB6F$_1$) mice and cultivated in hydrophobic Teflon bags (Biofolie 25; Heraeus, Hanau, FRG) according to the procedure of Munder et al [9]. The Mϕ were usually harvested at day 7 by gentle shaking of the culture bags. Cell viability was checked by trypan blue exclusion and was always 90% or more.

Single cell suspensions of normal spleen cells were obtained by passing isolated spleens from 8–12-week-old female CB6F$_1$ mice through a sterile stainless-steel sieve. The cells were centrifuged (500g, 10 min), washed two times, and resuspended in DMEM plus 10% FCS.

Ascites forms of 3-methylcholanthrene–induced fibrosarcoma cells (Meth A) were propagated IP in syngeneic CB6F$_1$ mice. Tumor cells were obtained from the peritoneal cavity 7 days after inoculation of 1×10^6 cells and washed two times with DMEM.

Cells of the metastasizing [3]Lewis-lung tumor were propagated in vivo in CB6F$_1$ mice essentially as previously described [10]. All other continuous cell lines investigated in this study were serially cultivated in the log phase of growth in our laboratory.

[3H]Thymidine Incorporation Assay

The antineoplastic effect of BM 41.440 was measured as a decrease of [3H]thymidine incorporation into the target cells. The cells were suspended in DMEM, supplemented with 10% inactivated FCS (56°C, 30 min), 5×10^{-5} M 2-mercaptoethanol (Roth, Karlsruhe,

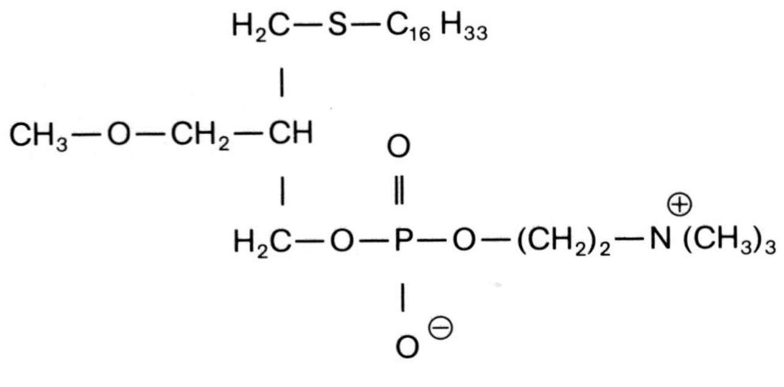

Fig. 1. Chemical structure of 1-hexadecylmercapto-2-methoxymethyl-rac-glycero-3-phosphocholine: BM 41.440.

FRG), 50 U penicillin/ml, and 50 μg streptomycin/ml (Boehringer Mannheim GmbH) at a final concentration of 5×10^3/ml in the absence or in the presence of various doses of BM 41.440. Quadruplicate cultures of 0.2 ml were incubated in a humidified atmosphere at 37°C, 10% CO_2, pH 7.4, for up to 3 days in microtiter plates (Nunc GmbH, Wiesbaden, FRG). After the times indicated in the legends to the tables and figures, the cultures were pulsed for 3 hr (cell lines) and 18 hr (human tumors) with 1 μCi [methyl-^{3}H]thymidine (specific activity, 21 Ci/mmol; New England Nuclear, Heidelberg, FRG). The cells were then harvested with a multisample harvester (Skatron AS, Lierbyen, Norway) on glass filter papers and washed repeatedly. The filter discs were dried and transferred to scintillation vials. Radioactivity was measured after addition of 2 ml Rotiszint (Roth) in a scintillation counter (Kontron MR 360; Kontron, Frankfurt, FRG).

Alkaline Phosphatase Assay

To measure target:effector cell interactions the alkaline phosphatase microtiter assay was carried out essentially as described by Ey and Ferber [11] and as modified by Munder et al [2]. This method takes advantage of the fact that the alkaline phosphatase activity (EC 3.1.3.1.) is an useful marker for tumor lines of the B lymphoid lineage and is enriched about 1,000-fold in the plasma membranes of these cells compared to membranes of macrophages and other effector cells [12].

Briefly, alkaline phosphatase-positive tumor cells ($1-5 \times 10^3$/well) were cocultured with murine, bone marrow-derived macrophages at target:effector ratios between 1:10 and 1:100 at 37°C, 10% CO_2, pH 7.4, in flat-bottomed microtiter plates in a final volume of 0.2 ml DMEM plus 10% FCS. In some experiments normal syngeneic, murine spleen cells were present in the incubations also (tumor cells:macrophages:spleen cells, 1:100:100). After the times indicated in the legends to tables and figures, the plates were centrifuged (500g, 10 min) and the pellets washed two times with PBS. Then the alkaline phosphatase was assayed in 0.1 ml/well of buffer containing 20 mM $MgCl_2$, 10% Triton X-100, 0.2 M diethanolamine HCl, pH 10.2, and 25 mM p-nitrophenylphosphate. After 1 hr incubation at room temperature the reaction was stopped with 0.1 ml 0.5 M NaOH per well, and the optical density was determined at 405 nm by means of a Titertek Multiskan (Flow Lab., Bonn, FRG). The absorbance change was linear with regard to time, for at least 4 hr, and with regard to tumor cell numbers up to 5×10^4 cells/well.

Growth Inhibition Assay

Cell viability was checked by the trypan blue exclusion assay according to Hudson and Hay [13].

Hemolysis Test

Human erythrocytes (5×10^6/ml) were incubated in PBS (pH 7.2) plus 10% FCS in the absence or presence of different concentrations of BM 41.440 at 37°C, 10% CO_2. At the times indicated aliquots of the suspensions were centrifuged, and hemoglobin was determined calorimetrically in the supernatants at 542 nm.

In Vivo Tumor Systems

Meth A fibrosarcoma. Viable cells of the Meth A transplantation tumor ($1-5 \times 10^5$ cells/mouse) were injected SC in 0.2 ml PBS into CB6F$_1$ mice. Tumor growth in control and BM 41.440-treated animals was determined by measuring two diameters (a and b) of the growing neoplasm and calculating the entire tumor volume of all mice per group by using the formula [2]:

$$V = \frac{\pi}{3} \cdot ab \cdot (a + b).$$

At the days indicated in the legends to figures and tables the experiments were terminated, and the tumor weights were determined.

[3]**Lewis-lung.** For in vivo treatment studies with BM 41.440, viable tumor cells (5–10 × 10^5/mouse) were injected into the right hind footpad of female CB6F[1] mice. Within 9 to 14 days the injected footpad reached a diameter of 0.6–0.8 cm. The primary tumors were removed at day 14 after tumor inoculation by amputating the right leg above the knee joint under phenobarbital anesthesia [10]. The [3]Lewis-lung tumor is highly malignant and metastasizes regularly to the lung [14]. The mice began to die from metastasis about 14 days after amputation. Therapeutic effects were evaluated by determining the weight of the lungs and by counting the number of metastases at the end of the experiments.

RESULTS

In a first set of experiments the direct antineoplastic activity of the thioether analog BM 41.440 on a variety of normal and malignant cell types of murine and human origin was tested concentration and time dependently in vitro using different assay systems including inhibition of [3H]thymidine incorporation, alkaline phosphatase activity, and trypan blue exclusion.

BM 41.440 had an inhibitory effect on the proliferation of three different human leukemic cell lines, K562, HL60, and Molt4 (Fig. 2). From this type of experiment C_{50} values, ie, the concentration of BM 41.400 that causes 50% tumor growth inhibition, were determined as a measurement of sensitivity/resistance of each cell type.

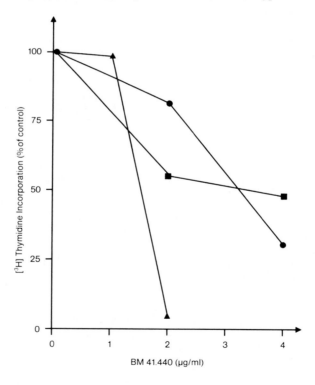

Fig. 2.   Effect of BM 41.440 on the proliferation of HL60, K562, and Molt 4 leukemia cells. Cells (1 × 10^4/ml) were incubated in DMEM + 10% FCS, pH 7.4, in 10% CO_2 at 37°C in microtiter plates for 48 hr. Then [3H]thymidine incorporation was determined as described in Materials and Methods. Mean of six cultures, SD < 15%. ▲, HL60; ●, K562; ■, Molt4.

For most tumor cell lines investigated, a C_{50} concentration between 0.5 to 2.0 μg/ml was found (Tables I and II). L929S and 3T3 fibroblasts, murine macrophages ($C_{50} > 35$ μg/ml), rat hepatocytes, and human erythrocytes (50% hemolytic concentration of BM 41.440: 42 μg/ml; 48 hr) were resistant within this concentration range and showed C_{50} values approximately 10- to 100-fold higher than those for sensitive tumor target cells. On the other hand, if 3T3 fibroblasts were transformed to malignant cells by SV40 virus (3T3 SV 40), these cells became susceptible to the cytotoxic attack of BM 41.440, with a C_{50} value of about 2 to 3 μg/ml (Table I).

Similar results were obtained from investigations on the antimalignant effect of BM 41.440 on seven different human esophageal tumor cell lines, five human acute and chronic myelogenous leukemias, and four human brain tumors (three glioblastomas, one meningioma) using the [3H]thymidine incorporation technique (data not shown).

In vivo, the antitumor activity of BM 41.440 has been documented in the methylcholanthrene-induced fibrosarcoma, L1210 leukemia and in the B16 melanoma tumor model.

Meth A tumor growth inhibition was observed in female CB6F$_1$ mice that were orally treated every second day from days 1 to 19 after tumor inoculation with a low dose of BM 41.440 (2.5 mg/kg bw) (Fig. 3.). A significant reduction of the tumor volume could be

TABLE I. Effect of BM 41.440 on the Proliferation of Different Cell Types of Murine Origin In Vitro

Cells or cell lines	Cell type	C_{50} (μg/ml)
Meth A	Methylcholanthrene-induced fibrosarcoma	0.7
L1210	Leukemia	1.1
ABLS-8.1	Abelson "pre-B" lymphoma	2.0
YAC	Moloney virus-induced lymphoma	1.3
P 815	Mastocytoma	1.7
[3]Lewis lung (metastasis)	Metastazing carcinoma	19.6
L929S	Chemically transformed embryo fibroblasts	24.3
3T3	Fibroblasts	>20
3T3-SV 40	SV 40-virus transformed 3T3 fibroblasts	~2–3

Cells, 5×10^3/ml DMEM plus 10% FCS, were incubated in the absence or presence of different concentrations of BM 41.440 at 37°C, 10% CO_2. After 48 hr [3H] thymidine incorporation was determined as described in Materials and Methods. C_{50}, 50% inhibition concentration of BM 41.440.

TABLE II. Effect of BM 41.440 on the Proliferation of Different Tumor Cell Lines of Human Origin In Vitro

Cells or cell lines	Cell type	C_{50} (μg/ml)
Raji	EBV B-cell lymphoma	1.0
Daudi	B-cell lymphoma	0.6
U 937	Histocytic lymphoma	1.4
HL 60	Promyelocytic leukemia	1.5
REH	Non-B, non-T-cell lymphoma	1.0
K 562	Erythroleukemia	5.5
Molt 4	T-cell leukemia	5.9

For experimental details, see legend to Table I and Materials and Methods. C_{50}, 50% inhibition concentration of BM 41.440.

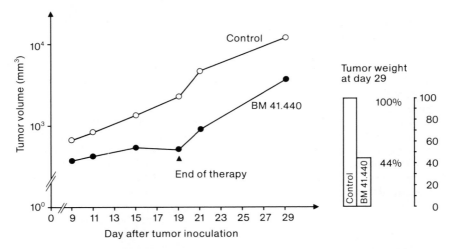

Fig. 3.   BM 41.440-induced inhibition of Meth A fibrosarcoma growth in CB6F$_1$ mice. Meth A sarcoma cells (1–5 × 10^5 cells/mouse) were injected SC in 0.2 ml PBS into female CB6F$_1$ mice (ten animals/group) at day 0. From days 1 to 19 after tumor inoculation treated animals received 2.5 mg BM 41.440/kg bw PO every second day. The tumor volumes were determined as described in Materials and Methods. At day 29 the experiments were terminated, and the tumors were weighed.

TABLE III. Antimetastatic Effect of BM 41.440 in the [3]Lewis-Lung Tumor Model

BM 41.440 (mg/kg)	Weight of the lungs (mg, means ± SD)	No. of metastases			
		0	1–2	2–5	>5
—	495 ± 47	0	1	2	14
0.005	364 ± 81	4	4	2	4
0.05	331 ± 65	7	0	4	4
0.5	221 ± 39	7	3	4	1
2.5	177 ± 27	10	3	2	0
5.0	231 ± 41	8	4	2	1

[3]Lewis-lung tumor cells (5 × 10^5 cells/mouse) were injected into the right hind footpad of female CB6F$_1$ mice (N = 14–20 mice/group). The hind leg was amputated as described in Materials and Methods at day 14. The animals in the treated groups received the appropriate dose of BM 41.440 PO every second day from days 14 to 28 after tumor inoculation. The experiments were terminated at day 28. The weights of the lungs and the numbers of metastases in the lungs were determined.

achieved as long as BM 41.440 was applied. Moreover, in treated animals the mean tumor weight was 44% that of controls at day 29.

The antimetastatic effect of BM 41.440 was studied in the [3]Lewis-lung tumor system in CB6F$_1$ mice. [3]Lewis-lung tumor cells regularly metastasize into the lungs if injected into the hind paw of mice. The grade of metastasis can be evaluated by determining the weights of the lungs and/or by counting the metastases in the lungs. Animals in the control group had a mean lung weight of 495 ± 47 (17)* mg at day 28 after tumor inoculation (Table III). In 14 out of 17 mice more than five metastases were found in the lungs. In treated groups a dose-dependent reduction of the weight of the lungs to 177 ± 27 (15) mg was observed, with an optimal concentration of BM 41.440 of 2.5 mg/kg bw given PO every second day. Furthermore, ten out of 15 animals in that group were absolutely free of lung metastases.

Alkyllysophospholipid analogs are known to activate immune-competent cells to cyto-toxic effector cells [6–8]. Therefore, in the following experiments the effect of BM 41.440 on murine bone marrow-derived macrophages (Mϕ) and normal spleen cells was studied in vitro.

A Meth A tumor growth inhibition was induced by Mϕ that had been preincubated for 24 hr together with 10 μg BM 41.440/ml (Fig. 4). While normal, nonactivated Mϕ essentially did not influence tumor proliferation, a significant inhibition of tumor growth was seen when target and preactivated effector cells were cocultured up to 3 days. In addition, data, not shown here, revealed that the inhibition of [^{3}H]thymidine incorporation into Meth A fibrosarcoma cells was dependent on the target to effector cell ratio and on the Mϕ preactivating dose of BM 41.440.

To examine the combined action of Mϕ and normal syngeneic spleen cells on tumor growth the alkaline phosphatase-positive tumor cell lines YAC, ABLS-8.1, L1210, and P815 were used as target cells. In this system, inhibition of target cell proliferation can be readily investigated by a decrease in the alkaline phosphatase activity, which is directly correlated to the actual tumor cell number in the cultures [2].

As shown by the optical density values (OD$_{405}$) coincubation of P815 cells together with normal Mϕ and spleen cells did not affect the proliferation of these neoplastic cells up to 72 hr (Fig. 5). When Mϕ were preactivated with BM 41.440 a significant reduction in the alkaline phosphatase activity (OD$_{405}$ = 9.8) compared to the control (OD$_{405}$ = 19.0) became obvious, probably indicating an inhibition of tumor cell growth mediated by the immune cells also present in the cultures. Addition of BM 41.440 in small amounts (2 μg/ml) to this system

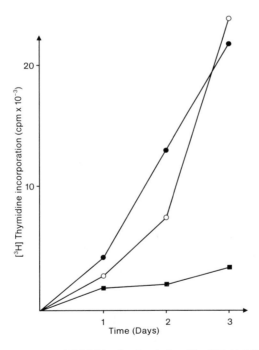

Fig. 4.   Meth A fibrosarcoma growth inhibition in vitro induced by BM 41.440-activated bone marrow-derived macrophages. Macrophages were grown from murine bone marrow cells and activated to cytotoxic effector cells by preincubation with 10 μg BM 41.440/ml DMEM plus 10% FCS. Then Meth A cells (1 $\times$ 10^3 cells/well) were coincubated with activated (aMϕ) or nonactivated (Mϕ) macrophages up to 3 days in microtiter plates at a target:effector ratio of 1:100. At the times indicated the experiments were terminated, and the [^{3}H]thymidine incorporation was determined. Mean of six cultures, SD < 15%. ●, controls; O, Mϕ; ■, aMϕ

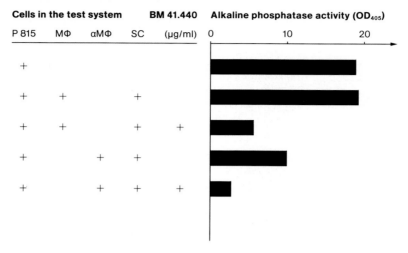

Fig. 5. Activation of murine bone marrow-derived macrophages and spleen cells to cytotoxic effector cells by BM 41.440. P815 target cells (5×10^3 cells/well) were cocultured, where indicated, with 1×10^5 nonactivated (Mϕ) and preactivated (aMϕ; 24 hr, 10 μg BM 41.440/ml) macrophages, respectively, and with 1×10^5 syngeneic spleen cells (SC) at 37°C in 10% CO_2 in microtiter plates in a final volume of 0.2 ml DMEM plus 10% FCS. In some cultures BM 41.440 was additionally present in a final concentration of 2 μg/ml. At the times indicated the alkaline phosphatase activity, expressed as optical density (OD_{405}), was determined as described in Materials and Methods. Data are given as means of quadruplicates, SD < 10%.

TABLE IV. Meth A Tumor Growth Inhibition Induced by BM 41.440-Activated Macrophages

Therapy	Tumor volume (mm^3)	Tumor weight (mg)	Tumor free/total
—	6.156 ± 1.569	1.080 ± 214	0/10
1×10^6 Mϕ/mouse	6.678 ± 1.721	1.142 ± 249	0/10
10×10^6 Mϕ/mouse	4.069 ± 1.095	876 ± 226	1/10
1×10^6 aMϕ/mouse	2.414 ± 0.784	535 ± 156	2/10
10×10^6 aMϕ/mouse	2.067 ± 0.606	573 ± 139	1/10

Meth A sarcoma cells (2×10^5 cells/mouse) were injected s.c. at day 0 in female CB6F$_1$ mice (N = 10). At days 3, 7, 14, and 17 after tumor inoculation, treated groups received 1×10^6 or 10×10^6 nonactivated (Mϕ) or activated (aMϕ) macrophages per mouse IV in a final volume of 0.2 ml PBS. Activated Mϕ were preincubated prior to injection in vitro for 24 hr in the presence of 10 μg BM 41.440/ ml DMEM plus 10% FCS. At day 22 the entire tumor volume of all animals per group (see Materials and Methods), the mean tumor weight, and the number of tumor-free animals per group were determined. Data are given as mean ± S.D.

further enhanced the inhibition of P815 proliferation. Similar results were obtained with YAC, ABLS-8.1, and L1210 as target cells (data not shown).

In a next series of experiments a possible therapeutic effect of IV applications of Mϕ that had been preactivated by BM 41.440 in vitro was investigated in the Meth A sarcoma model. Mean tumor volume and mean tumor weight were reduced 22 days after SC inoculation of 2×10^5 Meth A cells per mouse, dependent on both the number of Mϕ injected IV and their activation state (Table IV). Moreover, two out of ten animals were tumor free in the group in which each of the animals had received 1×10^6 preactivated Mϕ four times.

A prophylactic effect of BM 41.440 was seen in the L1210 leukemia system (Table V). When the thioether phospholipid was only applied once IP 4 days prior to L1210 injection into

TABLE V. Prophylactic Effect of BM 41.440 on the L1210 Leukemia Cells

BM 41.440 (mg/kg)	Mean survival time (days)	Range (days)	Survivors/ total
—	24	20–33	0/10
12.5	27	19–49	0/10
25.0	38	23–59	2/10

L1210 leukemia cells (1×10^3 cells/mouse) were injected IP in female DBA mice (N = 10). Animals in the treated groups received a single IP application of BM 41.440 4 days before L1210 challenge. The mean survival time and the number of tumor-free animals per group 60 days after L1210 inoculation were determined.

mice, the mean survival time increased dose dependently from 24 to 38 days in the treated groups. Two out of ten animals survived 60 days after L1210 inoculation.

DISCUSSION

This investigation is part of a research program aimed at elucidating the pharmacological effects of the 1-S-alkyl analog of lysophosphocholine (BM 41.440) on normal and neoplastic cells in vitro and in vivo. A panel of 35 different cell types, normal and malignant, proliferating and nonproliferating, continuous lines and spontaneous cells, of murine and of human origin, were screened for their sensitivity toward BM 41.440. The present data indicate that BM 41.440 is one of the most potent cytotoxic alkyllysophospholipids reported so far [2,15], with a high selectivity to neoplastic cells. This is demonstrated by the 10- to 100-fold higher C_{50} values of normal cells, including fibroblasts, macrophages, hepatocytes, and erythrocytes, compared to those of the susceptible tumor cell types (Tables I and II). In particular, the selective cytotoxicity of BM 41.440 was reflected by the differences in sensitivities of 3T3 and 3T3-SV 40 fibroblasts, respectively (Table I). Thus, our results are in agreement with the observations of others who described a direct and selective cytotoxic action of related 1-O-alkyl analogs on neoplastic cells [2,5,16,17].

The direct antitumor activity of BM 41.440 in vitro was not dependent on cellular proliferation as shown, for instance, by Meth A sarcoma cells and L929S fibroblasts (Table I). Although both cell lines have nearly the same doubling time (approximately 17–20 hr), the C_{50} concentration of BM 41.440 for L929S was about 28-fold higher compared to the C_{50} for Meth A, indicating sensitivity of Meth A and resistance of L929S to the cytotoxic attack of the thioether phospholipid. Thus, the present data confirm the recent observations with a closely related 1-O-alkyl derivative [17].

The molecular mechanism for selective cytocidal destruction of sensitive tumor cells is probably mediated by disturbances of the normal membrane phospholipid turnover [16–18], which may consecutively result in disruption of membrane integrity [19]. The answer to the question whether the lack of a 1-O-alkyl clevage enzyme in sensitive malignant cells [2,5,15] and/or different affinities of ALP to different cell types [20] could account for the selectivity of BM 41.440 and some other cytotoxic ALP remains controversial and is under investigation in our laboratory. Other mechanisms may also be involved in the direct cytolysis [21].

In a variety of animal tumor models, structurally closely related 1-O-alkyllysophospholipid analogs, have been shown to possess a therapeutic antineoplastic and antimetastatic effect in vivo [2,6]. The present investigations revealed a strong antimalignant activity of an oral treatment with BM 41.440 in vivo, as demonstrated with regard to weight and volume of tumors, prolongation of mean survival time, and increase of the number of tumor-free animals in the Meth A fibrosarcoma (Fig. 3), L1210 leukemia, and B16 melanoma tumor systems. Furthermore, oral application of BM 41.440 immediately after resection of the primary tumor at day 14 after tumor inoculation proved to be effective in inhibiting either the metastatic spread of [3]Lewis-lung cells from the implantation area or their local growth in the lungs (Table IV).

Because by the time of resection, tumor cells have already metastasized in the lung [22] inhibition of local metastatic growth may be possible. On the other hand, concerning the resistance of lung metastases to the direct cell destructive effect of BM 41.440 in vitro (Table I) inhibition of the metastatic spread seems more likely. An antiinvasive effect of the thioether phospholipid has been described by other investigators [23].

Numerous communications on ALP report its immune-stimulating effect [24]. The antitumor activity has frequently been interpreted as being partly mediated by the generation of tumoricidal immune-competent cells from the monocyte-macrophage lineage [2, 6–8].

The results from the experiments in which bone marrow-derived macrophages (Mϕ) alone or in combination with syngeneic spleen cells as a source of natural killers were used as effector cells (Fig. 4, Table V) also indicate that BM 41.440 was able at least in vitro to enhance tumor cell destruction. Moreover, low doses of the thioether phospholipid seemed to boost preactivated Mϕ (Table V). This finding is in agreement with data reported previously on 1-O-alkyl analogs [25].

In vivo, tumor growth of Meth A sarcoma was dose and time dependently reduced in CB6F$_1$ mice under therapeutic IV application of Mϕ preactivated by BM 41.440 in vitro (Table IV). BM 41.440 has a half-life in mice of about 30 hr (data not shown). The prophylactic effect of a single IP application of the compound 4 days prior to L1210 challenge may, therefore, also be explained by a stimulation of host-defense mechanisms. Peritoneal cells, mainly consisting of macrophages [2], have been shown to become activated by lysophosphocholine and ALP [2,24,25].

In conclusion, the data presented here indicate that the 1-S-alkyllysophospholipid BM 41.440 is a very potential antineoplastic, antimetastatic, and, at least in vitro, immune-stimulating compound. Clinical phase I and II trials, recently started in West Germany, will show whether these interesting biological activities will also hold true in human cancer therapy.

ACKNOWLEDGMENTS

We thank Mrs. M. Mosbacher for preparing the manuscript.

REFERENCES

1. Hill EE, Lands WEM. Phospholipid metabolism. In Wakil SJ Jr, ed: Lipid metabolism. New York: Academic Press, 1970: 185–277.
2. Munder PG, Modolell M, Bausert W, Oettgen HF, Westphal O. Alkyllysophospholipids in cancer therapy. In Hersh EM, Chirigos MA, Mastrangelo MJ, eds: Augmenting agents in cancer therapy. New York: Raven Press, 1981: 441–57.
3. Andreesen R, Modolell M, Weltzien HU, et al. Selective destruction of human leukemic cells by alkyllysophospholipids. Cancer Res. 1978; 38:3894–9.
4. Berdel WE. Antineoplastic activity of synthetic lysophospholipid analogs. Blut 1982; 44:71–8.
5. Andreesen R, Modolell M, Munder PG. Selective sensitivity of chronic myelogenous leukemia cell populations to alkyll-lysophospholipids. Blood 1979; 54:519–23.
6. Munder PG, Weltzien HU, Modolell M. Lysolecithin analogs: A new class of immunopotentiators. In Miescher PA, ed: Immunopathology. 7th Int Symp June 15–17, 1976. Basel:Schwabe & Co, 1976: 411–24.
7. Andreesen R, Osterholz J, Luckenbach A, et al. Tumor cytotoxicity of human macrophages after incubation with synthetic analogues of 2-lysophosphatidylcholine. JNCI 1984; 72:53–9.
8. Berdel WE, Fink U, Egger B, Reichert A, Munder PG, Rastetter J. Growth inhibition of malignant hypernephroma cells by autologous lysophospholipid incubated macrophages obtained by a new method. Anticancer Res 1981; 1:135–40.
9. Munder PG, Modolell M, Wallach DFH. Cell propagation on films of polymeric fluorocarbon as a means to regulate pericellular pH and pO$_2$ in cultured monolayers. FEBS Lett 1971; 15:191–6.
10. Treves AJ, Cohen IR, Feldman M. Brief communication: Immunotherapy of lethal metastases by lymphocytes sensitized against tumor cells in vitro. JNCI 1975; 54:777–9.

11. Ey PL, Ferber E. Calf thymus alkaline phosphatase. I. Properties of the membrane-bound enzyme. Biochim Biophys Acta 1977; 480:403–16.

12. Culvenor JG, Harris AW, Mandel TE, Whitelaw A, Ferber E. Alkaline phosphatase in hematopoetic tumor cell lines of the mouse: high activity in cells of the B lymphoid lineage. J Immunol 1981; 126:1974–7.

13. Hudson C, Hay FC. Viable lymphocyte count. In Hudson C, Hay FC, eds: Practical immunology. Oxford: Blackwell, 1976: 29–32.

14. Treves AJ, Carnaud C, Trainin N, Feldman M, Cohen IR. Enhancing T lymphocytes from tumor-bearing mice suppress host resistance to a syngeneic tumor. Eur J Immunol 1974; 4:722–7.

15. Hoffman DR, Hajdu J, Snyder F. Cytotoxicity of platelet activating factor and related alkyl-phospholipid analogs in human leukemic cells, polymorphonuclear neutrophils, and skin fibroblasts. Blood 1984; 63:545–52.

16. Modolell M, Andreesen R, Pahlke W, Brugger U, Munder PG. Disturbance of phospholipid metabolism during the selective destruction of tumor cells induced by alkyl-lysophospholipids. Cancer Res 1979; 39:4681–6.

17. Herrmann DBJ. Changes in cellular lipid synthesis of normal and neoplastic cells during cytolysis induced by alkyl lysophospholipid analogues. JNCI 1985; 75:423–30.

18. Vogler WR, Whigham E, Bennett WD, Olson AC. Effect of alkyl-lysophospholipids on phosphatidylcholine biosynthesis in leukemic cell lines. Exp Hematol 1985; 13:629–33.

19. Berdel WE, Fromm M, Fink U, et al. Cytotoxicity of thioether-lysophospholipids in leukemias and tumors of human origin. Cancer Res 1983; 43:5538–43.

20. Herrmann DBJ, Neumann HA. Cytotoxic ether phospholipids: Different affinities to lysophosphocholine acyltransferases in sensitive and resistant cells. J. Biol Chem 1986; 261:7742–47.

21. Helfman DM, Barnes KC, Kinkade JM Jr, Vogler WR, Shoji M, Kuo JF. Phospholipid-sensitive Ca^{2+}-dependent protein phosphorylation system in various types of leukemic cells from human patients and in human leukemic cell lines HL60 and K562, and its inhibition by alkyl-lysophospholipids. Cancer Res 1983; 43:2955–61.

22. James SE, Salsbury AJ. Effects of ($\pm$)-1,2-bis(3,5-dioxy-piperazin-l-yl)propane on tumour blood vessels and its relationship to the antimetastatic effect in the Lewis lung carcinoma. Cancer Res 1974; 34:839–44.

23. Storme, GA, Berdel WE, van Blitterswijk WJ, Bruyneel EA, DeBruyne GK, Marcel MM. Antiinvasive effect of racemic 1-0-octadecyl-2-0-methylglycero-3-phosphocholine on MO_4 mouse fibrosarcoma cells in vitro. Cancer Res 1985; 45:351–7.

24. Weltzien HU, Munder PG. Synthetic alkyl analogs of lysophosphocholine: Membrane activity, metabolic stability, and effects on immune response and tumor growth. In Mangold HK, Paltauf F, eds: Ether lipids. New York: Academic Press, 1983: 277–308.

25. Herrmann DBJ, Munder PG. Alterations in tumor cell lipid composition induced by activated macrophages. Cancer Detect Prev 1985; 8:597 (abstract).

26. Ngwenya BZ, Yamamoto N. Activation of peritoneal macrophages by lysophosphatidylcholine. Biochem Biophys Acta 1985; 839: 9–15.

Cancer Detection and Prevention Supplement 1:373–376 (1987)

Transfer Factor For Adjuvant Immunotherapy in Cervical Cancer

G. Wagner, MD
W. Knapp, MD
E. Gitsch, MD
S. Selander, MD

I^{st} (G.W., E.G.) and IInd (S.S.) Departments of Obstetrics and Gynecology and Institute of Immunology (W.K.), University of Vienna, Vienna, Austria

ABSTRACT In a prospective randomized double-blind study of 60 patients with invasive cervical cancer, 32 were treated with transfer factor (TF) derived from leukocytes of the patients' husbands, and 28 were treated with placebo. Within the first 2 years after radical hysterectomy, five out of 32 TF-treated patients and 11 out of 28 placebo-treated patients developed recurrence of malignancy. Excluding one further patient with intercurrent death this difference is significant ($\chi^2 = 3.9915$; $P < 0.05$). Subdividing the collectives, significant differences were found in patients aged below 35 years and in patients with stage I disease. Identical immune profiles were checked in leukocyte donors prior to leukophoresis and were serially checked in patients. Antigen-specific correlations were found between donors' and recipients' reactivities but not between donors' reactivity and recipient's course of the disease.

Key words: dialyzable leukocyte extracts, adjuvant cancer therapy, gynecologic malignancy

INTRODUCTION

Thirty years ago Lawrence [1] first described the transfer of delayed hypersensitivity by disrupted leukocytes. In subsequent studies this phenomenon was identified as a function of the low-molecular weight fraction, the so-called transfer factor (TF) [2]. Although much information on components, properties, and functions of TF were subsequently obtained [3–5], many questions about this substance, especially concerning its therapeutic value in clinical oncology, remain unresolved. To evaluate the clinical efficacy of TF for invasive cervical cancer a prospective randomized double-blind trial of TF versus placebo was initiated at the two gynecological clinics of the University of Vienna.

METHODS

Criteria for selection of patients were defined as cases of squamous cell carcinoma, with histologically proven tumor stage Ic (ie, tumor invasion into the outer third of the cervical

Address reprint requests to Dr. Gerhard Wagner, I. Univ. Frauenklinik, Spitalgasse 23, A-1090 Wien, Austria.

wall) or higher stages and/or pelvic lymph node involvement as well as complete standard therapy (i.e, radical hysterectomy according Latzko-Meigs or Wertheim followed by irradiation). Prior to randomization patients fulfilling the described criteria of selection were grouped according to the histological stage, their age, and the clinic responsible for standard therapy. The patients' husbands were selected as cell donors for TF preparation, which was carried out according to procedures described elsewhere [6]. Isotone saline mixed with vitamin B complex was used as placebo. According to the above-mentioned criteria 60 patients entered the study. Thiry-two patients were selected for treatment with TF and 28 were selected for placebo. The distribution of stage, lymph node involvement, and age was similar in both groups. About 3 weeeks after surgery, prior to radiation, adjuvant therapy was started with either 2 units of TF or 2 ml of placebo administered subcutaneously. This therapy was continued at monthly intervals for a period of 2 years except in cases of recurrence. Clinical and immunological investigations at 3 month intervals consisted of peripheral leukocyte, lymphocyte, and T lymphhocyte counts, skin tests with recall antigens and neoantigens, as well as mitogen- and antigen-induced lymphocyte blastogenesis. Identical immune profiles had been carried out in cell donors prior to cell separation. The rate of nonrecurrence within 2 years was evaluated as the main criterion of clinical efficacy of TF therapy. Because of lethal intercurrent disease one patient in the TF group had to be excluded from evaluation.

RESULTS

Five (16.1%) patients treated with TF and 11 (39.3%) patients treated with placebo were found to have developed recurrent disease within the 2 year period. This difference was found to be significant with the chi square test ($\chi^2 = 3.9915$; $P < 0.05$).This difference was even more pronounced when patients who were treated less than 3 months with TF or placebo were excluded ($\chi^2 = 6.0952$; $P < 0.05$) because early recurrence occurred in two patients in the TF group with a fatal outcome within a few weeks.

To determine which of the patients had most benefit from TF therapy, the rates of recurrence were evaluated in subclassified collectives of both treatment groups. In spite of small numbers, significant differences were found in patients with stage I disease ($\chi^2 = 5,5588$; $P < 0.05$) and in patients aged below 35 years ($\chi^2 = 4.4444$; $P < 0.05$), whereas the collectives with stage II disease and with ages over 35 years demonstrated only minimal differences ($\chi^2 = 0.4857$ and 0.9360, respectively). Patients with lymph node metastases had a markedly greater difference in recurrence rate than those without lymph node involvement ($\chi^2 = 3.2318$ and 1.1243, respectively).

Contrary to the well-defined differences that were observed in the clinical course of disease, most of the serially checked laboratory tests did not reveal considerable differences. The course of mean peripheral leukocyte counts was nearly identical in both groups, demonstrating a marked increase after surgery followed by a significant decrease after irradiation. Similarly no significant effects of adjuvant therapy on mean values of peripheral lymphocyte and T lymphocyte counts and of PHA-induced lymphocyte transformation were noted by analysis of variance for statistical calculation. In both collectives a significant decrease in these mean values was found after radiation therapy followed by an increase.

In contrast to this lack of any differences, the in vitro lymphocyte responses to several antigens (PPD, Varidase, KLH) were significantly reduced in the postoperative course of patients treated with placebo, whereas patients in the TF group demonstrated only minor variations in serial postoperative test results. A slight but not significant reduction in postoperative reactivity of skin tests with recall antigen (PPD, Varidase, Candidin) was found in the placebo group but not in the TF group possibly as a result of different recurrence rates. Patients with recurrence had significantly lower reactivity of skin tests than those who were free of disease at the time of this study.

No difference in postoperative reactivity was found in the skin tests with the neoantigen DNCB: In both groups only a small minority of patients demonstrated typical delayed hypersensitivity reactions when they were tested with a challenge dose prior as well as 2 weeks after sensitization. Contrary to this result, skin tests with KLH revealed a distinct difference between both treatment groups: Prior to sensitization the reactivity in the low dose test (20 mcg) was significantly better in the TF group compared to the Placebo group ($\chi^2 = 9.5050$; P < 0.01). After sensitization Placebo-treated patients had a similar reactivity and no evidence of a significant difference ($\chi^2 = 1.2451$).

Identical tests for evaluation of nonspecific cell-mediated immunity were also carried out in cell donors. To determine any possible transfer of immunity [3,5,7] postoperative reactivity to the tested antigens were compared in donors and recipients. By comparison of the total postoperative skin test results of TF-treated patients with skin test results of their cell donors a significant correlation was found in all antigen tests with the exception of DNCB. Direct dependency on donors' reactivity was evident in Varidase, Candidin, and KLH tests ($\chi^2 = 54.3444$, P < 0.001; $\chi^2 = 24.8028$, P < 0.001; $\chi^2 = 23.2425$, P < 0.001, respectively). In contrast to these findings, skin tests with PPD led to the highest rate of anergic reactions in patients treated with TF that was obtained from highly responding donors ($\chi^2 = 19.7218$; P < 0.001). Similar results were obtained by correlation of antigen-induced in vitro lymphocyte blastogenesis: A distinct, partially significant correlation, indicating direct dependency on donors' reactivity, was found in transformation tests with Candidin and Tetanus-Toxoid, whereas PPD transformation tests revealed a marked, partially significant negative correlation throughout the second year of TF treatment. No considerable dependency on donors' reactivity was found in lymphocyte transformation tests with Varidase and KLH. However, no influence of donors' reactivity on the recipients' course of disease was evident by either skin test or laboratory tests.

DISCUSSION

The results presented in this short communication lend support to the suggestion of a beneficial effect of TF in cervical cancer treatment, especially in younger patients with stage I disease. Similar results were reported in adjuvant TF therapy of lung cancer [8,9], malignant melanoma [10], osteogenic sarcoma [11], and other malignancies [5,12]. However, negative results of TF therapy were reported for malignancies as well as for other diseases [13–17]. Because the relationship between the clinical effect and the transfer of delayed-type hypersensitivity (DTH) or its suppression (PPD response) by TF was not evaluated, a different mechanisms of action must be assumed. Although the significant test results indicated transfer of DTH, the therapeutic mode of action of TF was not elucidated. A question of considerable importance deals with the selection of cell donors. At present no definitive conclusions can be drawn from past clinical studies about its influence on the beneficial clinial effects of TF, although reports on adjuvant TF treatment obtained from long-term survivors, relatives and household contacts seem to suggest satisfactory results. It remains unresolved in this article as to whether new laboratory methods may lead to improved prognosis and assessment of the clinical effect of TF. Therefore, further clinical and experimental studies are required to clarify some of the unresolved questions.

REFERENCES

1. Lawrence HS. The transfer in humans of delayed skin sensitivity to streptococcal M substance and to tuberculin with disrupted leukocytes. J Clin Invest 1955; 34:219–30.
2. Lawrence HS, Al-Askari S, David J, Franklin EC, Zweiman B. Transfer of immunological information in humans with dialysates of leukocyte extracts. Trans Assoc Am Physicians 1963; 76:84–9.
3. Spitler LE, Levin AS, Fudenberg HH. Human lymphocyte transfer factor. In Busch H, ed: Methods in cancer research, Vol 8. New York: Academic Press, 1973:59–106.
4. Khan A, Kirkpatrick CH, Hill NO, eds: Immune regulators in transfer factor. New York: Academic Press, 1979.
5. Kirkpatrick CH: Transfer factor. In Bastsakis J, Savory J, eds: Critical reviews in clinical laboratory sciences. West Palm Beach: CRC Press, 1980: 87–122.

6. Basten A, Pollard JD, Stewart GJ, et al. Transfer factor in treatment of multiple sclerosis. Lancet 1980; ii:931–4.

7. Wilson GB, Fudenberg HH. Is controversy about "transfer factor therapy" nearing an end? Immunol Today 1983; 4:157–61.

8. Fujisawa T, Yamaguchi Y, Kimura H, Arita M, Baba M, Shiba M. Adjuvant immunotherapy of primary resected lung cancer with transfer factor. Cancer 1984; 54:663–9.

9. Kirsh MM, Orringer MB, McAuliffe S, Schork MA, Katz B, Silva J Jr. Transfer factor in the treatment of carcinoma of the lung. Ann Thoracic Surg 1984; 38:140–5.

10. Blume MR, Rosenbaum EH, Cohen RJ, Gershow J, Glassberg AB, Shepley E. Adjuvant immunotherapy of high risk stage I melanoma with transfer factor. Cancer 1981; 47:882–8.

11. Ritts RE Jr, Pritchard DJ, Taylor WF, Gilchrist GS, Ivins JE. Comparison of transfer factor and combination chemotherapy as post surgical adjuvants in osteogenic sarcoma: results at three years. In Rainer H, Borberg H, Mishler JM, Schäfer U, eds: Immunotherapy of malignant diseases. Stuttgart: Schattauer, 1978: 343–52.

12. Grob PJ, Arrenbrecht S. Indications and limitations for transfer factor therapy. In Steffen C, Ludwig H, eds: Clinical immunology and allergology. Amsterdam: Elsevier, 1981: 207–18.

13. Goldenberg GJ, Brandes LJ, Lau WH, Miller AB, Wall C, Ho JH. Cooperative trial of immunotherapy for naso-pharyngeal carcinoma with transfer factor from donors with Epstein-Barr virus antibody activity. Cancer Treat Rep 1985; 69:761–7.

14. Gilchrist GS, Pritchard DJ, Dahlin DC, Ivins JC, Taylor WF, Edmonson JN. Management of osteogenic sarcoma. A perspective based on the Mayo clinic experience. Natl Cancer Inst Monogr 1981; 56:193–9.

15. Schwartz MA, Gutterman JU, Burgess MA. Chemoimmunotherapy of disseminated malignant melanoma with DTIC-BCG, transfer factor and melphalan. Cancer 1980; 45:2506–15.

16. Bukowski RM, Deodhar S, Hewlett JS, Greenstreet R. Randomized controlled trial of transfer factor in stage II malignant melanoma. Cancer 1983; 51:269–72.

17. Cramers M, Jensen JR, Kragballe K, Herlin T, Zachariae H, Thestrup-Pedersen K. Transfer factor in atopic dermatitis. Dermatologica 1982; 164:369–78.

Cancer Detection and Prevention Supplement 1:377–383 (1987)

Immunosuppressive Effects of Isoprinosine in Man:
A Comparison to Chlorambucil Effects in Multiple Sclerosis

Alain Pompidou, MD, PhD
Gérald Rancurel, MD
Marie-C. Delsaux, MD
Claude Meunier, MD

Louise Telvi, MD
Véronique Cour, MD
André Buge, MD

Laboratoire d'Anatomie-Pathologique, Hôpital Saint-Vincent de Paul (A.P., L.T., M.-C.D., C.M., V.C.) and Service de Neurologie, Hôpital Pitié-Salpétrière (G.R., A.B.), Paris, France

ABSTRACT Immunological and clinical functions were studied over a 2 year period in conjunction with a placebo controlled trial of isoprinosine and chlorambucil in 21 patients with exacerbating remitting multiple sclerosis. Laboratory and clinical evaluations were performed at 3 month intervals and during relapses. In placebo-treated patients, the decrease in circulating $T8^+$ cells was maximum during relapses, T lymphocyte function was impaired, and five of the six patients experienced clinical worsening. Chlorambucil treatment was responsible for a decrease in circulating $T4^+$ and $T8^+$ cells; nevertheless, T lymphocyte function was slightly improved during relapses. The alterations of delayed hypersensitivity responses were not accompanied by improvement in relapse rate or in intensity and major side effects: mainly infections with leukopenia and thrombocytopenia. During isoprinosine therapy, a regulation of circulating T lymphocytes and cell proliferation occurred. The higher level of circulating T cells was related to the increase in $T4^+$ and $T8^+$ cells, which did not decrease during relapses. The absence of Leu 7^+ cell modifications suggest that NK were numerically unaffected by isoprinosine therapy and that in vivo regulation of circulating T suppressor cells was performed by this treatment. Four out of seven patients did not experience any relapse during the duration of the trial. In relapsing patients, the frequency and duration of the relapses were significantly different from that of other patients. A reduction of the disease progression was observed without any side effects. While no conclusion can be drawn on the long-term effectiveness, the results of this pilot study are consistent indicators of the immunological and clinical beneficial effects of isoprinosine therapy in patients with exacerbating remitting multiple sclerosis.

Key words: multiple sclerosis, circulating T cells, isoprinosine

INTRODUCTION

Impairment of cellular immunity in multiple sclerosis (MS) has been reported [1], and abnormalities of immunoregulatory cells, more precisely a reduction of circulating T suppres-

---

Address reprint requests to Dr. Alain Pompidou, Laboratoire d'Anatomie-Pathologique, Hôpital Saint-Vincent de Paul, 74 avenue Denfert-Rochereau, 75014 Paris, France.

sor cells, have been observed in several studies [2–4]. Immunosuppressive treatment of patients with MS using cyclophosphamide was first suggested by Girard et al [5]. Since then, numerous trials have been carried out using azathioprine [6,7], antilymphocytic globulin [8], and ACTH [9,10]. The combined administration of antilymphocytic globulin, corticosteroids, and azathioprine resulted in a marginal beneficial effect [11]. In the present study, isoprinosine [12–14] was selected for one group of patients because, in relatively high concentrations, it can regulate T suppressor lymphocytes [15], and recent studies suggest beneficial effects in autoimmune diseases [16] as well as in viral infection [17,18]. Chlorambucil was selected as an immunosuppressive agent previously evaluated in MS therapy [19]. In this pilot trial, the clinical and immunological responses to these agents were compared to that obtained with a placebo over a 2 year period in patients with exacerbating remitting MS.

MATERIALS AND METHODS

Twenty-one patients with clinically definite exacerbating remitting MS [20] and oligoclonal IgG peak in their cerebrospinal fluid were enrolled in a randomized placebo controlled double-blind protocol. All patients, aged 25–45 years, had MS for a period of more than 5 years (7.6 $\pm$ 1.4 years) and more than one relapse a year (1.5 $\pm$ 0.6 per year). A group of seven patients receiving isoprinosine (25 mg/kg/day) and six patients receiving placebo were compared to another group of eight randomized patients who with their knowledge were treated with chlorambucil (0.1 mg/kg/day). This agent could not be blindly administered because of its side effects. In these patients, white blood cell counts were determined every 15 days during the first 3 months and monthly thereafter (chlorambucil dosage was lowered when the total lymphocyte count was $<400/mm^3$ or the number of platelets was $<90,000/mm^3$). The follow up evaluation of these patients was conducted by three physicians different from those who had initiated the treatment, and biological parameters were examined double blind by two different biologists.

The severity of neurological symptoms and overall disability were graded according to a scale based on McAlpine et al [21] and Krutzke [22] and a functional scale taking account of the daily living extent of a functional movement according to Sheikh et al [23]. A relapse was defined as the occurrence of one or more new symptoms or a pronounced worsening of existing symptoms lasting more than 5 days. The end of the relapse was defined by the absence of new symptoms during a period of 15 days. The treatment was began during an exacerbation of the disease. The handicap level was noted before and after treatment. Clinical score was assessed during relapse and remission periods and the number of relapses throughout the duration of the treatment. During exacerbation periods, all patients received ACTH (100 μ/day). This dosage was progressively diminished during remission.

Delayed hypersensitivity reaction (DHR) was performed by multipuncture skin test using a panel of seven recall antigens: tetanus, diphtheria, streptococcus, candidiasis, tuberculin, trychophyton, and proteus (Multitest ® [24]. A cumulative score was established by measurement of the extent of a positive reaction after 48 hr [25].

Peripheral blood mononuclear cells were separated from heparinized blood by density centrifugation gradient at 20°C on Ficoll-Hypaque (d = 1.076). The cells were adjusted at 10^6/ml in RPMI 1640 medium plus glutamine, antibiotics, and 10% heat-inactivated human AB serum. Lymphocyte proliferative response to PHA (PHA HA 16 5 μg/ml; Welcome) was measured in triplicate on 3 day cultures 18 hr after TH$_3$ incorporation, and cell number requirement was determined according to Knight et al [1]. The determination of T cell subsets was performed using mouse monoclonal antibodies OKT3, OKT4, OKT8 (Orthoclone), and Leu 7 (Becton Dickinson) [26]. Reactive cells identified by an indirect immunofluorescence assay using fluorescein-conjugated and affinity-purified goat antimouse immunoglobulin (Southern Biotechnology Associates) [27] were examined through a fluorescence microscope at ×400. Two hundred cells were counted for each peripheral blood samples.

The clinical and immunological status of the patients was assessed before the start of the treatment, during a period of disease exacerbation, at 3 month intervals thereafter, and during relapses before ACTH treatment.

The statistical significance of the different parameters was analyzed by the Wilcoxon matched pairs signed test [28], and Student chi square, and log rank tests [29].

RESULTS

Higher relative frequency of T cells (T3$^+$), increased proportion of suppressor/cytotoxic T cells (T8$^+$), and consequently lower helper/suppressor (T4$^+$/T8$^+$) ratios were observed during both remission and relapse phases in the group of patients receiving isoprinosine in comparison with placebo (Fig. 1). The frequencies of granular lymphocytes (Leu 7$^+$) were the same in both groups (13.7 $\pm$ 2.7 vs 14.6 $\pm$ 1.7), suggesting that NK cells were numerically unaffected by isoprinosine therapy and that in vivo regulation of circulating suppressor cells was performed by this treatment. In addition, the isoprinosine and chlorambucil-treated groups differed in that the later exhibited a significant reduction in relative frequency of cells with T helper phenotype (T4$^+$).

In terms of cell number requirement for PHA-induced proliferation, [1], a high depression was observed in placebo-treated patients during either relapse or remission (Fig. 2). Some 10^6 cells were necessary to obtain a response similar to that obtained in normal subjects with 1.25×10^5 cells. Similar findings were observed in the chlorambucil group except that the proliferative response to lower cell concentrations appeared to be somewhat increased during relapses. In contrast, isoprinosine-treated patients during remission had normal PHA responsiveness at lower cell concentrations, although impaired responsiveness could still be demonstrated at higher cell concentrations ($5-10 \times 10^5$ cells/ml) and for all concentrations during

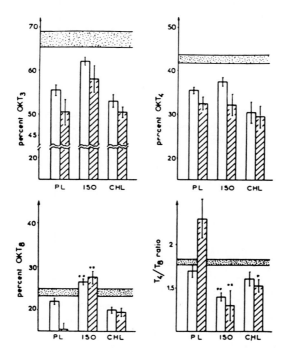

Fig. 1. Evaluation of circulating levels of total T cells (T3$^+$), helper T cells (T4$^+$), and suppressor/cytotoxic T cells (T8$^+$) during remission (open bars) or relapse (hatched bars) in 21 MS patients. Shaded areas indicate normal values $\pm$ standard deviation. *P $<$ 0.05 and **P $<$ 0.02 by Student test.

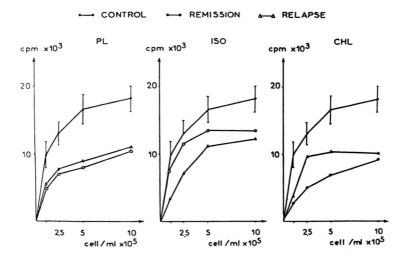

Fig. 2. Mean ^{3}H-thymidine uptake by peripheral blood mononuclear cells stimulated with PHA in triplicate cultures containing four different cell concentrations during remission ($\bigcirc$) or relapses ($\blacktriangle$) in MS patients (N = 21) treated in different ways. $\bullet$, Normal values in six healthy volunteers. Standard deviations depicted in controls are comparable to those of the patients (for details, see 1].

TABLE I. Delayed Hypersensitivity Responsiveness (DHR) in MS Patients Treated in Different Ways

	Clinical status	
Treatment group	Remission	Relapse
Placebo	13 ± 1.2	13.6 ± 1.7
Isoprinosine	8 ± 1.1*	9 ± 2.1*
Chlorambucil	5 ± 1.3*	6.5 ± 0.9*
Normal value	17 ± 2	

Multitest ® score was determined by measuring in millimeters the extent of DHR 48 hr after intradermal injections of a panel of seven recall antigens. The score is obtained by adding together the different measurements of the DHR extent (for details, see 24, 25).

relapses. These data were interpreted as a consequence of the functional improvement of T suppressor cells in the isoprinosine-treated group.

DHR was impaired in patients treated with isoprinosine (Table I) and significantly decreased during remission in the chlorambucil group. In all groups, no difference existed between the scores obtained during either remission or relapse.

All patients in the placebo or chlorambucil group had exacerbations of the disease during the 2 year observation period. In contrast, four out of seven individuals receiving isoprinosine had no evidence of any relapse while on this treatment. The clinical characteristics of relapses and remissions in all three groups during the observation period are presented in Table II. Among relapsing patients, the interval before the first relapse was significantly longer in the isoprinosine group, in which the frequency of the relapses but not the intensity of exacerbation was decreased. The number of relapses was significantly impaired in isoprinosine-treated patients compared to the placebo group (P < 0.05) using the chi square test and the Student test. This was confirmed by the use of the log rank test, which takes into account the number of frequency of relapses in relatively small samples [29]. All patients treated with either chlorambucil or isoprinosine exhibited a reduction of their handicap compared to the placebo group. However, chlorambucil therapy was not easily managed: Numerous bacterial and viral

TABLE II. Comparative Effects of Double-Blind Administration of Placebo, Isoprinosine, and Chlorambucil in 21 Randomized Patients With Exacerbating Remitting Multiple Scerlosis During the 2 Year Observation Period (mean ± SD)

Treatment	Patient No.	Interval before first relapse (months)	Remission, clinical score	Relapses			Handicap		Clinical results	
				Mean	Duration (months)	Clinical score	Before treatment	After treatment	Unchanged or worsened	Improved
Placebo	6	2.3 ± 1.1	3.8 ± 1.1	2.8 ± 0.9	3 ± 0.8	6.4 ± 1.8	2.7 ± 0.7	3.3 ± 0.7	5	1
Isoprinosine (25 mg/kg/day)	7	7.2 ± 1.2*	2.6 ± 0.7	0.5 ± 0.5*,†	0.5 ± 0.25‡,**	6.5 ± 1.2	2.5 ± 0.9	1.8 ± 0.7	3	4
Chlorambucil (1 mg/kg/day)	8	5.4 ± 1.9	2.8 ± 1.0	3.0 ± 0.9	2.7 ± 0.3	6 ± 1.3	3.1 ± 1.1	2.1 ± 0.7	4	4

†Over the 2 year observation.
‡For the three Iso-treated patients with relapses.
*P < 0.05.
**P < 0.02.

infections with leukopenia and thrombopenia requiring lowered dosages were observed during chlorambucil treatment, while no side effects were noted in isoprinosine-treated patients.

DISCUSSION

The results of this preliminary study have several interesting implications. Alterations in immune system parameters were seen in the isoprinosine-treated group, including near normal levels of total T cells (T3$^+$), helper T cells (T4$^+$), and T cells of the suppressor/cytotoxic phenotype (T8$^+$). The return toward normal of the level of T8$^+$ cells and the T lymphocytes partial functional restoration was especially impressive in this treatment group. At the same time, levels of NK cells (Leu 7$^+$) were not significantly affected in any of the treatment groups, which is noteworthy because the T8$^+$ subpopulation may include many Leu 7$^+$ granular lymphocytes. The integrity of DHR to a panel of recall antigens was impaired in both groups treated by isoprinosine or chlorambucil. Similar modifications of circulating T8$^+$ cells and DHR were observed in melanoma patients treated with isoprinosine (50 mg/kg, 5 days/15 days) [30].

In spite of the small number of patients, it appeared that isoprinosine had a significant effect on the relapse rate in active MS in reducing the number of both relapses and their duration. The severity of the individual relapses was not altered, but the degree of handicap was improved at the end of the treatment period, and four patients had not experienced any relapse. Chlorambucil treatment did not exhibit any beneficial effect on the relapse rate as compared to the placebo. Nevertheless, it does appear that there is a tendency for both isoprinosine and chlorambucil to be of some value in reducing the rate of progression in the disease. While the immunosuppressive drug chlorambucil led to frequent complicating infections and blood formula impairment, the immunomodulating agent isoprinosine was not associated with recognizable side effects.

These data indicate that continuous administration of isoprinosine exhibits regulatory activities on circulating T cells, more specifically on the T suppressor subset. This treatment over a 2 year period has not been accompanied by any side effects. These immunoregulatory properties of isoprinosine could be used for the treatment of autoimmune-related diseases in man after a short-term corticotherapy to block the initial stimulant effect of isoprinosine. The immunodepression of continuous or frequent administrations should be avoided in the treatment of immunocompromised cancer patients.

ACKNOWLEDGMENTS

We thank Max D. Cooper for his most helpful suggestions and critical comments; L. Gerbaud for testing patients' cerebrospinal fluid; P. Michel, D. Esnous, F. Coutance, and C. Bernard for technical assistance; and N. Maraud for preparing the manuscript.

REFERENCES

1. Knight SC, Harding B, Burman S, Mertin J. Cell number requirement for lymphocytes stimulation in vitro: Changes during the course of multiple sclerosis and effects of immunosuppression. Clin Exp Immunol 1981; 46:61–9.
2. Arnason BGW, Waksman BH. Immunoregulation in multiple sclerosis. Ann Neurol 1980; 8: 237–40.
3. Bach MA, Phan-Din-Tuy F, Tournier E, et al. Deficit of suppressor T cells in active multiple sclerosis. Lancet 1980; ii:1221–2.
4. Reinherz EL, Weiner HL, Hauser SL, et al. Loss of suppressor T cell in active multiple sclerosis: Analysis with monoclonal antibodies. N Engl J Med 1980; 303:125–9.
5. Girard P, Aimard G, Pellet H. Therapeutique immunosuppressive en Neurologie Presse Med 1967; 75:967–9.
6. Aimard G, Confavreux C, Trouillas P, Devic M. Own experience of Azathioprine treatment in multiple sclerosis. In Delmotte P, Hommes OR, Gonsette R, eds: Immunosuppressive treatment in multiple sclerosis. European Press, 1977:100–13.

7. Silberberg D, Lisak R, Zweiman B. Multiple sclerosis unaffected by Azathioprine in pilot study. Arch Neurol 1973;28:210-2.

8. Ring J, Seifert J, Angstwur H, et al. Pilot study with antilymphocytes globulin in the treatment of multiple sclerosis. Postgrad Med J 1976; 52(suppl 5):123-8.

9. Millar JHD, Vas CJ, Noronha MJ, et al. Long term treatment of multiple sclerosis with corticotrophin. Lancet 1967; ii:429-31.

10. Rose AS, Kuzma JW, Kurtzke JF, et al. Co-operative study in the evaluation of therapy in multiple sclerosis. ACTH vs placebo final report. Neurology 1970; 20:1-59.

11. Mertin J, Kremer M, Knight SC, et al. Double blind control trial of immunosuppression in the treatment of multiple sclerosis: Final report. Lancet 1982; ii:351-4.

12. Hadden JW, Englard A, Sadlik JR, et al. The comparative effect of inosiplex, levamisole, muramyl dipeptide and SM 12 13 on lymphocytes and macrophages proliferation and activation in vitro. Int J Immunopharmacol 1979; 1:17-27.

13. Renoux G, Renoux M, Degenne D. Suppressor cell activity after Inosiplex treatment of lymphocytes from normal mice. Int J Immunopharmacol 1979; 1:239-41.

14. Wybran J, Famaey JP, Appelboom T. Inosiplex, a new treatment in rhumatoid arthritis. J Rheumatol 1981; 8:643-4.

15. Pompidou A. In vitro effects of Methisoprinol on human peripheral blood lymphocytes. EOS 1984; 4:112-4.

16. Nakamura T, Miyasaka N, Pope RM, et al. Immunomodulation by Isoprinosine: Effects on in vitro immune functions of lymphocytes from human with autoimmune diseases. Clin Exp Immunol 1983; 52:67-74.

17. Jones CE, Hutten-Locher PR, Dyken PR, et al. Inosiplex therapy in subacute sclerosis panencephalitis. Lancet 1982; ii:1034-7.

18. Ohnishi H, Kosuzume H, Inaba H, et al. Mechanism of host defense suppression induced by viral infection: Mode of action of inosiplex as an antiviral agent. Infect Immun 1982; 38:243-50.

19. Sigwald J, Mazalton A, Raymondeau C, Piot C, Jacquillat C. Etude critique du traitement de la sclerose en plaque par le Chlorambucil et la corticothérapie intra-rachidienne. A propos de 100 cas suivis pendant une période comprise entre 2 et 9 ans. Rev Neurol (Paris) 1973; 128:72-7.

20. Poser CM, Paty DW, Scheinberg L, et al. New diagnostic criteria for multiple sclerosis: Guidelines for research protocoles. Ann Neurol 1983; 13:227-31.

21. McAlpine D, Lumsden CE, Acheson ED. Multiple sclerosis. A reappraisal. Edinburgh: Churchill Livingstone, 1972.

22. Kurtzke JF. Further notes on disability evaluation in multiple sclerosis with scale modifications. Neurology 1965; 15:654-61.

23. Sheikh K, Smith DS, Meade TW, Brennan PJ, Ide L. Assessment of motor function in study of chronic disability. Rheumatol Rehabil 1980; 19:83-90.

24. Kniker WT, Anderson CT, Roumiantzeff M. The multitest system: A standardized approach to evaluation of delayed hypersensitivity and cell mediated immunity. Ann Allergy 1979; 43:73-9.

25. Lesourd B, Winters WB. Specific immune response to skin test antigens following repeated multiple antigen in normal individuals. Clin Exp Immunol 1982; 50:635-43.

26. Abo T, Balch CM. A differentiation antigen of human NK and K cells identified by monoclonal antibody (HNK$_1$). J Immunol 1981; 127:1024-7.

27. Reinherz EL, Kung PC, Goldstein G, Schlossman SF. Separation of functional subsets of human T cells by a monoclonal antibody. Proc Natl Acad Sci USA 1979; 301:1018-22.

28. Moses LE, Emerson JD, Husseini H. Analyzing data from ordered categories. N Engl J Med 1984; 311:442-8.

29. Peto R, Pike MC, Armitage P, et al. Design and analysis of randomized clinical trials requiring prolonged observations of each patient. Br J Cancer 1976; 34:585-612.

30. Pompidou A, Telvi L, Soubrane C, et al. Immunological effects of Isoprinosine as a pulse immunotherapy in melanoma and ARC patients. Cancer Detect Prevent, Supplement 1, 1987; 457-62.

Cancer Detection and Prevention Supplement 1:385–397 (1987)

Immune Response by Biological Response Modifiers

Michael A. Chirigos, PhD, DSc
Erich Schlick, MD
Wladyslaw Budzynski, MD

Biological Therapeutics Branch, Biological Response Modifiers Program, Division of Cancer Treatment, National Cancer Institute, NIH, Frederick Cancer Research Facility, Frederick, MD

ABSTRACT   Several biological response modifiers (BRMs) were demonstrated to increase myelopoiesis and effector cell responses (Mϕ and natural killer cell activity) in vivo. The increased myelopoiesis was reflected by an increase in bone marrow cellularity and granulocyte-Mϕ colony-forming cells (GM-CFU-C). The increase in myelopoiesis appeared to be related to a concomitant increase in colony-stimulated factor (CSF) production and secretion by Mϕs and bone marrow cells. CSF induction by BRMs increased myelopoiesis and counteracted the myelosuppressive and immunosuppressive effects of cyclophosphamide. CSF induced in vivo by BRMs attained high titers and were maintained over a longer period than exogenously injected CSF, which was rapidly cleared from serum.

Key words: cyclophosphamide, colony-stimulating factor, macrophage, natural killer cell, bone marrow, myelopoiesis

INTRODUCTION

Major treatment modalities for various cancers are chemotherapy and radiotherapy. The treatment regimens often result in suppression of hematopoiesis, with a reduction in the number of hematopoietic stem cells and their progeny [1,2]. The depression of monocytes and macrophages (Mϕ) and granulocytopenia, which occur as a consequence of antineoplastic treatment, lead to infections that are a major cause of morbidity and mortality in cancer patients [3,4]. Cytoxan (CY) is considered one of the most potent anticancer agents available; however, its strong hematosuppressive and immunosuppressive properties has limited its usefulness. Treatment modalities that restore and/or counteract the suppressive effects of CY may therefore greatly enhance its effectiveness. Since the effector cells of the immune system are bone-marrow derived cells, such as Mϕ, and T and B cells, early and complete restoration of bone marrow function after CY is thus the first prerequisite for the restoration of normal immune functions [2,5,6,7].

It has been shown that spontaneous recovery of the depressed hematopoietic stem cell functions following primary antineoplastic therapy may occur only after a period of several

---

Dr. Michael A. Chirigos is now at USAMRIID, Fort Detrick, Frederick, MD 21701. Address reprint requests there.

days and may involve humoral factors, such as colony-stimulating factor (CSF) [2,8]. Biological response modifiers (BRMs), which are capable of stimulating proliferation and differentiation of hematopoietic progenitors, eg, through enhanced secretion of regulatory factors like CSF, may therefore be advantageous to the tumor-bearing host undergoing cytoreductive therapy.

Therefore, we were interested in testing the ability of selected, chemically defined BRMs to modulate in vivo growth and differentiation of myeloid progenitor cells after primary antineoplastic treatment with CY and to also reconstitute the functional activities of Mϕ. For that, we selected several BRMs to study based on their ability to augment Mϕ cytotoxicity and natural killer (NK) cell cytotoxicity [9] and to stimulate increased myelopoiesis in normal mice [10,11].

MATERIALS AND METHODS
Mice

Male BALB/c and female C57BL/6 mice were obtained from the Mammalian Genetics and Animal Production Section, Division of Cancer Treatment, National Cancer Institute—Frederick Cancer Research Facility, NIH (Frederick, MD). The animals were 6 to 8 weeks of age when used for experiments.

Biological Response Modifiers

MVE2 was a generous gift of Dr. R. Corrano (Adria Laboratories, Columbus, OH). Polyinosinic-polycytidylic acid poly-L-lysine (poly ICLC) was supplied by Dr. Hilton B. Levy (National Institute of Allergy and Infectious Diseases, National Institutes of Health, Bethesda, MD). Cyclophosphamide (Cytoxan [CY]) was obtained from the Division of Cancer Treatment, NCI (Bethesda, MD). Picibanil (OK432) was a generous gift of Dr. H. Nakano, Chugai Pharmaceuticals (Tokyo, Japan). Azimexone and BM 41.332 (Ciamexon) were generous gifts of Dr. U. Bicker, Boehringer-Mannheim (Mannheim, West Germany). Granulocyte macrophage–colony-stimulating factor (GM-CSF) preparations used were generated by injecting BALB/c mice with 5 μg/mouse of lipopolysaccharide (LPS). Sera and lung conditioned media from these mice were then subjected to concentration and ultrafiltration using Diaflo ultrafilters [12,13]. The molecular weight of the GM-CSF preparations used ranged between 15 and 35 Kd. Lipopolysaccharide from *Salmonella typhimurium* (LPS) was purchased from Difco Laboratories (Detroit, MI). The media and BRM preparations were tested for endotoxin contamination with the Limulus lysate assay and found to contain less than 0.125 ng/ml.

Tumor Cells

The tissue culture cell line of YAC-1, a Moloney virus-induced lymphoma of A/Sn origin, was used as the target for NK activity. MBL-2, a lymphoblastic leukemia cell line derived from C57BL/6, was used as the target for macrophage cytotoxic activity. Cell lines were maintained in tissue culture in RPMI 1640 supplemented with L-glutamine (Grand Island Biological Co., Grand Island, NY), 125 μg/ml of gentamycin (Microbiological Associates, Bethesda, MD), and 10% fetal bovine serum (Associated Biomedic Systems, Buffalo, NY).

Assays

Macrophage-mediated cytotoxicity. The assay for measuring the ability of BRMs to induce macrophage-mediated cytotoxicity against the MBL-2 cell line has been described previously [12].

Natural killer cells. A conventional ^{51}Cr-release assay was employed as previously described [13].

Prostaglandin E. Prostaglandin E$_1$ and E$_2$ was determined by radioimmunoassay as previously described [14].

Bone marrow cells. Sterile single cell suspensions from femoral bone marrow were prepared as previously described [15]. The total number of viable nucleated cells per femur was counted for each mouse by hemocytometer. Morphological characterization of the bone marrow cells was done by Giemsa and esterase staining. To determine the number of granulo-cyte-Mϕ–committed stem cells (GM-CFU-C), a previously described in vitro soft agar culture technique was used [16]. Briefly, 10^5 unfractionated bone marrow cells were suspended in 2 ml of 0.3% agar, supplemented with 15% horse serum (Gibco), 15% fetal calf serum (Gibco), 292 μg/ml L-glutamine (Gibco), and 100 μg/ml of gentamycin/ml (Sigma, St. Louis, MO), and were plated in 35 mm Petri dishes (Falcon, Oxnard, CA). A 0.2 ml volume of CSF was added. The cultures were incubated at 37°C in a fully humidified atmosphere of 70% CO_2 in air. Colonies (>40 cells) were scored and classified on the basis of their morphology at days 7 and 10 of the culture period. For determination of their CSF secretion, mononuclear bone marrow cells were separated by centrifugation on Ficoll-Hypaque (Lymphocyte Separation Medium, Litton Bionetics, MD). Approximately 10^7 mononuclear bone marrow cells were then incubated in 1 ml complete medium in 16 mm wells (Costar) for further experiments.

CSF assay. Cell-free supernatants from in vitro- or in vivo-activated Mϕ and mononu-clear bone marrow cells were harvested after 48 hr of subsequent in vitro culture (37°C and 5% CO_2) at a cell density of 10^6 Mϕ/ml or 10^7 BMC/ml and kept at -20°C until assayed. CSF concentrations were then determined using a bioassay as previously described [10]. Briefly, 0.2 to 0.6 ml of the supernatants from Mϕ and bone marrow cells or sera to be tested for CSF were added to each 35 mm Petri dish containing 10^5 nonadherent bone marrow cells from normal mice in 2 ml of 0.3% agar, supplemented with 15% horse serum, 15% fetal calf serum, 292 μg/ml of L-glutamine, and 100 μg/ml gentamycin. At the end of the culture period (10 days at 37°C and 7% CO_2), the colonies (>40 cells) were counted and classified on the basis of their morphology. CSF activity is expressed as units per milliliter [17]. Student's t test was used for statistical analysis.

RESULTS

Table I represents a summary of several individual studies designed to assess the various responses to MVE2 and poly ICLC. Both effector cell populations (NK cells and macrophages) responded significantly, as expected. Of particular interest was the correlation obtained be-tween the increase in CSF in serum and from incubated bone marrow cells from treated mice. The increase in CSF resulting from the treatment was reflected also by a significant increase in the number of nucleated bone marrow cells in the femur and GM-CFU-C. The myelopoietic growth inhibitor PGE was not increased in the serum of the BRM-treated mice, and bone marrow cells from the treated mice did not secrete PGE at levels above control values when incubated in vitro for 24 hr.

Antineoplastic treatment regimens consisting of chemotherapy and/or irradiation reduce the number of hematopoietic stem cells and their progeny, with a spontaneous recovery of the stem cell function occurring only after several days. In addition to their stimulatory effect on macrophages and NK cells, immunomodifiers can also have profound stimulatory effects on myelopoiesis. This combined effect would be advantageous to the tumor-bearing host undergo-ing cytoreductive therapy.

Since our studies (Table I) showed that MVE2 promotes growth and differentiation of myelomonocytic progenitors in mice (optimal effects occurred 3 days after treatment with MVE2), we wanted to test whether MVE2 could also be used to restore myelomonocytic dysfunctions caused by treatment with CY. This hypothesis was tested in mice that were treated with CY. Administration of 150 mg of CY/kg induced a time-dependent profound suppression of bone marrow cellularity, as measured by the number of granulocyte-macrophage–committed bone marrow stem cells and nucleated bone marrow cells per femur (Table II). One day after treatment with CY, the bone marrow cellularity was less than 10% of the control values (data not shown) and reached about 30% of the control values 4 days after CY (Table II). Bone

TABLE I. Regulation of Effector Cells and Secretory Products by BRMs

Group	Treatment*	Blood NK† (% cytotoxicity, 25:1)	Mφ† (% cytotoxicity)	CSF‡ (units/ml × 10^{-6}) Serum	CSF‡ BMC	Bone marrow cells per femur Mean × 10^{-6}	P§	PGE‡ per ml serum	PGE‡ per 10^6 BMC	GM-CFU-C from BMC × 10^{-5}
1	Placebo	5		10	2	9.2		48	200	27
2	Poly ICLC 2.0 mg/kg	18	92	74	24	12.8	< 0.01	40	180	54
3	Poly ICLC 0.5 mg/kg	14	94			11.6	< 0.05			
4	MVE-2 25 mg/kg	21	96	65	10	12.2	< 0.01	53	215	45
5	MVE-2 5.0 mg/kg	18	93			11.4	< 0.05			

*BALB/c mice injected with PBS (placebo) or BRM ip.

†MK and Mφ determined 3 days posttreatment.

‡CSF and PGE (picograms) determined at 24 hr after treatment (time based on results from previous studies).

§P values for differences from placebo group (Student's t test).

TABLE II. Combined Effects of Cytoxan and MVE-2 on Various Cellular Components

Cellular component examined	Normal and MVE2 values*	Treatment	Day of observation following cytoxan treatment†					
			4	6	7	10	13	16
Bone Marrow								
cells per femur	9.5	Cy	3.1	4.8	7.2	10.2	9.8	10.0
($\times 10^{-6}$)	13.5	Cy + MVE2	4.5	9.2	11.8	13.5	14.2	13.2
GM-CFU-C	100	Cy	24	41	62	108	95	98
per femur	144	Cy + MVE2	47	88	122	135	130	132
% Mφ	0	Cy	1	3	5	7	8	10
cytotoxicity	92	Cy + MVE2	49	74	90	78	57	12
% NK cell	10	Cy	3	5	6	9	10	10
cytotoxicity	34	Cy + MVE2	7	9	10	26	31	37
CSF†U/10^6	78	Cy	62	82	80	93		
Mφ cells	168	Cy + MVE2	91	196	185	183		

*Values for normal placebo treated mice (top value) and mice treated with MVE-2 (25 mg/kg) (bottom value) 3 days before sacrifice.

†MVE-2 (25 mg/kg) was administered at 3 days before sacrifice (day 0) to all Cytoxan (Cy)-pretreated groups (150 mg/kg).

‡Peritoneal exudate cells from treated mice were harvested by peritoneal lavage. CSF secretion by Mφs determined after 2 days of in vitro incubation of 10^6 Mφs/ml without stimulus.

marrow cellularity returned to control levels around 10 days after CY treatment. Administration of MVE2 (25 mg/kg) to CY-pretreated mice was able to ameliorate the bone marrow-suppressing effect of CY, with return to normal values within 6 days.

The granulocyte-macrophage–committed stem cells, similarly to the nucleated bone marrow cells, were also depressed below normal values for 7 to 10 days. MVE2 treatment led to an earlier recovery of GM-CFU-C. Macrophage and NK effector cell responses were depressed for 7 to 10 days. Following MVE2 treatment, NK cell activity reached normal values and was further augmented to levels obtained in mice treated with MVE2 alone. Macrophage activity was not affected by CY treatment. We have previously reported that CY and other chemotherapeutic agents as well as total body irradiation results in increases in Mφ activity [18,19]. Combined treatment led to an early response of Mφ tumor cell cytotoxicity.

Since it seemed likely that growth factors like CSF are involved in recovery of myelomonocytic cells from chemotherapy [2], we were interested in determining whether in vivo administration of MVE2 induced an increase in CSF secretion by CY-pretreated Mφs. We studied Mφs since they are a prominent source of CSF [20] and are less sensitive to CY than T lymphocytes, which also secrete CSF [21].

CY treatment resulted in a profound decrease in the number of peritoneal Mφs, which was about one third of the control value at 4 days after CY. The number of peritoneal Mφs recovered within 2 weeks after CY treatment (data not shown). CY treatment alone induced a transient increase in spontaneous CSF secretion by the residual Mφs 6 days following its injection (Table II). The Mφs from CY-pretreated mice were unable to increase their secretion of CSF in response to in vivo treatment 1 day later with MVE2 regardless of whether the interval between MVE2 and testing was 3 days (Table II) or 6 days (data not shown). In contrast, MVE2 given at ≥3 days after CY induced a significant increase in CSF secretion compared to untreated and CY-treated controls (Table II). MVE2 given 3 days after CY also stimulated recovery of the number of peritoneal Mφ to control levels by 7 days after CY treatment, ie, 7 days prior to recovery in mice given CY alone (data not shown).

Other BRMs were examined for their capacity to increase myelopoiesis when administered alone or following cytoreductive CY treatment. Picibanil has been reported to stimulate secretion of CSF and increase Mφ and NK cell activity [22]. This BRM was tested to assess its effect on boosting bone marrow cellularity and GM-CFU-C, since both cell populations appear to be dependent on CSF. A single treatment with Picibanil led to an increase in both bone marrow cellularity and GM-CFU-C (Table III). The depressive effect of CY on both cell populations was abrogated by Picibanil treatment, resulting in a more rapid recovery of bone marrow and GM-CFU-C.

Azimexone and BM 41.332, 2-cyanaziridine compounds, do not cause increases in Mϕ or NK cell activity. However, Azimexone has been reported to increase and/or protect bone marrow cellularity [16]. A single injection of either Azimexone or BM 41.332 resulted in a significant increase in serum CSF levels and in CSF secretion by Mϕ (Table IV). The increase in CSF in serum and in Mϕ-derived supernatants was followed by a significant augmentation of the number of granulocyte-macrophage–committed stem cells (GM-CFU-C) and the total number of nucleated bone marrow cells per femur. The response was dependent on the dose

TABLE III. Bone Marrow Reconstitution by Picibanil Following CYP Treatment

Treatment	Effector cell	Control Placebo	Control Picibanil	CYP ± Picibanil treatment* (day of observation) 4	7	10	13	16
PBS	BM†	9.5	12.3					
	GM-CFU-C‡	100	135					
CYP+PBS	BM			3.5	7.3	10.1	9.8	9.6
	GM-CFU-C			28	62	98	90	92
CYP+ Picibanil	BM			4.5	11.1§	12.4§	13.0§	10.1
	GM-CFU-C			42	110§	130§	127§	105

*BALB/c mice received a single ip injection of cyclophosphamide (CYP) 150 mg/kg on various days between day −16 to day −4, which was followed by a single ip injection of PBS or Picibanil (4 mg/kg) on day −3. All mice were sacrificed on day 0 for effector cell assay.
†Bone marrow cells per femur ($\times 10^6$).
‡GM-CFU-C per femur (% of placebo control).
§Statistical analysis (P < 0.01) between CYP + PBS and CYP + Picibanil.

TABLE IV. Effect of 2-Cyanaziridines on In Vivo Secretion of CSF, GM-CFU-C, and Nucleated Bone Marrow Cells: Dose Response

BRM* dosage (mg/kg)	CSF U/ml serum	CSF U/10^6 Mϕ	GM-CFU-C per femur ($\times 10^2$)	BMC per femur ($\times 10^6$)
Control	11†	72	31	9.8
Azimexone				
5	30	98	29	10.5
25	47‡	129‡	44‡	11.6‡
50	124‡	166‡	55‡	14.3‡
100	93‡	148‡	39‡	12.3‡
BM 41.332				
5	26	92	35	11.8‡
25	44‡	125‡	47‡	12.9‡
50	47‡	111‡	42‡	11.5
100	36‡	98	33	11.7‡
MVE2				
25	43‡	135‡	60‡	12.6‡

*BALB/c mice were injected with either PBS, different doses of the 2-cyanaziridine compounds, or 25 mg/kg of MVE2. The animals were sacrificed 3 days later for determination of serum CSF levels, CSF secretion by Mϕ, and GM-CFU-C and nucleated bone marrow cells per femur.
†Each value represents the mean of three separate experiments; SD was less than 20% of the mean.
‡P < 0.01 compared to control group.

employed, 50 mg/kg of Azimexone and 25 mg/kg of BM 41.332 producing the maximum effects. Optimal effects could be found 3 days after injection of either 2-cyanaziridine compound, with all parameters returning to control levels 7 days after injection of either compound (data not shown).

Since we have shown that 2-cyanaziridines may promote growth and differentiation of myelomonocytic progenitors in normal mice, we wanted to test whether they could also be of any value in restoring suppressed myelomonocytic functions in mice pretreated with CY. We selected Azimexone (50 mg/kg) for these studies based on its more pronounced effects on myelopoiesis in normal mice compared to BM 41.332 (Table V).

A single ip injection of 150 mg/kg CY resulted in a strong reduction in the number of granulocyte-Mϕ–committed bone marrow stem cells and the total number of nucleated bone marrow cells/per femur without decreasing the amount of circulating CSF (Table V, group 2). Three subsequent injections of Azimexone were able to stimulate in CY-pretreated mice a significant increase in serum CSF levels and in myelomonocytic bone marrow stem cells, which was followed by a near complete normalization of the total number of nucleated bone marrow cells per femur (Table V, group 3 vs group 2).

We investigated whether the in vivo modulation of CSF secretion by BRMs would lead to an increase in myeloid progenitor cells. We focused on MVE2 and poly ICLC, two potent stimulators of CSF production and secretion. Increased serum levels of CSF were detected in mice treated with either MVE2 (25 mg/kg) or poly ICLC (2 mg/kg). Serum levels of CSF began to increase as early as 1 hr after BRM injection and remained increased up to 5 days (Fig. 1). Peritoneal Mϕ and unfractionated bone marrow cells derived from those mice pretreated in vivo also secreted significantly higher amounts of CSF than controls on subsequent in vitro culture for 48 hr. The kinetics of in vitro secretion of CSF by these in vivo-stimulated Mϕ and bone marrow cells paralleled the changes in serum CSF levels.

Morphological analysis of the bone marrow colonies induced by CSF derived from the different tissue sources showed the following distribution of colony types: CSF derived from Mϕ induced $\approx 70\%$ pure Mϕ and $\approx 30\%$ pure granulocyte colonies; CSF from bone marrow cells induced $\approx 55\%$ pure Mϕ and $\approx 30\%$ pure granulocyte colonies and $\approx 15\%$ mixed granulocyte/Mϕ colonies. Serum-derived CSF induced colonies of all three types (Mϕ, granulocyte, mixed) in a proportion similar to that obtained with bone marrow-derived CSF.

The increases in serum CSF levels and in secretion of CSF by Mϕ and bone marrow cells were associated with an increase in granulocyte-Mϕ–committed stem cells and nucleated bone marrow cells per femur (Fig. 2). The increase in nucleated bone marrow cells was mainly due to an increased proliferation of cells of the myelomonocytic lineage, as shown by an increased myeloid/erythroid ratio (data not shown). Optimal effects occurred by day 3 follow-

TABLE V. Effect of Azimexone on Myelopoiesis in CY-Pretreated Mice

Group	Cyclophos-phamide* (150 mg/kg)	Azimexone† (50 mg/kg)	CSF‡ (U/ml serum)	GM-CFU-C per femur‡ (% of control)	BMC per femur‡ ($\times 10^6$)
1	−	−	11	100	9.7
2	+	−	14	36§	4.2§
3	+	Days −5, −3, −1	58§,‖	69‖	8.1‖
4	−	Days −5, −3, −1	108§	145§	12.4§

*BALB/c mice received on day −5 a single ip injection of either PBS or 150 mg/kg CY.
†Mice from groups 3 and 4 received additionally three ip injections of 50 mg/kg Azimexone at the days indicated; the first injection was given 4 hr after CY.
‡All mice were sacrificed on day 0 for determination of serum-CSF levels and bone marrow cellularity. Each value represents the mean of two separate experiments (N = 5 for each group per experiment); SD was less than 15% of the mean.
§P < 0.01 compared to group 1.
‖P < 0.01 compared to group 2.

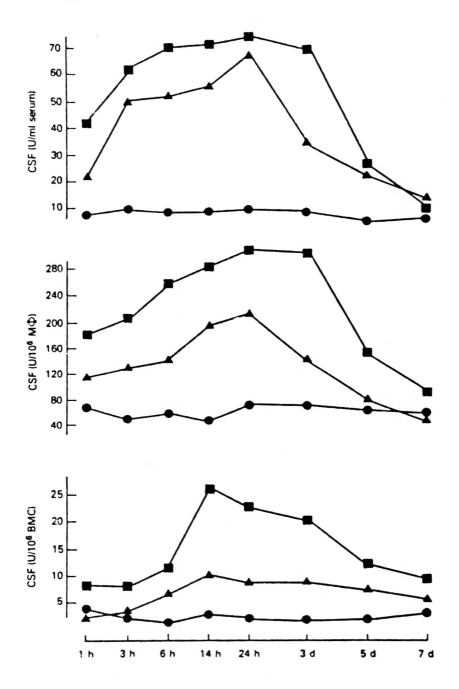

Fig. 1.   BALB/c mice received PBS (●), 25 mg/kg MVE-2 (▲), or 2 mg/kg poly ICLC (■) by ip injection. Mice were sacrificed on the days indicated for determination of CSF concentrations in serum and conditioned media (48 hr at 37°C and 5% CO_2) of peritoneal Mφ (10^6 Mφ/ml) and bone marrow cells (10^7 BMC/ml). Results are expressed as units of CSF/ml of serum or per 10^6 plated cells and are the averages of three experiments.

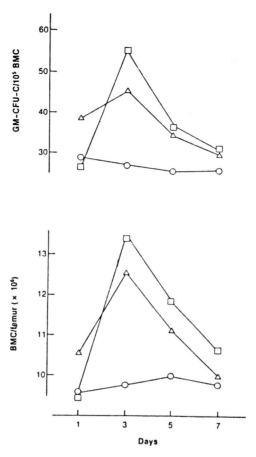

Fig. 2. BALB/c mice received PBS (○), 25 mg/kg MVE-2 (△), or 2 mg/kg poly ICLC (□) by ip injection. Mice were sacrificed on the days indicated for determination of GM-CFU-C and nucleated bone marrow cells. The results are the averages of three experiments.

ing BRM treatment and no significant differences between MVE2- and poly ICLC-induced effects could be observed. Both parameters fell back to near-normal levels by the seventh day after BRM treatment.

Since different BRMs can be used to stimulate secretion of CSF by Mϕ and bone marrow cells and thus increase myelopoietic growth and differentiation, we also wanted to test whether we could obtain similar results using CSF directly instead of CSF inducers. We injected mice iv either with a single injection of GM-CSF (1,000 U or 5,000 U per mouse) or with two injections of GM-CSF (each injection was 1,000 U or 5,000 U per mouse, given at a 24 hr interval). Immediately after the last GM-CSF injection, we determined serum CSF levels and 3 days later number and function of myelopoietic progenitor cells in bone marrow. The results in Figure 3 show that treatment of normal mice with GM-CSF (single vs double treatment) failed to enhance significantly myelopoiesis within the bone marrow compartment. The levels of CSF in serum decreased logarithmically after its injection, and estimates of the half-life of CSF in serum range between 6 and 9 min. The clearance of GM-CSF after the second injection seemed to be prolonged compared to the first injection.

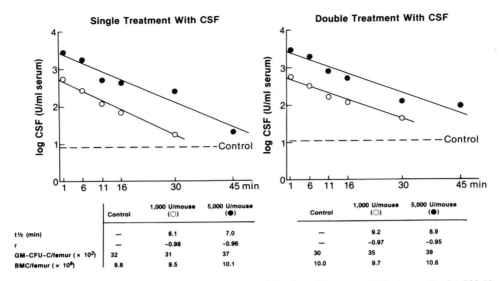

Fig. 3. BALB/c mice received either one or two iv injections (given at a 24 hr interval) of 1,000 U (○) or 5,000 U (●) of GM-CSF (lung-conditioned medium [12] with a molecular weight range between 15 and 30 Kd). Controls (dashed lines) received PBS. Mice were sacrificed at different times immediately after the last injection of CSF for determination of serum CSF levels and also 3 days after the last injection of CSF for determination of GM-CFU-C and nucleated bone marrow cells per femur. Results are the means of a typical experiment (N = 5 for each time point); SD was less than 20% of the mean. The experiment was repeated twice with similar results. r, correlation coefficient of regression curve.

DISCUSSION

The results of the studies presented here show that selected BRMs increase the in vivo proliferation of myelopoietic precursor cells and their progeny. Our studies further indicate that the effects of myelopoiesis are most likely related to the capacity of these BRMs to increase secretion of CSF by mononuclear bone marrow cells and peripheral macrophages rather than to a concomitant decrease in CSF inhibitors, since heating the sera and culture supernatants (56°C for 30 min), which abolishes inhibitors of CSF [23], did not change the bioactivity of CSF present in these fluids. Although we did not isolate the actual CSF molecules present in serum as well as in culture supernatants of Mφ and bone marrow cells of BRM-treated mice, the morphology of the colonies induced by these CSF molecules would indicate that peritoneal Mφ, whether treated in vitro or in vivo, secrete mainly CSF-1 and only minor amounts of CSF-3 [24,25].

The results of this study demonstrate that chemically defined BRMs (MVE2, poly ICLC, Azimexone, and BM 41.332) and a bacterial preparation (Picibanil) can counteract the myelo-suppressive effects of the anticancer drug CY, and, in addition, three BRMs (MVE2, poly ICLC, and Picibanil) had stimulatory effects on cytotoxic activity of Mφs and NK cells.

There have been reports suggesting that restoration of suppressed myelopoiesis involves growth factors, including CSF [2,16]. This is supported by our findings that the CY-induced functional impairment of Mφs and bone marrow cells to secrete CSF upon in vitro stimulation with a BRM seems to be directly related to the lag period in bone marrow recovery. MVE2, which we have predominantly focused on and which has been shown to induce increased myelopoiesis in normal mice presumably through stimulation of CSF secretion by Mφs and bone marrow cells [10], also plays a major role in bone marrow recovery after CY treatment. Our experiments show that MVE2 stimulates Mφs, as well as bone marrow cells of normal mice, to increase their CSF secretion. Both cell populations responded to in vitro, as well as in vivo, stimuli with normal CSF secretion after a lag period of about 3 days after CY treatment. The CSF secretion was then followed by an increase in the number of myelopoietic stem cells and progenitors. Based on our experiments, we propose the following chain of events: CY induces a reversible functional impairment of monocytes and Mϕs and the immediate death of myelopoietic stem cells, immature progenitors, and cycling Mϕs. After acquiring a normal functional status ($\sim$3 days after CY), the residual Mϕs increase their basal production of CSF, leading to spontaneous recovery of myelomonocytic cells. MVE2, given after Mϕs have acquired their normal function, induces increased secretion of CSF, which then causes earlier restoration of myelopoiesis and production of monocytes and Mϕs.

CSF secretion by activated T cells, an important source of CSF [21], may play a minor role only, compared to Mϕs in myelopoietic recovery after CY treatment, since CY is known to destroy the majority of T cells and since functional mature T cells can be demonstrated only a considerable time after CY treatment [26,27]. Only exogenous continuous administration of interleukin 2, as demonstrated recently, seems to have a significant stimulatory effect on T-cell recovery after CY [28].

Our studies thus show that BRMs can be divided into at least two classes on the basis of their effects on myelopoiesis and natural immunity: 1) BRMs, like the 2-cyanaziridines, which exert mainly (or only) a myelopoiesis modulating effect; and 2) BRMs, like MVE2, poly ICLC, and Picibanil, which modulate both natural immunity and myelopoiesis. These findings could be of clinical importance, since they might lead to the development of sequential treatment regimens for chemoimmunotherapy of cancer patients that take into consideration the status of the patients' myelopoietic and immune functions. Patients with symptoms of suppressed myeloid functions could first be treated with BRMs such as 2-cyanaziridines and then, after restoration of their myeloid functions, receive BRMs like MVE2 to activate natural immunity and to maintain myelopoietic growth and differentiation. Such a schedule would allow myeloid functions to be restored and natural immunity to be boosted separately.

The findings that single or multiple injections of low doses of GM-CSF alone into normal mice did not result in an increased myelopoiesis whereas injection of 2-cyanaziridines or other BRMs (eg, poly ICLC, MVE2, or Picibanil) increased serum CSF levels and CSF secretion by bone marrow cells followed by myelopoietic proliferation are not only of theoretical importance but could also be clinically relevant. This discrepancy between the effects of exogenous injections of CSF at low doses and endogenous CSF induction by BRMs is most likely attributable to the rapid clearance of CSF from serum, to distribution into different tissues, or to metabolic inactivation, all of which might prevent the maintenance of significant concentrations of CSF at the site of myelopoietic proliferation within the bone marrow compartment. Induction of contraregulatory mechanisms by CSF injections such as endogenous secretion of PGE [29,30], which could possibly prevent CSF-mediated stimulation of myelopoiesis, might also play a role, even though our experiments with combined treatment with indomethacin and 2-cyanaziridines or MVE2 [10] would argue against such a possibility. These findings also underline the importance of an intimate contact between myelopoietic stem cells as CSF responders and CSF secreting cells within the bone marrow compartment. The interaction between CSF responders and producers seems to be locally regulated under physiologic conditions and to require external activation signal(s) for increased proliferation above normal baseline levels (as shown in this study and in our previous study [10].). External activation signals could be either the BRM itself or another (BRM-) induced mediator, such as IFN.

ACKNOWLEDGMENTS

W.B. is a guest researcher from the Institute of Immunology and Experimental Therapy, Wroclaw, Poland.

REFERENCES

1. Blackett NM, Marsh JC, Gordon MY, Okell SF, Aguado M. Simultaneous assay by six methods of the effect on haemopoietic precursor cells of adriamycin, methyl-CCNU, ^{60}Co-γ-rays, vinblastine, and cytosine arabinoside. Exp Hematol 1978; 6:2–8.
2. Lohrman HP, Schreml W. Cytotoxic drugs and the granulopoietic system: Recent results. Cancer Res 1982; 81:1–22.
3. Bodey GP. Infections in cancer patients. Cancer Treat Rev 1975; 2:89–128.
4. Bodey GP, Buckley M, Sathe YS, Freireich E. Quantitative relationship between circulating leukocytes and infections in patients with acute leukemia. Ann Intern Med 1966; 64:328–40.
5. Cheever MA, Greenberg PD, Fefer A. Specificity of adoptive chemoimmunotherapy of established syngeneic tumors. J Immunol 1980; 125:711–4.
6. Lubet RA, Carlson DE. Therapy of the murine plasmacytoma MOPC 104 E: Role of the immune response. JNCI 1978; 61:897–903.
7. Moore M, Williams DE. Contribution of host immunity to cyclophosphamide therapy of a chemically induced murine sarcoma. Int J Cancer 1973; 11:358–68.
8. Schlick E, Bartocci A, Chirigos MA. Effect of azimexone on the bone marrow of normal and γ-irradiated mice. J Biol Resp Modif 1982; 1:179–86.
9. Bartocci A, Papademetriou V, Chirigos MA. Enhanced macrophage and natural killer cell antitumor activity by various molecular weight maleic anhydride-divinyl ethers. J Immunopharamcol 1980; 2:149–58.
10. Schlick E, Hartung K, Chirigos MA. Comparison of in vitro and in vivo modulation of myelopoiesis by biological response modifiers. Cancer Immunol Immunother 1984; 18:226–32.
11. Schlick E, Welker RD, Piccoli M, Ruffmann R, Chirigos MA. Biological characterization of MVE-2 and poly ICLC. In Kende M, Gainer J, Chirigos M, eds: Chemical regulation of immunity in veterinary medicine. New York: Alan R. Liss, Inc., 1983; 511–24.
12. Bartocci A, Papadiemtriou V, Chirigos MA. Enhanced macrophage and natural killer cell antitumor activity by various molecular weight maleic anhydride divinyl ethers. J Immunopharmacol 1980; 2:149–58.
13. Herberman RB, Nunn ME, Lavrin DH. Natural cytotoxic reactivity of mouse lymphoid cells against syngeneic and allogeneic tumors. I. Distribution, reactivity and specificity. Int J Cancer 1975; 16:216–29.
14. Hartung K, Schlick E, Stevenson HC, et al. Prostaglandin E by murine macrophages and human monocytes after in vitro treatment with biological response modifiers. J Immunopharmacol 1983; 5:129–46.
15. Schlick E, Friedberg KD. Bone marrow cells under the influence of low lead doses. Arch Toxicol 1982; 49:227.
16. Schlick E, Bartocci A, Chirigos MA. Effect of azimexone on the bone marrow of normal and γ-irradiated mice. J Biol Resp Modif 1982; 1:179.
17. Ladisch S, Reaman GH, Poplack GD. Bacillus Calmette-Guerin enhancement of colony stimulating activity and myeloid colony formation following administration of cyclophosphamide. Cancer Res 1979; 39:2544.
18. Stoychkov JN, Schultz RM, Chirigos MA, et al. Effects of adriamycin and cyclophosphamide treatment in induction of macrophage cytotoxic function in mice. Cancer Res 1979; 39:3014–7.
19. Schultz RM, Chirigos MA, Stoychkov JN, et al. Factors affecting macrophage cytotoxic activity with particular emphasis on corticosteroids and active stress. J Reticuloendothel Soc 1979; 26:83–92.
20. Sullivan R, Gans PJ, McCarroll LA. The synthesis and secretion of granulocyte-monocyte colony stimulating activity (CSA) by isolated human monocytes: Kinetics of the response to bacterial endotoxins. J Immunol 1983; 130:800–7.
21. Ruscetti FW, Chervenick PA. Release of colony stimulating activity from thymus-derived lymphocytes. J Clin Invest 1975; 55:520–7.
22. Chirigos MA, Saito T, Talmadge JE. The immunomodulatory activity of Picibanil (OK432). Amsterdam: Excerpta Medica, Ltd. 1984; 20–31.
23. Chan SH, Metcalf D, Stanley ER. Stimulation and inhibition of normal human serum of colony formation in vitro by bone marrow cells. Br J Immunol 1971; 20:329–40.
24. Das SK, Stanley ER, Guilbert LJ, Forman LW. Human colony-stimulating factor radioimmunoassay: Resolution of three subclasses of human colony-stimulating factors. Blood 1981; 58:630.

25. Stanley ER, Guilbert LJ. Methods for the purification, assay, characterization, and target cell binding of a colony stimulating factor (CSF). J. Immunol Methods 1981; 42:253.
26. Merluzzi VJ, Kenney RE, Schmid FA, Choi YS, Taanes RB. Recovery of the in vivo cytotoxic T-cell response in cyclophosphamide-treated mice by injection of mixed-lymphocyte culture supernatants. Cancer Res 1981; 41:3663–5.
27. Milton JD, Carpenter CB, Addision IE. Depressed T-cell reactivity and suppressor activity of lymphoid cells from cyclophosphamide-treated mice. Cell Immunol 1976; 24:308–17.
28. Merluzzi VJ, Welte K, Savage DM, Last-Barney K, Mertelsmann R. Expansion of cyclophosphamide-resistant cytotoxic precursors in vitro and in vivo by purified human interleukin 2. J Immunol 1983; 131:806–9.
29. Kurland JI, Broxmeyer HE, Pelus LM, et al. Role for monocyte-macrophage derived colony stimulating factor and prostaglandin E in the positive and negative feedback control of myeloid stem cell proliferation. Blood 1978; 52:388.
30. Kurland J, Pelus LM, Ralph P, et al. Induction of prostaglandin E synthesis in normal and neoplastic macrophages: Role for colony-stimulating factor(s) distinct from effects on myeloid progenitor cell proliferation. Proc Natl Acad Sci USA 1979; 76:2326.

Cancer Detection and Prevention Supplement 1:399–407 (1987)

Modulation of Antitumor Immune Responses

E. Mihich, MD

Grace Cancer Drug Center, Roswell Park Memorial Institute, New York State Department of Health, Buffalo, NY

ABSTRACT Based on experimentation in animal model systems it is reasonable to expect immunomodulation by anticancer drugs and biological response modifiers to be instrumental in at least some of the antitumor effects of such agents. Even in the defined animal models, however, the immunomodulating effects of any given agent are in most cases correlated only with the therapeutic response to that agent, whereas causal relationships still evade unequivocal demonstration. The difficulties in this respect are magnified in humans, in whom the very nature and regulation of antitumor immunity, taken in a broad sense, are not yet well defined; thus at this time the basis on which to interpret the therapeutic or toxicological causative relevance of an immunomodulating effect is insufficient. Despite these limitations and uncertainties, or perhaps responding to the challenge they provide, experimentation evaluating the potential of immunomodulation is being carried out in a number of diversified areas. Salient findings from selected investigations of the actions of 1) drugs, 2) cytokines, and 3) combinations of agents or effectors are discussed as examples of the realization of the potential of this overall approach as well as to outline the requirements for future development of biological response modifiers.

Key words: immunomodulation, interleukin 2, adriamycin, cyclophosphamide, interferons, tumor necrosis factor

INTRODUCTION

Despite the unquestionable therapeutic achievements in cancer chemotherapy and long-term survival without detectable disease that can be induced in patients by this modality of treatment with different types of neoplasias, it is evident that curative treatments are not yet available for the majority of the so-called solid tumors. Although continuing efforts are being made to develop new and better drugs and treatments with available drugs, in recent years attention has also been focussed on the possibility of establishing new modalities of treatment based on exploitation of host defenses against the tumor. Whereas the initial attempts in immunotherapy have been based essentially on immunomodulation through a relatively non-specific stimulation of host defenses by such agents as BCG [1–4], increasing knowledge of the multiple mechanisms of regulation of the immune response has led to the expectation that therapeutically advantageous imbalances of the immune response can be achieved through appropriate intervention and more ultimately yield more specific immune augmentation.

Address reprint requests to Dr. E. Mihich, Grace Cancer Drug Center, Roswell Park Memorial Institute, New York State Department of Health, Buffalo, NY 14263.

Immunomodulation may be achieved through the use of chemicals, including anticancer drugs, or natural products, through the administration of cytokines, of antibodies directed against regulatory components of the immune system, or of restorative agents such as thymic factors [1]. The administration of exogenous effectors of the immune response such as immune cells, antibodies directed against epitopes present in greater quantities on tumor cells than on normal cells, or cytotoxic cytokines normally mediating the action of host defense cells is another current approach. Active immunization with tumor-associated antigens (TAA), whether natural or modified by chemicals, viruses, or enzyme action, is also an important potential component of this area of therapeutics. Most of these approaches have been discussed recently by this author from different points of view [1–8], and it would be beyond the scope of this paper to review them extensively. Instead, only a few topics and concepts of current interest are considered herein, which are projected towards future developments in clinical experimentation more than being based on established clinical achievements. Consequently, most of the data discussed in this paper have been obtained in animal experimentation.

The types of immune interaction briefly considered are immunomodulation by anticancer drugs, antitumor effects of cytokines, and therapeutic potential of immune cell transfer. Requirements for the development of biological repsonse modifiers (BRM) like those just mentioned, and difficulties in meeting these requirements, are also outlined.

Based on the evidence that TAAs exist in humans [4] and that they are capable of eliciting a response in the autochthonous patient [4], it is reasonable to expect that immunomodulation through host or exogenous effectors or mediators will ultimately cause antitumor effects [4,9]. In most cases, immunomodulation involves a multiplicity of cells of the immune systems and a cascade of effects through multiple and often sequential actions of specific mediators and regulatory mechanisms. Moreover, it is becoming increasingly clear that tumor has multiple influences on host defenses, some of them resulting in an escape from those defenses [10]; indeed, it would be reasonable to expect that therapeutically advantageous immunomodulation could also be exerted through an intervention against the tumor escape mechanisms. From these all too sketchy remarks, it is already evident that the optimal design of therapeutically effective immune intervention requires a thorough knowledge of the immune status of a patient in specific relation to the tumor as well as to the antihost effects of the tumor. Moreover, although consistencies between immunomodulation and biological effects can usually be identified, direct causal relationships between immunomodification and antitumor actions are in most cases elusive. Thus, although efforts should be intensified to achieve the basic knowledge in clinical immunology required for the optimal design of immunomodulation in cancer therapeutics, at present a measure of empiricism in cancer immunotherapy must still unavoidably be accepted.

IMMUNOMODULATION BY DRUGS: ADRIAMYCIN (ADM) AND CYCLOPHOSPHAMIDE (Cy)

That certain anticancer drugs can exert immunomodulating activities has been repeatedly documented in recent years [6–8,11,12]. Some of the effects of ADM and Cy are discussed herein as examples of such drug action. Whereas the immunomodulation induced by these drugs has been demonstrated in animal model systems, the exploitation of their action in the treatment of human cancer has not yet been extensively attempted.

Studies in animals by others had suggested that the therapeutic effects of ADM against experimental tumors are in part mediated by cooperating mechanisms of host defenses. In fact, the antitumor effects of ADM are greater than those of daunorubicin in normal but not in immunocompromised mice [13,14]; these effects parallel the degree of tumor immunogenicity both in the Moloney virus tumor system [15] and in the leukemic L1210 system [16], and the drug is synergistic with *Corynebacterium Parvum* in normal but not in nude mice [17]. Based on these suggestions from in vivo experimentation, detailed studies of the potential immunomodulating activity of ADM were initiated in this laboratory. It was found that in an allogeneic tumor system ADM augments the differentiation of macrophages [18], inhibits selectively T-regulatory cells adherent to glass or plastic [19], stimulates interleukin-2 (IL-2) production from spleen cell population [20], stimulated PGE_2 production from macrophages [20,21], inhibits NK cells [21], stimulates lymphokine-activated killer (LAK) cell responses [21], and augments cytotoxic T-lymphocytes (CTL) responses [12,12,22]. From the overall evidence obtained it seems that macrophages and CTL and LAK cell responses are instrumental in the host-dependent therapeutic effects of ADM in mouse tumor model systems. The increased production of IL-2 by cells exposed to ADM represents an example of the potential modulation by an anticancer agent of a regulatory lymphokine, and it may be instrumental in the augmented CTL and/or LAK cell responses seen upon drug administration.

In investigations carried out using the Meth A sarcoma mouse model system [23], evidence has been found in support of the notion that tumor escape mechanisms are put into motion consequent to tumor growth. In fact, after the tumor reaches a certain critical size, TAAs elicit the development of Ly $1-2^+$ CTL. However, upon further growth, the tumor presence promotes the development of Ly 1^+2^--suppressor (Ts) cells that inhibit the CTL response. These pioneering investigations by North and his group were confirmed in different tumor model systems and provided information on which to base attempts at a therapeutic modification of the suppressor response. The opportunity to verify the feasibility of this approach was offered by the finding that at low doses Cy selectively inhibits Ts cell function. In the MOPC-315 mouse tumor model system, it was indeed found that the delayed administration of low doses of Cy induced tumor regression in contrast to the lack of effects of high doses of Cy or of low doses of the drug given early after tumor implantation [24]. The timing of low-dose Cy effectiveness was quite consistent with the timing of peak Ts development described by North [23] and suggests that therapeutic advantages can be obtained through a selective inhibition of Ts function. This suggestion was also supported by the observation made in the Meth A tumor system that Cy treatments in combination with T-cell adoptive transfer can exert therapeutic effects at the time of Ts development [23].

The exquisite selectivity of Cy on subsets of T cells was further demonstrated using both mouse [25] and human [26,27] T-cell systems in vitro. These experiments were made possible by the availability of 4-hydroperoxycyclophosphamide (4OOH-CY), a compound that in aqueous medium converts into active Cy metabolites without the need for hepatic biotransformation [28]. In a mouse Lyt 123^+ cell population, it was found that at certain concentrations 400H-CY selectively kills precursors of Ts cells without affecting Ts or either precursor of or mature T-killer cells [25]. Likewise, in a human OKT4$^+$8$^-$ cell population, the compound selectively eliminated precursor of Ts without affecting either precursor or mature T-killer cells [27]. Whereas these results indicate the ultimate selectivity of action of Cy in T-cell systems and the potential for selective therapeutic intervention, they also point to the fact that this drug was more discriminating than available monoclonal antibodies in selecting out subsets of T-cells within the same Lyt 123^+ or OKT4$^+$8$^-$ phenotype.

In conclusion, as indicated by the examples of ADM and Cy discussed, anticancer drugs have significant potentiality for immunomodulation and as such may provide useful tools for the dissection of immune responses and the identification of new functional cell types or of specific subsets of cells within a phenotype otherwise recognized as homogenous by the same monoclonal antibody. The utilization of drug-induced immunomodulation in cancer therapeutics seems promising, especially during remission-maintenance treatments or otherwise after tumor burden has been reduced by other therapeutic means; the design of clinical protocols to verify this promise is urgently needed.

ANTITUMOR EFFECTS OF CYTOKINES: INTERFERONS (IFN), TUMOR NECROSIS FACTOR (TNF), AND INTERLEUKIN 2 (IL-2) PLUS CELL TRANSFER

Considered in a rather broad sense, cytokines are cell products with activity on another cell or on self, which are made following different endogenous or exogenous stimuli. As a diversified group of biological products, cytokines undoubtedly have great potential for utilization in cancer therapeutics. They can exert direct antitumor action mimicking the action of physiological effectors, can act as immunomodulating agents to induce host-mediated antitumor effects, and can exert effects such as expansion and maintenance of host cells participating host defense mechanisms or induction of terminal differentiation in tumor cells. With the advent of recombinant DNA technology, the potential of cytokines can now be verified; indeed, until recently the main obstacle in this field was the difficulty of obtaining these biological products in sufficient quantity and purity. In this paper only certain aspects of the potential of IFNs, of TNF, and of IL-2 plus LAK cells transfer are briefly discussed as these cytokines have reached the level of clinical investigation.

The activity of IFNs, particularly IFNα, against human tumors is well known. It is sufficient to mention here than IFNα has activity against some human tumors when tested as a single agent. Objective responses have occurred in 10–15% of patients with renal cell carcinoma, melanoma, myeloma, and Kaposi's sarcoma; they have also been seen in about 40% of patients with different lymphomas and in 80–90% of patients with hairy cell leukemia and mycosis fungoides [4]. Initial trials with IFNβ and IFNγ suggest that these agents are also of therapeutic interest; in fact, IFNγ seems to have greater immunomodulating and antiproliferative activity than IFNα or INFβ [29]. As a whole, it seems reasonable to state that IFNs have shown activity against some forms of human cancer comparable to those exerted by certain cytotoxic agents at a similar stage of development. Moreover, it is likely that the antitumor action of IFNs will be better exploited when clinical investigations can be carried out with an increased knowledge of pertinent mechansims of response: The pursuit of basic and clinical investigations of IFNs seems not only amply justified but also urgently needed.

Numerous immunomodulating effects have been ascribed to the IFNs. IFNs have been reported to induce augmentation of CML to allogeneic cells, of ADCC, and of NK and to induce macrophage phagocytic and cytotoxic actions. Inhibition of mitogen-induced proliferation and DH reactions and, depending on conditions, either augmentation or depression of anti-SRBC antibody, GVH disease, and allograft rejection have also been found [5]. Recently, it was proposed that IFN plays a role in the activation of LAK cells [30]. Among these effects, augmentation of NK activity and of ADCC and activation of cells of the monocyte-macrophage type have received more attention as possible correlates of antitumor action. Until now, however, no correlation has been unequivocally demonstrated, this failure providing an example of the basic difficulties encountered in clinical investigations of BRMs when attempts are made to identify a BRM action that would be casuatively related to antitumor action [4]. The multiplicity of immunomodulating effects exerted by most BRMs studied to date further increases the difficulties in this regard.

Of the known activities of IFNs, namely, antiviral, direct antitumor cells, immunomodulating, and cell differentiating, each could have a role in the action of IFN against different tumor types. To date, many uncertainties still exist about the mode of action of the IFNs in patients with cancer. In particular, the role of immunomodulating vs antiproliferative effects has not yet been clarified, nor have the optimal dose and regimen been definitely established. It cannot be excluded that, depending on tumor type and dose, immunomodulation or direct anticell effect will prevail in determining antitumor action [4].

TNF is a glycoprotein produced by macrophages conditioned by BCG and triggered by endotoxin; it has now been obtained by recombinant DNA technology and is currently undergoing phase I clinical trials. It is too early to say whether the promise of laboratory experimentation will reach fruition in humans. As extensively studied by Old and his group [31–33], TNF induces hemorrhagic necrosis of tumor in rodent and selective cytotoxicity of certain tumor cell types in culture without effects on normal cells or other tumor cells. Sensitivity to lytic activity appears to be related to the presence of specific receptors on the target cell surface [33–35] and seems to be mediated through binding of the molecule to such receptors; TNF introduced directly into sensitive cells by micromanipulation is without effect

[35]. In addition to its direct cytotoxic effects, TNF also exerts immunomodulation as evidenced by the augmentation of CTL and LAK cells and macrophage functions induced in mouse model systems (unpublished results). It is not yet known whether the immunomodulating effects of TNF play a role in the antitumor action of the agent in mouse tumor model systems nor in humans. The 30% identity of TNF with lymphotoxin [36] poses questions about the relationships among cytotoxic cytokines and is consistent with the highly conserved nature of these molecules [36,37].

Increasing evidence is being obtained indicating that certain biological agents with BRM action when used in combination exert synergistic anticell action in culture, this suggesting the potential for in vivo synergisms. Although undoubtedly the examples of antitumor synergism will rapidly increase in the future, also including effects of biologicals combined with drugs having either BRM or cytotoxic action, at present several examples have already been reported in the case of IFNγ. IFNγ has been shown to synergize with IFNα [38], lymphotoxin [39], TFN [40], and the membrane-active agent tunicamycin [41] in causing the lysis of certain tumor cells, some of them insensitive to the action of either combinant alone. Synergism with MDP in augmenting macrophage activation [42] and with IL-2 in inducing LAK cells [30,43] has also been reported. As has been the case with cytotoxic drugs, there is little doubt that, also in the case of BRMS, their ultimate clinical utilization will be in combination, among themselves and/or with antiproliferative and cytotoxic agents. The facts that immunosuppression by anticancer drugs is generally of short duration [44] and that cytoreduction of tumor burden appears to facilitate BRM antitumor action are also consistent with the development of exploitable sequential combinations of cytotoxic drugs or cytotoxic BRMs with immunomodulating BRMs.

Clinical investigations of recombinant DNA IL-2 are at an early stage, and the therapeutic value of this lymphokine used alone cannot yet be assessed. Substantial evidence has been obtained in mice suggesting the potential value of IL-2 as an agent expanding and supporting the generation and function of T-effector and/or T-helper cells [45,46] and one that might be usefully employed in conjunction with adoptive transfer of immune lymphocytes [45–47]. Following the exhaustive pioneering investigations of the Seattle group, in recent years it was found that high concentrations of IL-2 induce the generation of antigen-independent lymphokine-activated killer (LAK) cells in culture of mouse spleen cells [48]. These cells are relatively specific against primary and metastatic mouse tumors in vivo but are clearly antigen-independent. IL-2 administration is required to sustain the proliferation and/or function of LAK cells developed in culture and transferred adoptively to tumor-bearing mice. These findings have been confirmed recently by Rosenberg and his group [49,50] in humans, in whom it was found that LAK cells can be generated from peripheral blood cells of the monocytic type. In phase I clinical studies, it has been demonstrated that IL-2 plus LAK cells can be safely administered to patients with advanced cancer [50]. In studies currently underway to test the anticancer efficacy of this combined treatment, objective responses were seen in 11 of 25 patients [51].

From the brief comments made above, it becomes evident that cytokines as a group may offer diversified opportunities for exploitation in cancer therapies based on their cytotoxic, immunomodulating, or differentiating action, including the possibility of using agents such as IL-2 to support the action of cells transferred adoptively to cancer patients. It is estimated that more than 100 different cytokines exist in nature; this large pool of biological factors with specificities of action is bound to represent a source of useful new anticancer agents, a hope consistent with the promise of those members of the group that have reached the stage of clinical trial [4].

GENERAL REQUIREMENTS OF BRM DEVELOPMENT

The examples of immunomodulation with potential therapeutic applications discussed herein are representative of some of the approaches currently the subject of intensive and focussed investigations. Approaches based on diversified uses of monoclonal antibodies were not mentioned, even though this is an area of considerable activity focussing on a variety of promising leads.

The use of anticancer drugs as immunomodulating agents may acquire importance in the future both in eliciting augmentation of effector responses and in facilitating these responses through an inhibition of immune suppressor and other mechanisms of tumor escape. Anticancer drugs were selected as an example of chemically induced immunomodulation because of their importance in oncology and the lack of sufficient recognition among clinical chemotherapists of their potential uses as BRMs. This is not to exclude from consideration other immunomodulating agents purified from fungi or microorganisms or synthesized chemically; these were extensively dicussed in recent reviews [1–5], as were their limitations and potentalities.

A difficulty that most immunomodulating chemicals and other agents have in common is the fact that they modify a variety of response mechanisms such that it is difficult to identify and verify the therapeutic potential of a unique modification of the immune effector system. This is an important deficiency; one of the major pre-requisites for optimal BRM development is, in fact, the identification of BRM action relevant to the antitumor action and the correlation between the two. Only through the establishment of such a correlation is it possible to determine a relevant optimal BRM dose (OBRMD), which, in appropriate relation to the maximum tolerated dose (MTD), could provide a basis for the design of phase II trials during which antitumor and BRM action would be rigorously correlated.

In the case of the cytokines, a distinction should be made between a true BRM effect and direct cytotoxicity of tumor cells. IFN and TNF are endowed with both types of activities. For their immunomodulating activity, the same considerations are valid in terms of the limitations related to the multiplicity of effects elicited by the agent. In contrast, for their cytotoxic activity, the well known concepts of selectivity of antitumor action established for cytotoxic agents would pertain.

Contrary to initial assumptions and optimistic expectations, BRMs have been shown to elicit toxicity both in preclinical systems and in humans [9], although in most cases this toxicity is not necessarily related to the mechanism of antitumor action as is usually the case for cytotoxic agents. Even for cytotoxic effectors such as IFN and TNF, toxicity does not seem to be primarily related to their antitumor cytotoxic action. In some cases, biological products of human origin are species-specific, and this may pose problems for a meaningful preclinical toxicological evaluation. Indeed, it is important that toxicological studies be carried out in relevant species and that relevant end points be measured with respect to the intrinsic characteristics of the BRM under development.

In conclusion, fundamental requirements for optimal BRM develoment are closely integrated with the need for increases in basic knowledge, in animals as well as in humans, about such fundamental phenomena as 1) tumor antigenicity and its role in determining immune responses and in effecting their regulation 2) pleiotropic mechanisms of regulation of antitumor host defenses, 3) mode of action of every BRM under study with specific focus on those actions that may be relevant to antitumor action, and 4) dynamic status of antitumor host defenses at the time of treatment, a major factor in determining the effectiveness and sometimes the direction of responses to BRMs [4]. It is fair to acknowledge that the fulfillment of these requirements is in most cases fraught with major difficulties, particularly in the face of the paucity of knowledge of tumor immunity in man. Althoguh these difficulties can be discouraging to some, they should also provide a stimulus towards intensifying investigations aimed at securing needed fundamental information on the action of BRMs and the biology of cancer such that this type of agent can be optimally developed with consequent realization of the therapeutic promise they represent.

REFERENCES

1. Mihich E. Biological response modifiers in cancer therapeutics. In Burchenal JH, Oettgan HF, eds: Cancer achievements, challenges and prospects for the 1980s, New York: Grune and Stratton, 1981, Vol 27 135–46.

2. Mihich E, Fefer A (eds): Report on the biological response modifiers by the subcommittee of the DCT Board of Scientific Advisors. J Ntl Cancer Inst Monogr No 63, 1983.

3. Mihich E. Biologial response modifiers: Their potential and limitations in cancer therapeutics. Cancer Invest 1985; 3:71–83.

4. Mihich E. Future perspectives for biological response modifiers: A viewpoint. Semin Oncol. In Pinsky C, Yarbro J, eds: New York: Grune Stratton, 1986; 13:234–254.

5. Mihich E. Relationships between chemotherapy and immunotherapy: A brief overview. In Tsubura E, Urushizaki I, Aoki T, eds: Rationale of biological response modifiers in cancer treatment (Int Cong Series 690). Amsterdam; Excerpta Medica, 1985; 105–15.

6. Ehrke MJ, Mihich E. Immunoregulation by cancer chemotherapeutic agents. In Hadden JW, Szentivanyi A, eds: The reticuloendothelial system: A comprehensive treatise. Vol 8, Pharmacology, New York: Plenum Press, 1985; 309–47.

7. Ehrke MJ, Mihich E. Immunological effects of anticancer drugs. In Berkarda B, Karrer K, Mathe G, eds: Clinical Chemotherapy. Vol III, Antineoplastic chemotherapy. Stuttgart: Thieme-Stratton, Inc. 1984; 475–99.

8. Ehrke MJ, Mihich E. Effects of anticancer agents on immune responses. Trends Pharmacol Sci 1985; 6:412–417

9. Mihich E, Kanter PM: The toxicology of biological response modifiers. In: Proc Int Seminar on the Immunotoxicological System as a Target for Toxic Damage, Luxembourg, November, 1984, London: Oxford Press, (in press).

10. Ozer H. Tumor immunity and escape mechansims in humans. In Mihich E, ed: Immunological approaches to cancer therapeutics. New York: John Wiley and Sons 1982; 39–73.

11. Ehrke MJ, Mihich E. Adriamycin and other anthracyclines. In Mitchell MS, Fahey JL, eds: Clinics in immunology and allergy. Vol 4, Immune Suppression and Modulation. London: WB Saunders Co, 1984; 259–77.

12. Mihich E, Ehrky MJ, Ishizuka M. Immunomodulations by antibiotics. In Mihich E, Sakurai Y, eds: Biological responses in cancer. Vol, 3 Immunodulation by anticancer drugs. New York: Plenum Press, 1985; 71–94.

13. Schwartz HS, Grindey GB. Adriamycin and daunorbuicin: A comparison of antitumor activities and tissue uptake in mice following immunosuppression. Cancer Res 1973; 33:1837–44.

14. Schwartz H, Kanter P. Cell interactions: Determinants of selective toxicity of adriamycin and daunorubicin. Cancer chemother Rep 1975; 6:107–14.

15. Giuliani F, Casazza AM, DiMarco A. Virologic and immunologic properties and response to daunomycin and adriamycin of a non-regressing mouse tumor derived from MSV-induced sarcoma. Biomedicine 1974; 21:435–39.

16. Mantovani A, Candiani P, Luini W, Saloma M, Spreafico F, Garattini S. Effects of chemotherapuetic agents on host defense mechanisms: Its possible relevance for the antitumoral activity of these drugs. In Ferrone S, Gorini S, Herberman RB, Reisfeld RA, eds: Current trends in tumor immunology. New York: Garland Press, 1979; 139–54.

17. Houchens DP, Johnson RK, Ovejera A, Gaston MR, Goldin A. Effects of *Corynebacterium parvum* alone and in combination with adriamycin in experimental tumor systems. Cancer Treat Rep 1976; 60:823–28.

18. Cohen SA, Ehrke MJ, Ryoyama K, Mihich E. Augmentation of the phagocytic activity of murine spleen cell populations induced by adriamycin. Immunopharmacology 1982; 5:75–83.

19. Ehrke MJ, Ryoyama K, Cohen SA. Cellular basis for adriamycin-induced augmentation of cell-mediated cytotoxicity in culture. Cancer Res 1984; 44:2497–504.

20. Ehrke MJ, Maccubbin D, Ryoyama K, et al. Correlation between adriamycin-induced augmentation of interleukin 2 production and of cell mediated cytotoxicity. Cancer Res 1986; 46:54–60.

21. Ehrke MJ, Maccubbin D, Salazar D, Mihich, E, Cohen SA. Evaluation of the link between adriamycin-induced effects of NJ or LAK activities and modulation of soluble mediators. Int J Immunopharmacol 1985; 7:307.

22. Ehrke MJ, Cohen SA, Mihich E. Selective effects of adriamycin on murine host defense systems. Immunol Rev 1982; 65:55–78,

23. North RJ. The murine antitumor immune responses and its therapeutic manipulation. Adv Immunol 1984; 35:-89–105.

24. Mokyr MB, Hengst JCD, Dray S. Role of antitumor immunity in cyclophosphamide-induced rejection of subcutaneous nonpalpable MOPC-315 tumors. Cancer Res 1982; 42:974–9.

25. Cowens JW, Ozer H, Ehrke MJ, Colvin M, Mihich E. Inhibition of the development of suppressor cells in culture by 4-hydroperoxycyclophosphamide. J Immunology 1983; 132:95–100.

26. Ozer H. Effects of alkylating agents on immunoregulatory mechanisms. In Mihich E, Sakurai Y, eds: Biological responses in cancer. Vol 3, Immunomodulations by anticancer drugs. New York: Plenum Press, 1985; 95–130.

27. Smith J, Cowens W, Nussbaum-Blumenson A, Sheedy D, Mihich E, Ozer H. Functional separation of human suppressor and cytotoxic T subsets defined in vitro by 4-hydroperoxycyclophosphamide (4-HC). Fed Proc 1982; 41:797.

28. Colvin M, Padgett A, Fenselou C. A biologically active metabolite of cyclophosphamide. Cancer Res 1973; 33:915.

29. Oldham RK. Biologicals and biological response modifiers: New approaches to cancer treatment. Cancer Invest 1985; 3:53–70.

30. Shiiba K, Suzuki R, Kawakami K, et al. Interleukin 2-activated killer cells: Generation in collaboration with interferon γ and its suppression in cancer patients. Cancer Immunol Immunother 1986; 21:119–128.

31. Carswell EA, Old LJ, Kassel RL, Green S, Fiore N, Williaman B. An endotoxin-induced serum factor that causes necrosis of tumors. Proc Natl Acad Sci USA 1975; 25:3666–73.

32. Hoffman MK, Oettgen HF, Old LJ, Mittler RS and Hammerling U. Induction and immunological properties of tumor necrosis factor. J Reticuloendothel Soc 1978; 23:307–19.

33. Rubin BY, Anderson SL, Sullivan SA, Williamson BD, Carswell EA, Old LJ High affinity binding of ^{125}I-labeled human tumor necrosis factor (LuKII) to specific cell surface receptors. J Exp Med 1985; 162:1099–104.

34. Kull FC Jr, Jacobs S, Cuatrecasas P. Cellular receptor for ^{125}I-labeled tumor necrosis factor: Specific binding, affinity labeling and relationship to sensitivity. Proc Natl Acad Sci USA 1985; 82:5756–60.

35. Niitsu Y, Urushizaki I and Hayashi H. Antitumor effects of TNF. Abstracts, 14th Int Cong Chemother, Kyoto, Japan, 1985. Abst. SY6-6, page 14.

36. Pennica D, Nedwin GE, Hayflick JS, et al. Human tumor necrosis factor: Precursor structure, expression and homology to lymphotoxin, Nature 1984; 312:724–9.

37. Beutler B, Greenwald D, Hulmes JD, et al. Identity of tumor necrosis factor and the macrophage-secreted factor cachectin. Nature 1985; 316:552–4.

38. Fleischmann WR Jr. Potentiation of the direct anticellular activity of mouse interferons: Mutual synergism and interferon concentration dependence. Cancer Res 1982; 42:869–75.

39. Lee SH, Aggarwal BB, Rinderknecht E, Assisi, F, Chiu H. The synergistic anti-proliferative effect of γ-interferon and human lymphotoxin. J Immunol 1984; 133:1083–6.

40. Williamson BD, Carswell EA, Rubin By, et al. Human tumor necrosis factor produced by human B-cell lines: Synergistic cytotoxic interaction with human interferon. Proc Natl Acad Sci USA 1983; 80:5397–401.

41. Maheshwari RK, Sreevalsan T, Silverman RH, Hay J, Friedman RM. Tunicamycin enhances the antiviral and anticellular activity of interferon. Science 1983; 219:1339–41.

42. Saiki I, Fidler IJ, Synergistic activation by recombinant mouse interferon-γ and muramyl dipeptide of tumoricidal properties in mouse marophages. J. Immunol 1985; 135:684–8.

43. Itoh K, Shiiba K, Shimizu Y, Suzuki R, Kumagai K. Generation of activated killer (AK) cells by recombinant interleukin 2 (rIL2) in collaboration with interferon-γ (IFN-γ). J Immunol 1985; 134:3124–9.

44. Mihich E. Chemotherapy and immunotherapy as a combined modality of cancer treatment. In: Advances in tumor preventions (Int Cong Series 420). Amsterdam: Excerpta Medica, 1978; 113–21.

45. Cheever MA, Greenberg PD, Fefer A. Lymphocyte transfer for cancer therapy: Prerequisites for efficacy and the use of long-term cultured T lymphocytes. In Mihich E, ed: Biological responses in cancer: Progress toward potential applications. New York, Plenum Press, 1984; Vol 2, 145–83.

46. Cheever MA, Greenberg PD, Fefer A. Potential for specific cancer therapy with immune T lymphocytes. J Biol Response Modif 1984; 3:113–27.

47. Cheever MA, Thompson JA, Kern DE, Greenberg PD, Interleukin-2 administered in vivo induces the growth and augments the function of cultured T cells in vivo. J Biol Response Modif 1984; 3:462–7.

48. Rosenstein M, Yron I, Kaufmann Y, Rosenberg SA, Lymphokine-activated killer cells: Lysis of fresh syngeneic natural killer-resistant murine tumor cells by lymphocytes cultured in interleukin-2. Cancer Res 1984; 44:1946–53.

49. Grimm EA, Mazumder A, Zhang HZ, Rosenberg SA. Lymphokine-activated killer cell phenomenon, lysis of natural killer-resistant fresh solid tumor cells by interleukin 2-activated autologous human peripheral blood lymphocytes. J Exp Med 1982; 155:1823–41.

50. Rosenberg SA. Immunotherapy of cancer by systemic administration of lymphoid cells plus interleukin-2. J Biol Response Modif 1984; 3:501–11.

51. Rosenberg SA, et al. Observations on the systemic administration of autologous lymphokine activated killer cells and recombinant Interleukin 2 to patients with metastatic cancer. N Engl J Med 1985; 313:1485–1492.

Cancer Detection and Prevention Supplement 1:409–421 (1987)

Correction of Secondary T-Cell Immunodeficiencies With Biological Substances and Drugs

John W. Hadden, MD

*Program of Immunopharmacology, University of South Florida
Medical College, Tampa, FL*

ABSTRACT   Secondary T-lymphocyte deficiencies are common in cancer, aging, malnutrition, chronic infection, and AIDS. Reconstitution with thymic hormones has not been successful. The various thymic hormone preparations induce prothymocyte differentiation and promote the differentiated functions of mature T cells, but they do not regulate intrathymic maturation. In contrast, interleukin 2, endotoxin, thymic epithelial cell products, but not interleukin 1 were found to promote functional maturation of immature thymocytes. Logically, thymic hormones may have synergistic interaction with inducers of intrathymic maturation, and preliminary evidence in athymic nude mice supports this notion. Two classes of drugs show thymomimetic actions. Levamisole, diethyl dithiocarbamate, and other sulfur-containing compounds restore T-cell function via induction of a thymic hormone-like factor. Isoprinosine, NPT 15392, and related hypoxanthine derivatives induce T-cell maturation directly and promote T-cell function in vitro and in vivo. An assessment of the combined actions of these drugs and biologicals should improve immunorestoration in T-cell deficiencies.

Key words: thymic hormones, interleukin 2, thymomimetic drugs, synergy

INTRODUCTION

Secondary immunodeficiencies involving the thymus-dependent T cell are more common than previously recognized. They result in a failure of cell-mediated immunity (CMI) with increased frequency and severity of infections and with an increased incidence of cancer and autoimmune phenomena. The clinical sequelae are generally only observed when the system becomes significantly compromised (eg, >50% loss of function). In the cancer patient the severity of the defects increase with the stage of the cancer, with poor nutrition and with multidrug cytoreductive therapy. As a result, infections are the most frequent cause of morbidity and mortality in cancer. Secondary T cell immunodeficiencies are also common to aging, malnutrition, parasitosis, chronic bacterial infection, and acute and chronic viral infections. Such deficiencies are also produced by immunosuppressive agents used in transplantation and inflammatory diseases or by accidental immunotoxicant exposure.

Perhaps the most dramatic example of secondary T-cell deficiency is the acquired immunodeficiency syndrome (AIDS) and its prodrome, the AIDS-related complex (ARC). In

Address reprint requests to Dr. John W. Hadden, Director, Program of Immunopharmacology, University of Southern Florida Medical College, 12901 North 30th St., Tampa, FL 33612.

these disorders the loss of number and function of T cells, particularly helper T cells, is progressive. Associated are defects of thymic hormone production and destruction of both the lymphoid and epithelial components of the thymus. The cause of the destruction is not clear. Infection of T cells with human T cell lymphotrophic virus (HTLV-III) also called *lymphade-nopathy-associated virus* (LAV) is a central feature; however, infection alone is not sufficient since the syndrome can be associated with specific immunity and the absence of immune deficiency. As a result of constitutional issues or concomitant infection with other lympho-trophic or immunosuppressive viruses, like herpes simplex virus, hepatitis B virus, cytomega-lovirus (CMV), or Epstein Barr virus (EBV), the T-cell destruction becomes progressive and irreversible, and complications by infections (particularly *Pneumocystis carinii* and *Mycobac-terium avium*) or cancer (particularly Kaposi sarcoma) develop. The rapid progression of this uniformly lethal disease and its epidemic nature in high risk populations has created a sense of urgency, and clinical immunologists and immunopharmacologists are being called upon to initiate, as quickly as possible, therapies to reverse the disease in AIDS patients and to prevent the progression of the AIDS-related complex into AIDS. The complexities involved in this problem have recently been reviewed [1]. I would like to review in a more general perspective what is known about the cellular and molecular components that regulate the T-cell system and discuss what the therapeutic prospects are for regulating the system with biologicals and drugs in the prevention or treatment of disease.

The expression of cellular immunity involves mainly a cooperation between thymus-derived T cells and monocyte-derived macrophages. In fact, the predominant cell in a CMI response in the macrophage. It will not be the purpose of this article to discuss those defects that derive from defective numbers or functions of the macrophage but rather to focus exclusively on the T cells. It is also notable that most severe T-cell defects result in dysregu-lation of the humoral immune, or B-cell, system with hyperglobulinemia, paraproteinemia, autoantibodies, and so forth. However, the B cell will not be discussed in any detail either.

The T-cell population is made up of two main and probably interchangeable components. The major population (approximately 5×10^{10} to 5×10^{11}) circulates in blood, percolates through the body's tissues, and circulates through lymphatics back into the blood. The second major population of approximately the same size resides in discrete areas of lymph nodes (deep cortex and paracortical areas), of spleen (periarteriolar region of the white pulp), and of Peyer patches and tonsils. The system is populated from the thymus primarily during late fetal life and early childhood and once populated can expand (two to 100 times) in relation to specific antigenic challenge. Normally, the system is a balanced and effective one capable of meeting a large variety of challenges quickly and efficiently and, once resolved, retaining resistance and memory for decades thereafter.

Defects of the T-cell system are variously but generally associated with decreased numbers of circulating T cells. Virtually all lymphocytopenias are T-cell lymphopenias since T cells constitute about 80% of peripheral blood lymphocytes (eg, cancer and AIDS). In other disorders T cells are present in near-normal numbers but are dysfunctional or nonfunctional (eg, aging and drug-induced immunosuppression for transplantation). Dysfunction of T cells may result from extrinsic causes such as suppressor factors or drugs, or intrinsic causes such as cellular senescence or viral infection. Other causes of dysfunction are deficiency of specific nutrients (eg, zinc or biotin), endocrine hormone deficiencies (eg, growth hormone, thyroid hormone, and insulin), and, perhaps most importantly, thymic hormone deficiency (to be elaborated on later). In other disorders a combination of the two types of defects are manifest (eg, AIDS-related complex).

In most clinical settings T-cell deficiencies can be diagnosed by a variety of techniques using T-cell counts, lymphoproliferative assays, and skin test responses. More specific diag-nostics and subset enumeration using more complex T-cell subset functional analysis, serum inhibitor analyses, anti-T-cell antibodies, lymphokine production, IL-2 receptors, thymulin or thymosin α_1 serum levels, and so forth, represent experimental tests reserved for the research laboratory.

So far, treatment specifically designed to correct T-cell deficiencies has been restricted to the following: 1) fetal thymus transplantation in certain patients with severe combined immunodeficiency disease (SCID); 2) thymic hormone therapy in primary immunodeficiency, particularly DiGeorge syndrome and SCID with B cells [2]; 3) thymic hormones and transfer factor treatment in collected acquired deficiencies [2–4]; 4) levamisole and thymosin treatment of cancer patients [3,5]; and 5) a variety of substances (isoprinosine, azimexon, imreg, thymosin, thymopoietin, thymulin, and interleukin 2 (IL-2) in AIDS and the AIDS-related complex [1]. All of these treatments are presently considered experimental in the United States. All have shown some degree of efficacy, and it is reasonable to expect that as our clinical efforts, both diagnostically and therapeutically, became more precise these treatments will become accepted in clinical practice. The ensuing discussion will focus briefly on the preclinical immunopharmacologies of the biologicals and drugs that are likely candidates for future clinical use in the correction of T-cell deficiencies.

THYMIC HORMONES [2,3,6]

A large variety of substances have been extracted from the thymus gland and termed *thymic hormones*. These substances are thought to be extracted from the hormone-producing cells of the thymus, the thymic epithelial cells. Unfortunately, the entire thymus has been used in their preparation so that in the partially purified preparations (like thymosin fraction V and thymostimulin TP-1) lymphocyte and epithelial constituents abound in addition to thymic hormones (see Table I).

Three thymic hormone preparations have been purified to homogeneity and synthesized either by chemical synthesis or by genetic engineering. These are thymopoietin, thymosin α_1, and thymulin (previously FTS). All of these thymic hormones have been shown to modulate prothymocyte and thymocyte function in one or another assay; however, few direct comparisons have been made to allow a proper assessment of differences in their actions. By way of general statement it can be said that several different substances show activity and can be considered to meet the criteria of a thymic hormone. The capacity to modulate thymocyte development is consistent with events that are known to occur in the thymus and in the periphery in the presence of a thymus (ie, a source of thymic hormone); however, none of these preparations are sufficiently potent to restore cell-mediated immunity in the absence of a thymus or when the defect is well established and severe.

INTERLEUKIN 2 [3,7]

IL-2 is a product of mature T cells and immature large granular lymphocytes (probably pre-T cells). The production by mature T cells results from the action of a monocyte/macrophage product called *interleukin 1* (IL-1). IL-2 acts to allow antigen-primed, mature T cells (triggered to synthesize RNA and protein) to enter DNA synthesis and to replicate

TABLE I. Thymic Hormone Characterization

	Source	M.W. isoelectric point	Sequenced	Demonstrated epithelial origin	In vitro induction of markers	Active on CMI in vivo
Thymosin Fraction V	Bovine Thymus	>35 Peptides	−	+	+	+
Thymostimulin (TP-1)	Thymus	Variable Multiple	−	ND	+	+
Thymosin α_1	Thymus	3107	+	+	+	+
Thymopoietin	Thymus	5662	+	+	+	+
Thymulin (FTS)	Pig Serum	$857 + Zn^{2+}$	+	+	+	+

clonally. Only mature T cells respond to IL-1 to make IL-2; however, immature T cells have recently been described to have IL-2 receptors [8,9]. Their possible role in T-cell development will be discussed later in this article.

TRANSFER FACTOR/DIALYZED LEUKOCYTE EXTRACT/IMREG [4,10]

A variety of small, dialyzable factors have been extracted from T cells and given various names. All have been described to modulate nonspecifically the T cell-mediated immunity. Transfer factor has been ascribed specificity in that it can transfer sensitivity from a sensitized to a nonsensitized donor. It is important to note, for purposes that will become apparent, that while the structure of transfer factor has not been elucidated, it is thought to contain inosine as part of its structure. If one accepts both the specific and the nonspecific aspects of the transfer factor phenomena, the logical postulate is that lymphocytes when killed or perhaps following antigen challenge release transfer factor. It then circulates in the blood and acts on immature or precommitted cells to make them responsive to the particular antigen and acts to prime or precommitted cells to make them responsive to the particular antigen and acts to prime generally the T-cell system to be more active. How these postulated events occur is not clear.

ENDOTOXIN [11,12]

Lipopolysaccharide (LPS) components of gram-negative bacteria have long been known to be active to modulate cellular immune responses. The actions of LPS on T cells have generally been considered secondary to its effects as a polyclonal B lymphocyte mitogen and as a macrophage activator; however, a variety of effects on T cells have been described [12].

Scheid et al [13] have shown that LPS induces prothymocytes to differentiate in culture into cells bearing the markers of intrathymic lymphocytes. We have shown that LPS induces immature thymocytes to mature into mitogen-responsive T cells [12]. Several investigators [14–17] have shown that, while LPS does not induce polyclonal activation of thymocytes or T cells, it does synergize with concanavalin A (Con A) to increase T-cell proliferation, particularly at low doses of Con A [18]. Whether this latter effect is mediated by IL-1 produced by thymic macrophages is not clear, since unfractionated thymocyte populations were used in these studies. Others [19] have shown that LPS can stimulate growth of the T-cell line and a small population (3%) of splenic T cells. These studies indicate that T cells at various stages of development are sensitive to LPS action.

These effects are important to consider here for several reasons: Endotoxins act to induce T-cell maturation at several steps, and the effect, in so far as examined, is mediated by lipid A; lipid A has recently been detoxified by Ribi et al. [20] as monophosphoryl lipid A (MPLA) and is being introduced into clinical trails in humans. MPLA may be useful in certain circumstances to modulate safely T-cell development and immunity.

THYMOMIMETIC DRUGS [21]

The two main classes of compounds having thymomimetic action are represented by levamisole and isoprinosine (Table II). They act directly or indirectly via induced factors to induce the differentiation of prothymocytes and to modulate mature T-cell receptors and functions. Each class is also represented by structurally similar compounds that, in so far as have been examined, share similar immunopharmacologies. Representatives of both classes of agents augment cell-mediated immune responses as measured both in vitro and in vivo.

Not all of the activities of the two compounds can be termed thymomimetic. Additional features of levamisole's in vitro actions that are not strictly thymomimetic include augmentation of lymphokine-induced macrophage phagocytosis and activation, augmentation of macrophage and granulocyte motility, and induction of interferon. Similarly, additional features of isoprinosine's in vitro action that are not strictly thymomimetic include induction of B-cell differentiation, potentiation of γ interferon and interleukin 2 production by T cells, increase in natural killer cell activity, increased monocyte phagocytosis, potentiation of lymphokine-induced

TABLE II. Classification of Thymomimetic Drugs

Class 1: sulfur-containing compounds	Indirect T- cell induction*	Active rosettes	CMI	T-dependent B-cell response
Levamisole	+	+	+	+
Diethyl dithiocarbamate	+	NT	+	+
NPT 16416	NT	+	NT	+
Thiabendazole	+ (antigen)	NT	+	NT
Thiazolobenzimidazole	NT	+	+	+
Cimetidine	NT	+	+	+
Class 2: purine-containing compounds	Direct T- cell induction	Active rosettes	CMI	T-dependent B-cell response
Isoprinosine	+	+	+	+
NPT 15392	+	+	+	+
NPT 16416	+	+	NT	+
Transfer factor	+	+	NT	NT

NT, not tested.
*Via a serum factor induced in vitro.

macrophage proliferation and activation, and increased antibody-dependent cytotoxicity by eosinophils.

Many of the immune functions shown to be affected by levamisole, isoprinosine, and the thymic hormones in vitro have been confirmed in vivo following administration to experimental animals and human subjects. The in vivo results in animals and man are summarized qualitatively in Table III. For the purposes of simplicity, the actions of the various thymic hormone preparations have been grouped collectively to indicate that these are general actions of thymic hormones. Not all of the preparations have been demonstrated to be active in each assay. Individual preparations shown to be active have been noted. Table III makes the general point that, to the extent tested, levamisole and isoprinosine share the immunopharmacologic actions of the thymic hormones as assessed by in vitro parameters, DTH, and resistance to viral infection, cancer, and autoimmunity.

REGULATION OF T-CELL ONTOGENY

Much of the foregoing and the reviews cited described the action of the biologicals and drugs discussed on mature T cells. While association of thymic hormones with T-cell differentiation is known, the roles of the endocrine thymus and, for that matter, other possible mediators in the regulation of T-cell ontogeny remain unclear. The successful therapeutic correction of these T-cell deficiencies depends on a more complete understanding of the regulation of T-cell maturation. To understand the potential for these substances to reconstitute T-cell number as well as T-cell function, I will review some of our recent studies on their actions at various levels of T-cell ontogeny [22]. Figure 1 depicts one version of the ontogeny of T cells in the mouse; similar schema have been presented for the human [23].

The first step of T-cell development is determined in the Komuro-Boyse assay [13]. The Komuro-Boyse assay employs prothymocytes obtained from athymic nude mouse spleens in a 2 hr incubation with various inducers. The induction of Thy-1 (formerly Θ) is assessed as a measure of one of the earliest steps of T-cell differentiation.

A number of thymic hormone preparations are active in the induction of T-cell differentiation in this assay (Fig. 2A). These include thymosin fraction V, thymosin α_1, thymulin, and thymopoietin. Thymic epithelial cell supernatants prepared by A. Galy and J.-L. Touraine are also active (Fig. 2B). We have recently found that IL-2 (electronucleonics) and cloned IL-2 (kindly provided by Steven Gillis, Immunex) are active between 2 and 32 units/ml to induce maturation in this assay (Fig. 2C). We have also found that Il-2 regulates the basal proliferation

TABLE III. In Vivo Effects of Levamisole, Isoprinosine, and Thymic Hormones on Immune Function of Experimental Animals* and Man

Immune function	Levamisole	Isoprinosine	Thymic hormones†
Experimental animals			
T cell-marker induction in athymic or thymectomized mice	+	+	+
T-cell mitogen responses	+	+	+
Lymphokine production	+	+	+
Cytotoxicity of T cells	+	+	+
Cell-mediated immunity			
DTH or graft rejection	+	+	+
T-dependent antibody production	+ (variable)	+	+
Natural killer cell activity	?	+	?
Macrophage function	+	+	0
Resistance to pathogen challenge	+	+	+
Resistance to tumor recurrence			
Following cytoreductive therapy	+	NT	+
Without cytoreductive therapy	0	0	0
Reduction of autoimmunity	+	+	+
Reversal of effects of aging on immune response	+	+	+
Man			
Active rosettes of T cells	+	+	+
T-cell mitogen response	±	+	+
Lymphocyte counts	±	±	±
DNCB or skin tests	+	+	+
Resistance to cancer	+ (after chemotherapy)	NT	+ (thymosin)
Resistance to virus infection	+	+	+ (THF)
Decreased autoimmunity	+	+	+ (FTS, TP5)

*Particularly in immunosuppressed mice.
†Particularly in thymectomized mice.
NT, not tested.

of this cell population. These represent the first observations delineating a functional role for IL-2 on prothymocytes of the mouse and indicate that these cells have IL-2 receptors.

Inosine-like compounds isoprinosine and NPT 15392 have been previously shown by Ikehara et al [24] to induce prothymocyte maturation (Fig. 2D) leading to the description of these compounds as thymomimetic drugs [21]. We previously postulated that these drugs act to induce T-cell differentiation via a purine (nonadenosine) receptor, perhaps the same receptor acted on by transfer factor since the latter has been shown to contain inosine [25]. Figure 2E shows the effect of a transfer factor prepared by Chen et al [26] to induce prothymocyte differentiation, strengthening the postulate that the action of transfer factor and thymomimetic purines may be related phenomena. Figure 2F summarizes the observations of Scheid et al [13], showing that endotoxin and polyA:polyU also induce T-cell maturation. Figure 2F presents studies by Specter and Hadden in the mouse showing that a new thymomimetic drug, LF 1695 [2 (methyl-1-pyperidinyl)-5 aminophenyl (4-chlorophenyl)-methanone], induces Thy-1, thus confirming the work of Othmane et al [27] in the human. Also active in this system are sera from athymic mice treated with sulfur-containing drugs such as levamisole and diethyl dithiocarbamate (DTC), which, according to Renoux et al [28,29], contains a factor derived from liver called *hepatosine*.

The validity with which one can extrapolate from these in vitro data to the in vivo setting is open to question; however, the following substances, in addition to thymosin and the other thymic hormone preparations, have been shown to induce Thy-1–bearing cells in vivo:

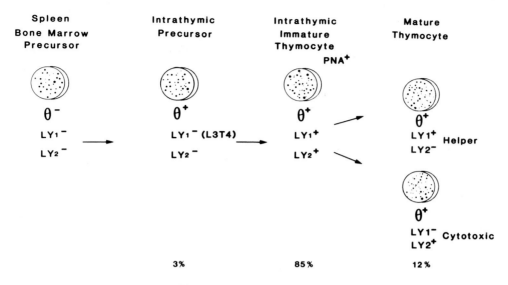

Fig. 1.   Mouse T-cell ontogeny.

Interleukin-2 [30], isoprinosine and NPT 15392 [31] (Ikehara, Pahawa, and Hadden, unpublished data), and levamisole and DTC [28].

The second assay in the study of thymocyte ontogeny [32] involves the use of peanut agglutinin-positive (PNA$^+$), immature cortical thymocytes in a 16–24 hr incubation with various inducers. The induction of Con A responsiveness is measured by thymidine incorporation after 72 hr of culture. Since only PNA$^-$ mature, medullary thymocytes are Con A responsive, this assay measures the maturation of PNA$^+$ cells to acquire functional traits of PNA$^-$ cells. The receptor correlates of these intrathymic maturation steps have been previously reported by us and others [12,13,32] and are summarized in Figure 1.

The maturation of PNA$^+$ immature cells (ie, Thy-1$^+$, Ly$^-$ and/or Thy-1$^+$, Ly$^+$ [L3T4$^+$, Ly2$^+$] cells) to mature subsets of Thy-1$^+$, L3T4$^+$, Ly2$^-$ or L3T4$^-$, and Ly2$^+$ cells depicted on the right side of Figure 1 are the steps presumed to be influenced in the PNA$^+$ thymocyte induction assay. The induction of maturation of Thy-1$^-$ cells to Thy-1$^+$ cells is not known to be associated with the acquisition of any of the functions characteristic of mature T lymphocytes, and it has not been shown that any of the aforementioned substances alone can induce function of Thy-1$^+$ lymphocytes in vivo in the athymic nude mouse in the absence of antigen. Therefore, it becomes important to assess the question as to what are the appropriate inducers of intrathymic maturation for mature phenotype and function. We showed that IL-2 induces PNA$^+$ thymocytes to undergo surface receptor changes of H2 and TL antigens corresponding to the acquisition of the mature phenotype [32]. Conlon et al [33] and Oppenheim et al [34] showed that IL-2 induces mitogen responsiveness in the otherwise Con A-unresponsive PNA$^+$ thymocytes. Irle et al [35] previously showed that lymphokine preparations plus mitogen also induce these functions. Kruisbeek and Astaldi [36] and Beardsley et al [37] have reported that thymic epithelial cells produce factors acting to induce PNA$^+$ immature thymocytes to become responsive to mitogen and to the mixed leukocyte reaction with the production of IL-2, cytotoxic T cells, and T cell-replacing factor.

Using two protocols for incubating PNA$^+$ thymocytes with various inducers we attempted to ascertain how IL-2 induced the functional maturation of these cells. In the first procedure the cells were preincubated with IL-2 for 24 hr followed by the addition of concanvalin A (Con A), a further 72 hr of culture, and terminated by a 4 hr pulse to assess thymidine incorporation; one control for this assay included the addition of IL-2 with Con A

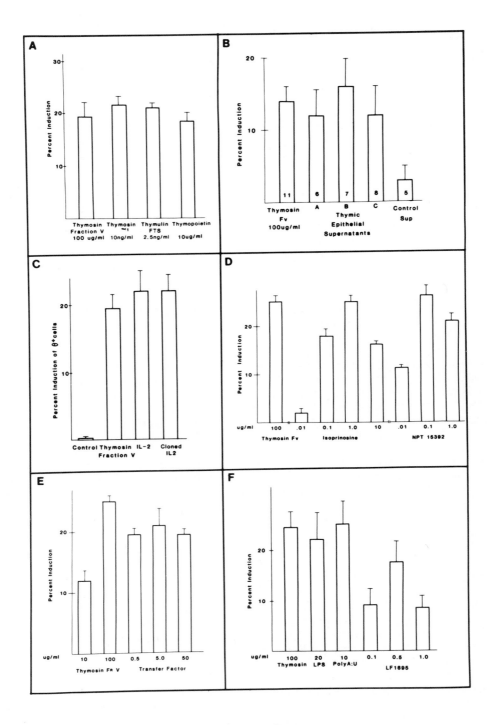

Fig. 2.   The Komuro-Boyse assay.

at 24 hr after culture initiation to assess what portion of the action of the inducer temporally proceeded the action of Con A. In the second protocol the cells were washed thoroughly after 24 hr preincubation with IL-2 but prior to the addition of Con A to remove inducer. Figure 3A shows the effect of IL-2 on PNA$^-$ mature T cells and PNA$^+$ immature T cells using the first protocol. As expected, PNA$^-$ cells are very responsive to Con A, IL-2 alone causes a small increase in thymidine incorporation, and the two added together show an increased response. The preincubation of these cells with IL-2 followed by its removal does not increase their intrinsic Con A responsiveness. In contrast, the PNA$^+$ thymocytes (26% yield of the total cells in these experiments) showed a negligible resonse to Con A. They did show a small but significant increase in thymidine incorporation with IL-2 (1 to 32 units) in the absence of Con A. If preincubated with IL-2 a sizeable Con A response developed, approaching 30–50% of that of the PNA$^-$ matue cells. This reponse was not observed when IL-2 was added at the same time as Con A, presumably because of the temporal restrictions of exposure to IL-2 in the assay (72 hr for the coincubation and 96 hr for the preincubation) or because of a fragility of the inducible population (R. Scollay, personal communication). Importantly (as shown in Fig. 3B), preincubation followed by washing to remove the Il-2 also induced a comparable Con A response in PNA$^+$ cells. Under both circumstances cloned IL-2 at similar concentra-

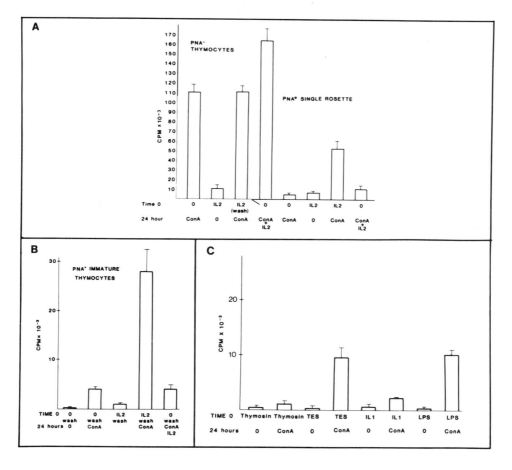

Fig. 3 Results of experiments attempting to show how IL-2 induces the functional maturation of thymocytes.

tions was equally active (data not shown). These data indicate further that IL-2 is a regulator of immature thymocyte maturation.

The source of intrathymic Il-2 remains to be determined, and an extrathymic source derived from activated mature T cells or from large granular lymphocytes in the periphery remains a possibility to be confirmed. Such a possibility offers an explanation for how activation of T cells could lead to an IL-2 signal calling for intrathymic maturation of immature cells and their exodus to replenish and magnify a response. Thymosin fraction V (known to contain thymosin α_1, thymulin, and thymopoietin, as well as other active peptides) did not induce Con A responses in PNA$^+$ cells (Fig. 3C). Coincubation of thymosin fraction V and IL-2 neither increased nor decreased the IL-2 effect, thus ruling out the presence of inhibitors or a synergistic interaction. IL-1 (kindly provided by C. Dinarello) was also inactive in this assay. Endotoxin (LPS) (0.1–10 μg) and the thymic epithelial supernatants (TES) were also active. Both the endotoxin and the TES were free of IL-2–like activity as tested in the IL-2–dependent CTLL cell assay. The TES preparations were sufficiently free of endotoxin (<20 ng/ml) to disallow endotoxin contamination as an explanation for their effect. The effects of LPS in this system (E. Hadden and A. Galy, unpublished data) are additive with those of IL-2, are mimicked by monophosphoryl lipid A (Detox, kindly provided by E. Ribi, Ribi Immunochem), blocked by polymyxin B, and occur in thymocytes from C57Bl/6 but to a lesser extent in C3H/HeJ mice. It is notable that TES contain active molecules not present in thymosin fraction V.

In summarizing these results, it is clear that IL-2, endotoxin, and thymic epithelial factors promote Con A responses of PNA$^+$ thymocytes. The significance of the acquisition of Con A responsiveness in PNA$^+$ cells is presumably that the cells also acquire the other functional and surface marker attributes of mature cells.

Recent experiments using thymus populations separated by a fluorescence-activated cell sorter (FACS) have raised questions about the target cells responsive in the PNA$^+$ thymocyte assay [38–40]. Raulet [9] has shown that the intrathymic precursor population (3%; see Fig. 1) is responsive to IL-2$^+$ and Con A with proliferation. Shortman and Scollay [38] and Chen et al [39] have argued that PNA$^-$ mature cells contaminating the PNA$^+$ population account for the results. The recent results of Andrews et al. [40] confirm our results that thymic hormones do not act on the PNA$^+$ immature population. Zatz and Goldstein [41] have recently shown effects of thymosin fraction V to augment IL-2 production by PNA$^-$ mature thymocytes; however, Andrews et al were unable to show effects of TES to stimulate PNA—mature thymocytes [40]. In the unfractionated thymocytes, thymosin, LPS, IL-2, IL-1, and TES all augment mitogen resonses. It thus remains unclear whether the biologics under discussion act on immature nonfunctional cortical cells and/or prefunctional medullary cells, as well as mature T cells. Further work using cell separation in conjunction with marker induction and function assay is needed. It will be important not to overlook cell-cell interactions, perhaps evident in the responses of unfractionated T cells.

Many studies indicate that mature T cells in the periphery are modulated by thymic hormones, TES, as well as the thymomimetic drugs isoprinosine and levamisole and their various analogs. Table IV summarizes the actions of various regulators discussed here on various parameters of T-cell maturation.

CONCLUSION

From the immunopharmacologist's standpoint, the significance of these observations lies in their potential to increase the effectiveness of thymic reconstitution using molecular means. The attempts at functional reconstitution in athymic humans and mice have been somewhat limited with thymic hormone treatment alone. The observations reported herein would indicate that current thymic hormone preparations do not display all of the activities manifest in TES and the current thymic hormone preparations will act synergistically with IL-2 and/or endotoxin in reconstituting T cell-dependent individuals. The prospects of molecular reconstitution

TABLE IV. Immunopharmacologic Attributes of Various Biologicals and Drugs

	Prothymocyte induction Komuro-Boyse assay	PNA$^+$ thymocyte induction	PNA$^-$ thymocyte and mature T-cell modulation	Active on CMI in vivo
Thymic hormones	+	0	+	+
TES	+	+	+*	ND
IL-2	+	+	+	+*
IL-1	0	0	+	ND
LPS	+	+	+	+
Isoprinosine and/or related compounds	+	0	+	+
Levamisole and/or related related compounds	+	ND	+	+

*Unpublished results.

of both the humoral function of the thymus in the athymic individual and the positive therapeutic regulation of the ontogeny of T cells in individuals bearing a thymus but otherwise deficient in T cells appear to be realizable goals. To achieve such goals further dissection of the action of the various biologicals on the component steps of the system is needed. Theoretically, as one can reconstitute cell-mediated immunity in the neonatally thymectomized mouse using a thymic transplant in a cell impermeable millepore chamber, one should be able to reconstitute with the appropriate soluble mediators involved, ie, thymic hormones, TES, IL-1, and IL-2, and so forth. it is known that gnotobiotic animals show significant T-cell deficiencies, so it is thus relevant to consider whether the absence of LPS as well as the absence of antigen is important. We have recently postulated that the development of the T-cell system may be dependent on endotoxin interacting with other molecualr components of the system [12,22]; therefore, it may be important to include detoxified endotoxin as part of the effort to reconsitute the immune system. Other extrathymic factors of central nervous system, hepatic, or endocrine origin need also to be considered. The foregoing assumes that the thymus can be replaced with molecular therapy; it ignores the role of the thymus in major histocompatability (MHC)-defined self-recognition. The lack of intrathymic education may pose limitations such as incomplete reconstitution or autoimmunity. To explore these strategies the athymic nude mouse represents an ideal model for the efforts. Several reports document T-cell maturation with thymic hormones, IL-2, levamisole, DTC, isoprinosine, virus infection, and aging [28–31,35,42,43]. I have confidence that if we are able consistently and effectively to reconstitute T-cell number and function in the athymic nude mouse by molecular means we will be able to develop the most appropriate therapy for secondary T-cell deficiencies, including AIDS.

REFERENCES

1. Hadden JW. Perspectives on the Immunotherapy of AIDS. NY Acad Sci 1985; 437:76–84.
2. Byrom NA, Hobbs JR. Thymic factor therapy. Serono Symposium, Vol 16. New York: Raven Press, 1984.
3. Goldstein A. Thymic hormones and lymphokines. New York: Plenum Press, 1984.
4. Spitler LE. Immunopharmacologic therapy of immunodeficiency. In Hadden JW, Chedid L, Mullen P, Spreafico F, eds. Advances in immunopharmacology. Oxford: Pergamon Press, 1981; 149–56.
5. Amery WK, Hörig C. Levamisole. In Fenichel RL, Chirigos MA, eds. Immune modulation agents and their mechanisms. New York: Marcel Dekker, Inc., 1984; 383–408.
6. Goldstein G, Lau C. Thymopoietin and immunoregulation. In Beers, F, Basset EG, eds. Polypeptide hormones. New York: Raven Press, 1980; 459–64.
7. Smith KA, Wang, H-M, Cantrell DA. The varibles regulating T cell growth. In Yamamura Y, Tada T, eds. Progress in Immunology V. Tokyo: Academic Press, 1984; 259–71.

8. Ceredig R, Lowenthal JW, Nahholz M, MacDonald HR. Expression of interleukin-2 receptors as a differentiation marker on intrathymic stem cells. Nature 1985; 314:98–100.

9. Raulet DH. Expression and function of interleukin-2 receptors on immature thymocytes. Nature 1985; 314:101–3.

10. Fudenberg H, Wilson G, Tsang K. Evaluation of transfer factor potency and prediction of clinical response. In Fudenberg H, Whitten H, Ambrogi F, eds. Immunomodulation. New York: Plenum Press, 1984; 115–30.

11. Nowotny A. Beneficial effects of endotoxin, New York: Plenum Press, 1983.

12. Hadden JW, Galy A, Hadden E, Touraine J-L, Coffey RG. Cyclic nucleotides in the immunopharmacology of lipopolysaccharide endotoxins. In Nowotny A, Friedman H, Szentivanyi A, eds. The immunobiology and immunopharmacology of bacterial endotoxins. New York. Plenum Press (in press).

13. Scheid MP, Goldstein G, Boyse EA. The generations and regulation of lymphocyte populations. J Exp Med 1978; 147:1727–32.

14. Forbes J, Nakao Y, Smith R. T mitogens trigger LPS responsiveness in mouse thymus cells. J Immunol 1975; 114:1004–8.

15. Ozato K, Adler W, Ebert J Synergism of bacterial lipopolysaccharides and concavalin A in the activation of thymic lymphocytes. Cell Immunol 1975; 17:532–7.

16. Watson J. The influence of intracellular levels of cyclic nucleotides on cell proliferation and the induction of antibody synthesis. J Exp Med 1975; 141:97–102.

17. Watson J. The involvement of cyclic nucleotide metabolism in the initiation of lymphocyte proliferation induced by mitogens. J Immunol 1976; 117:1656–61.

18. Schmidtke J, Najarian J Synergistic effects on DNA synthesis of phytohemagglutinin or concanavalin A and lipopolysaccaride in human peripheral blood lymphocytes. J Immunol 1975; 104:742–7.

19. Vogel S, Hilfiker M, Caulfield M. Endotoxin-induced T-lymphocyte proliferation. J Immunol 1983; 130:1774–9.

20. Ribi EE, Amano K, Cantrell J, Schwartzman S, Parker R, Takayama K. Preparation and antitumor activity of nontoxic lipid A. Cancer Immunol Immunother 1982; 12:91–6.

21. Hadden JW. Thymomimetic drugs. In Miescher P, Bolis L, Ghione M, eds. Immunopharmacology. New York: Serono Symposium Press, 1985; 183–92.

22. Hadden JW, Spector S, Galy A, Touraine L-L, Hadden EM. Thymic hormones, interleukins, endotoxin and thymomimetic drugs. In Chedid L, Hadden J, Spreafico F, Dukor P, Willoughby D, eds. Immunopharmacology III. Oxford: Pergamon Press 1986; 487–97.

23. Umiel T, Schlossman D, Reinherz E. A functionally unique IL-2 responsive human cortical thymocyte subpopulation epxresses mature T cell antigens. In Serrou B, Rosenfeld C, Daniels JC, Saunders JP, eds. Current concepts in human immunology and cancer immunomodulation. The Netherlands: Elsevier Biomedical Press, 1982; Vol 17, 31–47.

24. Ikehara S, Hadden JW, Good RA, Pahwa R. In vitro effects of two immunopotentiators, isoprinosine and NPT 15392 on murine T-cell differentiation and function. Thymus 1981; 3:97–106.

25. Hadden JW, Cornaglia-Ferraris P, Coffey RG. Purine analogs as immunomodulators. In Yamamura Y, Tada T, eds. Progress in immunology V. Tokyo: Academic Press, 1983; 1393–408.

26. Chen SS, Tung JS, Gillis S, Good RA, Hadden JW. Changes in surface antigens of immature thymocytes under the influence of interleukin II and thymic factors. Int J Immunopharmacol 1982; 4:381.

27. Othmane O, Touraine L-L, Sanhadji K, Pascal M. Evaluation of a new immunomodulator, LF 1695, on human and murine lymphocytes. EOS 1984; 4:151–3.

28. Renoux G, Renoux M, Guillaumin J-M, Gouzien C. Differentiation and regulation of lymphocyte populations: Evidence for immunopotentiator-induced T cell recruitment. J Immunopharmacol 1979; 1:415–22.

29. Renoux G. The mode of action of imuthiol (sodium dieihyldithiocarbamate): A new role for the brain neocortex and the endocrine liver in the regulation of the T cell lineage. In Fenichel R, Chirigos MA, eds. Immune modulation agents and their mechanisms. New York: Marcel Dekker, Inc., 1984; 607–26.

30. Stötter H, Rude E, Wagner H. T cell factor (interleukin 2) allows in vivo induction of T helper cells against heterologous erythrocytes in athymic (nu/nu) mice. Eur J Immunol 1980; 10:719–22.

31. Renoux G, Renoux M, Gillaumin JM. Isoprinosine as an immunopotentiator. J Immunopharmacol 1979; 1:337–56.

32. Chen SS, Tung JS, Gillis S, Good RA, Hadden JW. Changes in surface antigens of immatue thymocytes under the influence of T cell growth factor and thymic factors. Proc Natl Acad Sci USA 1983; 80:5980–4.

33. Conlon PJ, Henney CS, Gillis S. Cytokine-dependent thymocyte responses: Characterization of IL-1 and IL-2 target subpopulations and mechanism of action. J Immunol 1982; 128:797–801.

34. Oppenheim JJ, Stadler MD, Seraganian RP, Mage M, Mathieson B. Lymphokines: Their role in lymphocyte responses. Fed Proc 1982; 41:257–60.

35. Irlé C, Piguet P-F, Vassalli P. In vitro maturation of immature thymocytes into immunocompetent T cells in the absence of direct thymic influence. J Exp Med 1978; 32–44.

36. Kruisbeek AM, Astaldi GCB. Distinct effects of thymic epithelial culture supernatants on T cell properties of mouse thymocytes separated by the use of peanut agglutinin. J Immunol 1979; 123:984–91.

37. Beardsley TR, Pierschbacher M, Wetzel GD, Hays EF. Induction of T cell maturation by a cloned line of thymic epithelium (TEPI). Proc Natl Acad Sci USA 1983; 80:6005–9.

38. Shortman K, Scollay R. Cortical and medullary thymocytes. In Watson J, Marbrook J, eds. Recognition and regulation in cell-mediated immunity. 1985; 31–60.

39. Chen W-F, Scollay R, Shortman K, Skinner M, Marbrook J. T cell development in the absence of a thymus: The number, the phenotype, and the functional capacity of T lymphocytes in nude mice. Am J Anat 1984; 170:339–47.

40. Andrews P, Shortman K, Scollay R, et al. Thymus hormones do not induce proliferative ability or cytolytic function in PNA$^+$ cortical thymocyte. Cell Immunol 1985; 91:455–66.

41. Zatz M, Goldstein A. Mechanism of action of thymosin. I. Thymosin fraction 5 increases lymphokine production by mature murine T cells responding in a mixed lymphocyte reaction. J Immunol 1985; 134:1032–8.

42. Scheid M, Goldstein G, Boyse E. Differentiation of T cells in nude mice. Science 1975; 190:1211–3.

43. Ikehara S, Pahwa R, Fernandez G, Hansen C, Good RA. Functional T cells in athymic nude mice. Proc Natl Acad Sci USA 1984; 81:886–8.

Cancer Detection and Prevention Supplement 1:423–443 (1987)

Antitumor and Metastasis-Inhibitory Activities of Lentinan as an Immunomodulator:
An Overview

Goro Chihara, DP
Junji Hamuro, DEng
Yukiko Y. Maeda, DP
Tsuyoshi Shiio, DAgr

Tetsuya Suga, MP
Nobuo Takasuka, MP
Takuma Sasaki, DP

National Cancer Center Research Institute (G.C., T.Su., N.T., T.S.), The Tokyo Metropolitan Institute of Medical Sciences (Y.Y.M.), Tokyo and Ajinomoto Central Laboratory, Yokohama (J.H., T.Sh.), Japan

ABSTRACT   The antitumor and metastasis-inhibitory activities, mode of action, and clinical application of lentinan, a strictly purified β-1,6:β-1,3-glucan, are reviewed. Lentinan exerts a prominent antitumor effect and prevents chemical and viral oncogeneses. The antitumor action of lentinan is host-mediated. Compared to other well-known immunostimulants, such as bacille Calmette Guérin (BCG), *Corynebacterium parvum*, and lipopolysaccharide (LPS), lentinan appears to represent a unique class of immunopotentiator, a T cell-oriented adjuvant. Lentinan triggers the increased production of various kinds of bioactive serum factors associated with immunity and inflammation, such as IL-1, CSF, IL-3, vascular dilation inducer, and acute-phase protein inducer, by the direct impact of macrophages or indirectly via lentinan-stimulated T cells, which results in the induction of many immunobiological changes in the host. Augmented IL-1 production amplifies the maturation of immature effector cells to mature cells capable of responding to lymphokines such as IL-2 and T cell-replacing factors. Because of this mode of action, intact T cell compartments for antitumor activity of lentinan are required. Lentinan has little toxic side effects. Excellent results were obtained in a 4 year follow-up of the randomized control study of lentinan in phase III on patients with advanced and recurrent stomach and colorectal cancer.

Key words: lentinan, anticancer drug, oncogenesis prevention, immunostimulant

INTRODUCTION

In oriental medicine practiced in Asian countries, some kinds of fungi belonging to basidiomycetes have been used since olden times as folk remedies for cancer. Based on such a concept, we isolated a polysaccharide with marked antitumor activity from *Lentinus edodes* (Berk.) Sing., the most popular edible mushroom in Japan, and named it *lentinan* about 20 years ago [1,2]. Lentinan is a neutral polysaccharide, a fully purified β-1,3-D-glucan with β-

Address reprint requests to Dr. Goro Chihara, National Cancer Center Research Institute, Tsukiji 5-1-1, Chuo-ku, Tokyo 104, Japan.

TABLE I. Structure and Physicochemical Properties of Lentinan

1. Primary structure

2. Higher structure
   Right-handed triple helical structure (by X-ray analysis)
   Lattice constant: hexagonal, a = b = 15 Å, c = 6 Å
3. Molecular formula (by elementary analysis)
   $(C_6H_{10}O_5)_n$: Culcd, C: 44.44%, H: 6.22%
   Found, C: 44.16%, H: 6.27%
   N, P, and S: Negative
4. Sugar component
   Glucose only (by gas chromatography)
5. Molecular weight
   Distribution in a range between $4 \times 10^5 - 8 \times 10^5$ daltons
   (by gel permeation chromatography and Laser Raman light scattering)
6. Physical constants
   Specific rotation: $[\alpha]_D^{20}$, $13.5 - 14.5°$ (in 2% NaOH), $19.5 - 21.5°$ (in 10% NaOH)
   UV spectra: No peak
   IR spectra: 890 cm^{-1} (β-glucose)
   Ultracentrifugation: One peak
   High voltage electrophoresis: One spot
   Solubility: Slightly soluble in water (0.1%)

1,6 branches having a triple helical structure, and its physical and chemical properties are strictly characterized [3,4] (Table I). This is the most important point of lentinan for immunopharmacological studies and clinical use.

Lentinan exerts a prominent antitumor activity in allogeneic, syngeneic, and autochthonous tumor-host systems, prevents chemical and viral oncogenesis [1,2,5–7], and increases host resistance to bacterial, viral, and parasitic infections [8,9]. Its immunopharmacological properties are well characterized as a T cell-oriented adjuvant in which macrophages play some part [10–18].

Lentinan caused little toxic side effects in in vivo application in animal models and human [19,20]. A four year follow-up of the phase III randomized control study of lentinan resulted in prolongation of life span of patients with advanced and recurrent stomach and colorectal cancer [21]. This review concerns the current status and perspectives on the antitumor and metastasis-inhibitory effects and mode of action of lentinan as an immunomodulator.

ANTITUMOR ACTIVITIES OF LENTINAN

The antitumor and metastasis-inhibitory effects of lentinan are summarized in Table II. It was initially found that lentinan caused complete regression of sarcoma 180 transplanted SC in Swiss albino or CD-1 mice at a dose of 1 mg/kg IP daily for 10 days [2].

TABLE II. Antitumor and Metastasis-Inhibitory Effects of Lentinan

Tumors*	Hosts	Dose of lentinan (1 mg/kg × days)	Route	Days of lentinan injection†	Tumor inhibition Ratio (%)‡	Complete regression of tumor
Allogeneic						
Sarcoma 180	CD-1/ICR	1 × 10	IP	1–10	100	10/10
	A/J	5 × 4	IP	1–4	96.5	9/10
	DBA/2N	5 × 4	IP	1–4	100	10/10
	SWM/Ms	1 × 10	IP	1–10	100	10/10
Ehrlich carcinoma	CD-1/ICR	1 × 10	IP	1–10	54.7	0/5
CCM adenocarcinoma	SWM/Ms	1 × 10	IP	1–10	65.3	0/10
Syngeneic						
A/Ph.MC.S1 fibrosarcoma	A/J	1 × 10	IP	1–10	100	18/18
DBA/2.MC.CS-1 fibrosarcoma	DBA/2N	1 × 10	IP	1–10	76.5	2/7
P-815 mastocytoma	DBA/2N	5 × 4	IV	8, 10, 15, 17	89.0	2/8
L-5178Y lymphoma	DBA/2N	10 × 3	IV	7, 14, 21	84.0	3/9
MM-46 carcinoma	C3H/HeN	5 × 2	IV	13, 15	100	9/9
Madison 109 carcinoma	BALB/c	25 × 2	IP	15, 18		8/22
Autochthonous						
MC-induced primary tumor§	DBA/2N	1 × 10	IP	1–10	80.5	2/5
Inhibition of metastasis						
DBA/2.MC.CS-1 fibrosarcoma	DBA/2N	1 × 10	IP	−11 to −1	94.2‖	
MH-134 hepatoma	C3H/HeN	1 × 14	IP	21–40	100¶	
Madison 109 carcinoma	BALB/c	25 × 2	IP	15, 18		10/14
Prevention of oncogenesis						Tumor occurrence
Methylcholanthrene-induced	SWM/Ms	1 × 10	IP	21–31		83 - 33%
Methylcholanthrene-induced	DBA/2N	1 × 10	IP	14–24		78 - 37%
Adenovirus type 12-induced	C3H/HeN	10 × 3	IP	14, 16, 18		79 - 40%

*All tumors were solid forms implanted s.c.

†Tumors were implanted on day 0.

‡Tumor inhibition ratio = (C − T)/C × 100. (C = average tumor weight of control mice: T = that of lentinan treated mice).

§Tumor grown to 5 mm diameter was day-0.

‖Colony inhibition in lung.

¶Survival after surgery.

Allogeneic Tumor-Host System

Several characteristics of the antitumor action of lentinan were observed. Its action was host-mediated without cytotoxicity against tumor cells when tested in cell culture systems. Lentinan generally had no antitumor effect in vivo against ascites tumor cells. Use of lentinan revealed an interesting phenomenon of optimal dose. A higher dose of lentinan injection showed considerably decreased antitumor effects. This phenomenon of optimal dose was also observed in various immune reactions induced by lentinan. Therefore, dose, frequency, timing, and route of lentinan administration are essential. There was also a marked difference in the antitumor effects of lentinan among various mouse strains.

The results of an antitumor assay of lentinan against sarcoma 180 in different inbred mice and their F1 hybrids are shown in Table III. Lentinan showed strong inhibitory effects on tumor growth in A/J, DBA/2, and SWM/Ms mice. When lentinan was used at the dose of 4 mg/kg IP daily for 5 days starting 1 day after SC tumor transplantation, almost all tumors underwent complete regression, and the inhibition ratios of tumor growth were 96.5, 100, and 100%, respectively. In contrast, C3H/He and C57BL/6 were low responder mice to lentinan treatment, and no complete regression was observed. BALB/c and CBA mice were moderately responsive. The susceptibility of tumors in the F1 hybrids to lentinan treatment seemed to be regulated by their parentage.

These results raise the question of why DBA/2, A/J, and SWM/Ms mice are high responders and C57BL/6 and C3H/He mice are low responders to the antitumor action of lentinan. The H-2 haplotypes, fur color genes of mouse strains, and allogenicity between tumor and host had no relationship to lentinan action. Therefore, certain host factors whose immune reactivity is regulated by lentinan may be the underlying cause of strain differences in lentinan action.

The relationship between the tumor susceptibility to lentinan treatment and the host immune response such as delayed-type hypersensitivity reaction (DTH), cytotoxic T lymphocytes (CTL), natural killer (NK) cells, and phagocytic macrophages, in inbred mouse strains

TABLE III. Effects of Lentinan Against Sarcoma 180 on Different Inbred Strains and Their F1 Hybrids

	Parent strains (H-2 haplotypes)						
	DBA/2 (dd)	A/J (aa)	BALB/c (dd)	CBA (kk)	C3H/He (kk)	C57BL/6 (bb)	SWM/Ms (?)
DBA/2							
IR (%)	100	98.7	96.6	90.7	64.3	87.5	
CR	5/5	4/6	2/6	3/6	1/6	0/8	
Response	High	High	High	High	Moderate	Moderate	
A/J							
IR		96.5	91.5	91.5	41.6	68.2	
CR		6/7	1/5	0/6	0/7	0/6	
Response		High	High	High	Low	Moderate	
BALB/c							
IR			80.6	75.7	36.6	43.4	
CR			3/6	2/7	0/7	0/6	
Response			Moderate	Moderate	Low	Low	
CBA							
IR				74.1	71.9	71.8	
CR				0/6	0/5	0/6	
Response				Moderate	Moderate	Moderate	
C3H/He							
IR					36.2	58.8	
CR					0/6	0/6	
Response					Low	Low	
C57BL/6							
IR						51.8	
CR						0/6	
Response						Low	
SWM/Ms							
IR							100
CR							6/6
Response							High

IR, Inhibition ratio of tumor growth; CR, complete regression of tumors. Antitumor assay: Dose of lentinan was 4 mg/kg IP daily for 5 days. Tumor transplantation was SC.

is summarized in Table IV. In general, multiple changes were detected in lentinan-treated animals, depending on the experimental system used. The DTH and/or CTL responses seemed to be the most important mechanism in these tumor-host systems, in which DBA/2, A/J and SWM/Ms mice were the most suitable strains.

Syngeneic Tumor-Host System

Because A/J, DBA/2, and SWM/Ms mice were suitable hosts for lentinan action, the effect of lentinan against syngeneic and autochthonous tumors was examined by use of these strains of mice. Lentinan injected IP at doses of 1 mg/kg daily for 10 days starting 1 day after tumor transplantation led to complete regression of methylcholanthrene(MC)-induced A/Ph.MC.S1 fibrosarcoma in A/Ph(A/J) syngeneic host. A/Ph mice in which this tumor had regressed were also able to reject a secondary challenge with the same tumor [5] (Fig. 1).

TABLE IV. Relationship Between the Antitumor Susceptibility to Lentinan Treatment and the Capability of Host Immune Factors

	ATS	DTH	CTL	NK	Mϕ
DBA/2	High		High		Low
A/J	High	High		Low	Low
SWM/Ms	High	High		Low	Low
BALB/c	Moderate			Low	
C3H/He	Low	Low		High	High
C57BL/6	Low			Moderate	High

ATS, antitumor susceptibility to lentinan treatment; DTH, delayed-type hypersensitivity reaction; CTL, cytotoxic T lymphocyte activity; NK, natural killer cell activity; Mϕ, macrophage phagocytic activity.

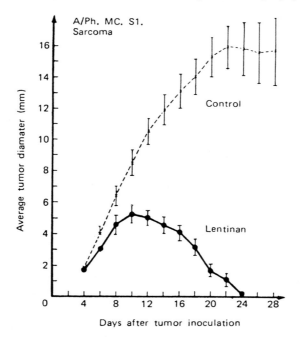

Fig. 1. Growth of syngeneic A/Ph.MC.S1 fibrosarcoma in control and lentinan-treated A/Ph mice. Both groups of mice (15 and 18, respectively) received 2.5×10^4 tumor cells ID and treatment with lentinan or control [5].

Lentinan showed a marked antitumor effect against the native and trypsinized DBA/2.MC.CS-1 fibosarcoma established in our laboratory for these experiments (Table V) [6]. As a trypsinized tumor should not be called a true syngeneic in the strict sense of the word, the native DBA/2.MC.CS-1 sarcoma was mainly used. When 0.1 ml of tumor cell suspension of native DBA/2.MC.CS-1 sarcoma was transplanted SC into syngeneic DBA/2 mice, the inhibition ratios of tumor growth induced by lentinan were 54.0 or 47.3% with a dose of 1 mg/kg $\times$ 10 or 10 mg/kg $\times$ 1, respectively. Lentinan was more effective against this tumor when DBA/2 mice were implanted with a smaller dose (1×10^4 cells) of tumor cells. The tumor inhibition ratio was 57.4%, and complete regression of tumor was observed in two out of five mice with 4 mg/kg $\times$ 4 by IP injection of lentinan. In the case of trypsinized DBA/2.MC.CS-1 sarcoma, the tumor inhibitory effect of lentinan was striking. With lentinan given in ten doses of 1 mg/kg each, tumor inhibition ratio was 76.5%, and tumors underwent complete regression in two out of seven mice.

Lentinan was also effective against various kinds of semisyngeneic tumors, such as P-815 mastocytoma and L-5178Y lymphoma in DBA/2 mice, virus-induced MM-46 and MM-102 carcinomas in C3H/He mice, and others (Table II). In these cases, timing of lentinan administration was very important. One hundred percent regression of MM-46 carcinoma was observed when 5 mg/kg of lentinan was injected twice, at 13 and 15 days after tumor transplantation.

Autochthonous Tumor-Host System

When DBA/2 mice were used, the IP injection of lentinan inhibited the growth of methylcholanthrene (MC)-induced autochthonous primary tumors [6] (Table VI). The tumors grew to 5 mm diameter within 15 weeks after MC treatment and were markedly inhibited by the IP injection of 1 mg/kg lentinan daily for 10 days starting at day 0 (grown to 5 mm diameter). The inhibition ratio of tumor was 80.5%, and the primary tumors underwent complete regression in two out of five mice. On the other hand, the tumor inhibitory effect of lentinan during 16 to 30 weeks after the MC inoculation was 50.4%, and no complete regression was observed, possibly because of a higher antigenicity of an earlier-occurring tumor than of a later-occurring one [22].

METASTASIS-INHIBITORY ACTIVITY OF LENTINAN

The correlation between spread of lymph node metastasis and prognosis after surgical resection of lung cancer was summarized by Watanabe and Suemasu [23] of the National

TABLE V. Effects of Lentinan on Growth of Native and Trypsinized DBA/2.MC.CS-1 Fibrosarcomas in DBA/2 Mice

DBA/2. MC.CS-1 fibrosarcoma	Treatment	Dose	D/T	Average tumor weight (gm)*	Tumor inhibition ratio (%)	No. of complete regressions
Native tumor†	Lentinan	1 mg/kg $\times$ 10	0/6	2.19	54.0	0/6
	Control		0/6	4.76		0/6
Native tumor†	Lentinan	10 mg/kg $\times$ 1	0/6	2.99	47.3	0/6
	Control		0/6	5.67		0/6
Native tumor‡	Lentinan	5 mg/kg $\times$ 4	0/5	0.84	57.4	2/5
	Control		0/6	1.97		0/6
Trypsinized tumor§	Lentinan	1 mg/kg $\times$ 10	0/7	0.47	76.5	2/7
	Control		0/7	2.00		0/7

†Tumor cell suspension 0.1 ml (1 gm of tumor tissue per 1 ml of saline); probably over 10^7 cells were transplanted SC.
‡Approximately 1×10^4 tumor cells were transplanted SC.
§Tumor cells 2.4×10^6 were transplanted SC.
*$P < 0.01$; Student t test compared to the control group.

TABLE VI. Antitumor Activity of Lentinan Against Methylcholanthrene-Induced Primary Tumors in DBA/2 and BALB/c Mice

Time of occurrence of MC-induced primary tumor	Lentinan treatment*	Dose	Average tumor weight (gm)	Tumor inhibition ratio (%)†	No. of complete regressions
DBA/2					
Within 15 weeks	Lentinan	1 mg/kg × 10	0.58	80.5	2/5
after MC treatment	Control		2.98		0/5
During 16 to 36	Lentinan	1 mg/kg × 10	2.75	40.5	0/4
weeks after MC	Control		4.79		0/4
BALB/c					
Within 15 weeks	Lentinan	1 mg/kg × 10	0.21	77.7	1/6
after MC treatment	Control		0.94		0/9

*When every primary tumor had grown to 5 mm diameter, treatment of lentinan was started.
†$P < 0.01$ by Student t test compared to the control group.

TABLE VII. Spread of Lymph Node Metastases and Prognosis After Surgical Operation in Lung Cancer

Spread of lymph node metastasis	Case	Over-5-year survival cases/total operation cases	5-Year survival ratio (%)
No metastasis in lung	$n^0(-)$	88/172	51.1
Metastasis inner lung	$n^0(+)$	8/15	53.3
Metastasis: Hilus LN	n^1	32/95	33.7
Metastasis: Mediastinum	n^2	14/154	9.0
Metastasis: Other places	M1	0/33	0
Total		142/472	30.1

Data are from Watanabe and Suemasu [23] of the National Cancer Center Hospital, Tokyo.

Cancer Center Hospital, Tokyo (Table VII). In the cases of $n^0 (-)$ lung cancer without any metastases in lung, the 5 year survival ratio of the patients was only 51.1% after surgical resection.

A fundamental concept in the clinical treatment of cancer metastasis is regression of a small number of autochthonous tumor cells scattering in the host. Because immunosuppressive anticancer drugs have a detrimental effect on cancer patients, the application of strong immunopotentiators such as lentinan should be suitable for adjuvant therapy after surgical resection.

Hematogenous Metastasis

Lentinan inhibited hematogenous pulmonary metastasis of syngeneic DBA/2.MC.CS-1 fibrosarcoma (Table VIII). After the IP injection of 1 mg/kg of lentinan daily for 10 days, 3×10^7 cells of this tumor were injected IV into the teil vein of DBA/2 mice. The lung metastases of this tumor were markedly inhibited by lentinan, and the metastasis inhibition ratio, calculated by the colony numbers of lung metastasis, was 94.2%.

Lymph Node Metastasis

Lentinan was also effective in lymph node metastases of MH-134 hepatoma. After SC inoculation of MH-134 hepatoma into syngeneic C3H/He mice, metastases occurred to lung, liver, heart, and other organs via lymph nodes. Lentinan prevented the recurrence of MH-134 hepatoma after tumor resection, and all mice survived when 1 mg/kg of lentinan was injected IP daily for 10 days after surgical resection (Fig. 2).

TABLE VIII. Inhibition of Hematogenous Pulmonary Metastases of Syngeneic DBA/2.MC.CS-1 Fibrosarcomas by Lentinan

No. of tumor cells*	Lentinan injections (1 mg/kg × 10)†	Average colony No. of lung metastasis	Metastasis inhibitory ratio (%)
1×10^5	−	7.0	−
1×10^5	+	0.6	91.4
3×10^5	−	27.8	−
3×10^5	+	1.6	94.2
1×10^6	−	34.0	−
1×10^6	+	5.3	84.4

*IV injection from teil vein.
†IP injection from 10 days before tumor implantation.

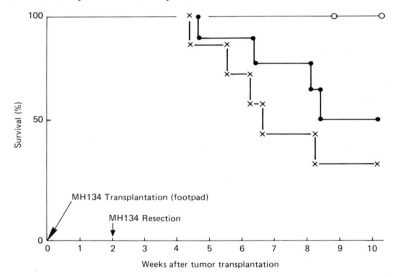

Fig. 2.   Inhibition of postoperative MH-134 hepatoma metastasis by lentinan administration. ✗, Control (surgery only); ●, surgery plus lentinan 1 mg/kg/day IP × 14 from 1 to 14 days after tumor transplantation; ○, surgery plus lentinan 1 mg/kg/day IP × 14 from 15 to 28 days after tumor transplantation; MH-134 transplantation, foodpad SC; MH-134 resection, 2 weeks after tumor transplantation.

Similar results using Madison 109 lung carcinoma and lentinan were obtained by Rose et al. [24]. They reported that lentinan prevented death from metastases after surgical resection of this tumor. The effects of surgery alone and surgery followed by an injection of 25 mg/kg of lentinan compared with untreated control are demonstrated in Figure 3.

PREVENTION OF ONCOGENESIS BY LENTINAN

Lentinan prevented chemical and viral oncogenesis [6,7]. Hamada [7] reported that lentinan inhibited adenovirus-induced oncogenesis. When newborn C3H/He mice were infected with 10^7 TCID$_{50}$ of adenovirus type 12, the tumor incidence was about 80% at day 80 after the infection, whereas the tumor incidence in mice given triple injections of 10 mg/kg of lentinan at 14, 16, and 18 days after the infection was about 40% (Fig. 4). Prevention of oncogenesis may be considered as an experimental method for inhibition of metastasis because of the control of small amounts of autochthonous tumor cells in the host.

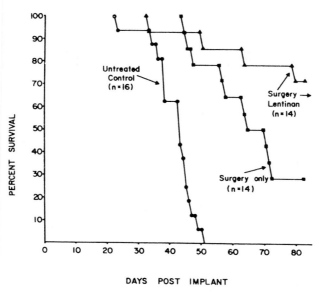

Fig. 3. Inhibition of postoperative syngeneic Madison 109 lung carcinoma metastases in BALB/c mice by lentinan injection. Data from untreated controls, surgery only, and surgery plus lentinan 25 mg/kg/day IP × 2 from 1 and 4 days after tumor resection are compared. Madison 109 implantation, foodpad SC; Madison 109 resection, 13 or 14 days after tumor implantation. Data are from Rose et al [24].

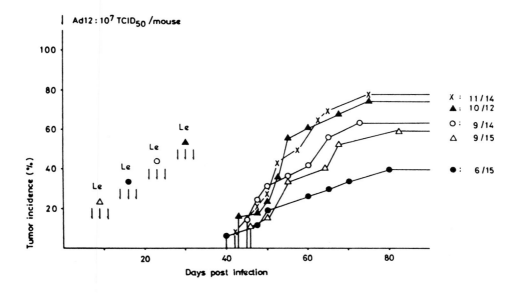

Fig. 4. Inhibition of the development of adenovirus type 12-induced tumor by lentinan. Newborn C3H/He mice were infected with 1×10^7 $TCID_{50}$ of adenovirus type 12. Lentinan treatment (10 mg/kg) was given on days 7, 9, and 11 ($\triangle$); 14, 16, and 18 ($\bullet$); 21, 23, and 25 ($\bigcirc$); and 28, 30, and 32 ($\blacktriangle$) postinfection, respectively. Control mice were infected but untreated ($\times$). Data are from Hamada [7].

We found that lentinan suppressed chemical carcinogenesis [6]. When 1 mg/kg of lentinan was injected IP daily for 10 days into DBA/2 mice from 2 weeks after MC treatment, the tumor occurrence ratio was about 30% after week 40 compared to about 80% in untreated control mice (Fig. 5).

In another experiment, timing of lentinan administration for prevention of chemical carcinogenesis was examined using the high responder SWM/Ms mice. Tumor incidence was strikingly suppressed in the mice that were given lentinan 3 weeks after MC inoculation. However, lentinan given 6 weeks after MC treatment was less effective (Fig. 6). This suggests a possible effectiveness of lentinan on micrometastasis after surgical resection in cancer patients, because the small number of autochthonous tumor cells that may have occurred in the host within 3 weeks after MC inoculation had regressed through immunopotentiation by lentinan.

MODE OF ACTION OF LENTINAN AS A T-CELL ADJUVANT

Lentinan has no direct cytotoxicity against tumor cells, and its antitumor action is host-mediated. The immunological activities of lentinan are listed in Table IX. The antitumor activity of lentinan was absent in neonatally thymectomized mice [11] and was decreased by the administration of antilymphocyte serum [25]. These results suggest that the antitumor action of lentinan requires an immunocompetent T-cell compartment and that the activity is mediated through thymus-dependent immune mechanisms. Antitumor effects of lentinan were also inhibited by pretreatment with the antimacrophage agents carrageenan and silica. Thus, lentinan is a T cell-oriented adjuvant in which macrophages play some parts. Among the well-known immunostimulants, such as BCG, *C. parvum*, and LPS, lentinan appears to represent an unique class of immune adjuvant.

It is, however, not clear how lentinan affects the host at a stage before the induction of many immunological changes. It is suggested that the biological activities of lentinan may depend on the presence of certain substances or cells in the host that interact with lentinan.

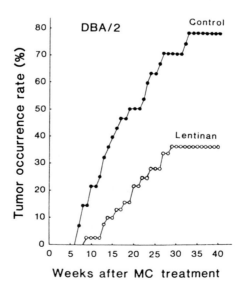

Fig. 5.   Preventive effect of lentinan on 3-methylcholanthrene-induced carcinogenesis in DBA/2 mice. Data from controls (no lentinan treatment) and mice receiving lentinan injections (1 mg/kg IP daily for 10 days) started 2 weeks after MC treatment are shown.

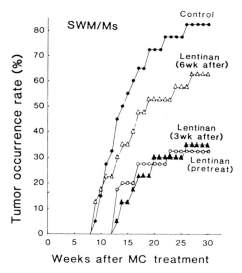

Fig. 6.   Significance of timing of lentinan injections in prevention of 3-methylcholanthrene-induced carcinogenesis. ●, Control (no lentinan treatment); ○, lentinan injection begun 10 days before MC inoculation; ▲, lentinan injections begun 3 weeks after MC inoculation; △, lentinan injections begun 6 weeks after MC inoculation. Dose of lentinan was 1 mg/kg IP daily for 10 days.

Appearance of Serum Bioactive Factors Soon After Lentinan Injection

We found a transitory increase in various serum protein components and bioactive serum factors soon after lentinan administration (Table X). These are IL-1 production-inducing factor (IL1-IF), IL-3, and colony-stimulating factors (CSF) [26], vascular dilatation and hemorrhage-inducing factor (VDHIF) [27], and acute-phase transport protein-inducing factor (APPIF) [28]. These factors were produced by mainly accessary macrophages or lentinan-stimulated T cells, and the increase in these factors resulted in the activation of lymphocytes, hepatocytes, and probably mastocytes and the development of many biological reactions in the host. Complement components also increased in the lentinan-treated mice.

Acute-Phase Transport Protein-Inducing Factor

Several protein components increased markedly in the mouse serum 4 to 7 days after lentinan injection [29]. These were identified by the two-dimensional electrophoretic method as acute-phase transport proteins such as haptoglobin, hemopexin, and ceruloplasmin [30].

We recently found a factor that regulates the increase of acute-phase transport proteins in the serum (L10-6h serum) that was obtained from mice 6 hours after an injection of 10 mg/kg of lentinan [28]. The acute-phase transport proteins were markedly increased 4 days after the IV injection of L10-6h serum, and this increase was inhibited by pretreatment with the antimacrophage agents carrageenan and anti-Ia antiserum of donor mice (Fig. 7). Therefore, APPIF appears to be a product of macrophages, and it may stimulate hepatocytes to prepare the acute-phase proteins.

Vascular Dilation and Hemorrhage-Inducing Factor

L10-6h serum was found to induce vascular dilatation and hemorrhage [27]. This factor also appeared to be a product of macrophages, because the injection of carrageenan before lentinan treatment inhibited its production. This reaction, however, was thymus-dependent, because L10-6h serum did not induce the vascular dilatation reaction in nude mice. L10-6h

TABLE IX. Immunological Activities of Lentinan

1. T cell participation

Neonatal thymectomy	Abolished antitumor effect
Antilymphocyte serum	Decreased antitumor effect
Helper T cell in vitro	No observed effect
Helper T cell in vivo	Activation or restoration
Cytotoxic T cell in vitro	Augmentation of IL-2 responsibility
Cytotoxic T cell in vivo	Increased responsibility to IL-2
Suppressor T cells	No induction
Migration inhibitory factor- producing T cells	Activation
IL-3	Increased production
T cell-derived CSF	Increased production

2. Natural killer cell participation

NK cells in vitro	No effect
NK cells in vivo	Activation in C3H/He, but not BALB/c mice

Augmented NK activity
  by poly I:C or IL-2 in vitro
	More activation when used in
	  lentinan-treated mouse spleen cells

3. Macrophage participation

Antimacrophage agent	Decreased tumor suppressive effect by carrageenan and silica
Macrophage: Phagocytic in vitro	No effect
Macrophage: Phagocytic in vivo	Very weak effect
Macrophage: Cytotoxic in vitro	Not observed
Macrophage: Cytotoxic in vivo	Activation
Macrophage: Suppressive in vivo	Decreased prostaglandin E release from macrophages
IL-1	Increased production in vitro and in vivo

4. Antibody formation

Antibody for SRBC	Increased production with T cells
Antibody-dependent cell-mediated cytotoxicity	Activation

5. Cellular reactions

Delayed hypersensitivity in vivo	Stimulation or restoration
Local cellular reaction	Increase around tumor
Granuloma formation	Increase around Shistosoma

6. Complement participation

Alternative pathway	Activation
C3 splitting activity	Activation
C3 absolute value	Increased production
Total complement value	Increased production
Classical pathway	Activation

serum may contain a histamine-producing cell stimulating factor. Interestingly, there is a close correlation between antitumor activity and vascular dilatation-stimulating activity of lentinan.

IL-1 Production-Inducing Factor, Colony-Stimulating Factor, and IL-3

Lentinan triggers the increased production of IL-1 by a direct impact on macrophages or indirectly via colony-stimulating factor (CSF) from lentinan-stimulated T cells.

After lentinan injection two peaks of increased CSF were observed (Fig. 8). Three hours after lentinan injection the appearance of CSF in the serum was found to be generated from alveolar macrophages that were stimulated by lentinan. However, the CSF that appeared several days after lentinan injection was found to have originated from T lymphocytes, because this increase was not present in nude mice. Similarly, IL-1 production-inducing activity in the

TABLE X. Increase of Protein Components and Bioactive Factors in Mouse Serum After Lentinan Administration

Activities (peak, 2–24 hours after)	Components (peak, 3–7 days after)
IL-1 production-inducing factor	Interleukin-1
Interleukin-3	Colony-stimulating factor (T cell-derived)
Colony-stimulating factor (directly from macrophages)	Haptoglobin
Acute-phase protein-inducing factor	Hemopexin
Vascular dilatation and hemorrhage-inducing factor	Ceruloplasmin
Lysozyme activity	Serum amyloid P
	Complement C3
	Complement C5
	Complement factor B

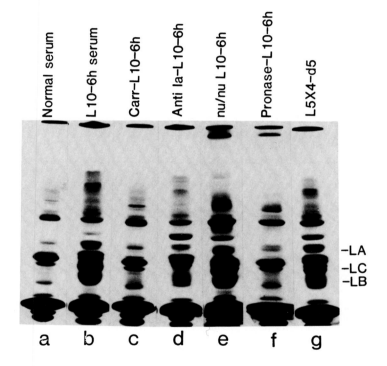

Fig. 7. Polyacrylamide gel electrophoresis patterns of serum samples obtained from mice 4 days after the injection of 0.2 ml per mouse of various serum samples: **a:** Normal CD-1 mouse serum; **b:** L10-6h serum; serum obtained from CD-1 mice 6 hours after IP injection of 10 mg/kg of lentinan; **c:** Carr-L10-6h; L10-6h serum obtained from the mice that received 100 mg/kg of carrageenan 24 hours before lentinan injection; **d:** Anti-Ia L10-6h; L10-6h serum obtained from mice that received 0.1 ml of anti-Ia antiserum 5 to 10 minutes before lentinan injection; **e:** nu/nu L10-6h; L10-6h serum obtained from athymic nu/nu CD-1 mice; **f:** Pronase-L10-6h; pronase E-treated L10-6h serum; **g:** L5×4-d5: Serum sample obtained from CD-1 mice on day 4 after the final injection of 5 mg/kg of lentinan daily for 4 days.

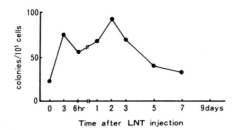

Fig. 8. Colony-stimulating activity (CSA) in the serum of lentinan-injected DBA/2 mice. Serum was harvested at 0, 3, and 6 hours and 1, 2, 3, 5, and 7 days after an IV injection of 10 mg/kg of lentinan. CSA assay was a soft-gel system; 10^5 C57BL/6 bone marrow cells per dish were cultured for 7 days.

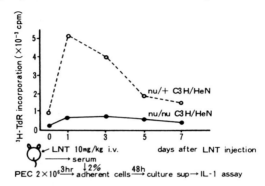

Fig. 9. IL-1 production-inducing activity in the serum of lentinan-injected mice.

	ILI (Δcpm)	CSA (colonies/10^5 cells)
normal serum (2 %)	− 10	159
LNT serum (2 %)	245	821
medium	23	31

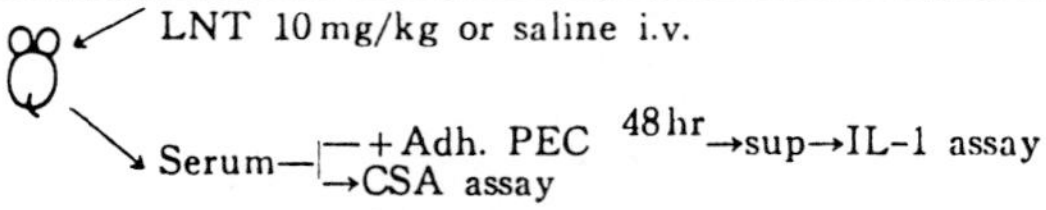

LNT 10 mg/kg or saline i.v.

Serum—|—+Adh. PEC $\xrightarrow{48\,hr}$sup→IL-1 assay
         └→CSA assay

Fig. 10. Correlation between IL-1 producing activity and colony-stimulating activity induced by lentinan. IL-1 (Δcpm) was determined by tritium incorporation into thymocytes. Δcpm = (+ serum or medium) − (− serum or medium). CSA increased in early phase augments IL-1 production by macrophages.

serum of lentinan-injected mice was also absent in nude mice (Fig. 9). Thus, T cells seem to play a relevant role in the generation of IL-1 production-inducing factor and of CSF. There is a correlation between IL-1 producing activity and CSF activity induced by lentinan (Fig. 10). Increased CSF in the early phase augments IL-1 production of macrophages. The augmented effect was also demonstrated by use of chromatographically purified CSF [26].

Direct Production of IL-1 From Monocytes and Macrophages

On the other hand, augmented production of IL-1 was observed when human monocytes [31], murine peritoneal cells, or macrophage cell line P388D1 were cocultivated with lentinan in vitro. The peritoneal adherent cells obtained from the lentinan-treated mice produced increased amounts of IL-1 in cultured supernatant (Fig. 11).

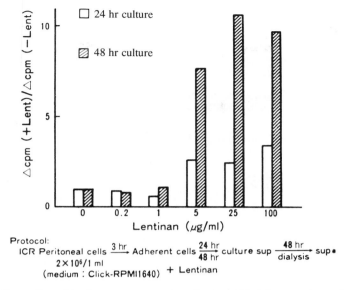

Fig. 11. Direct effect of lentinan on augmented production of IL-1 from murine peritoneal cells.

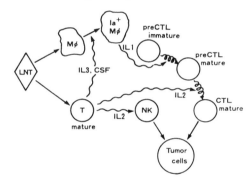

Fig. 12. Cytokine(s) production and induction of effector cells by lentinan. Straight lines show direct action, wavy lines show factors, and coiled lines show differentiation.

Cytotoxic T Lymphocytes and Lentinan

In view of the fact that IL-1 is capable of differentiating thymic premature T cells into immunocompetent mature T cells, the findings presented here suggest that lentinan promotes the differentiation of premature T cells into immunocompetent mature T cells. The augmented cytokine production, induced by lentinan, apparently stimulates generation of effector cells against tumor cells (Fig. 12). This mode of action suggests the requirement of an intact T cell compartment for the antitumor activity of lentinan. To evaluate the validity of the explanation, the generation of allokiller cells from thymocytes was tested. Thymocytes, harvested from BALB/c mice and treated with lentinan, induced augmented generation of allokiller cells in the presence of IL-2 (Fig. 13). This demonstrates that thymocytes of lentinan-treated mice had an increased reactivity to IL-2.

In a syngeneic tumor-bearing system such as P815-DBA/2, the generation of allokiller cells from thymocytes is considerably suppressed even in the presence of IL-2. After injection of lentinan, however, the generation of allokiller cells was restored to the level of control mice. The generation of allokiller cells from splenocytes was also restored by lentinan injection

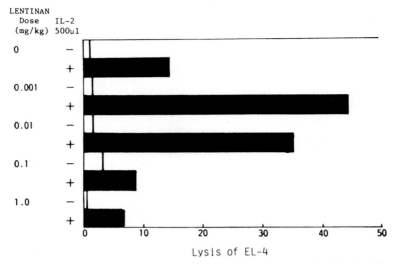

Fig. 13.   Lentinan augments sensitivity of thymocytes to IL-2. Augmented allokiller T cell induction by lentinan from thymocytes in the presence of IL-2. Mixed lymphocyte culture: BALB/c C57BL/6; E:T = 3:1.

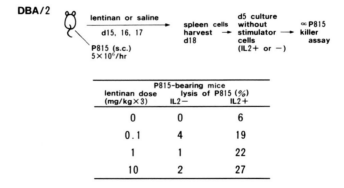

lentinan dose (mg/kg×3)	P815-bearing mice lysis of P815 (%)	
	IL2−	IL2+
0	0	6
0.1	4	19
1	1	22
10	2	27

Fig. 14.   Augmented allokiller T cell generation by lentinan in a P-815 syngeneic tumor-bearing DBA/2 mouse system. Effector:Target = 50:1 (culture base). Killer assay, 3 hours, ^{51}Cr release.

from 0 to 40%. These results may explain the increase in the formation of mature T cells reactive to IL-2. Furthermore, spleen cells harvested from syngeneic tumor-bearing mice that had received triple IP injections of lentinan were able to generate significant levels of antisyngeneic tumor killer cells in the presence of IL-2 (Fig. 14). This suggests that lentinan may restore decreased immune reactivity in cancer and AIDS by the combination therapy with recombinant IL-2.

Delayed Hypersensitivity Reaction and Lentinan

Delayed-type hypersensitivity (DTH) reaction is an important mechanism of lentinan action. Lentinan restored the decreased DTH reaction in tumor-bearing hosts. Furthermore, DTH reaction was markedly enhanced by the administration of lentinan, when the syngeneic A/Ph.MC.S1 fibrosarcoma had completely regressed [32,33]. This augmenting effect produced by lentinan injection may be explained also by the augmenting effect of lentinan on the reactivity of macrophages to macrophage-activating factor (MAF) as demonstrated in tumor antigen-directed DTH [18].

Natural Killer Cells and Lentinan

Concerning the other important nonspecific effector, natural killer (NK) cells, it was found that lentinan could augment NK activity in spleen cells and peritoneal exudate cells when administered into NK high responder C3H/He mice, contrary to its administration into BALB/c mice. However, lentinan did not activate NK cells when incubated in vitro, as poly I:C and zymosan do [18].

Augmented NK cell generation was observed when spleen cells obtained from lentinan-treated mice were cultured with poly I:C or IL-2 (Fig. 15). Because lentinan does not activate NK cells in vitro, it seems likely that in vivo application of lentinan results in the augmentation of NK cell reactivity to IL-2.

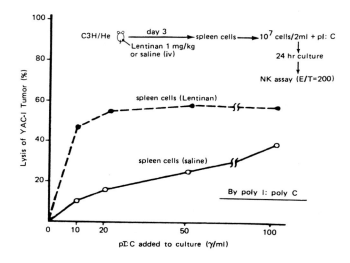

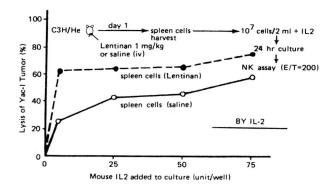

Fig. 15. Synergistic augmentation of natural killer cells by lentinan with poly I:C and with IL-2 in vitro. Natural killer activity was assayed using ^{51}Cr-labeled YAC-1 cells as target cells in a 4 hour ^{51}Cr-release assay at a ratio of effector:target = 200:1.

Complement and Nonspecific Cytotoxicity of Macrophages

Lentinan not only augments antigen-specific cellular immune responses by increased responsibility to IL-2 and cytokines, but is also capable of triggering nonspecific immune responses against neoplastic cells. Lentinan activated the alternative pathway of complement system [34,35]. Lentinan splits C3 into C3a and C3b in vitro, resulting in augmented generation of nonspecific cytotoxicity of macrophages. Peritoneal exudate cells obtained from lentinan-treated mice showed considerable nonspecific cytotoxicity against sarcoma 180, Ehrlich carcinoma, and L5178Y lymphoma [36]. The cytotoxicity of peritoneal macrophages harvested from lentinan-treated CBA mice was over 80% lysis against P-815 mastocytoma, while the lysis with control mice was only 2.5% [18]. Lentinan, however, did not have any cytotoxicity in in vitro experiments.

Lentinan, nevertheless, did not enhance the phagocytic activity of macrophages in vitro and in vivo as assessed by a carbon clearance test [11]. Therefore, lentinan seems to be distinct from most immune stimulants, so-called RES stimulants.

Conclusion Regarding Mechanism of Action

Lentinan appears to be a unique immunological adjuvant with nontoxic side effects from in vivo application. In light of the various described immunological characteristics of lentinan, the possible mode of action of lentinan is tentatively suggested although there are still many points to be elucidated (Fig. 16).

CLINICAL APPLICATION AND POSSIBLE FUTURE TRENDS

Lentinan was found to have a distinct antitumor and metastasis-inhibiting effect in allogeneic, syngeneic, and autochthonous hosts, and its unique mode of action has been evaluated. Many acute, semiacute, and chronic toxicological studies have been completed in animal models, and the LD_{50} is over 2,500 mg/kg IP and 250–500 mg/kg IV in mice and rats. Therefore, lentinan is worthy of consideration for effective therapy of cancer patients.

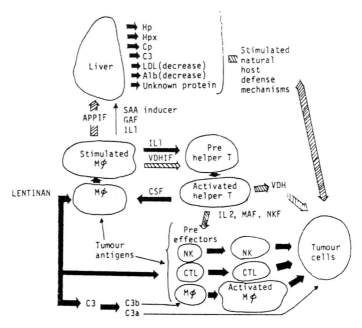

Fig. 16.   Possible mode of action of lentinan.

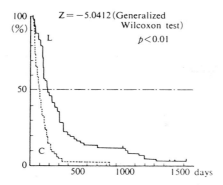

Fig. 17. Clinical application of lentinan on survival curves from patients with advanced and recurrent gastric cancer—4 year follow-up results of a randomized control study of lentinan in phase III. L, lentinan-treated group, 2 mg/person/week of lentinan plus 400–1200 mg/person/day of Tegaful; C, control group, 400–1200 mg/kg of Tegaful alone. Drawn by Kaplan-Maier's method and examined by generalized Wilcoxon's test. Control group, 68 cases, 50% survival 92 days. Lentinan group, 77 cases, 50% survival 173 days. Data are from Taguchi et al [21].

Taguchi and cooperative clinical study groups investigating lentinan have carried out phase I, II, and III studies of randomized control clinical trials of lentinan [20]. Recent results of a 4 year follow-up phase III randomized control study of lentinan patients with advanced and recurrent stomach and colorectal cancer revealed that the combination therapy of lentinan with Tegaful led to prolongation of their lifespan (Fig. 17) [21]. In the case of stomach cancer, the percent survival ratios of the lentinan-treated patients were 24.32, 12.97, 9.51, and 3.81%, while those of the control group (Tegaful only) were only 3.70, 3.70, 0, and 0% in 1, 2, 3, and 4 year results, respectively.

These results suggest that the use of lentinan may increase the survival time and cause the complete cure of micrometastases after surgical resection in cancer patients. Human cancer is a disease with great diversities comparable to all infectious diseases. Tumor-host relationships may differ depending on the stage of tumor growth and on the course of treatments. Therefore, the use of lentinan for human cancer should be based on strict injection times and dose schedules in compliance with the immunological and biological changes that were observed in lentinan-treated animals. The effect of lentinan in the treatment of human cancer is increased when used in conjunction with other therapies, especially after surgical resection. An important task for clinical immunologists is to determine parameters for tumor-host relationships which serve as indicators for protocols on the use of immunopotentiators such as lentinan.

REFERENCES

1. Chihara G, Maeda YY, Hamuro J, Sasaki T, Fukuoka F. Inhibition of mouse sarcoma 180 by polysaccharides from *Lentinus edodes* (Berk.) Sing. Nature 1969; 222:687–8.
2. Chihara G, Hamuro J, Maeda YY, Arai Y, Fukuoka F. Fractionation and purification of the polysaccharides with marked antitumor activity, especially lentinan, from *Lentinus edodes* (Berk.) Sing., an edible mushroom. Cancer Res 1970; 30:2776–81.
3. Sasaki T, Takasuka N. Further study of the structure of lentinan, an antitumor polysaccharide from *Lentinus edodes*. Carbohydrate Res 1976; 47:99–104.
4. Bluhm TL, Sarco A. The triple helical structure of lentinan, β-(1-3)-D-glucan. Can J Chem 1977; 55:293–9.
5. Zákány J, Chihara G, Fachet J. Effect of lentinan on tumor growth in murine allogeneic and syngeneic hosts. Int J Cancer 1980; 25:371–6.
6. Suga T, Shiio T, Maeda YY, Chihara G. Antitumor activity of lentinan in murine syngeneic and autochthonous hosts and its suppressive effect on 3-methylcholanthrene induced carcinogenesis. Cancer Res 1984; 44:5132–7.

7. Hamada C. Inhibition effect of lentinan on the tumorigenesis of adenovirus type 12 in mice. In Aoki T, Urushizaki I, Tsubura E, eds: Manipulation of host defence mechanisms. Amsterdam: Excerpta Medica, 1981; 76–87.

8. Kanai K, Kondo E, Jacques PJ, Chihara G. Immunopotentiating effect of fungal glucans as revealed by frequency limitation of post-chemotherapy relapse in experimental mouse tuberculosis. Jpn J Med Sci Biol 1980; 33:283–93.

9. Byram JE, Sher A, DiPietro J, von Lichtenberg F. Potentiation of schistosome granuloma formation by lentinan—A T-cell adjuvant. Am J Pathol 1979; 94:201–18.

10. Maeda YY, Chihara G. Lentinan, a new immunoaccelerator of cell-mediated responses. Nature 1971; 229:634.

11. Maeda Y, Chihara G. The effect of neonatal thymectomy on the antitumor activity of lentinan, carboxymethylpachymaran and zymosan, and their effects on various immune responses. Int J Cancer 1973; 11:153–61.

12. Dennert G, Tacker D. Antitumor polysaccharide lentinan—A T-cell adjuvant. JNCI 1973; 51:1727–9.

13. Dresser DW, Phillips JM. The orientation of the adjuvant activities of *Salmonella typhosa* lipopolysaccharide and lentinan. Immunology 1974; 27:895–902.

14. Haba S, Hamaoka T, Takatsu K, Kitagawa M. Selective suppression of T-cell activity in tumor bearing mice and its improvement by lentinan, a potent antitumor polysaccharide. Int J Cancer 1976; 18:93–104.

15. Hamuro J, Wagner H, Röllinghoff M. β-1,3-Glucans as probe for T-cell specific immune adjuvants. Enhanced in vitro generation of cytotoxic T-lymphocytes. Cell Immunol 1978; 38:328–35.

16. Hamuro J, Röllinghoff M, Wagner H. β-1,3-Glucans mediated augmentation of alloreactive murine cytotoxic T-lymphocytes in vivo. Cancer Res 1978; 38:3080–5.

17. Hamuro J, Röllinghoff M, Wagner H. Induction of cytotoxic peritoneal exudate cells by T-cell immune adjuvants of β-1,3-glucan type lentinan and its analogues. Immunology 1980; 39:551–9.

18. Hamuro J, Chihara G. Lentinan, a T-cell oriented immunopotentiator: Its experimental and clinical applications and possible mechanism of immune modulation. In Fenichel RL, Chirigos MA, eds: Immune modulation agents and their mechanisms. New York: Marcel Dekker, 1985: 409–36.

19. Sortwell RJ, Dawe S, Allen DG, et al. Chronic intravenous administration of lentinan to the rhesus monkey. Toxicol Lett 1981; 9:81–5.

20. Taguchi T, Furue H, Kimura T, Kondo T, Hattori T, Ogawa N. Clinical efficacy of lentinan on neoplastic disease. In Klein K, Spector S, Friedman H, Szentivanyi A, eds: Biological response modifiers in human oncology and immunology. New York: Plenum Press, 1983; 181–7.

21. Taguchi T, Furue H, Kimura T, et al. End-point results of phase III study of lentinan. Gan to Kagakuryoho [Jpn J Cancer Chemother] 1985; 12:366–78.

22. Klein G, Sjögren O, Klein E, Hellström KE. Demonstration of resistance against methylcholanthrene-induced sarcoma in the primary autochthonous host. Cancer Res 1960; 20:1561–72.

23. Watanabe H, Suemasu K. Cancer surgical therapy and lymph node metastases. Oncologia 1982; 1:83–9.

24. Rose WC, Reed III FC, Siminoff P, Bradner WT. Immunotherapy of Madison 109 lung carcinoma and other murine cancer using lentinan. Cancer Res 1984; 44:1368–73.

25. Maeda YY, Hamuro J, Chihara G. The mechanisms of action of antitumor polysaccharide: The effect of antilymphocyte serum on the antitumor activity of lentinan. Int J Cancer 1971; 8:41–6.

26. Izawa M, Ohno K, Amikura K, Hamuro J. Lentinan augments the production of Interleukin 3 and colony stimulating factor(s) by T-cells. In Aoki T, Tsubura E, Urushizaki I, eds: Manipulation of host defence mechanisms. Amsterdam: Excerpta Medica, 1984; 59–69.

27. Maeda YY, Watanabe ST, Chihara G, Rokutanda M. T-cell mediated vascular dilatation and hemorrhage induced by antitumor polysaccharides. Int J Immunopharmacol 1984; 5:493–501.

28. Suga T, Maeda YY, Uchida H, Rokutanda M, Chihara G. Macrophage-mediated acute-phase transport protein production induced by lentinan. Int J Immunopharmacol 1986; 8:691–9.

29. Maeda YY, Chihara G, Ishimura K. Unique increase of serum proteins and action of antitumor polysaccharides. Nature 1974; 252:250–2.

30. Manabe T, Takahashi Y, Okuyama T, Maeda YY, Chihara G. Identification of mouse serum proteins increased by the antitumor polysaccharide lentinan by micro two dimensional electrophoresis. Electrophoreses 1983; 4:242–6.

31. Fruehauf JP, Bonnard GD, Herberman RB. The effect of lentinan on production of Interleukin-1 by human monocytes. Immunopharmacology 1982; 5:65–74.

32. Zákány J, Chihara G, Fachet J. Effect of lentinan on the production of migration inhibitory factor induced by syngeneic tumor in mice. Int J Cancer 1980; 26:783–8.

33. Spika S, Ábel G, Csongor J, Chihara G, Fachet J. Effect of lentinan on the chemiluminescence produced by human neutrophils and the murine macrophage cell line C4MØ. Int J Immunopharmacol 1985; 7:745–51.

34. Okuda T, Yoshioka Y, Ikekawa T, Chihara G, Nishioka K. Anticomplementary activity of antitumor polysaccharides. Nature [New Biol] 1972; 238:59–60.

35. Hamuro J, Hadding U, Bitter-Seuermann D. Solid phase activation of alternative pathway of complement by β-1,3-glucans and its possible role for tumor regressing activity. Immunology 1978; 34:695–705.

36. Maeda YY, Chihara G. Periodical consideration on the establishment of antitumor action in host and activation of peritoneal exudate cells by lentinan. Gann [Jpn J Cancer Res] 1973; 64:351–7.

Cancer Detection and Prevention Supplement 1:445–455 (1987)

Do Tuftsin and Bestatin Constitute a Biopharmacological Immunoregulatory System?

G. Mathé, MD

Institut de Cancérologie et d'Immunogénétique (Univ. Paris—Sud, CNRS UA 04-1163; Assoc. Claude-Bernard and ARC), Hôpital Paul-Brousse, 94804 Villejuif, France

ABSTRACT   Tuftsin is the tetrapeptide Thr-Lys-Pro-Arg. It is spontaneously released from the Fc fragment of IgG by two specific enzymes. One 25-μg dose administered to mice in good immunologic status stimulated phagocytosis, macrophage killing of tumor cells, delayed hypersensitivity, cytolytic T-cell activity, antibody production, antibody-dependent cell-mediated cytotoxicity (ADCC), and natural killer (NK) cell activity. Administered for 6 months at the dose of 10 μg once a week to old, immunodepressed mice, tuftsin restored macrophage and T-cell cytotoxic activities. At this dosage, tuftsin prevented spontaneous tumor development. Tuftsin was also well tolerated in phase I studies in humans in increased polymorphonuclear leukocytes and OKT4-positive lymphocytes. Bestatin is extracted from *Streptomyces olivoreticuli*. One 100-μg dose of bestatin injected in young mice with normal immunologic status increased macrophage cytotoxicity, antibody production, ADCC, and NK cell activities. Long-term administration of bestatin (100 μg once a week) corrected macrophage and T-cell cytotoxicity and prevented age-related spontaneous tumors. Bestatin inhibited lymphocyte membrane aminopeptidase, which degrades tuftsin into a tripeptide that is an antagonist competing with it for receptors. Tuftsin and bestatin constitute a biopharmacologic system that can be developed as other aminopeptidase inhibitors are available for study.

Key words: tuftsin, bestatin, biological response modifiers, T-cell subjects

INTRODUCTION

Among the many pharmacologically available molecules we have studied for their immunomodifying capabilities [1–9], tuftsin and bestatin appear to be particularly useful because of their immunorestorative capabilities [10–12].

TUFTSIN

The binding of an autologous IgG, and accessorily IgM, with isohemagglutinin activity to human erythrocytes was observed by Harshman and Najjar in 1963 [13] and shown by Fidalgo et al [14, 15] and Lahiri et al [16] to be important for the viability of these cells. Constantopoulos and Najjar [17] demonstrated the binding of IgG and IgM to thrombocytes as

---

Address reprint requests to Dr. G. Mathé, Institut de Cancérologie et d'Immunogénétique, Hôpital Paul-Brousse, 12-16 av. Paul-Vaillant-Couturier, 94804 Villejuif, Cédex, France.

well as their role in platelet respiration [18]. The binding of one type of IgG to blood monocytes and neutrophils was also seen by Fildalgo and Najjar [19]; this type of IgG was called *leukokinin* [20]. The main effect observed in these cells was a stimulation of in vitro phagocytosis [21]. When leukokinin was first incubated with autologous phagocytic cells for 30 min without particles, it failed to stimulate phagocytosis. The reason was sought in a possible enzymatic action of the cell membrane, and it was shown that such an action affected an oligopeptide responsible for the activity of the parent carrier leukokinin molecule [22,23].

The oligopeptide was isolated, sequenced [22,23], and synthesized [24, 25] and called *tuftsin* (TFST). It is the tetrapeptide Thr-Lys-Pro-Arg.

It has been shown that TFST is produced spontaneously from the IgG molecule in two enzymatic steps: 1) the splenic TFST-endocarboxypeptidase cleaves IgG at its carboxy-terminal arginine, and 2) leukokinase cleaves it at its amino-terminal threonine. The TFST molecule is also a part of the Fc fragment of the IgA chain [26].

It has been observed that TFST is degraded by leukokininase, pronase, subtilisin, carboxypeptidase B, and leucine aminopeptidase and that TFST is resistant to trypsin, chymotrypsin, pepsin, papain, clostripain, and alkaline phosphatase [24,26,27]. Some peptides behave as TFST inhibitors, especially the tripeptide Lys-Pro-Arg and the pentapeptide Thr-Lys-Pro-Pro-Arg [24,28].

Receptors for TFST and for active analogs have been demonstrated on phagocytes. Studies using fluorescent analogs of TFST have shown that the formation of clusters and internalization of peptide-receptor complexes is a rapid process [29,30]. The level of TFST in blood is measured by a biological test [31] or by radioimmunoassay [32,33].

Pathology

Splenectomy. Studies have shown phagocytosis and the half-life of erythrocytes to be affected by splenectomy [34], and the disorder was corrected by administration of plasma γ-globulin [35,36]. The TFST serum level was decreased after splenectomy and in several types of splenic impairment [32].

Hyposplenia. In Hodgkin disease, Gaucher disease, and idiopathic thrombocytopenic purpura, hyposplenia was complicated by TFST deficiency [34]. The spleen acts on TFST production by endocarboxypeptidase; in its absence, TFST remained bound at the arginine end [37].

Acquired TFST deficiency. A deficiency has been described; it was related to a point mutation resulting in the replacement of lysine by glutamic acid in TFST structure and was due to the replacement of adenine by guanine in the lysine triplets (AAA→AAG). This abnormal tetrapeptide is a TFST antagonist [38–40]. The patients affected have had frequent skin eczemas, respiratory infections, and adenitis. Najjar [35], Inada et al [38], and Constantopoulos [39] described families of TFST-deficient patients. The clinical response to γ-globulin was excellent [39].

Immunophysiology and Pharmacology

Phagocytosis activation. It has been shown that the first and main effect of TFST, which was the guide for controlling its preparation, is phagocytosis stimulation [40]. Sialic acid is necessary for TFST stimulation of phagocytosis [41]. It may function as a binding site for the three positively charged residues. The TFST mobilizes intracellular calcium and modulates cAMP and cGMP levels.

Phagocyte migration, chemotaxis, and differentiation. The TFST accelerates granulocyte and macrophage differentiation, increases the formation of bone marrow colonies in vitro [42], and stimulates blood granulocytes and peritoneal macrophage immunogenic activity, namely, the processing of antigen [43].

Macrophage killing of tumor cells. We showed that macrophage killing of tumor cells was strongly stimulated after TFST administration [5]. This effect has been confirmed by others [44–47]. In macrophages, TFST increased the quantity of superoxide and the adenosine deaminase activity [48]. We have also observed an increase in delayed hypersensitivity, cytolytic T-cell activity, antibody production, antibody-dependent cell-mediated cytotoxicity (ADCC), and natural killer (NK) cell activity (Fig. 1) [5].

Bactericidal direct effect. A direct bacteria-killing effect similar to that of the bipeptide Lys-l-Lys has been suggested [49].

Viral expression effect. The exposure to TFST of Balb/c mouse cells transformed by Kirsten sarcoma virus enhanced the expression of the endogenous xenotropic retrovirus [50].

Immunorestoration and spontaneous tumor prevention. In aged, immunodepressed mice that had decreased macrophage cytostatic activity, T-cell helper and killer activities, antibody production, and NK cell activity, (Fig. 2) [6], we observed that TFST injected weekly for 6 months at a dose of 10 μg restored the macrophage killing effect on tumor cells and the cytolytic T-cell activity (Fig. 3) [12]. The TFST did not change the NK cell activity or ADCC [12] but completely suppressed the appearance of spontaneous tumors, especially lymphomas, in old, immunodepressed mice (Table I).

Other antitumor effects. In another study, TFST exerted antitumor activity on several grafted tumors and inhibited the development of Cloudman S-91 melanoma and CH1 B-cell lymphoma metastasis in mice. It increased the tumor latent period and reduced tumor incidence after viral (Rous sarcoma virus) and chemical (3-methylcholanthrene) carcinogenesis [51].

Neurologic effects. An analgesic effect has been observed after TFST injection into the lateral ventricle [52]. The macrophages have been shown to possess high- and low-affinity sites for substance P and for neurotensin, which are known to stimulate their phagocytosis [53]. In addition, TFST stimulated phagocytosis of the retinal pigmented epithelium [54]. When injected into the cerebral ventricles, TFST induced biphasic changes of locomotor activity: first depression, then stimulation. It also increased blood pressure. These effects were antagonized by pretreatment with bradykinin but not by pretreatment with naxolone [55]. Thus TFST may represent a new class of nonopiate analgesics, and these neurologic effects should be monitored in clinical applications.

Other Effects

Preclinical study. There were no toxic effects when TFST was given to mice in doses up to 1 mg. The LD$_{50}$ was 2,400 mg/kg. In dogs, the dose of 1 mg/kg was not toxic [56]. We

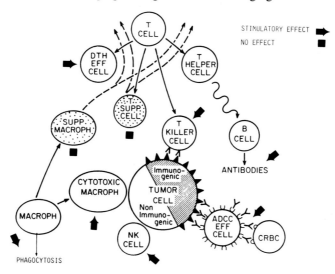

Fig. 1.   Effect of tuftsin (one injection of 25 μg/mouse) on the main immunologic functions in young mice.

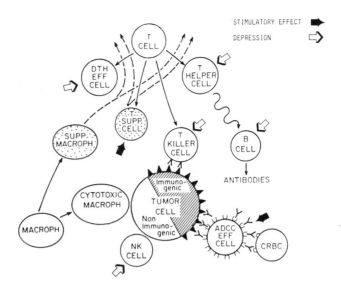

Fig. 2.   Effect of aging on main immunologic functions.

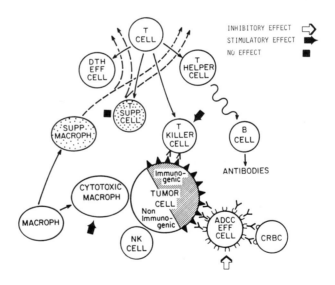

Fig. 3.   Effect of tuftsin (one injection of 10 μg/mouse applied weekly for 6 months) in old, immuno-depressed mice.

have studied the action of TFST in baboons and observed 1) no lethal toxicity and 2) a dose-related neutrophilic amplification (unpublished data).

   Human studies. In humans, we have given TFST at a dose of 50 mg/m^2 without toxic effects and with a significant increase in the number of polymorphonuclear leukocytes and OKT4-positive lymphocytes in peripheral blood. A phase II study is in progress. Catane et al [57] have given doses ≤0.96 mg/kg; 50% of the patients showed an increase in leukocytosis. Doses of 0.08–0.48 mg/kg increased NK cell activity in 80% of the subjects.

TABLE I. Effect of Tuftsin on the Incidence of Spontaneous Tumors Appearing in F1 (C$_{57}$BL/6 × DBA2) Mice Between 16 and 28 Months of Age

	Treatment applied		
	Saline		Tuftsin (10 μg/mouse)
No. of tumor-bearing mice	6/27	P < 0.01	0/22
Total No. of mice in group (%)	(22%)		(0%)

Histologic forms of the tumors included one unclassified malignant lymphoma, two undifferentiated malignant lymphomas, one immunoblastic lymphoma, and two adenocarcinomas.

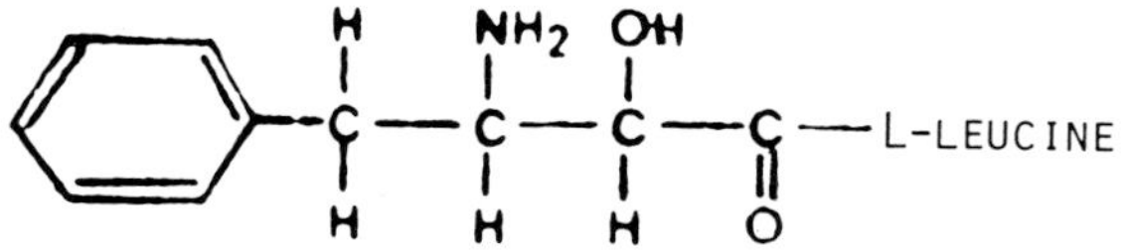

Fig. 4.   Structure of bestatin. (After Suda et al [64] and Nakamura et al [65]).

Analogs

Martinez and Winternitz [58] have prepared TFST analogs that have been found to be active [9]. Of the analogs synthesized by Konopinska et al [59], the following may be useful: Thr-Lys-Pro-Lys-Thr-Lys-Pro-Arg; Thr-Lys-Pro-Lys-Thr-Lys-Pro-Lys; Ala-Lys-Thr-Lys-Pro-Arg-Glu-Gln; Arg-Thr-Lys-Pro-Arg; Pro-Arg-Thr-Lys-Pro-Arg; and Lys-Pro-Arg-Thr-Lys-Pro-Arg. The octapeptide tuftsinyl-tuftsin has been shown to be active on L1210 leukemia and melanoma B16/5B [60].

BESTATIN

Umezawa [61,62] isolated a product of small molecular weight from *Streptomyces olivoreticuli* that permits the accumulation of peptidases in cell-free extracts and in intact reticulocytes [63]. It was named *bestatin* (BST). Suda et al [64] and Nakamura et al [65] established its structure (Fig. 4) and subsequently synthesized it [66]. Studies have shown that BST is an inhibitor of leucine aminopeptidase and aminopeptidase B but does not inhibit aminopeptidase A, trypsin, chymotrypsin, elastase, papain, or pepsin [67–70].

Immunopharmacology

The basic mechanism of action of BST is not limited to protease inhibition. It has also been shown that BST works directly on DNA metabolism [71,72] and protein breakdown in T cells [73]. It enhances delayed hypersensitivity [70]. In addition, it amplifies the activation by concanavalin A of small lymphocytes [74] and other types of blastogenesis [75–77].

Like TFST, BST injected once at the dose of 100 μg stimulated the macrophage killing of tumor cells in our study. At this dose, it enhanced ADCC, and at 10 and 100 μg, antibody production and NK cell activity were enhanced (Fig. 5) (unpublished data). Administered at the dosage of 100 μg once a week for 6 months from the age of 16 months, it enhanced or restored macrophage cytotoxicity, T-cell toxicity, and delayed hypersensitivity (Fig. 6). It restored antibody production at the dosage of 10 μg once a week. At 100 μg once a week, it prevented spontaneous lymphomas from appearing after the age of 14 months (Table II) [10].

Other Effects

Cytologic effects. The chemical induction of sister chromatin exchanges has also been inhibited by BST [78].

Neurologic effects. It has been shown that BST inhibits several neuroenzymatic processes, ie, the degradation of acetylocholine and other receptors in the muscle cells [79], the

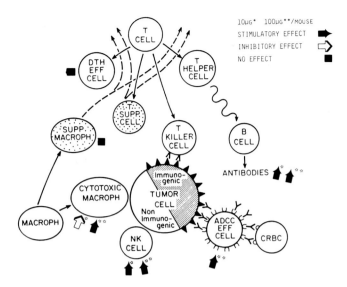

Fig. 5.   Action of bestatin on the main immunologic functions in young mice.

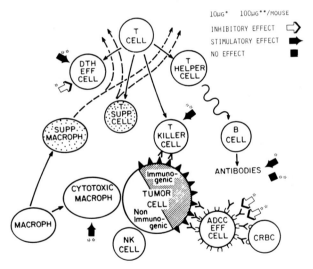

Fig. 6. Effect of bestatin according to dose on the immunologic functions in old mice.

degradation of cerebral prolidases EC 3.4.13.9 [80], the degradation by the brain of the melanotropin inhibiting factor [81], and the degradation of ACTH 1–4 by the brain cytosol [82].

Animal toxicology. In mice, BST exerted different effects according to the dose administered (10–100 μg). We also found different effects on the spontaneous tumor incidence and, according to the mouse age, for long-term administration. While BST corrects immunodepression, administration at ages 7–21 months aggravates it.

Human studies. With Serrou et al [83], we conducted a phase I study that determined the tolerated and immunoactive dose in humans to be 30 mg/m^2/day. The preliminary results of trials conducted by Ota [84] on acute myeloid leukemia, by Ikeda and Ishihara [85] on melanoma, and by Edsmyr et al [86] on prostate carcinoma are favorable.

TABLE II. Prevention by Bestatin of the Incidence of Spontaneous Tumors Appearing in F1 (C57BL/6 × BALB/c) Mice Between 16 and 28 Months of Age

	Untreated group	100 μg Bestatin-treated group
Histological type of the tumors	6	
Malignant lymphoma	1	
Hepatoma	1	
Leukemic lymphoma		
Lymphoma		1
No. of tumor-bearing animals per total No. of animals per group (%)	8/22* (36)	1/20* (5)

*P = 0.01.

CONCLUSIONS

As shown in this comparative study, TFST and BST exert almost the same pharmacologic effects on immunologic functions. Under certain conditions, they are both able to restore immune function in animals with depressed immunity and simultaneously prevent the appearance of spontaneous tumors. Do TFST and BST constitute a complementary system, BST partially working by protecting TFST? TFST is sensitive to aminopeptidase [25,26], an enzyme that is inhibited by BST [67]. This question is under study. The answer will be of major therapeutic importance, because BST could be administered in clinical situations of immunodepression when the blood level of TFST is normal, and BST could be given when the TFST level is low.

ACKNOWLEDGMENTS

I am thankful to N. Vriz and E. Couvé for their help in the preparation of the manuscript.

REFERENCES

1. Olsson L, Florentin I, Kiger N, Mathé G. Cellular and humoral immunity to leukemia in BCG-induced controlled growth of a murine leukemia. JNCI 1977; 59:1297–306.
2. Bruley-Rosset M, Florentin I, Kiger N, Davigny M, Mathé G. Effects of BCG and levamisole on immune responses in young adult and age-immunodepressed mice. Cancer Treat Rep 1978; 62:1641–50.
3. Florentin I, Kiger N, Bruley-Rosset M, Schultz J, Mathé G. Effect of seven immunomodulators on different types of immune responses in mice. In: Serrou B, Rosenfield R, eds: Human lymphocyte differentiation: Its application to cancer. Amsterdam: North Holland, 1978: 299–303.
4. Florentin I, Bruley-Rosset M, Davigny M, Mathé G. Comparison of the effects of BCG and a preparation of heat-killed Pseudomonas aeruginosa on the immune response in mice. In: Werner GH, Floch F, eds: The pharmacology of immunoregulation. New York: Academic Press, 1978: 335–51.
5. Florentin I, Bruley-Rossett M, Kiger N, Imbach JL, Winternitz F, Mathé G. In vivo immunostimulation by tustsin. Cancer Immunol Immunother 1978; 5:211–6.
6. Bruley-Rosset M, Florentin I, Kiger N, Schulz J, Davigny M, Mathé G. Age related changes of the immune response and immunorestoration by stimulating agents. In: Doria G, Eshkol A, The immune system: Functions and therapy of dysfunction. New York: Academic Press, 1980: 171–87.
7. Bruley-Rosset M, Hercend T, Martinez J, Rappaport H, Mathé G. Prevention of spontaneous tumors of aged mice by immunopharmacologic manipulation: Study of immune antitumor mechanism. JNCI 1981; 66:1113–9.
8. Bruley-Rosset M, Rappaport H. Natural killer cell activity and spontaneous development of lymphoma. Effects of single and multiple injections of interferon into young and aged $C_{57}B1/6$ mice. Int J Cancer 1983; 31:381–9.
9. Florentin I, Martinez J, Maral J, et al. Immunopharmacological properties of tuftsin and of some analogs. Ann NY Acad Sci 1983; 419:177–91.

10. Bruley-Rosset M, Florentin I, Kiger N, Schulz J, Mathé G. Restoration of impaired immune functions of aged animals by chronic bestatin treatment. Immunology 1979; 38:75–83.

11. Bruley-Rosset M, Florentin I, Kiger N, Schulz JI, Mathé G. Correction of immunodeficiency in aged mice by levamisole and bestatin administration. In: Mathé G, Muggia FM, eds: Cancer chemo- and immunopharmacology. 2. Immunopharmacology, relations and general problems. Heidelberg: Springer Verlag, 1980: 139–46.

12. Bruley-Rosset M, Hercend T, Rappaport H, Mathé G. Immunorestorative capacity of tuftsin after long-term administration to aging mice. Ann NY Acad Sci 1983; 419:242–50.

13. Harshman S, Najjar VA. The binding of autologous γ-globulin with isohemagglutinin activity to human red blood cells. Biochem Biophys Res Commun 1963; 11:411–5.

14. Fidalgo BV, Najjar VA, Zukoski CF, Katayama Y. The physiological role of the lymphoid system. II. Erythrophilic γ-globulin and the survival of the erythrocyte. Proc Natl Acad Sci USA 1967; 57:665–72.

15. Fidalgo BV, Katayama Y, Najjar VA. The physiological role of the lymphoid system. V. The binding of autologous (erythrophilic) γ-globulin to human red blood cells. Biochemistry 1967; 6:3378–85.

16. Lahiri AK, Mitchell WM, Najjar VA. The physiological role of the lymphoid system. VIII. The nature of the in vitro binding of the erythrophilic γ-globulin and its effect on the configuration of the erythrocyte. J Biol Chem 1970; 245:3906–10.

17. Constantopoulos A, Najjar VA. The physiological role of the lymphoid system. The binding of autologous thrombophilic γ-globulin to human platelets. Eur J Biochem 1974; 41:135–8.

18. Sandberg-Hansen M, Bang NU. Plasma protein regulation. Mol Cell Biochem 1979; 24:143–58.

19. Fidalgo BV, Najjar VA. The physiological role of the lymphoid system. III. Leucophilic γ-globulin and the phagocytic activity of the polymorphonuclear leucocyte. Proc Natl Acad Sci USA 1967; 57:957–64.

20. Fidalgo BV, Najjar VA. The Physiological role of the lymphoid system. VI. The stimulatory effect of leucophilic γ-globulin (leucokinin) on the phagocytic activity of human polymorphonuclear leucocyte. Biochemistry 1967; 6:3385–92.

21. Najjar VA, Nishioka K. Tuftsin: A physiological phagocytosis-stimulating peptide. Nature 1970; 228:672–3.

22. Nishioka K, Constantopoulos A, Satoh P, Najjar VA. The characteristics, isolation and synthesis of the phagocytosis stimulating peptide tuftsin. Biochem Biophys Res Commun 1972; 47:172–9.

23. Nishioka K, Constantopoulos A, Satoh PS, Mitchell WM, Najjar VA. Characteristics and isolation of the phagocytosis-stimulating peptide tuftsin. Biochem Biophys Acta 1973; 310:217–29.

24. Nishioka K, Satoh PS, Constantopoulos A, Najjar VA. The chemical synthesis of the phagocytosis tetrapeptide tuftsin (Thr-Lys-Pro-Arg) and its biological properties. Biochem Biophys Acta 1973; 310:230–7.

25. Najjar VA, Constantopoulos A. A new phagocytosis-stimulating tetrapeptide hormone, tuftsin, and its role in disease. J Reticuloendoth Soc 1972; 12:197–215.

26. Satoh PS, Constantopoulos A, Nishioka K, Najjar VA. Tuftsin, threonyl-lysyl-prolyl-arginine, the phagocytosis stimulating messenger of the carrier cytophillic γ-globulin leukokinin. In: Meinhoffer J, ed: Chemistry and biology of peptides. Ann Arbor: Ann Arbor Science Publ, 1972: 403–8.

27. Najjar VA. The physiological role of γ-globulin. In: Meister A, ed: Advances in enzymology. New York: John Wiley & Sons, Inc., 1974: 129–78.

28. Blumenstein M, Layne PP, Najjar VA. Nuclear magnetic resonance studies on the structure of the tetrapeptide tuftsin, L-threonyl-L-lysyl-L-propyl-L-arginine, and its pentapeptide analogue L-threonyl-L-lysyl-L-propyl-L-propyl-L-arginine. Biochemistry 1979; 18:5247–53.

29. Gottlieb P, Stabinsky Y, Hazum E, et al Tuftsin receptors. In Anon: Abstracts Conf antineoplastic, immunogenic and other effects of the tetrapeptide tuftsin: A natural macrophage activator. New York, February 16–17, 1983 (abstract No. 9).

30. Amoscato AA, Davies PJA, Babcock GF, Nishioka K. Receptor-mediated internalization of tuftsin. In Anon: Abstracts Conf antineoplastic, immunogenic and other effects of the tetrapeptide tuftsin: A natural macrophage activator. New York, February 16–17, 1983 (abstract No. 11).

31. Constantopoulos A, Likhite V, Crosby WH, Najjar VA. Phagocytic activity of the leukemic cell and its response to the phagocytosis stimulating tetrapeptide, tuftsin. Cancer Res 1973; 33:1230–4.

32. Spirer Z, Zakuth V, Bogair N, Fridkin M. Radioimmunoassay of the phagocytosis stimulating peptide tuftsin in normal and splenectomized subjects. Eur J Immunol 1977; 7:69–74.

33. Gottlieb P, Stabinsky Y, Zakuth V, Spirer Z, Fridkin M. Synthetic pathways to tuftsin and radioimmunoassay. In Anon: Abstracts Conf antineoplastic, immunogenic and other effects of the tetrapeptide tuftsin: A natural macrophage activator. New York, February 16–17, 1983 (abstract No. 2).

34. Spirer Z, Zakuth V, Orda R, Wiznitzer T. Acquired tuftsin deficiency. In Anon: Abstracts Conf antineoplastic, immunogenic and other effects of the tetrapeptide tuftsin: A natural macrophage activator. New York, February 16–17, 1983 (abstract No. 21).

35. Najjar VA. The clinical and physiological aspects of tuftsin deficiency syndromes exhibiting defective phagocytosis. Klin Wochenschr 1979; 57:751–6.

36. Najjar VA, Nishioka K, Constantopoulos A, Satoh PS. The function and interaction of erythrophilic γ-globulin with autologous erythrocytes. In Rapoport S, Jung M eds: VI Int Sym über Struktur und Funktion der Erythrozyten. Berlin: Akademi-Verlag, 1972; 355–62.

37. Najjar VA, Konopinska D, Chaudhuri MK, Schmidt DE, Linehan L. Tuftsin, a natural activator of phagocytic functions including tumoricidal activity. Mol Cell Biochem 1981; 41:3–12.

38. Inada K, Nemeto N, Nishijima A, Wada S, Hirata M, Yoshida M. A case suspected of tuftsin deficiency. In: Kokobun, Yoshida. Phagocytosis: Its physiology and pathology. Baltimore: University Park Press, 1979; 158–74.

39. Constantopoulos A. Congenital tuftsin deficiency. Ann NY Acad Sci 1983; 419:214–9.

40. Constantopoulos A, Najjar VA, Smith JW. Tuftsin deficiency: A new syndrome with defective phagocytosis. J Pediatr 1972; 80:564–72.

41. Constantopoulos A, Najjar VA. The requirement for membrane sialic acid in the stimulation of phagocytosis by the natural tetrapeptide. J Biol Chem 1973; 248:3819–22.

42. Babcock GF, Amoscato AA, Nishioka K. Effect of tuftsin on the migration, chemotaxis and differentiation of macrophages and granulocytes. Ann NY Acad Sci 1983; 419:64–74.

43. Najjar VA. Tuftsin: A natural activator of phagocyte cells, an overview. Ann NY Acad Sci 1983; 419:1–11.

44. Nishioka K. Anti-tumour effect of the physiological tetrapeptide tuftsin. Br J Cancer 1979; 39: 342–5.

45. Najjar VA, Chadhuri MK, Konopinska D, Beck BD, Layne PP, Linehan L. Tuftsin (Thr-Lys-Pro-Arg) a physiological activator of phagocytic cells: A possible role in cancer suppression and therapy. In: Hersh EJ, Chirigo MS, Mastrangelo G. eds: Augmenting agents in cancer therapy. New York: Raven Press, 1981; 459–78.

46. Nishioka K, Babcock GF, Phillips JH, Noyes RD. Antitumor effect of tuftsin. Mol Cell Biochem 1981; 41; 13–8.

47. Catane R, Schlanger S, Gottlieb P, et al. Toxicology and antitumor activity of tuftsin in mice. Proc Am Soc Clin Oncol 1981; 22:371 (abstract C-152).

48. Tritsch GL. Purine salvage pathway enzyme activity in tuftsin stimulated macrophages. In Anon: Abstracts Conf antineoplastic, immunogenic and other effects of the tetrapeptide tuftsin: A natural macrophage activator. New York, February 16–17, 1983 (abstract No. 8).

49. Dabrowska M, Kupryszewski G, Musalewski F, Kochanowski J. Derivatives of the L-lysine-peptides with antibacterial activity. Pol J Pharmacol Pharm 1976; 28:77–88.

50. Suk WA, Long CW. Enhancement of endogenous xenotrophic murine retrovirus expression by tuftsin. Ann NY Acad Sci 1983; 419:75–86.

51. Nishioka K, Babcock GF, Phillips JH, Banks RA. In vivo and in vitro antitumor activities of tuftsin. Ann NY Acad Sci 1983; 419:234–41.

52. Herman ZS, Stachura Z, Opielka L, Siemion IZ, Nawrocka E. Tuftsin and D-Arg³-tuftsin possess analgesic action. Experientia 1981; 37:76–7.

53. Goldman R, Bar-Shavit Z. On the mechanism of the augmentation of the phagocytic capability of phagocytic cells by tuftsin, neurotensin and kentsin and the interrelationship between their receptors. Ann NY Acad Sci 1983; 419:143–55.

54. Fisher LJ, Stevens G Jr, McCann P. Tuftsin stimulation of phagocytosis by the retinal pigment epithelium. Ann NY Acad Sci 1983; 419–30.

55. Herman ZS, Stachaura Z, Kreminski T. Central effects of tuftsin. Ann NY Acad Sci 1983; 419: 156–63.

56. Catane R, Schlanger SW, Weiss L. Toxicology and antitumor activity of tuftsin in animals. Ann NY Acad Sci 1983; 419:251–60.

57. Catane R, Treves AJ, Weiss L, et al. Clinical phase I study of tuftsin. Proc Amer Soc Clin Oncol 1983; 2:45 (abstract C-175).

58. Martinez J, Winternitz F. New synthetic and natural tuftsin related compounds and evaluation of their phagocytosis stimulating activity. Ann NY Acad Sci 1983; 419:23–34.
59. Konopinska D, Luczak M, Wlekuk M. Elongated tuftsin analogues: Synthesis and biological investigations. Ann NY Acad Sci 1983; 419: 35–43.
60. Najjar VA, Linehan L, Konopinska D. The antineoplastic effects of tuftsin and tuftsinyltuftsin on B16/5B melanoma and L1210 cells. Ann NY Acad Sci 1983; 419:261–8.
61. Umezawa H. Small molecular microbial products enhancing immune response. Antibiot Chemother 1978; 24:9–18.
62. Umezawa H. Advances in microbial secondary metabolites: Enzyme inhibitors. In Anon: Abstr papers Centen Mtg. Am Chem Soc, 1976: MEDI 3.
63. Botbol V, Scornick OA. Intermediates in the degradation of abnormal globin. Bestatin permits the accumulation of the same peptidase in cell-free extracts as in intact reticulocytes. J Biol Chem 1979; 254:11254–57.
64. Suda H, Takita T, Umezawa H. The structure of bestatin. J Antibiot 1976; 29:100–1.
65. Nakamura H, Suda H, Takita T, Aoyagi T, Umezawa H, Iitaka Y. X-ray structure determination of (2S, 3R)-3-amino-2-hydroxy-4-phenylbutanoic acid, a new amino acid component of bestatin. J Antibiot 1976; 29:102–3.
66. Suda H, Takita T, Aoyagi T, Umezawa H. The chemical synthesis of bestatin. J Antibiot 1976; 29:600–1.
67. Nishizawa R, Saino T, Takita T, Suda H, Aoyagi T, Umezawa H. Synthesis and structure-activity relationship of bestatin analogues, inhibitors of aminopeptidase B. J Med Chem 1977; 20:510–15.
68. Suda H, Aoyagi T, Takeuchi T, Umezawa H. Inhibition of aminopeptidase B and leucine aminopeptidase by betsatin and its atereoisomer. Arch Biochem Biophys 1976; 177:196–200.
69. Umezawa H, Aoyagi T, Suda H, Hamada T, Takeuchi T. Bestatin, an inhibitor of aminopeptidase B, produced by actinomycetes. J Antibiot 1976; 29:97–9.
70. Umezawa H, Ishizuka M, Aoyagi T, Takeuchi T. Enhancement of delayed-type hypersensitivity by bestatin, an inhibitor of aminopeptidase B and leucine aminopeptidase. J Antibiot 1976; 29:857–9.
71. Arendes J. Activation of DNA metabolism in T-cells by bestatin. Arch Pharmacol 1980; 311:R7.
72. Mullar WEG, Zahn RK, Arendes J, Munsch N, Umezawa H. Activation of DNA metabolism in T-Cells by bestatin. Biochem Pharmacol 1979; 28:3131–7.
73. Libby P, Goldberg AL. Effects of chymostatin and other proteinase inhibitors on protein breakdown and proteolytic activities in muscle. Biochem J Cell Aspects 1980; 188:213–20.
74. Saito M, Aoyagi T, Umezawa H, Nagai YY. Bestatin, a new specific inhibitor of aminopeptidases, enhances activation of small lymphocytes by concanavalin A. Biochem Biophys Res Commun 1977; 76:526–33.
75. Saito M, Takegoshi K, Aoyagi T, Umezawa H, Nagai Y. Stimulatory effect of bestatin, a new specific inhibitor of aminopeptidases, on the blastogenesis of guinea pig lymphocytes. Cell Immunol 1978; 40:247–62.
76. Ishizuka M, Masuda T, Kanbayashi N, et al. Effect of bestatin on mouse immune system and experimental murine tumors. J Antibiot 1980; 33:642–52.
77. Ishizuka M, Sato H, Sugiyama Y, Takeuchi T, Umezawa H. Mitogenic effects of bestatin on lymphocytes. J Antibiot 1980; 33:653–62.
78. Umezawa H, Sawamura M, Matshushima T, Sugimura T. Inhibition of chemically indiced sister chromatid EXH exchanges by protease inhibitors from streptomyces. Chem Biol Interact 1980; 30:247–51.
79. Libby P, Bursztajn S, Goldberg AL. Degradation of the acetylcholine receptors in cultured muscle cells: Selective inhibitors and the fate of undergraded receptors. Cell 1980; 19:481–91.
80. Hui KS, Lajtha A. Activation and inhibition of cerebral prolidase EC-3.4.13.9. J Neurochem 1980; 35:489–94.
81. Hui KS, Cheng KP, Wong KH, Salschutz M, Lajtha A. Degradation of melanotropin inhibiting factor by brain. J Neurochem 1980; 35:471–8.
82. Neidle A, Reith MEA. Degradation of ACTH 1-4, by mouse brain cytosol. Arch Biochem Biophys 1980; 203:288–95.
83. Serrou B, Cupissol D, Flad H, et al. Phase I evaluation in patients bearing advanced solid tumors. In Anon: Abstracts 1st Int Conf Immunopharmacol. Brighton, 29 July–1 August, 1980; (abstract 36, p 168).
84. Ota K. Randomized control clinical studies of bestatin treatment leukemia. In: Umezawa H, Edsmyr F, Sedlacek HH, eds: Chemo-immunotherapy (bestatin). Proc 13th Int Congr Chemother. Vienna, 28 August–2 September 1983. Vienna, 1983: SY67-7:31–5.

85. Ikeda S, Ishihara K. Randomized controlled study or immunochemotherapy with bestatin. A new small-molecular immunomodulator and chemotherapy as adjuvant to surgery for stage IB and II malignant melanoma. In: Umezawa H, Edsmyr F, Seclacek HH, eds: Chemo-immunotherapy (bestatin). Proc 13th Int Congr Chemother. Vienna, 28th August–2nd September 1983. Vienna, 1983; SY67-5:21-4.

86. Edsmyr F, Esposti PL, Andersson L, Naslund I, Blomgren H. Clinical study on bestatin and peplomycin in treatment of prostatic carcinoma. In: Carter SK, Ultmann J, eds: Peplomycin Proc 13th Int Congr Chemother. Vienna 28 August–2 September 1983. Vienna, 1983; SY87-2:5.

Cancer Detection and Prevention Supplement 1:457–462 (1987)

Immunological Effects of Isoprinosine as a Pulse Immunotherapy in Melanoma and ARC Patients

Alain Pompidou, MD, PhD
Claude Soubrane, MD
Véronique Cour, MD

Louise Telvi, MD
Claude Meunier, MD
Claude Jacquillat, MD

Hôpital Saint-Vincent de Paul (A.P., L.T., C.M.) and Hôpital Pitié-Salpétrière (C.S., V.C., C.J.), Paris

ABSTRACT Immunomodulatory effect of Isoprinosine are presented in melanoma and HTLV-III/LAV infected patients. Isoprinosine® (50 mg/kg) was used as a pulse immunotherapy according to two different schedules: A) 5 days every 15 days and B) 5 days every 15 days for 2 months, then 5 days every 2 months. The patients' immunological profiles were tested before and during the treatment in terms of T-cell subsets, cell number requirement for PHA-induced proliferation, and delayed hypersensitivity reaction to recall antigens. Primary malignant melanoma patients are randomized between surgery alone or associated to isotherapy (schedule A or B). Schedule A, after an initial improvement of surgery-induced immune deficiency, is responsible for an immunodepression, whereas schedule B determines a prolonged restoration in immune responses in melanoma and AIDS related complex or Kaposi sarcoma patients as well. In vitro effects of Isoprinosine on HTLV-III/LAV infection are presented. These data exhibit 1) the need of an immunological follow-up during isotherapy and 2) the immunological benefit of a pulse immunotherapy during acquired immunodeficiences related to cancer surgery or to HTLV-III/LAV infection in man.

Key words: immunomodulation, T-cell subsets, T-cell functions

INTRODUCTION

The impairment of circulating T-helper cells has been reported in cancer patients [1,2] and more recently before the onset of acquired immunodeficiency syndrome (AIDS) [3]. The strategies of developing immunomodulatory agents are becoming the subject of intensive investigation. One of these agents is Isoprinosine (ISO), and its immunopotentiating activity has already been reported. ISO, the p-acetamidobenzoic acid salt of inosine dimethylamino-isopropanol, induces in man an in vitro T-cell maturation in terms of precursor T-cell differentiation [4] and $T_4^+ DR^+$ phenotypic expression in peripheral blood lymphocytes [5,6]. In this study, we present the modulation of T-cell subsets and functions in melanoma and

Address reprint requests to Dr. A. Pompidou, Hôpital Saint-Vincent de Paul, 74, avenue Denfert-Rochereau 75014 Paris, France.

AIDS-related complex (ARC) patients after in vivo administration of ISO according to different schedules of pulse immunotherapy.

PATIENTS AND METHODS

ISO (50 mg/kg) was given as a pulse immunotherapy according to two different schedules: A) 5 days every 15 days or B) 5 days every 15 days for 2 months, then 5 days every 2 months. Fifty primary malignant melanoma patients were randomized into three groups: surgery alone, surgery + ISO on schedule A, and surgery + ISO on schedule B. Seven HTLV-III/LAV infected patients (three ARC, two AIDS, two Kaposi sarcoma [KS]) were treated according to schedule B. All patients were treated for 1 year, and immunological parameters were examined at days 30 and 60, and then every 2 months.

Lymphocytes from venous heparinized blood were purified by Ficoll-Hypaque (Pharmacia Laboratories) gradient centrifugation. Cells were washed in RPMI 1640 (Flow Laboratories) and final cell preparations adjusted for cultures to 10^6 cells/ml. They were more than 98% pure mononuclear cells (85% lymphocytes by morphological criteria). Short-term cultures were performed in RPMI 1640 with 10% heat-inactivated human AB serum, specillin G (100 IU/ml; Specia Laboratories), and streptomycin (100 μg/ml; Specia). The cells were distributed at 200 ul/well in flat-bottomed microplates (Costar, Cambridge, MA) after adjustment to 1.25, 2.5, 5, and 10.10^5 cells/ml. Equal values of PHA (5 μg/ml) (PHA HA16, Welcome Laboratories) or medium were added in triplicate wells, and ^{3}H-thymidine (0.5 μCi/well) was added 18 hr before a 72-hr culture. Radioactivity was counted using a scintillation counter and the cell number requirement for proliferative response were evaluated as previously described [7].

Cells washed in phosphate buffer (pH 7.2) supplemented with 5% FCS and 0.1% sodium azide were used for fluorescent evaluation of T-cell subsets using monoclonal antibodies (OKT3, OKT4 and OKT8) (Orthoclone; Ortho, Raritan, NJ) and flourescein labeled with serum affinity-purified goat antirat immunoglobulin (Southern Biotechnology Associates, Birmingham, AL) as described previously [8].

Delayed hypersensitivity reaction (DHR) to recall antigens was performed by skin test using a panel of seven antigens: tetanus, diphtheria, *Streptococcus,* trychophyton, *Proteus,* candidiasis, and tuberculin (Multitest, Institut Mérieux). A cumulative score was established by measurement of the extent of positive reactions 48 hr after intradermal injection [9,10].

RESULTS
Influence of Isotherapy in Melanoma Patients

In the group treated with surgery alone, a significant decrease in circulating $T4^+$ cells was observed within 3 months (Fig. 1). In patients immunodepressed by surgery, isotherapy determined within 1 month an acute peak in $T4^+$ cells and a decrease in $T8^+$ cells. When the first four courses of ISO were followed by closely related courses, a rapid decrease in $T4^+$ cells was observed in the schedule A-treated group, whereas in the control group the $T4^+$ cell defect is spontaneously improved. An increase in $T8^+$ cells is observed concurrently with the circulating T4 impairment. This regulation of T-suppressor cells did not last more than 2 months after the interruption of the treatment. On the contrary, interruption of treatment after the fourth course and the administration of Isoprinosine at wide intervals kept circulating $T4^+$ cells at a normal level and did not induce any rise in $T8^+$ cells.

The evaluation of cell number requirement for PHA-induced proliferation response is depicted in Figure 2, which shows the impairment of the response 3 months after surgery and its restoration at the beginning of isotherapy. The prolongation of isotherapy according to schedule A was responsible for a significant impairment of the response after 12 months treatment.

The variations of DHR in terms of the Multitest scores were very similar to those of circulating T-lymphocyte subsets (Fig. 3): the initial DHR impairment observed in patients

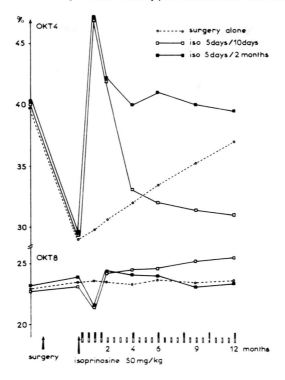

Fig. 1.   Influence of pulse isotherapy (schedules A and B) on T lymphocyte subsets in primary malignant melanoma.

treated by surgery alone was improved after 2 months isotherapy. The administration of ISO at wide intervals maintained the normalization of DHR, whereas closely related courses were responsible for a significant impairment of the response.

Influence of Isotherapy HTLV-III/LAV Infected Patients

Isotherapy was used in these patients for 1 year according to schedule B. Within 4 months two KS and three ARC patients exhibited 50% and 30% increases respectively, in circulating $T4^+$ cells (Fig. 4). The $T8^+$ cell count, not impaired in KS patients, was not modified, whereas in ARC patients the initial high level of circulating $T8^+$ cells was normalized within 10 months. No beneficial effects have been obtained in evolved AIDS patients with this schedule of administration for isotherapy.

DISCUSSION

In melanoma patients, we must emphasize the correlation between the different immunological parameters tested. The T-helper cell induction is accompanied by a restoration of T-lymphocyte function and DHR; the decrease in T-helper cells with T-suppressor induction is concomitant with an impairment of proliferative responses and DHR.

These data indicate the value of follow-up of patients treated with a long-term pulse isotherapy in order to assess rapidly any immunosuppressive effect reversible after the interruption of the treatment. The immunosuppressive effect of schedule A could be related to the close intervals between the different courses; moreover, the induction of $T8^+$ cells by in vitro treatment with high concentrations of ISO has been reported [5]. Schedule B does not induce immunodepression and does not determine a high level of circulating $T4^+$ cells. Thus, the best schedule for pulse isotherapy still needs to be drawn.

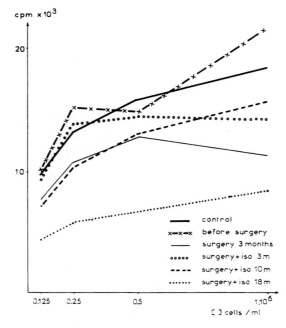

Fig. 2. Influence of pulse isotherapy (schedule A) on cell number requirement for PHA-induced proliferation in primary malignant melanoma.

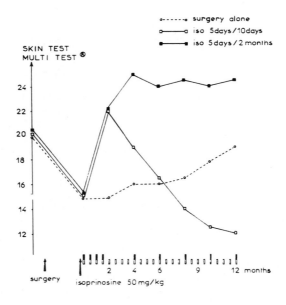

Fig. 3. Influence of pulse isotherapy (schedules A and B) on DHR (Multitest score) in primary malignant melanoma.

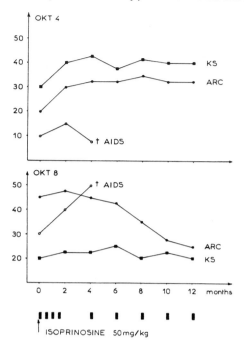

Fig. 4.   Influence of pulse isotherapy (schedule B) on T lymphocytes subsets in HTLV-III/LAV-infected patients.

In melanoma patients, the third course of isotherapy is responsible after the initial peak for a decrease in T4$^+$ cells, which would be avoided if the treatment were temporarily stopped after the first two courses. This allows us to propose a new regimen for pulse isotherapy: two 5-day courses every 10 days, repeated each 3 months; this is currently being tested in melanoma patients. This schedule should have a positive effect in terms of maintaining a high level of circulating T-helper cells. The influence of the different schedules of isotherapy on the relapse rate of the disease is now being tested.

In ARC patients, the induction of T4$^+$ cells has been reported after in vitro immunomodulation with ISO [6], and this can explain the regulation of T-helper cells after in vitro treatment. In HTLV-III/LAV-infected patients, it must be emphasized that besides the increase in T4$^+$ target cells, no acuteness of the viral infection has been observed after treatment. This could be related to the immunomodulating properties of the nonmitogenic agent [11,12]. A clinical improvement of the disease occurred in terms of disparition of polyadenopathies in ARC and diminution of skin lesions in KS patients. This could be explained by our recent in vitro results, obtained in collaboration with P. Sarin (Laboratory of Tumor Cell Biology, National Cancer Institute, Bethesda, MD), showing a 50% decrease in reverse transcriptase activity and p15 and p24 protein expression of human PBL infected with 10^8 viral particles and *simultaneously* treated with 200 µg/ml ISO [13]. The absence of any beneficial effects when human lymphocytes or viral particles are pretreated with the immunomodulator suggests that, besides the absence of direct antiviral effect, ISO inhibits at least partially the penetration of viral particles in target cells and/or their integration in the cell genome.

The recent demonstration [14] of the presence of circulating viral particles in the plasma of ARC patients and the data presented here support the utilisation of pulse isotherapy in ARC patients. The absence of any deleterious effect, the rapid restoration of surgery-induced immunological impairment in melanoma patients and the immunomodulating effects in KS and ARC patients exhibit the beneficial effect of pulse isotherapy provided that immunological parameters are tested during long-term treatments. The best schedule still needs to be drawn in order to obtain a better control of circulating T-cell subsets in immunocompromised patients.

ACKNOWLEDGMENTS

This work was supported by Ligue Nationale contre le Cancer (Comité de Paris), Association pour la Recherche contre le Cancer (ARC), and Fondation pour la Recherche Médicale. We thank F. Fouquet, Ch. Bernard, and M.C. Risal for technical assistance and N. Maraud and D. Esnous for preparing the manuscript.

REFERENCES

1. Kaszubowski PA, Husby G, Tung KSK, Williams RC. T lymphocyte subpopulation in peripheral blood and tissue of cancer patients. Cancer Res 1980; 40:4645–57.
2. Renoux G, Renoux M, Lemarie E, et al. Sodium diethyldithiocarbamate (Imuthiol) and cancer. In Klein T, Specter S, Friedman H, Szentivanyi A, eds: Biological response modifiers in human oncology and immunology. New York: Plenum Publishing Corporation, 1983; 223–39.
3. Schroff RW, Gottlieb MS, Prince HE, Chai L, Fahey JL. Immunological studies of homosexual men with immunodeficiency and Kaposi's sarcoma. Clin Immunol Immunopathol 1983; 27:300–13.
4. Touraine JL, Hadden JW, Touraine F. Isoprinosine induced T cell differentiation and T cell suppressor activity in humans. Curr Chem Infect Dis 1980; 2:1735–8.
5. Pompidou A. In vitro effects of Methisoprinol on human peripheral blood lymphocytes. EOS 1984; 2:112–4.
6. Pompidou A, Delsaux MC, Telvi L, et al. Isoprinosine and Imuthiol, two potentially active compounds in patients with AIDS related complex symptoms. Cancer Res 1985; 45:4671s–3s.
7. Knight SC, Harding B, Burman S, Mertin J. Cell number requirement for lymphocyte stimulation in vitro: Changes during the course of multiple sclerosis and effects of immunosuppression. Clin Exp Immunol 1981; 46:61–9.
8. Reinherz EL, Kung PC, Goldstein G, Schlossman SF. Separation of functional subsets of human T cells by a monoclonal antibody. Proc Natl Acad Sci USA 1979; 301:1018–22.
9. Kniker, WT, Anderson CT, Roumiantzeff M. The multitest system: A standardized approach to evaluation of delayed hypersensitivity and cell mediated immunity. Ann Allerg 1979; 43:73–9.
10. Lesourd B, Winters WB. Specific immune response to skin test antigens following repeated multiple antigen in normal individuals. Clin Exp Immunol 1982; 50:635–43.
11. Hadden JW, Hadden EM, Coffey RG. Isoprinosine augmentation of PHA induced lymphocyte proliferation. Infect Immun 1976; 13:382–5.
12. Tsang P, Lew F, O'Brien G, Selikoff IJ, Bekesi JG. Immunopotentiation of impaired lymphocyte functions in vitro by isoprinosine in prodromal subjects and AIDS patients. Int J Immunopharmacol 1985; 7:511–4.
13. Pompidou A, Zagury D, Gallo RC, Sun D, Thornton MS, Sarin PS. Inhibition of LAV/HTLV III infections in normal human lymphocytes and H$_9$ cell in presence of imuthiol or isoprinosine. Lancet (in press), 1985.
14. Zagury D, Fouchard M, Vol JC, et al. Detection of infections by HTLV III/LAV virus in cell free plasma from AIDS patients. Lancet 1985; 2:505–6.

Cancer Detection and Prevention Supplement 1:463–475 (1987)

Modulation of NK Activity in Regional Lymph Nodes by Preoperative Immunotherapy With OK-432 in Patients With Cancer of the Oral Cavity

K. Vinzenz, MD
M. Matejka, MD
G. Watzek, MD

H. Porteder, MD
N. Neuhold, MD
M. Micksche, MD

Clinic for Maxillo-Facial Surgery (K.V., H.P.), Division of Oral Surgery, Dental School (M.Ma., G.W.), Department of Pathology, Medical School (N.N.), and Institute of Applied and Experimental Oncology (M.Mi.), Vienna University, Vienna, Austria

ABSTRACT   The influence of preoperative perilesional therapy with the potent bacterial biological response modifier (BRM) OK-432 on natural killer (NK) cell activity in peripheral blood and tumor draining lymph nodes (LNs) of patients with head and neck cancer (HNC) has been investigated. Pretreatment NK activity in peripheral blood (PB) was comparable within the group of HNC patients. However, after perilesional OK-432 therapy, a significant increase in cytotoxicity was observed by day 8. Furthermore, postoperative suppression of PB NK activity was less pronounced in patients with OK-432 therapy. In tumor draining LNs, NK activity was significantly higher in patients receiving OK-432 therapy than in those treated by surgery alone. No differences were detected concerning the in vitro stimulatory capacity of interferon (IFN) and/or *Staphylococcus* protein A (SPA) on LN NK activity in both the OK-432 treated and untreated group. Furthermore, by immunoperoxidase technique, LNs of OK-432 treated patients were found to express a higher number of cells reacting with the monoclonal antibody HNK-1 compared to LNs of the untreated group. Both these results suggest that perilesional OK-432 therapy leads to an increase in number and function of NK cells in regional LNs, together with an increase in NK activity in PB in some but not all patients.

Key words: NK activity, lymphnodes, immunotherapy, oral cavity cancer, OK-432

INTRODUCTION

Cancer of the head and neck region comprises a variety of malignant tumors that, though mostly squamous cell carcinomas, differ in regional extent and metastatic spread. Curability by radical surgery and/or radiotherapy mainly depends on the localization of the primary tumor and on the presence or absence of lymph node metastases [1]. Despite the possibility of radical local interventions for erradicating the malignant disease, cancer of the head and neck

---

Address reprint requests to Dr. K. Vinzenz, University Clinic for Maxillo-Facial Surgery, Vienna University, Alserstraße 4, 1090 Vienna, Austria.

region tends to recur locally [2], indicating that local defense mechanisms are ineffective in producing an immune response against the remaining tumor cells. Several studies revealed an impairment of cell-mediated immunity, especially of T-lymphocyte function in the peripheral blood of head and neck cancer patients [3]. These immune dysfunctions were shown to be closely correlated with tumor burden, clinical stage, and response to therapy; patients with impaired response to skin test antigens also had the poorest prognosis [4,5]. These results suggest that stimulation of the immune response in immunosuppressed patients by therapeutic measures, such as immunotherapy, may lead to an improved response to conventional therapy and a reduction in recurrence rate. However, all attempts to demonstrate that immune restoration in this type of cancer is clinically beneficial for the patients have not been successful [6]. Neither application of bacterial preparations such as BCG or *Corynebacterium parvum*, nor tumor cell vaccines improved the results achieved by conventional therapies [7–9]. Considering the results of these studies it may be assumed that laboratory tests of immunomodulation attempted by use of various agents may not reflect the immune reactions that are actively involved in the patients' defense mechanisms against cancer cells [6,10,11].

Recently, considerable studies were devoted to a lymphocyte subpopulation that is active in the destruction of circulating tumor emboly, thus preventing metastatic spread [12]. These cells have been designated natural killer (NK) cells because of their capacity to kill a variety of tumor targets in vitro without presensitization [13]. It has been demonstrated that NK activity in cancer patients was suppressed in peripheral blood in advanced stages of the disease [14]. Significant augmentation of NK activity was achieved by in vitro and in vivo treatments with biological response modifiers such as bacterial products, Interferon (IFN), and Interleukin-2 (IL-2) [15]. There is evidence that growing tumors exert a negative influence on the NK activity of effector cells isolated from peripheral blood [16], intra- and peritumoral areas [17], and tumor draining lymph nodes [18,19]. Although isolates obtained from the above sources contained large granular lymphocytes (LGL)—the major cell population mediating NK activity—NK activity was found to be reduced or even absent. The same observation was made in lymphoid cells isolated from malignant pleural and peritoneal exudates of cancer, pointing to a depression of NK activity by malignant tumor [19,20].

We have recently demonstrated that NK activity of tumor draining lymph nodes obtained from patients with head and neck cancer was significantly lower compared to that in the peripheral blood of autochthonous donors [21]. Significant cytotoxicity was detected in nine of 19 lymph nodes, demonstrating an impairment of NK activity in more than 50% of samples. In vitro incubation with IFN-α led to a significant increase of killing activity in 33% of lymph nodes [21]. Both these results suggest that local defense mechanisms are depressed by primary tumors. In tumor draining lymph nodes immunosuppression might be a prerequisite for the spread of tumor cells.

We have shown previously that in vitro preincubation of human lymphocytes derived from peripheral blood, malignant effusions, lymph nodes, and separated LGL with OK-432, a streptococcal preparation, resulted in a significant augmentation of NK activity [22]. Furthermore, in phase I studies we have demonstrated that the major toxic side effects of OK-432 therapy were fever and local inflammatory reactions at the injection site. At the same time a significant augmentation of NK activity in peripheral blood and pleural effusion was detected subsequent to either systemic or intrapleural injection of OK-432 that in some patients was found to correlate with the course of the disease [23].

In the present study we investigated the effects of preoperative perilesional OK-432 therapy in patients with locally advanced cancer of the oral cavity on NK activity in peripheral blood and regional lymph nodes. Moreover, the expression of HNK-1 phenotype of cells in tumor draining lymph nodes after OK-432 therapy was investigated.

MATERIALS AND METHODS
Patients

Thirteen patients (12 males, one female, age range from 44–70 years, mean 55 years) with cancer of the mouth floor or tongue were included into this study. According to histopathological staging, each of three patients were classified T_2N_0, T_3N_0, and T_2N_1, six patients were T_3N_1, and four patients T_4N_1. After clinical staging and confirmation of malignant disease by biopsy, patients were informed and, their consent given, admitted to therapy.

OK-432 Pharmaceutical Preparation

OK-432 is a heat-killed and penicillin-treated preparation of the Su stain of *Streptococcus pyogenes* (generously supplied by Chugai Pharmaceutical Co., Tokyo, Japan) in vials containing 0.1 mg (=1 KE; Klinische Einheit, used to express the strength of the preparation) of lyophilized streptococci powder [22]. Before use, the content of the vial was dissolved in sterile saline and adjusted to the respective dose and injection volume.

Regional Therapy

Patients were given increasing doses of OK-432, ie, 0.2, 0.5, 1.0, 1.5, 2.0, and 2.5 KE, injected by a hypodermic needle into small perilesional deposits around the tumor. Injection volumes were 0.1 ml at each site, and the total volume was 1.0 ml. Doses were individually adapted according to side effects observed.

Record of Side Effects

Local inflammatory response regional lymph node swelling, and fluctuations in body temperature were evaluated during and after therapy for determination of side effects.

Preparation of Effector Cells

Heparinized peripheral blood (PB) was diluted, and mononuclear cell fraction was separated by Ficoll-Hypaque (Lymphoprep, Nyegaard, Oslo, Norway) gradient centrifugation. Cells in the interphase were washed and resuspended in RPMI 1640 supplemented with 25 mM Hepes, 2 mM L-glutamine, 100 U penicilline/ml, 100 µg streptomycin/ml, and 10% heat-inactivated fetal calf serum (Gibco Biocult, Glasgow, UK) (complete medium), and subsequently adjusted to the required cell number as previously described [20].

Lymph nodes were obtained during surgery of the primary tumor by radical neck dissection, trimmed of connective tissue and fat, and single cell suspensions were prepared as previously described [19,21]. Mononuclear cell fraction was obtained by gradient separation as described for PB. Preparations of individual lymph nodes (LNs) were never pooled and were used for further studies only when viability (trypan blue exclusion) exceeded 90%. Lymph nodes were free of metastases, as verified by histology and/or cytology.

Treatment With Interferon and *Staphylococcus* Protein A (SPA)

Mononuclear cells (5×10^5) were incubated for 18 hours in complete medium with or without addition of 1,000 IU/ml of purified natural IFN-α (kindly supplied by Dr. Bodo, E. Boehringer Institute, Vienna, Austria) and/or 50 µl/ml *Staphylococcus aureus* protein A (SPA" Pharamacia, Upsala, Sweden). After incubation, cells were washed and resuspended in complete medium and tested in the cytotoxicity assay in the respective E:T ratios.

Cytotoxicity Assay

NK activity was determined in a 4 hour ^{51}Cr release assay using K562 targets as described previously [19–21]. Briefly, 100 µl (1×10^4) of ^{51}Cr-labeled (Na$_2$ $^{51}CrO_4$, specific activity 100–350 µCi/µg; Amersham, UK) K562 cells and 100 µl effector cells were transferred to microwells of round-bottomed microtiter plates (NUNC 1482, Denmark), centrifuged, and incubated for 4 hours at 37°C in a humidified CO_2 atmosphere. After incubation, plates were centrifuged, and supernatants (100 µl) were transferred to counter vials; radioactivity was counted in an autogamma scintillation counter (Beckman Instruments, Vienna, Austria). Spontaneous release (never exceeding 15%) was determined in wells containing targets alone and maximum release by addition of Triton X-100.

The percentage of specific cytotoxicity for triplicate samples was calculated by the formula

$$\text{specific cytotoxicity} = \frac{\text{mean cpm test} - \text{mean cpm spont.}}{\text{mean cpm max} - \text{mean cpm spont.}} \times 100$$

Statistical analysis was performed by the Student t test and the chi square test.

Immunohistochemistry

LN samples obtained from patients with head and neck cancer receiving OK-432 therapy preoperatively were also investigated for the expression of HNK-1 phenotypes, detected on a certain proportion of NK cells by the immunoperoxidase method. Paraffin-embedded LNs from both OK-432 treated and untreated patients had been coded and prepared for analysis by an independent pathologist as follows.

Sections 3–5 μm thick were deparaffinated by xylol and, after dehydration by decreasing concentrations of ethyl alcohol, endogenous peroxidase was quenched by treatment with 3% hydrogen peroxide for 30 minutes. Subsequent to washing, the slides were incubated with human serum (1:5 diluted in Tris-HCI buffer 0.05 m, pH 7.4) and 1% bovine serum albumin (Behring Werke, Marburg, FRG) for 15 minutes, and rinsed again with Tris buffer. Then Leu-7 (HNK-1 monoclonal antibody; Beckton Dickinson nr 7390, USA), 1:60 diluted in Tris buffer, was applied to the sections. After an incubation period of 2 hours, rabbit antimouse Ig (Dako, Bender, Vienna); dilution 1:100, in human serum 1:20 and 1% BSA) was added, followed by an incubation period of 30 minutes. Finally, sections were treated with mouse PAP (Arnel 2604 1:100, human serum 1:20, and BSA 1%). The reaction was developed by diaminobenzidine solution (0.05%) in 0.01% hydrogen peroxide. The slides were cleansed under running tap water, dipped into distilled water, and counterstained by hemotoxylin.

Slides were covered with a coverglass and read within 24 hours. To express the cell number reacting with HNK-1, a scale (+1, +2, +3) roughly corresponding to the cell counts was used.

RESULTS

Thirteen patients were included in this therapy trial. In the majority of patients, the treatment period with OK-432 was 8 days. Patients received an initial dose of O. 2 KE which was subsequently increased every other day (Table I). The last injection was given 2 to 3 days before surgery.

Side Effects

In 11 patients local inflammatory reactions were observed at the injection site, ie, the peritumoral area; in seven of these patients there was also swelling of regional (submandibular) lymph nodes (Table I). A moderate increase in body temperature (37°C) was found in six patients, and seven patients developed fever reaction 6–12 hours after injection, returning to normal within 6 hours without medication. Slight difficulties in swallowing were noted in nine and more pronounced difficulties in three patients, probably as a result of the inflammatory reactions in the injection area. Side effects were most pronounced after the first two injections. In none of the patients did OK-432 therapy have to be interrupted or surgery delayed because of side effects.

NK Activity in Peripheral Blood

Investigations performed before surgery revealed a stage-dependence of NK activity in PB; patients with tumor stages T1–2 had a reactivity comparable to that of healthy controls, whereas those in stages T3–4 had significantly lower levels [21]. Compared to pretreatment

TABLE I. Preoperative OK-432 Therapy: Patients' Characteristics, OK-432 Dose and Side Effects

Patient	Age (years)	Sex	TNM	Total dose OK (KE)	Side effects			
					LIR	LS	DS	F
A	44	M	T_3N_1M0	2.7	+++	++	+	+
B	49	M	T_4N_1M0	2.7	+	+	+	++
C	51	M	T_4N_1M0	2.7	++	++	+	+
D	57	M	T_2N_1M0	2.7	++	++	+	+
E	57	M	T_2N_0M0	3.7	+	+	+	+
F	45	M	T_3N_1M0	4.0	++	++	+++	+++
G	58	M	T_3N_0M0	4.2	+++	+++	+++	++
H	46	M	T_3N_1M0	4.2	++	++	+	++
I	67	F	T_4N_1M1	4.2	++	+	+	++
J	52	M	T_3N_1M0	4.5	++	+	+	+
K	79	M	T_4N_1M0	5.7	++	++	+++	++
L	50	M	T_3N_1M0	5.7	++	+	++	++
M	60	M	T_3N_1M0	5.7	++	+	+	+

LIR, local inflammatory reactions; LS, lymphnode swelling; DS, difficulty in swallowing; F, fever; T, tumor; N, nodes; M, metastases.

TABLE II. NK Activity in Peripheral Blood

Therapy status	N	% Cytotoxicity (E:T 20:1)
Preoperative	40	30.0 ± 18.2
Preoperative	13*	42.6 ± 22.0
		†
Postoperative		23.0 ± 16.3
Preop. d 0 OK-432	13*	32.2 ± 14.8
		†
Postop. d 7 OK-432		51.0 ± 16.8
Preop. d 0 OK-432	6‡	35.2 ± 12.2
		†
Preop. d 7 OK-432		49.3 ± 16.5
		NS
Postop. OK-432		40.2 ± 15.1

NS, not significant.
*Identical patients without OK-432 therapy.
†$P < 0.05$.
‡Identical patients receiving preoperative OK-432 therapy.

levels, NK activity was significantly decreased in patients tested in the immediate postoperative period (Table II).

Patients were tested at the times indicated before and during OK-432 therapy. A drop of NK activity present in three out of eight patients on day 4 was followed by a significant increase in reactivity compared to pretreatment levels in three out of 11 patients tested on day 6 and in nine of 13 on day 8 (Figs. 1, 2).

After surgery, six patients were investigated; compared to those received no preoperative immunotherapy, immunosuppression was less pronounced (Table II).

NK Activity in Lymph Nodes

We found in previous investigations that tumor draining LNs obtained during surgery from patients with head and neck cancer had low but significant NK activity [21]. In the

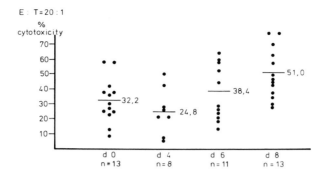

Fig. 1.   NK activity (E:T = 20:1) of patients receiving OK-432 therapy. Day 0, pretreatment value; d 4, d 6, d 8 indicate days of therapy. Significant increase in NK activity was seen by day 8 (P > 0.01).

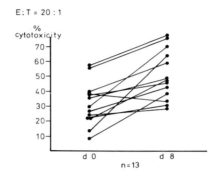

Fig. 2.   NK activity of patients receiving preoperative OK-432 therapy (N = 13). Day 0 (pretreatment) values are compared with day 8 values. Significant increase in reactivity was observed in nine patients.

present study, we extended our investigations and confirmed our previous findings. At an E:T ratio of 40:1 in ten out of 23 (43%) LN samples, significant cytotoxicity (>10% specific cytotoxicity) with a mean value of 11.2 ± 7.6% (Fig. 3a) was detected. LNs of patients (n = 13) who had received preoperative OK-432 therapy (Table III) had a mean value of cytotoxicity of 20.8 ± 14.7% at E:T = 40:1; 11 out of 13 (84%) showed significant levels of cytotoxicity. The difference between treated and untreated LNs was significant (P < 0.01), suggesting that OK-432 therapy resulted in an augmentation of local NK activity.

Influence of IFN and SPA

To test the state of reactivity of LNs after OK-432 therapy, LN cells of six individual patients were incubated overnight with IFN and tested for NK activity. Without IFN (incubation in medium) and at E:T = 40.1, mean levels were 23.2 ± 16.2%, whereas after the addition of IFN the mean cytotoxicity was 28.2 ± 16.1% (Table IV). A significant increase was detected in three out of nine samples, no change was observed in four, and a decrease was seen in two LN; the latter samples had higher spontaneous reactivity compared to those that could be augmented (Fig. 3b; Table IV).

After five individual LN samples were incubated with SPA, four displayed a significant increase in reactivity compared to control cultures. Mean values rose from 23.7 ± 10.1% (% cytotoxicity at E:T 40:1) to 43.8 ± 10.6% (Fig. 3c; Table V).

Follicular Reaction

With regard to the follicular reactions, no differences were detected in both groups.

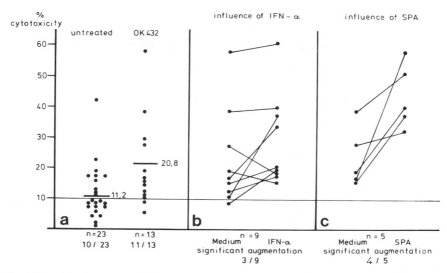

Fig. 3. NK activity in tumor draining LNs of patients with head and neck cancer. **a:** Twenty-three LNs from 14 patients without preoperative therapy were evaluated for NK activity. Mean value is 11.2 ± 7.6% cytotoxicity (E:T = 40:1). Thirteen LNs of six patients with preoperative OK-432 therapy were tested for NK activity (E:T = 40:1): $\bar{X}$ = 20.8 ± 14.7%; significantly (P < 0.01) higher compared to the control group. **b:** In vitro incubation of LNs (N = 9) of patients treated with medium or interferon (IFN-α) for 18 hours (for details, see Materials and Methods). Significant increase of NK activity was present in three out of nine samples. See also Table IV. **c:** In vitro incubation of LNs (N = 5; patients treated with OK-432) with medium or SPA (see Materials and Methods). Significant increase of NK activity was seen in four of five samples. See also Table V.

TABLE III. Preoperative OK-432 Therapy: NK Activity of Draining LNS

		Spontaneous cytotoxicity	
Treatment	LN/Pts.	Mean % cytotoxicity (E:T 40:1)	No. with positive cytotoxicity (%)
None	23/14	11.2 ± 7.6*	10/23 (43)
OK-432	13/6	20.8 ± 14.7*	11/13 (84)

*P < 0.01.

TABLE IV. Influence of IFN

Treatment	LN/Pts.	Mean		Mean % cytotoxicity, IFN		Significant augmentation (%)
None	23/14	11.2 ± 7.6*	P < 0.01	20.0 ± 12.6*	P < 0.005	9 (39)
OK-432	9/6	23.2 ± 16.2 †		28.2 ± 16.1 †		3 (33)

*P < 0.01.
†P < 0.1.

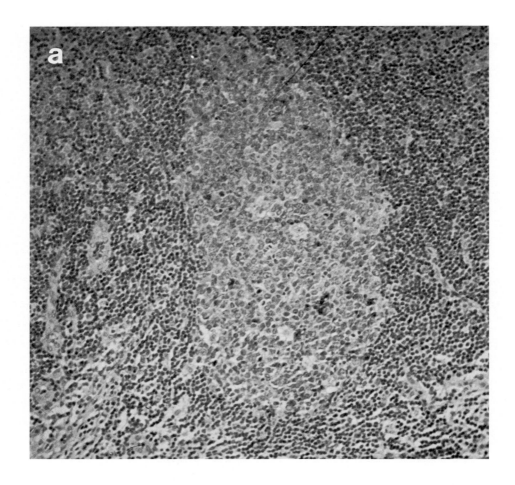

Fig. 4.   Immunoperoxidase technique for LN cells reacting with the mononuclear antibody HNK-1. **a:** Untreated LN. HNK-1[+] cells are scarcely seen; almost all are confined to the follicular areas. **b:** LN of patients treated with OK-432. HNK-1[+] cells are increased in number, again mostly confined to follicular areas.

TABLE V. Influence of SPA

Treatment	LN/Pts.	Mean		SPA		Significant augmentation
None	5/4	9.6 ± 1.9*	$P<0.025$	19.6 ± 8.9*	$P < 0.01$	3/5
OK-432	5/3	23.7 ± 10.1†		43.8 ± 10.6†		4/5

*$P < 0.025$.
†$P < 0.01$.

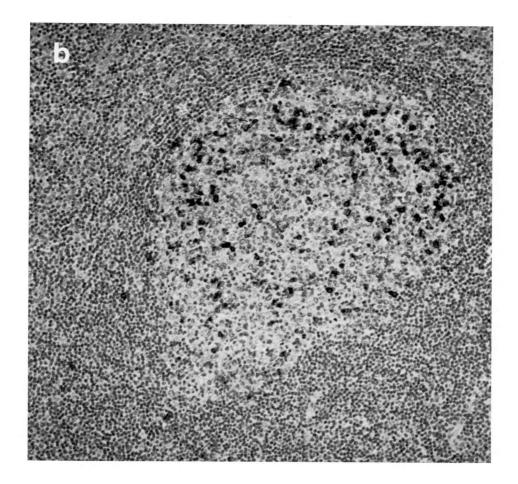

Figure 4

HNK-1 Immunohistochemistry

We demonstrated previously that cell suspensions of LNs draining cancer of the oral cavity had about $8.0 \pm 1.4\%$ of cells reacting with the monoclonal antibody HNK-1$^+$, which identified a certain proportion of cells that mediate NK activity. Using immunoperoxidase staining, we investigated fixed and embedded LN material obtained from 11 patients who had received OK-432 therapy and compared it to samples from 11 patients treated by surgery alone (Fig. 4). Investigations were performed in coded samples by an independent pathologist. According to the garding applied, eight LN samples were found to contain an increased number of HNK-1$^+$ (grade $+3$) (Table VI) in the OK-432 therapy group in contrast to none in the untreated group. The latter had staining patterns in the LNs classified grade 1 in seven LNs and grade 2 in four LNs. Examples of untreated (Fig. 4a) and OK-432 treated LNs (Fig. 4b) showed the distribution pattern of HNK-1$^+$ cells in LNS. These results suggest that OK-432 therapy leads to an increase in a population of cells in regional LNs that is able to mediate NK killing, as has also been observed in cytotoxicity assays.

TABLE VI. Preoperative OK-432 Therapy

Treatment	N	Follicular reaction			HNK-1$^+$ cells		
		+1	+2	+3	+1	+2	+3
None	11	8	3	0	7	4	0
OK-432	11	7	4	0	2*	1	8†

Chi square test: *P < 0.1; † P < 0.005.

DISCUSSION

Despite numerous reports showing that NK activity in peripheral blood of cancer patients decreases with tumor burden and that therapy with biological response modifiers significantly augments NK activity, precise knowledge on the biological significance of NK activity in cancer in still lacking [4]. The NK activity in peripheral blood does not seem to reflect closely the immune reaction that may be induced and/or is involved in the defense mechanisms against locally developing and growing neoplasms. Evidence for this fact is strengthened by the observation that patients with low tumor burden display normal NK activity in PB. This suggests that low NK activity in PB of patients with a larger tumor burden is not a prerequisite for local tumor development. These studies revealed the importance of investigating defense mechanisms in the vicinity of the tumor. In recent studies it was demonstrated that LGL within isolated tumor-infiltrating lymphocytes of cancer patients lacked killing activity [17]. This suggests that the growing tumor itself exerts a negative influence on the expression of spontaneous cytotoxicity. Low or absent NK activity has also been found in lymphocyte populations isolated from milignant pleural and peritoneal effusions [20,25]. Furthermore, LNs removed from tumor draining areas have been found to express low and/or vairable levels of NK activity that can be stimulated only to a certain extent by IFN in vitro [18,19]. This is another indication of a functional defect in NK cells, mediated probably by the tumor tissue itself. Prostaglandin E$_2$, which is produced by some tumors, has been found to suppress NK activity [26]. Preincubation of LN cells with indomethacin led to increased levels of cytotoxicity [27].

In the present investigations we extended our clinical experiences with local OK-432 immunotherapy. Previously we had demonstrated that intrapleural OK-432 therapy in patients with milignant pleural effusions resulted in a significant increase of NK activity together with a reduction of suppressor cell activity for NK cells [28]. Moreover, we found that LGL also contribute to cytotoxic reactions against autologous effusions derived from fresh tumor cells, offering at least some explanation for the biological role of these cells [29]. Furthermore, we have demonstrated that intrapleural injection of OK-432 resulted in a significant increase in lymphocyte cytotoxicity against autologous tumor cells [30].

In the present study we produced evidence that preoperative perilesional OK-432 therapy led to increased levels of cytotoxicity in tumor draining LNs compared to those obtained in patients without immunotherapy. These results are in agreement with findings from animal studies showing the injection of C. parvum into the footpad increased NK activity in LNs when injected into the draining area, but produced no effect when injected into the contralateral site. Additionally, splenic and blood NK activity was augmented independent of the route of injection [31].

Similarly, in our therapy study we found that NK activity was augmented not only in regional LNs but also in PB. This is in contrast to our previous findings on the effects of intraperitoneal OK-432 therapy; despite strong augmenting effects on effusion NK activity, no increase in PB was found in the same patients [28]. This was recently observed also in patients receiving intraperitoneal IFN [32]. Probably there are different levels of communication and cellular exchange existing between PB, LNs, and peritoneal and pleural cavities, as reflected by different systemic responses to BRM, depending on route of application, [11,20,31].

The mechanism of OK-432 activating NK activity has not yet been fully elucidated. There is evidence for OK-432 acting directly on LGL [22], which are the predominant population of cells mediating natural cytotoxicity. Moreover, it has been demonstrated that LGL by themselves produce certain cytokines such as interferons (IFN-α, IFN-γ), Interleukin (IL-1, -2), and natural killer cell activating factor (NKAF) [33] that might also contibute to an increased cytotoxicity induced by OK-432, as found in our previous in vitro [22] and in vivo [21] studies in cancer patients. Furthermore, OK-432 also seems to stimulate other cell populations such as T lymphocytes and monocytes/macrophages, thus leading to the production of mediators such as IFN-γ, IL-1, and IL-2 [34], which may contribute to the increased cytotoxic activity in LNs observed in the present study. In this context we found that only 30% of untreated LN cells could be stimulated by preincubation with IFN, suggesting some defect in the response in IFN [21]. This hyporesponsiveness in LNs, in comparison to PB in which NK activity could be augmented in up to 80% of the samples by IFN was eliminated by overnight preincubation of LN cells, as has been demonstrated with LNs obtained from patients with breast cancer [27]. After this preincubation, lymphocytes were found to show higher sensitivity to the stimulating effect of IFN.

After OK-432 therapy we found that 30% of samples could be stimulated by addition of IFN, suggesting that OK-432 treated cells were already activated and that addition of IFN resulted in an augmented stimulation of some samples only. An interesting observation was the fact that LNs with high activity of OK-432 therapy could either not be stimulated or showed a decrease by preincubation with IFN. However, when LN cells were preincubated with SPA, which has been found to induce at least IFN-γ and/or IFN-α production by human mononuclear blood cells, four out of five samples were found to be stimulated independently of the spontaneous levels of activity.

With regard to the distribution of NK cells in regional LNs, several studies using HNK-1 monoclonal antibody have demonstrated that LNs have low numbers of cells expressing the phenotype of cells mediating NK activity [21]. In immunohistochemical studies HNK-1[+] cells were found mainly in the germinal center [35], as has been demonstrated also in our present investigation. However, after OK-432 therapy a significant increase in the number of cells that were positive with monoclonal antibody HNK-1 was detected in regional LNs, indicating that the therapy probably had induced a maturation step from immature cells not expressing this phenotype. Another possiblity is that a shift in compartmentalization was induced by OK- 432 therapy, ie, NK cells from PB or other compartments were attracted to migrate toward the draining LNs.

Further evidence for a distribution of NK cells from circulation into other organs is derived from studies in rats, showing that local application of BRM results in a decrease of PB NK activity accompanied by an increase in both number and function of NK cells in certain organs, eg, in the liver [11]. In our own studies, in some patients we detected an initial decrease in PB NK activity, suggesting that such a decrease in number of LGL in PB might be responsible; however, we did not determine the absolute numbers in LGL in PB. At present, we are unable to determine the role of preoperative perilesional therapy for the final clinical outcome of the patients, because the number of patients is small and other variables such as postoperative chemo- or radiotherapy have to be taken into consideration. As immune reactions are weak in tumor draining LNs, our findings on the augmentation of regional defense mechanisms by preoperative OK- 432 therapy might be a valuable tool for delaying local recurrence in patients with head and neck cancer.

ACKNOWLEDGMENTS

The skillful technical assistance of Ing. Eva Sandor and Cornelia Kahler is gratefully acknowledged. This work was partly supported by Bürgermeister-Fonds, City of Vienna.

REFERENCES

1. Kramer S. Combined surgery and radiation therapy in management of locally advanced head and neck squamous carcinoma. In Chretien PB, Johns ME, Shedd DP, Strong EW, Ward PH, eds: Head and Neck Cancer. Philadelphia: BC Decker Inc, 1985; 1:48–54.

2. Harrison BFN. Head and neck surgery in the 1980s: The role of more or less. In Chretien PB, Johns ME, Shedd DP, Strong, EW, Ward PH, eds: Heak and Neck Cancer. Philadelphia: BC Decker Inc, 1985; 1:27–37.

3. Silverman NA, Alexander JC, Hollinshead AC, Chretien PB. Correlation of tumor burden with in vitro lymphocyte reactivity and antibodies to Herpes virus tumor associated antigens in head and neck squamous carcinoma. Cancer 1976; 37:135–9.

4. Catalona KJ, Chretien PB. Abnormalities of quantitative Dinitrochlorobenzene sensitisation in cancer patients: Correlation with tumor stage and histology. Cancer 1970; 31:353–8.

5. Eilber FR, Morton DL, Ketcham AS. Immunologic abnormalities in head and neck cancer. Am J Surg 1974; 128:534–7.

6. Vinzenz K, Micksche M. Immunotherapy in patients with head and neck cancer. Int J Immunother 1986 (in press).

7. Johns ME. Immunological considerations of head and neck cancer. In Batsakis W, ed: Tumors of the head and neck, clinical and pathological considerations. Baltimore: Williams & Wilkins Co, 1979: 503.

8. Mihich E, Fefr A. Clinical aspects of biological response modifiers: Current status and future prospects. In Anon.: Biological response modifiers: Sub-committee report. NCI Monogr 63. Washington DC: USGPO, 1983: 35–64

9. Hersh, EM. Immunotherapy of human cancer: Current status and prospect for future development. In Hadden JW, Chedid L, Dukar P, Spreafico F, eds: Advances in Immunopharmacology. Oxford: Pergamon Press, 1983: 487–500.

10. Bier J, Nicklisch U, Platz H. The doubtful relevance of nonspecific immune reactivity in patients with squamous cells carcinoma of the head and neck region. Cancer 1983; 52:1165–72.

11. Wiltrout RH, Herberman RB, Chirigos MA, Ortaldo JR, Green K, Talmadge JE. Role of organ associated NK cells in decreased formation of experimental metastases in lung and liver. J Immunol 1985; 134:426–30.

12. Gorelik E, Wilhout K, Okamura K, Mebu S, Herberman RB. Role of NK cells in the control of metastatic spread and growth of tumor cells in mice. Int J Cancer 1982; 30:107–12.

13. Herberman RB, ed. Natural cell mediated immunity against tumors. New York: Academic Press, 1980.

14. Pross HF, Brains MG. Spontaneous human lymphocyte mediated cytotoxicity against tumor targets. I. Effect of malignant disease. Int J Cancer 1976; 18:593–604.

15. Herberman RB, Timonen T, Ortaldo JR. Characteristics of NK cells and their possible role in vivo in mediation of cellular immunity in cancer by immune modifiers. In Chirigos MA, Mitchell M, Mastrangelo MJ, Krim M, eds: Prog Cancer Res. New York: Raven Press, 1981: 19

16. Kadisch AS, Doule AT, Steinhauer EH, Ghossein NA. Natural cytotoxicity and interferon production in human cancer: Deficient natural killer cell activity and normal interferon production in patients with advanced disease. J Immunol 1981; 127:1817–22.

17. Moore M, Vose BM. Extravascular natural cytotoxicity in man: Anti K562 activity of lymph node and tumor-infiltrating lymphocytes. Int J Cancer 1981; 27:265–72.

18. Cunningham-Rundles S, Filippa PA, Braun PW, Antonelli H, Ashikari H. Natural cytotoxicity of peripheral blood lymphocytes and regional lymph node cells in breast cancer women. JNCI 1981; 67:585–90.

19. Yanagawa E, Uchida A, Micksche M. Natural cytotoxicity of lymphocytes from lymph nodes draining breast carcinoma and its augmentation by interferon and OK-432. Cancer Immunol Immunother 1984; 17:1–6.

20. Uchida A, Micksche M. Natural killer cells in carcinomatous pleural effusions. Cancer Immunol Immunother 1981; 11:131–8.

21. Micksche M, Vinzenz K, Kokoschka EM, Kokoschka R. Natural killer cell activity in tumor draining lymph nodes. Investigations in patients with malignant melanoma and head and neck cancer. Nat Immun Cell Growth Regul 1985; 4:315–27.

22. Uchida A, Micksche M. In vitro augmentation of natural killer cell activity by OK-432. Int J Immunopharmacol 1981; 3:365–75.

23. Uchida A, Micksche M. Augmentation of NK cell activity in cancer patients by OK-432: Activation of NK cells and reduction of suppressor cells. In Herberman RB, ed: NK cells and other natural effector cells. New York: Academic Press 1982: 1303–8.

24. Lotzová E. Effector immune mechanisms in cancer. Nat Immun Cell Growth Regul 1985; 4:293–304.

25. Mantovani A, Allavena P, Sessa C, Balis G, Magioni, Natural killer cell activity of lymphoid cells isolated from human ascitic ovarian tumors. Int J Cancer 1980; 25:573–82.

26. Goodwin, JS, Hushby, G, Williams, RC. Prostaglandin and cancer growth. Cancer Immunol Immunother 1980; 8:3–7.

27. Cunningham-Rundles S. Control of natural cytotoxicity in regional lymph node in breast cancer. In Herberman RB, ed: NK cells and other natural effector cells. New York: Academic Press, 1982: 1133–40.

28. Uchida A, Micksche M. Intrapleural administration of OK-432 in cancer patients: Activation of NK cells and reduction of suppressor cells. Int J Cancer 1983; 21:1–5.

29. Uchida A, Micksche M. Lysis of fresh human tumor cells by autologous large granular lymphocytes from peripheral blood and pleural effusions. Int J Cancer 1983; 32:37–44.

30. Uchida A, Yanagawa E, Micksche M. In vivo and in vitro augmentation of natural killing and auto-tumor killing activity by OK-432. In Hoshino T, Uchida A, eds: Clinical and experimental studies in immunotherapy. Amsterdam: Excerpta Medica, 1984: 75–94.

31. Hisano G, Hanna G. Murine lymph node natural killer cells. Regulating mechanisms of activation or suppression. JNCI 1982; 69:665–71.

32. Berek JS, Hacker NF, Lichtenstein A, et al. Intraperitoneal recombinant alpha-interferon for "salvage" immunotherapy in stage III epithelial ovarian cancer: A gynecologic oncology group study. Cancer Res 1985; 45:4447–53.

33. Allavena P, Scala G, Djeu J, et al. Production of multiple cytokines by clones of human large granular lymphocytes. Cancer Immunol Immunother 1985; 19:121–6.

34. Ichimura O, Suzuki S, Saito M, Sugawara Y, Ishida N. Augmentation of interleukin 1 and interleukin 2 production by OK-432. Int J Immunopharmacol 1985; 7:263–70

35. Ritchie AWS, James K, Micklem HS. The distribution and possible significance of cells identified in human lymphoid tissue by the monoclonal antibody HNK-1. Clin Exp Immunol 1983; 51:439–47.

Cancer Detection and Prevention Supplement 1:477–486 (1987)

Effects of Immunization Against Human Choriogonadotropin on the Growth of Transplanted Lewis Lung Carcinoma and Spontaneous Mammary Adenocarcinoma in Mice

Hernan F. Acevedo, PhD
Radmila B. Raikow, PhD
John E. Powell, BS
Vernon C. Stevens, PhD

Department of Laboratory Medicine, Allegheny-Singer Research Institute, Allegheny General Hospital, Pittsburgh, PA (H.F.A., R.B.R.); Department of Obstetrics and Gynecology, The Ohio State University, Columbus, OH (J.E.P., V.C.S.)

ABSTRACT   We studied the effects of preimmunization with a synthetic carboxy-terminal peptide of the β-subunit of human choriogonadotropin (hCG) conjugated to diphtheria toxoid on the growth of two tumor models, the transplantable Lewis lung carcinoma in C57BL/6J mice and the spontaneous mammary carcinoma in C3H/OuJ mice. Immunization with the conjugate prior to Lewis lung tumor implantation significantly (P < 0.05) retarded the growth of tumors as measured by tumor weight 18 days following transplantation. The weights of Lewis lung tumors in animals preimmunized with the hCG immunogen were inversely correlated (r = 0.61) with the levels of circulating antibodies against human chorionic gonadotropin, whereas no statistical correlation was found between tumor weights and the levels of antibodies reactive to diphtheria toxoid. The number of conjugate-treated C3H/OuJ mice that developed mammary tumors was significantly (P < 0.05) reduced compared to their vehicle-treated cohorts. Pretreatment with the synthetic muramyl dipeptide analog utilized as an adjuvant with both immunogens did not show any effect on the tumor growth in either tumor system.

Key words: cancer immunoprophylaxis, antibodies against hCG, synthetic hCG peptide conjugate, C57BL/6J mice, C3H/OuJ mice

INTRODUCTION

Material similar to human choriogonadotropin (hCG), a sialoglycoprotein synthesized by human trophoblasts, has been shown to be produced by many types of human malignant cells [1,2]. Although production of hCG by rodent placental cells has not been fully established, reactivity of a substance(s) immunologically similar to hCG on the cell membrane of

Address reprint requests to Dr. Hernan F. Acevedo, Department of Laboratory Medicine, Allegheny General Hospital, Pittsburgh, PA 15212.

murine neoplastic cells has been demonstrated by immunochemistry and flow cytofluorometry using antisera raised against hCG and its β-subunit (hCGβ) [3–5]. It has been suggested that the expression of hCG-like material by transformed and/or malignant cells may be an essential feature of malignant transformation [4,6]. The material may be immunoprotective [7–9] and act as a specific growth factor for malignant cells [10].

Kellen et al [11] demonstrated that the addition of antisera against hCGβ to rat R3230AC adenocarcinoma cells in tissue culture diminished the metastatic potential of the cells (Winn assay). Investigations were undertaken to test whether preimmunization with hCG immunogens could alter tumor growth in vivo. Kellen et al [12] demonstrated that immunization of female Fischer rats with a conjugate of hCGβ and tetanus toxoid (hCGβ-tt) prior to the IV administration of R3230AC adenocarcinoma cells essentially prevented the development of lung metastases that normally occur following such treatment. Using the same vaccine, Cianci et al [13] reported similar results in Wistar rats with the ascites form of Yoshida sarcoma, a tumor that is not known to express hCG-like material. Data on the inhibitory effects of preimmunization of rats with the hCGβ-tt conjugate on the growth of SC implants of two solid tumors, R3230AC adenocarcinoma and 5123 1-1 hepatoma, have also been published [14].

Another anti-hCG vaccine consisting of a synthetic COOH-terminal fragment of hCGβ, sequence 109–145, which appears to be unique to the hCG molecule, conjugated with diphtheria toxoid (hCGβ-CTP:DT) and mixed with a synthetic adjuvant has been developed and tested as a potential method of birth control in women [15]. The present study was designed to determine whether preimmunization with this vaccine would 1) affect the subsequent growth of inplants of Lewis lung carcinoma in C57BL/6J mice and 2) affect the spontaneous development of mammary adenocarcinomas in C3H/OuJ mice. Cells from both neoplasms have previously been shown to express hCG-like material in their cell membranes [3].

MATERIALS AND METHODS
Reagents

Highly purified hCG, CR 119, was a gift from the Center for Population Research of NICHHD. 125-Iodine was purchased from New England Nuclear Corp. (Boston, MA). The hCGβ-CTP:DT conjugate was prepared according to Lee et al [16] and contained 25 peptides/100 K daltons of DT. Synthetic adjuvant CGP 11637 (nor-MDP, N-acetyl-nor-muramyl-L-alanyl-D-isoglutamine) was a gift from Ciba-Geigy Ltd. (Basel, Switzerland). Squalene and Arlacel A were purchased from Sigma Chemical Co. (St. Louis, MO) and mixed 4:1 w/w, respectively. RPMI 1640 medium was purchased from MA Bioproducts (Walkersville, MD). Fetal calf serum was obtained from Sterile Systems (Logan, UT) and dimethyl sulfoxide from Fisher Scientific (Pittsburgh, PA). All other reagents were reagent grade quality.

Experimental Animals

Forty-two-day-old C57BL/6J male mice and C3H/OuJ female mice, obtained from Jackson Laboratory (Bar Harbor, ME) were housed in plastic cages with sterilized wood chip bedding, in rooms with controlled temperature, humidity, and light cycle. The mice were fed autoclaved Purina Lab Chow and sterilized acidified water ad libitum. The animals were acclimatized in our facility for 2 weeks before starting the experiments.

C3H/OuJ mice develop mammary tumors in approximately 100% of multiparous females by the time they are around 308 days old (personal communication from Jackson Laboratories) and in about 80% of virgin females around the age of 240 days [17]. These mice are derived from C3H/HeJ mice and are known to harbor the Bittner mammary tumor virus.

Immunization of Mice

In a first experiment, C57BL/6J mice were divided into three groups; a group of 17 mice to be immunized with the hCGβ-CTP:DT immunogen (test group), a group of 18 animals to be immunized with DT only (first control group), and a group of 20 mice to be left untreated (second control group).

Two hundred micrograms of hCGβ-CTP:DT or 100 μg of DT alone was used for the first immunization. Details of the preparation of the immunogen, adjuvant and vehicle into an emulsion are described elsewhere [18–20]. Briefly, hCGβ-CTP:DT or DT only was mixed with 100 μg of nor-MDP, dissolved in saline, and emulsified with an equal volume of squalene:Arlacel A (4:1 w/w). The mice were injected SC in the dorsal area with 0.3 ml of the emulsion. Booster immunization using 100 μg and 50 μg of conjugate and of DT, respectively, were given at 1, 2, and 4 months.

Two additional control groups were run in a separate experiment, one group consisting of 17 mice injected with nor-MDP only and the other group of 15 mice given the saline/squalene:Arlacel A emulsion (vehicle) only. Treatment was repeated 1 month later. In both experiments, the animals were 56 days old at the time of the first injection.

Two studies were done using C3H/OuJ mice. In the first, 13 of these mice were injected with the hCGβ-CTP:DT conjugate in the same way and at the same dose as described above, while 14 were injected with the vehicle only. In the second study, 20 C3H/OuJ mice were injected only with nor-MDP (100 μg/injection), and 19 were injected with vehicle alone. In both experiments the first injection was made when all of the mice were 137 days old, then repeated every 28 days until the end of the experiment. When using hCG immunogen this injection regime is expected to maintain a constant, high level of anti-hCG antibodies [19].

Tumor Transplants and Tumor Growth Assessment

The Lewis lung carcinoma cells that are maintained in our laboratories frozen in liquid nitrogen in RPMI medium containing 25% calf serum and 8% dimethyl sulfoxide, were originally obtained from the Mason Research Institute (Worcester, MA). To obtain enough cells for transplantation, 10,000 viable cells (trypan blue assessment) in 0.2 ml of saline were inoculated into the hind limb of each of four C57BL/6J donor mice. After 15 days the tumors obtained were removed from these mice, and using sterile conditions the outer portion of the neoplasms, excluding necrotic areas, were minced and dispersed, and single cells were then collected. In the first experiment, all of the mice were injected IV with 10^4 viable Lewis lung cells obtained from a trypsin-dispersed tumor 2 weeks after the first booster injection. No signs of tumors could be found as a result of this inoculation in any of the three groups. Because of the ineffectiveness of the first inoculation of trypsin-dispersed cells, a second transplant consisting of 10^6 viable, mechanically dispersed cells was injected into all mice of the three groups 94 days later and 3 days after injection of a third booster. This injection was made SC into their lower back, previously shaved to allow easier volume measurements of the tumor.

At the time of cell implants, the mice were individually marked by ear punch and cage number and transferred to small cages of five or fewer per cage. The cages were numbered randomly, and the persons measuring and handling the mice did not know which cage contained which preimplantation treatment. External tumor volumes were measured with calipers in all mice on days 10, 14, 15, and 17 after tumor inoculation. On day 18 all of the mice were anesthetized with ether, bled from the brachial plexus for determination of antibody levels, and sacrificed by cervical dislocation. Carcass weight was determined before and after tumor removal. Tumor weights were made to the nearest 10 mg.

In the second experiment, all mice were given 10^5 viable Lewis lung carcinoma cells 2 weeks after the two injections of nor-MDP administered on days 0 and 28, respectively. The animals were killed 20 days after tumor transplantation, and the tumor weights were determined as above.

For the studies of the effects of the hCG immunogen on the spontaneous mammary carcinoma of C3H/OuJ mice, the animals were palpated each week for tumors after reaching 200 days of age. Mice with suspected tumors were killed 1–2 weeks after these were first noted, and each tumor was confirmed at autopsy.

Determination of Antibody Levels

The levels of antibodies reactive to hCG and to diphtheria toxoid were measured by isotopically labeling hCG (CR-119) and/or DT with 125-Iodine and reacting it with various dilutions of the antisera. Incorporation of 125-Iodine into the antigen was done by the chloramine-T method described by Greenwood et al [21]. Purification of the labeled protein from free iodine was done by gel filtration using Bio Gel P-60. The eluted protein was diluted in phosphate-buffered saline (PBS) containing 1% bovine serum albumin for use in assays [18].

The sera to be tested were serially diluted in PBS-0.05 M EDTA-20% normal calf serum buffer, pH 7.4. Each tube contained 0.2 ml of diluted serum and 0.1 ml of labeled antigen. When testing for hCG antibodies, the serial dilutions were incubated for 120 hr at 4°C with 1.3 pM of ^{125}I-hCG mixed with three amounts of unlabeled antigen (1 to 50 ng) to ensure antibody separation. Bound and unbound hCG were separated by adding 1.0 ml of 25% polyethylene glycol 6000 and centrifuging. The precipitate containing the bound hCG was counted in a gamma spectrometer. Antibody binding was calculated as moles of hCG bound per liter of serum, based on a molecular weight of 38,000 for hCG. In the case of diphtheria toxoid the binding was calculated as milligrams of DT bound per liter of serum.

Statistical Analysis

Analysis of variance followed by the Dunnet's test was conducted on the data for Lewis lung tumor volume and weight by the Biometrics Laboratory, Department of Preventive Medicine, Ohio State University (Columbus, OH). The data in Table II were analyzed by Student's t test and the curves in Figure 3 by Colton life table statistics [22]. Correlation coefficients (r) for tumor weight vs antibody levels were determined according to the method indicated by Ostle [23].

RESULTS

In the first study with Lewis lung carcinoma, only 15 of the 17 mice preimmunized with the hCG immunogen (test mice) were evaluated for tumor volume and weight; one died of unknown causes shortly after challenge, and there was no tumor take in another. Also, only 18 of the 20 untreated mice could be evaluated for tumor weight because two of this control group died with large tumors before tumor weight could be obtained. Because of extensive variability in the measurement of external tumor volumes, differences in tumor volumes between the animals pretreated with the hCG immunogen and those of the control groups were not statistically significant. However, as seen in Table I, when the mean weight of the tumors of the animals pretreated with the hCG immunogen was compared to the mean weight of the tumors of the nonimmunized group, which represents the natural development of the transplanted neoplasm, a significant difference (P < 0.05) was found. The difference between the mean tumor weight of the animals preimmunized with DT only and the mean tumor weight of the nonimmunized control group was not statistically significant.

We attempted to minimize initial variability by selecting on day 10 those mice whose tumor volumes fell within one half of the standard deviation from the overall mean of all the 53 mice in the experiment. The justification for this selection was that the variability seen on day 10 after challenge was probably mostly due to variations in the tumor inocula since the

TABLE I. Comparison of the Mean Tumor Weights (g) of Test and Control C57BL/6J Mice 18 Days After Inoculation With 10^6 Lewis Lung Cells

	N	Tumor weight ± SEM	P
Nonimmunized control	18	7.00 ± 0.86	—
Immunized with diphtheria toxoid	18	4.80 ± 0.48	NS*
Immunized with hCG immunogen	15	4.13 ± 0.48	<0.05

*Not significant.

treatment had apparently no significant effect at that early time. By this criterion, seven mice were included in the nonimmunized control group, six in the group immunized with diphtheria toxoid, and four in the group immunized with the hCG immunogen. Table II, which compares the mean tumor volumes of these selected mice on days 10 and 17 and their mean tumor weights on day 18, shows that, while on day 10 the three groups are indistinguishable, by day 17 the group immunized with the hCG immunogen, and only this group, differed significantly ($P < 0.05$) from the other two.

The results of the second experiment with Lewis lung carcinoma in which a comparison was made between the mean tumor weight of the mice pretreated with nor-MDP (N = 17) and the animals injected only with the vehicle (N = 15) demonstrated no difference of their tumor weights (g $\pm$ SEM), this being 2.81 $\pm$ 0.23 and 2.98 $\pm$ 0.33, respectively.

The relationships between individual tumor weights and the serum levels of the antibodies elicited by the hCG immunogen and the DT immunogen are illustrated in Figures 1 and 2, respectively. In the animals preimmunized with the hCG immunogen, the serum levels of hCG antibodies were inversely correlated with tumor weight (r = 0.61), while no statistical correlation was found between the serum levels of antibodies against DT in the animals preimmun-

TABLE II. Comparison of the Mean Tumor Volumes (cm³) and Tumor Weights (g) of C57BL/6J Mice of the Two Treated Groups and the Nonimmunized Control Group

	Day 10 (vol $\pm$ SEM)	P	Day 17 (vol $\pm$ SEM)	P	Day 18 (Wt $\pm$ SEM)	P
Nonimmunized control group (N = 7)	1.38 $\pm$ 0.09	—	7.86 $\pm$ 1.33	—	5.11 $\pm$ 0.80	—
Immunized with diphtheria toxoid (N = 6)	1.36 $\pm$ 0.06	NS*	7.20 $\pm$ 0.54	NS	5.55 $\pm$ 0.66	NS
Immunized with hCG immunogen (N = 4)	1.31 $\pm$ 0.12	NS	4.80 $\pm$ 0.81	<0.05	2.95 $\pm$ 0.86	<0.05

The mice included here were selected from those in Table I for having tumor volumes no more than one half of a standard deviation from the overall mean volume on day 10 after tumor inoculation.
*Not significant.

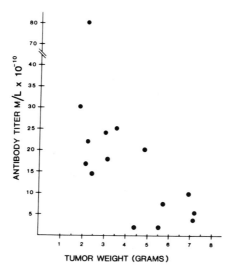

Fig. 1.   Relation between tumor weight (g) and hCG antibody titer (moles/liter of serum $\times$ 10^{-10}) in mice preimmunized with the hCG immunogen. The coefficient of correlation was 0.61, indicating an inverse correlation ($>0.5<1.0$).

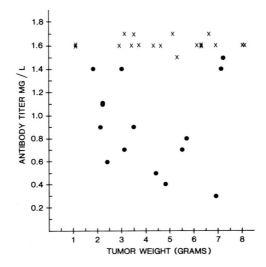

Fig. 2. Relation between tumor weight (g) and diphtheria toxoid antibodies (mg/liter of serum) in individual mice. ●, preimmunized with the hCG immunogen (n = 15); ✗, preimmunized with diphtheria toxoid immunogen (N = 18). Coefficients of correlation were 0.092 and 0.076 respectively, indicating no correlation.

ized with the hCG immunogen or with DT only, their r values being 0.092 and 0.076, respectively.

Figure 3 shows the results obtained with C3H/OuJ mice, which developed spontaneous mammary adenocarcinomas. We plotted the percentage of mice with tumors versus their age. As can be seen in Figure 3A, the mice that received the hCG immunogen had significantly fewer tumors than those that received only the vehicle. This difference was significant at the 0.05 level between days 296 and 355 and at the 0.01 level between days 300 and 318. As was also the case with the Lewis lung tumor, nor-MDP injected alone had no effect on the development of this mammary tumor (Fig. 3B).

DISCUSSION

Previous reports of inhibitory effects on tumor growth resulting from active immunization with hCG immunogens involved studies employing the intact β-subunit of hCG conjugated with tt as the primary immunogen in rats [11–13]. In those experiments, because of the high immunogenicity of hCGβ-tt conjugate in rats, no adjuvant was utilized. A recent study using a preparation of killed bacteria that expresses an hCG-like material as immunogen [24] has also demonstrated antigrowth effects in a transplantable transitional cell carcinoma [24]. Furthermore, results reported by Bagshawe [26] using the same hCGβ-CTP:DT but Freund adjuvant instead of the synthetic nor-MDP, indicated that preimmunization of mice with this vaccine and subsequent challenge with Ridgeway osteogenic sarcoma, a tumor that is not known to express hCG-like material, also produced a significant growth delay.

The studies reported here have demonstrated that antitumor effects can also be obtained with a synthetic peptide representing the COOH-terminal 37 amino acids of hCGβ. This fragment of hCGβ was coupled to DT to enhance antigenicity, mixed with nor-MDP, and given in a slow-release subcutaneous depot injection. Since the synthetic peptide contains an hCG sequence not found in other glycoprotein hormone molecules, it is probable that this preparation does not elicit antibodies that react with molecules other than hCG, and for this reason it may be applicable to human use.

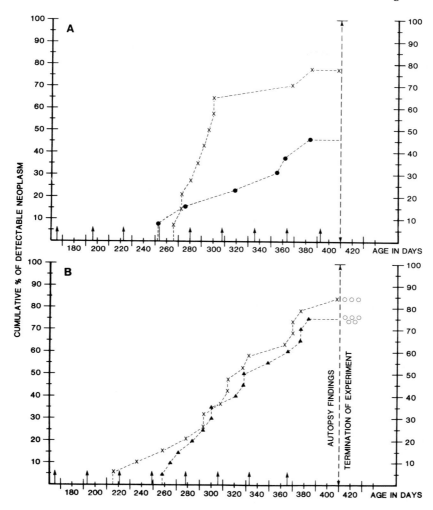

Fig. 3. Age of C3H/OuJ mice vs percentage of mice with palpable tumors. Panel **A:** ●, C3H/OuJ mice immunized with hCG-immunogen (N = 13); ✗, mice injected with vehicle only (N = 14). Arrows indicate booster immunizations. No tumors were found at autopsy at termination of experiment. **B:** ▲ C3H/OuJ mice injected with nor-muramyl dipeptide adjuvant (N = 20); ✗, mice injected with vehicle only (N = 19); ○, no tumor found at autopsy. Arrows indicate nor-MDP injections.

The present results also demonstrated that the adjuvant, nor-MDP, used alone has no effect on the growth of the transplantable Lewis lung carcinoma or the spontaneous C3H mammary tumor. Results of our previous investigations [17] have demonstrated that under the experimental conditions used, nor-MDP elicits a significant antiviral activity and has no effect on tumor growth unless the growth of the neoplasm requires viral replication and subsequent infection of normal cells.

In respect to possible effects of diphtheria toxoid alone, previous work has shown that a toxoid or any detoxified toxin by itself had no effect on transplanted or spontaneous solid tumors [14,27] even though bacterial toxoids, which are devoid of cytotoxic or cytolytic activities, can produce nonspecific stimulation of the reticuloendothelial system. We found no statistically significant effects from immunization with DT. The results obtained by our manipulation of the data to eliminate variability indicated that the apparent but not significant effect of immunization with the DT adjuvant mixture occurred during the early stages of tumor growth. The effect of the hCG immunogen, in contrast, seemed most significant when older tumors were measured.

The IV injections of 10^4 trypsin-treated Lewis lung carcinoma cells injected on day 42 of the first experiment appeared to be totally devoid of any immunogenic effect. Possible undetected influences of this inocula on the immune system, however, could not account for the differences obtained between groups, since the same inocula were given to all of the mice.

The inverse correlation observed between individual Lewis lung tumor weights and antibodies elicited against hCG (Fig. 1) may represent an effect of the antibodies on the neoplastic cells. It is also possible that this inverse correlation may be due to a specific binding of the hCG antibodies to the hCG epitopes of the neoplastic cells expressing the hCG-like material; thus large tumors may be expected to bind more antibody than the small ones.

The relative constancy of the DT antibodies produced by DT-immunogen (Fig. 2) may be a reflection of the effects of the slow release type of administration of the antigen and of the synthetic adjuvant used. We have observed that this method of injection tends to minimize individual differences in the production of antibodies with this particular hCG immunogen in normal animals [19,20]. On the other hand, the greater variation of the DT antibodies elicited by the hCG immunogen may be due to different characteristics of these antibodies because of conformational changes of the DT molecule when it is conjugated to the synthetic peptide.

Well-known problems with experimental solid tumors used to study effects of immunological manipulations include heterogeneity of the antigenic expression by the neoplastic cells [1,4,5], in this case, expression of hCG and lack of antibody access to the malignant cells, particularly in those neoplasms with a dense connective tissue component. Because of this and because of our recent findings showing that the expression of hCG-like material in malignant cells correlates with the metastatic phenotype [28], it is remarkable that preimmunization of rats and mice with different vaccines eliciting antibodies reacting with different hCG epitopes have shown a statistically significant antigrowth effect in the transplantable solid neoplasms that have been investigated, considering that in most primary transplantable tumors these cells appear to constitute the minority of the viable population [4,5].

The hCGβ carboxy-terminal vaccine also inhibited significantly the development of mammary tumors in C3H/OuJ mice. Since these mice were not observed for the duration of their entire life span we cannot be certain whether the vaccine reduces the percentage of mice that develop tumors or delays the time of onset of these tumors. The mammary tumor in C3H/OuJ mice is caused by an RNA virus (Bittner) that infects neonates via the mother's milk, integrates into their DNA, and produces tumors approximately 8 months later [29]. The long incubation period resembles that in human tumor development and therefore may be a more valid experimental model than those using transplanted solid tumors.

The data from this study are inadequate to suggest exact mechanism(s) by which preimmunization against hCG affects tumor growth. Complement-mediated cytotoxicity of hCG antisera on normal and malignant trophoblasts in vitro and cytotoxic activity of rabbit hCG antibodies on early human trophoblasts cultured in diffusion chambers in the intraperitoneal cavity of rabbits have been reported [30,31]. The role of cell-mediated effects from hCG immunizations cannot be ruled out. While further investigation is needed before the possible utility of this particular anti-hCG vaccine for tumor prevention or growth retardation can be ascertained, the data obtained in this study justify further research.

ACKNOWLEDGMENTS

This work was supported by a donation to H.F.A. in memory of B.D. Cadwallader, by a General Research Support Grant from NIH (grant 2 S07-RR5801) to Allegheny-Singer Research Institute, and by a grant from the Cancer Federation, Inc.

REFERENCES

1. McManus LM, Naughton MA, Martinez-Hernandez A. Human chorionic gonadotropin in human neoplastic cells. Cancer Res 1976; 36:3476–81.
2. Wilson TS, McDowell EM, McIntyre KR, Trump BF. Elaboration of human chorionic gonadotropin by lung tumors. Arch Pathol Lab Med 1981; 105:169–73.
3. Acevedo HF, Campbell-Acevedo EA, Pardo M, Slifkin M. Immunohistochemical localization of choriogonadotropin-like antigen in animal malignant cells. In Burchiel S, Rhodes BA, eds. Tumor imaging: The radioimmunochemical detection of cancer. New York: Masson, 1981: 73–88.
4. Acevedo HF, Slifkin M, Pouchet GR, Rakhshan M. Human chorionic gonadotropin in cancer cells. I. Identification in in vitro and in vivo cancer cell systems. In Nieburgs H, ed: Detection and prevention of cancer, part 2. New York: Marcel Dekker, 1978; 1:937–63.
5. Raikow RB, Fogarty PA, Buffo MJ, Acevedo HF. Flow cytometric analysis of human choriogonadotropin-like material in human and rodent malignant cells. Proc Int Symp Immunobiol Cancer Allied Immune Dysfunctions November 4–7, 1985, Copenhagen, Denmark. Cancer Detect Prev 1985; 8:591 (abstract 151).
6. Stanbridge EJ, Rosen SW, Sussman HH. Expression of the α-subunit of human chorionic gonadotropin is specifically correlated with human cell hybrids. Proc Natl Acad Sci USA 1982; 79:6242–5.
7. Fauve RM, Hevin B, Jacob H, Gailland JA, Jacob F. Antiinflammatory effects of murine malignant cells. Proc Natl Acad Sci USA 1974; 71:4052–6.
8. Hammerstrom L, Fuchs T, Smith CIE. The immunodepressive effect of human glucoproteins and their possible role in the nonrejection process during pregnancy. Acta Obstet Gynaecol Scand 1979; 58:417–22.
9. Bartocci A, Welker RD, Schlick E, Chirigos MA, Nisula BC, Immunosuppressive activity of human chorionic gonadotropin preparation in vivo: Evidence for gonadal dependence. Cell Immunol 1983; 82:334–42.
10. Melmed S, Braunstein GD. Human chorionic gonadotropin stimulates proliferation of Nb2 rat lymphoma cells. J Clin Endocrinol Metab 1983; 56:1068–70.
11. Kellen JA, Kolin A, Teodorczyk-Injeyan JA, Malkin A. Effect of pre-treatment with antisera against choriogonadotropin on the metastatic potential of a rat adenocarcinoma. In Hellman K, Hilgard P, Eccles S, eds. Developments in oncology. The Hague: Martinus Nijhoff, 1980; 4:237–41.
12. Kellen JA, Kolin A, Acevedo HF. Effects of antibodies to choriogonadotropin in malignant growth. I. Rat 3230 AC mammary adenocarcinoma. Cancer 1981; 49:2300–4.
13. Cianci S, Corbino N, Palumbo G, Bernardini A, Cianci A. hCG and neoplastic disease. Proc 3rd World Congr Hum Reprod, Berlin, March 22–26, 1981:379 (abstract).
14. Kellen JA, Kolin A, Mirakian A, Acevedo HF. Effects of antibodies to choriogonadotropin in malignant growth. II. Solid transplantable rat tumors. Cancer Immunol Immunother 1982; 13:2–4.
15. Stevens VC, Powell JE, Lee AC, Griffin D. Antifertility effects of immunization of female baboons with C-terminal peptides of the β-subunit of human chorionic gonadotropin. Fertil Steril 1981; 36:98–105.
16. Lee AC, Powell JE, Tregear GW, Niall HD, Stevens VC. A method for preparing β-hCG peptide carrier conjugates of predictable composition. Mol Immunol 1980; 17:749–56.
17. Acevedo HF, Raikow RB, Acevedo HO, Delgado TF, Pardo M. Prevention of oncogenic viral infections in mice with CGP 11637, a synthetic muramyl dipeptide analog. Antimicrob Agents Chemother 1985; 28:589–96.
18. Powell JE, Lee AC, Tregear GJ, Niall HD, Stevens VC. Characteristics of antibodies raised to carboxy-terminal peptides of hCG beta subunit. J Reprod Immunol 1980; 2:1–13.
19. Stevens VC, Cinader B, Powell JE, Lee AC, Koh SW. Preparation and formulation of a human chorionic gonadotropin antifertility vaccine: Selection of a peptide immunogen. Am J Reprod Immunol 1981; 1:307–14.
20. Stevens VC, Cinader B, Powell JE, Lee AC, Koh SW. Preparation and formulation of a human chorionic gonadotropin antifertility vaccine: Selection of adjuvant and vehicle. Am J Reprod Immunol 1981; 1:315–21.
21. Greenwood FC, Hunter WM, Glover JS. The preparation of ^{131}I-labeled human growth hormone of high specific activity. Biochem J 1963; 80:114–23.
22. Colton T. Statistics in medicine. Boston: Brown, 1974.
23. Ostle B. Statistics in research. Ames: Iowa State Press, 1954: 182.

24. Domingue GJ, Acevedo HF, Powell JE, Stevens VC. Antibodies to bacterial vaccines demonstrating specificity for human choriogonadotropin (hCG) and immunochemical detection of hCG-like factor in subcellular bacterial fractions. Infect Immun 1986; 53:95–8.

25. Domingue GJ, Wicker HS, Frentz GD, Acevedo HF, Powell JE, Stevens VC. Effects of antibodies to bacteria containing choriogonadotropin-like protein on growth of a transplantable tumor. Proc Am Assoc Cancer Res 1983; 24:812 (abstract).

26. Bagshawe KD. Human chorionic gonadotropin as a model for a fetal antigen. In Evered D, Whelan J, eds: Fetal antigens and cancer. Ciba Foundation Symposia. London: Pitman, 1983: 76:146–59.

27. Ribi E, Amano K, Cantrell J, Schwartzman S, Parker R, Takayama K. Preparation and antitumor activity of nontoxic lipid A. Cancer Immunol Immunother 1982; 12:91–6.

28. Kellen JA, Wong A, Gardner HA, Raikow RB, Acevedo HF. Expression of hCG-like material correlates with invasive phenotype of R3230 rat carcinoma. Proc Am Assoc Cancer Res 1986; 27:222 (abstract).

29. Moore DH, Holben JA. Effect of parity regimen on the rate of occurrence of mammary tumors in A, C3H and RIII mice. Int J Cancer 1979; 24:161–4.

30. Currie GA. Immunological studies of trophoblast in vitro II. The effects of anti-hCG antisera on normal and malignant trophoblast in vitro. J Obstet Gynaecol Br Commonw 1967; 74:845–8.

31. Morisada M, Yamaguchi H, Iizuka R. Toxic action of anti-hCG antibody to human trophoblast. Int J Fertil 1972; 17:65–71.

Cancer Detection and Prevention Supplement 1:487–491 (1987)

AIDS in Subsaharan Africa

R.J. Biggar, MD

Environmental Epidemiology Branch, National Cancer Institute, Bethesda, MD

ABSTRACT   AIDS has existed in subsaharan Africa at least since 1980. However, the genesis of this condition and its emergence as a health problem remain obscured by lack of data and by antibody data that are now questionable. In Africa, as elsewhere, AIDS is associated with an immunodeficiency associated with the LAV/HTLV-III retrovirus. The clinical manifestations vary somewhat because of the different range of opportunistic pathogens in that environment. Although the "classical," more indolent, endemic form of African Kaposi sarcoma is not associated with this virus or with immunodeficiency, a new, aggressive variety of Kaposi sarcoma in Africa appears to be. The origin of LAV/HTLV-III remains unclear, but the clinical syndrome of AIDS has emerged in Africa only in the past decade. A pattern of geographic spread can be recognized, in which AIDS was seen earliest in Kinshasa, Zaïre, and then emerged in Zambia, Rwanda, and Uganda. Recently, reports indicate spread into Tanzania and Kenya. Transmission appears to be primarily heterosexual, but the factors enhancing heterosexual spread in Africa to a greater extent than in the U.S. and Europe need to be further studied.

Key words: Africa, AIDS, epidemiology

The acquired immunodeficiency syndrome (AIDS) has been an epidemic problem in the United States and Europe for at least the past 5 years [1,2]. As of September, 1985, more than 13,000 cases had been diagnosed in the United States and more than a thousand cases in Europe[3]. Unless an effective treatment is found, the majority of these people will die within 2 years [4,5]. In addition to the personal tragedy of these victims, there is the staggering cost of medical care for their illnesses, estimated to be more than one-half billion dollars [6]. With the number of cases expected to double by the end of 1986, the dimensions of this tragedy will be even larger.

With the description of AIDS cases from the United States in 1981 [7,8], clinicians in Europe, particularly Belgium and France, recognized a similarity between these cases and patients arriving for medical evaluation from the central region of Africa [9–12]. These patients had infections of an opportunistic nature that strongly suggested an abnormality of their immune system, and when direct measurements of the T-lymphocyte helper and suppressor cells were made, the type of abnormality was found to be similar to that seen in AIDS [13]. Patients with similar illnesses were soon found in Zaïre and Rwanda, the sources of many of the African patients with AIDS-like illness seen in Europe [14,15]. There was initial scepticism, because the epidemic profile of the patients (1.2 male:1.0 female) was greatly different from

Address reprint requests to Dr. Robert J. Biggar, Head, International AIDS Epidemiology Environmental Epidemiology Branch, Landow Building 3C19, National Cancer Institute, Bethesda, MD 20205.

that of the European and U.S. experience (19 male:1.0 female), but, with the discovery of the causative agent of AIDS, the human T-lymphotropic virus type III (HTLV-III) [16] or an almost identical agent, the lymphadenopathy-associated virus (LAV) [17], it has been possible to demonstrate that the cause of this syndrome is the same virus in Africa and in the U.S. and Europe [18–20].

The emergence of AIDS in Africa is obscured by the lack of data. The available evidence supports a relatively recent onset of AIDS, beginning perhaps in the mid–1970s and certainly by 1980. Patients with AIDS-like diseases who had been living in Africa were seen in Europe in 1976 [21] and 1977 [22], but there are no specimens available to prove that these patients had AIDS. African AIDS cases diagnosed in Europe began to increase alarmingly only in 1980 [23]. Records available from Kinshasa, Zaïre, indicate that cryptococcosis, a disease associated with HTLV-III/LAV-related immunodeficiency in Africans, increased in frequency greatly beginning in 1980 [13]. Record review in Zambia and Uganda indicates that other AIDS-related diseases (aggressive Kaposi sarcoma and enteropathic AIDS) became notably more frequent in those countries in 1982 [24,25], and, since then, in all of these areas AIDS cases have dramatically increased. By April, 1985, more than 300 cases had been diagnosed in Kinshasa, Zaïre, and the number was increasing weekly [26].

Attempts to determine the prevalence of antibody against this virus in historic collections of sera from Africa have been frustrated by reactivity that appears to be nonspecific for HTLV-III/LAV in many instances. This reactivity is statistically associated with recurrent parasitic diseases, especially malaria [27], but the cause of the problem is not yet clear. The effect has, however, led to publication of results that may be misleading in that reactivity was found to be common in children in the early 1970s [28] and to be widespread [29–31]. This was interpreted to indicate an endemic focus of HTLV-III/LAV or a related virus in Africa, but it may be that the reactivity detected was not specific [27]. If these results were truly negative, this adds to evidence that HTLV-III/LAV is likely to be new and a problem that is currently spreading in the African environment.

Clinically, AIDS in Africa has been most often manifest by opportunistic infections. In contrast to the experience among AIDS cases in the U.S. and Europe [1,2], *Pneumocystis carinii* pneumonia appears to be uncommon, although this might be due in part to lack of recognition of this difficult-to-diagnose disease. More common have been cryptococcosis, oral and esophageal candidiasis, disseminated cytomegalovirus, herpes infections, tuberculosis, and a condition known as enteropathic AIDS, in which the etiology of a syndrome of diarrhea and wasting is not yet certain [10–13,25]. About half of the U.S. AIDS cases have had Kaposi sarcoma [1], an otherwise rare tumor in the United States [32]. In a long belt along East Africa, Kaposi sarcoma has been known for decades to be one of the more common tumors. However, this form of Kaposi sarcoma, an indolent, nodular disease affecting the distal limbs, is not associated with HTLV-III [33] or immunodeficiency [34]. Since 1982, another form of Kaposi sarcoma, histologically the same as the indolent form, has been observed in increasing numbers in Zambia and Uganda [26,35]. This form is similar to that seen in U.S. AIDS cases, having plaque lesions and internal involvement at an early stage with rapid progression to death [26,35]. Termed *aggressive* or *epidemic* Kaposi sarcoma, this disease is associated with HTLV-III infection [36] and probably immunodeficiency [35]. So far, no other malignancies have been observed to be associated with AIDS in Africa, but a statistical association with Burkitt-like lymphomas (a tumor common in Africa) and AIDS has been observed in the U.S. [37], leaving open the possibility.

The source of the HTLV-III/LAV is unclear. There have been suggestions that this virus emerged in Africa, based on similarities between HTLV-III/LAV and a similar virus found in African green monkeys [38]. A comparison of the molecular structures of these two viruses is underway to determine if they are closely related. If the virus did emerge from Africa, it must have rapidly spread to the U.S., since disease appeared there at nearly the same time. AIDS in the homosexual population of Europe was associated with sexual exposure to U.S. homosexuals [39], but, with the establishment of a focus of HTLV-III/LAV within the European homosexual community [40], continuing contact is no longer needed. Spread between continents might also have occurred by the use of internationally distributed, commercially prepared factor VIII concentrate, which is made from the pooled plasma of thousands of donors [41].

It is not clear how the agent is spreading in Africa, however. Among most African societies, homosexuality and heterosexual acts involving oral or anal sex are unusual and generally denied by African patients with AIDS. The equal male:female sex ratio and the age of the cases (18–50 years) suggest that heterosexual vaginal sex is important. Additional evidence favoring this is the observation of a high prevalence of antibodies against HTLV-III/LAV in prostitutes and in men who frequent prostitutes [42,43]. In at least one instance, a chain of male to female to male AIDS cases was observed [15]. In other areas of the world, both male-to-female and female-to-male transmission have been observed, but it seems likely that this is not commonplace [44–47]. Thus the factors that permit frequent spread by this route in Africa need to be understood, and additional routes need to be investigated.

The implications of these findings are important. If AIDS is new in Africa, there remains a possibility that its spread can be limited. Many areas of Africa, particularly in the west and south have so far reported no or very few cases [2]. Thus understanding the factors related to spread becomes urgent. The most reliable evidence of HTLV-III has been the presence AIDS, but, given the long period between infection, immune abnormality, and disease outcome [48,49], monitoring this outcome will provide data too late for practical intervention. Instead, it is critical to understand the problems of specificity in Africa and to find serological assays that can reliably and cheaply screen populations in Africa to determine the margins of the virus distribution.

For health planners, monitoring the status of the population will help to assess the magnitude of the current problem and to evaluate the entry of the agent into their environment. For this purpose, screening of patients presenting in venereal disease clinics will be the most expeditious system, since it is probably among the sexually active populations that antibodies against this agent will first appear. If European and U.S. experiences apply in Africa, between 10% and 20% of those with antibody will develop AIDS, a proportion likely to increase over time. Most of these will ultimately die. Therefore, prevention efforts are of enormous importance.

In the U.S. setting, health education has been effective in reducing the promiscuity of the group contributing the greatest number of cases, homosexual men. However, it came too late to be very effective in limiting disease spread, since by the time behavior had modified, disease was already very widespread. In Africa, health education is probably most effective through the news media, and, indeed, the reading population of most areas is already conversant with the subject of AIDS. Thus, studies to confirm the importance of heterosexual spread in Africa need to be completed and the results, if suggesting an effective means of limiting disease, should be widely disseminated in the news media.

Health-allocated resources in Africa are limited, and the burden that AIDS adds to an already strained budget seems unfair. AIDS is a real problem in Africa, however, and one that will steadily grow worse in the near future. Affecting the young working population, and perhaps disproportionately frequent among the affluent and educated portion of this group, it could have a marked impact on development in these countries, since it is these people who will be most economically productive in developing countries. Ignoring AIDS or prohibiting research about HTLV-III/LAV will only aggravate an emerging crisis. If there is to be any hope for containment in Africa, collaborative research efforts involving Africa health professionals and outside investigators with experience in AIDS and HTLV-III/LAV should be encouraged as a high priority.

REFERENCES

1. Allen JR. Epidemiology—United States. In Ebbesen P, Biggar RJ, Melbye M, eds: AIDS, a guide to clinicians. Munksgaard, Copenhagen: Munksgaard/Saunders, 1984.

2. Melbye M, Biggar RJ, Ebbesen P. Epidemiology—Europe and Africa. In Ebbesen P, Biggar RJ, Melbye M, eds: AIDS, a guide to clinicians. Munksgaard, Copenhagen: Munksgaard/Saunders, 1984.

3. Centers for Disease Control Update: Acquired immunodeficiency syndrome—Europe. Morbid Mortal Weekly Rep 1985; 34:583-9.

4. Goedert JJ, Blattner WA. In DeVita VT, Hellman S, Rosenberg SA, eds: The epidemiology of AIDS and related conditions. Philadelphia: JB Lippincott Company, 1985.

5. Curran JW, Morgan WM, Hardy A, Jaffe HW, Darrow WW, Dowdle WR: The epidemiology of AIDS: Current status and future prospects. Science 1985; 229:1352-7.

6. Landesman SH, Ginzberg HM, Weiss SH. The AIDS epidemic. N Engl J Med 1985; 312:512-25.

7. Centers for Disease Control: Pneumocystis pneumonia—Los Angeles. Morbid Mortal Weekly Rep 1981; 30:250.

8. Centers for Disease Control: Kaposi's sarcoma and pneumocystis pneumonia among homosexual men. New York City and California. Morbid Mortal Weekly Rep 1981: 30:305-8.

9. Biggar RJ, Bouvet E, Ebbesen P, Faber V, Koch M, Melbye M, Velimirovic B. The clinical features of AIDS in Europe. Eur J Cancer Clin Oncol 1984; 20:164-70.

10. Clumeck N, Mascart-Lemone F, de Maulbeuge J, Brenez D, Marcellis L. Acquired immune deficiency syndrome in black Africans. Lancet 1983; i:642.

11. Sonnet J, De Bruyere M. Syndrome de deficit acquis de l'immunite—acquired immunodeficiency syndrome (AIDS): Etat de la question. Donnees personnelles de la pathologie observee chez de Zairois. Louvain Med 1983; i:102:297-307.

12. Brunet JB, Bouvet E, Chaperon J, et al. Acquired immunodeficiency syndrome in France. Lancet 1983; i:700-1.

13. Clumeck N, Sonnet J, Taelman H, et al. Acquired immune deficiency syndrome in African patients. N Engl J Med 1984; 310-492-7.

14. Perre P, Rouvroy D, Lepage P, Bogaerts J, Kestelyn P, Kayihigi J, Hekker AC, Butzler JP, Clumeck N. Acquired immunodeficiency syndrome in Rwanda. Lancet 1984; ii:62-5.

15. Piot P, Quinn TC, Taelman H, Feinsod FM, Minlangu KB, Wobin O, et al. Acquired immunodeficiency syndrome in a heterosexual population in Zaire. Lancet 1984; ii:65-9.

16. Schupbach J, Popovic M, Gilden RV, Gonda MA, Sarngadharan MG, Gallo RC. Serological analysis of a subgroup of human T-lymphotropic retroviruses (HTLV-III) associated with AIDS. Science 1984; 224:503-5.

17. Brun-Vezinet F, Rouzioux C, Barré-Sinoussi F, Klatzmann D, Saimot AG, Rozenbaum W, Christol D, Gluckman JC, Montagnier L, Chermann JC: Detection of IgG antibodied to lymphadenopathy-associated virus in patients with AIDS or lymphadenopathy syndrome. Lancet 1984; i:1253-6.

18. Ellrodt A, Barré-Sinoussi F, Le Bras P, et al. Isolation of human T-lymphotropic retrovirus (LAV) from Zairian married couple, one with AIDS, one with prodromes. Lancet 1984; i:1383-5.

19. Brun-Vezinet F, Rouxioux C, Montagnier L, Chameret S, Gruest J, Barre-Sinoussi F, Geroldi D, et al. Prevalence of antibodies to lymphadenopathy associated retrovirus in African patients with AIDS. Science 1985; 226:453-6.

20. McCormick JB, Krebs JW, Mitchell SW, Feorino PM, Getchell JP, Odio W, Kapita B, Quinn TC, Piot P. Isolation of LAV-HTLV-III virus from African AIDS patients and from persons without AIDS or IgG antibody to LAV/HTLV-III. Science (in press).

21. Bygbjerg IC. AIDS in a Danish surgeon (Zaire, 1976). Lancet, 1983; i:925.

22. Vandepitte J, Verwilghen R, Zachee P. AIDS and cryptococcosis (Zaire, 1977). Lancet 1983; i:925-6.

23. Biggar RJ, Bouvet E, Ebbesen P, Faber V, Koch M, Melbye M, Velimirovic B. The epidemiology of AIDS in Europe. Eur J Cancer Clin Oncol 1984; 20:157-64.

24. Bayley AC. Aggressive Kaposi's sarcoma in Zambia, 1983. Lancet 1984; i:1318-20.

25. Serwadda D, Mugerwa RD, Sewankambo NK, Lwegara A, Carswell JW, Kirya GB, Bayley AC, Downing RG, Tedder RS, Clayden SA, Weiss RA, Dalgleish AG. Slim disease: A new disease in Uganda and its association with HTLV-III infection. Lancet 1985; ii:849-52.

26. Francis H, Mann J, Quinn T, Curran J, Kapita BM, et al. Immunologic profile of AIDS and other parasitic infections in Africa and their relationship to HTLV-III infection. Paper presented at the International Conference on Acquired Immunodeficiency Syndrome (AIDS) in Atlanta, April 14-17, 1985.

27. Biggar RJ, Gigase PL, Melbye M, Kestens L, Sarin P, Bodner AJ, Demedts P, Stevens WJ, Paluku L, Delacollette C, Blattner WA: ELISA HTLV retrovirus antibody reactivity associated with malaria and immune complexes in healthy Africans. Lancet 1985; ii:520-3.

28. Saxinger WC, Levine PH, Dean AG, de The G, Sarngadharan MG, Gallo RC. Evidence for exposure to HTLV-III in Uganda prior to 1973. 1984; 225:1473–6.

29. Biggar, RJ, Melbye M, Kestens L, deFeyter M, Saxinger C, Bodner AJ, Blattner WA, Gigase PL. The seroepidemiology of HTLV-III antibodies in a remote population of eastern Zaire. Br Med J 1985; 290:808–10.

30. Biggar RJ, Johnson BK, Oster C, Sarin PS, Ocheng D, Tukei P, Nsanze H, Alexander S, Bodner AJ, Siongok TA, Gallo RC, Blattner WA. Regional variation in prevalence of antibody against human T-lymphotropic virus types I and III in Kenya, East Africa. Int J Cancer 1985; 35:763–7.

31. Van de Perre P, Munyambuga D, Zissis G, Butlzer JB, Nzaramba D, Clumeck N. Antibody to HTLV-III in blood donors in Central Africa. Lancet 1985; i:336–7.

32. Biggar RJ, Horm J, Fraumeni JF Jr, Greene MH, Goedert JJ. Incidence of Kaposi's sarcoma and mycosis fungoides in the United States including Puerto Rico, 1973–81. JNCI 1984; 73:89–94.

33. Biggar RJ, Melbye M, Kestens L, Sarngadharan MG, de Feyter M, Blattner WA, Gallo RC, Gigase P. Kaposi's sarcoma in Zaire is not associated with HTLV-III infection. N Engl J Med 1984; 311:1051–2.

34. Kestens L, Biggar RJ, Melbye M, Bodner AJ, De Feyter AJ, Gigase PL. Absence of immuno-suppression in healthy subjects from eastern Zaire who are positive for HTLV-III antibodies. N Engl J Med 1985; 312:1517–8.

35. Dowing RG, Eglin RP, Bayley AC. African Kaposi's sarcoma and AIDS. Lancet 1984; i:478–80.

36. Bayley AC, Downing RG, Cheingsong-Popov R, Tedder RS, Dalgleish AG, Weiss RA. HTLV-III distinguishes atypical and endemic Kaposi's sarcoma in Africa. Lancet 1985; i:359–61.

37. Biggar RJ, Horm J, Lubin JH, Goedert JJ, Greene MH, Fraumeni JF. Cancer trends in a population at risk of AIDS. JNCI 1985; 74:793–7.

38. Kanki PJ, Alroy J, Essex M. Isolation of a T-lymphotropic retrovirus related to HTLV-III from wild-caught African green monkeys. Science (in press).

39. Biggar RJ, Ebbesen P, Melbye M, Weinstock R, Mann DL, Goedert JJ, Strong DM, Blattner WA. Low T-lymphocyte ratios in homosexual men: Epidemiological evidence of a transmissible agent. JAMA 1984; 251:1441–6.

40. Melbye M, Biggar RJ, Ebbesen P, et al. Seroepidemiology of HTLV-III antibody in Danish homosexual men: Prevalence, transmission, and disease outcome. Br Med J 1984; 289:573–5.

41. Melbye M, Froebel KS, Madhok R, et al. HTLV-III seropositivity in European haemophiliacs exposed to factor VIII concentrate imported from the USA. Lancet 1984; ii:1444–6.

42. Van de Perre P, Clumeck N, Carael M, Nzabihimana E, Robert-Guroff M, de Mol P, Freyens R, Butzler JP, Gallo RC, Kanyanmupira JB. Female prostitutes: a risk group for infection with human T-cell lymphotropic virus type III. Lancet 1985; ii:524–6.

43. Kreiss JK, Koech DK, Plummer F, Holmes KK, Piot P, Ronald AR, Ndinya-Achola JO, D'Costa LJ, Quinn T. HTLV-III infection in Kenyan prostitutes (abstract 227). 25th Interscience Conference on Antimicrobial Agents and Chemotherapy, Minneapolis, 29 Sept–2 Oct, 1985.

44. Centers for Disease Control. Heterosexual transmission of human T-lymphotropic virus type III/ lymphadenopathy-associated virus. Morbid Mortal Weekly Rep 1985; 34:561–3.

45. Melbye M, Ingersley J, Biggar RJ, Alexander S, Sarin P, Goedert JJ, Zachariae E, Ebbesen P, Stenbjerg S. Anal intercourse as a possible factor in heterosexual transmission of HTLV-III to spouses of hemophiliacs. N Engl J Med 1985; 312:857.

46. Kreiss JK, Kitchen LW, Prince HE, Kasper CK, Essex M. Antibody to human T-lymphotropic virus type III in wives of hemophiliacs. Ann Intern Med 1985; 102:623–6.

47. Stewart GT, Tyler JPP, Cunningham AL, et al. Transmission of human T-cell lymphotropic virus type III (HTLV-III) by artificial insemination by donor. Lancet 1985; ii:581–4.

48. Goedert JJ, Biggar RJ, Weiss SH, et al. Three-year incidence of AIDS among HTLV-III infected risk group members: A comparison of five cohorts. Submitted.

49. Melbye M. The natural history of human T-lymphotropic virus III infection—The cause of AIDS. Submitted.

Cancer Detection and Prevention Supplement 1:493–499 (1987)

Genetic Comparison of LAV-Related Isolates

Samuel Magasiny
Bruno Spire, MD
Francoise Rey, PhD
Francoise Barre-Sinoussi, PhD
Jean-Claude Chermann, PhD

Viral Oncology Unit, Institut Pasteur, Paris, France (S.M., B.S., F.R., F.B-S., J.-C.C.), Division de Radiobiologie et de Radioprotection, Centre de Recherches du Service de Santé des Armées, Clamart, France (B.S.)

ABSTRACT LAV/HTLV-III has been found to be the etiological cause of AIDS. This new human retrovirus has a selective tropism for T lymphocytes of the OKT4/leu 3 subset, in which it induces a cytopathic effect. We have compared Southern blot patterns of integrated proviral DNAs from different individuals at risk or not using a nick-translated LAV probe. We find that LAV/HTLV-III is very similar to our Haitian isolate and close to an isolate from an early-recognized (in 1982) AIDS case in New York. More variation is apparent with Zaïrian isolates as well as an isolate from a nonhigh-risk group when we used Hind III or Bgl II Sac-digested fragments. We also looked at virus isolated from a Sicilian child who developed AIDS after allogenic bone marrow transplant and transfusion. This isolate shows two forms: One is similar to the prototype LAV, the second much different.

Key words: AIDS virus, genomic variability, retrovirus

INTRODUCTION

It is now known that AIDS is caused by a human retrovirus. This retrovirus has been studied in several laboratories and is named LAV [1], HTLV-III [2], or ARV [3]. This virus is characterized by a selective tropism for T4 lymphocytes, in which it induces a cytopathic effect [4]. Our interest has been in the genomic variability of such viruses. Genetic heterogeneity has already been suspected [5,6], and previous studies tend to indicate that this would be at two levels: 1) There is a variability among isolates; for example, there is a 5% difference between the nucleotide sequences of LAV/HTLV-III and ARV [7–9], and 2) variability can also be found within an isolate itself; one isolate contains different molecular clones that differ at one restriction enzyme site [5,10].

In our laboratory, we obtained more than 100 viral isolates. Having such a number of viruses, it was worth investigating some in depth. Therefore, we decided to compare seven isolates with one another, according to the risk factor or the geographical origin.

Address reprint requests to Jean-Claude Chermann, Viral Oncology Unit, Institut Pasteur, 25 rue du Dr. Roux, 75724 Paris CEDEX 15, France.

PATIENTS AND METHODS
Patients

We chose to compare six isolates to LAV-1, which was first isolated in 1983 from a French homosexual patient who had travelled to New York and who presented with lympha-denopathy syndrome [1]. All other patients were serologically positive for LAV/HTLV-III. Viral isolation was obtained from all of them. Among these six isolates one had been found in a Haitian female who presented with opportunistic infections, one had been isolated from a New York homosexual who was one of the first recognized AIDS cases, one came from a bone marrow transplant recipient who developed clinical symptoms of AIDS after the transplanta-tion, two were obtained from Zaïrian patients (the first one had many opportunistic infections [11]; the second presented with Kaposi's sarcoma. This last patient had never travelled out of Zaïre before becoming ill), and the last virus had been isolated from and AIDS patient in New York who did not belong to a conventional high risk group. These epidemiological character-istics are summarized on Table I.

Methods

The viruses were isolated from peripheral lymphocytes [1], and they were then propa-gated by coculture on the continuous permissive H9 cell line [12]. The H9 cell line was chosen because of its ability to be highly infected with all viral strains and, essentially, because differences in the intensity of the cytopathic effect could be observed among isolates on this cell line. Infected H9 cell DNAs were extracted and then digested with restriction enzymes, and an analysis of the differences between the proviral DNAs was then carried out using the Southern blot technique [13] with a full LAV probe.

LAV/HTLV-III being integrated into the cellular genome at random, it was necessary to use enyzmes that could cut in the LTR of all isolates. Therefore, Sac I digestion was systematically used on all DNAs, because this enzyme is known to cut in the LTR of all described prototypical isolates like LAV, HTLV-III, and different ARV strains [5,6,10]. Then, other enzymes were also used in order to compare our isolates.

RESULTS
Sac I Digestion

DNAs were first digested with the restriction enzyme Sac I. This digestion makes it possible to measure the approximate size of each provirus and to determine the number of molecular clones in each isolate. The results are indicated on Figure 1. They confirm the presence of two molecular clones in the LAV/HTLV-III prototype: a clone A with an internal Sac I site and a clone B with Sac I sites in the LTR only.

Our Haitian isolate corresponds to clone A, as does the virus isolated from the New York homosexual. Zaïrian strains correspond to clone B without an internal Sac I site. The virus isolated from a bone marrow transplant recipient who developed AIDS contains both forms, but A seems to be predominant. This result was confirmed by using other single digestions such as Bgl II alone, and the restriction pattern observed with this enzyme also shows bands of different intensities. The virus isolated from the nonhigh-risk patient contains an internal Sac I site, but its size seems to be about 0.5 kb shorter than the other proviruses.

Comparison of Isolates

We also digested the proviral DNAs with Sac I followed by a second digestion with another restriction enzyme. These results are shown in Figure 2. Hind III and Bgl II cut the LAV/HTLV-III prototype at different points of the genome, including the ENV gene, which is the region most suspected of being variable [6,10]. Results of the digestions with these enzymes show that all isolates have a restriction pattern differing from the LAV/HTLV-III pattern. However, the Haitian isolate and the virus isolated from the early New York homosexual case seem similar to clone A of LAV with these enzymes; besides, they do not contain any clone B.

TABLE I. Epidemiological Characteristics

Isolate	Group at risk	Sex	Geographical origins	Symptoms	Remarks
LAV	Homosexual	M	France	Lymphadeno-pathy	Travelled widely, including the U.S.
1	Haitian	F	Haiti	Opportunistic infections	—
2	Homosexual	M	New York	Opportunistic infections	One of the first known AIDS cases
3	Bone marrow transplant + transfusion recipient	M	Sicily	Opportunistic infections	
4	Central African	M	Zaïre	Opportunistic infections	Heterosexual; developed AIDS while living in France for 1 year
5	Central African	M	Zaïre	Kaposi sarcoma	Heterosexual; had never been outside Zaïre before his admission to the hospital
6	None	M	New York	Kaposi sarcoma	Heterosexual; does not use drugs; no blood transfusions; never travelled outside U.S.

The other viruses are much different: Zaïrian strains look clearly different from LAV, but no particular relationship between these two African viruses can be detected. The first Zaïrian isolate has at least one modified Bgl II site in the ENV gene. The virus isolated from the nonhigh-risk patient is also very different: it was found to be shorter, and it has two Hind III sites more than LAV, one in the 3′ terminal part of the genome and the other in the POL region. The bone marrow transplant recipient isolate contains two molecular clones, as has been suggested in Figure 1. It has lost one of the Hind III site of the ENV region.

The DNAs were then analyzed by a digestion with Sac I and Eco RI. Eco RI cuts the LAV prototype in the POL region, and also in the noncoding region betweem Q and S (see Fig. 1). The three fragments, which could be, according to the restriction map of LAV, 4.1, 1, and 3.9 kb, were detected in LAV-infected cell DNA, but a supplementary band was also observed: Its size is 4.9 kb. This suggests a polymorphism inside the LAV isolate for the Eco RI sites, such as has already been described for other enzymes, like Hind III and Sac I [5,10]. It looks like there are two kinds of clones: clones with two Eco RI sites and clones with one Eco RI site only.

Analyzing the various isolates, it appears that the only clone the Haitian isolate contains is the clone with two sites. However, the New York homosexual virus differs from the Haitian isolate here in having only the one Eco RI site clone. The Eco RI site seems to be the one between Q and S, because DNAs are systematically digested with Sac I (see Fig. 1). The first Zaïrian strain contains both types of clones; the second Zaïrian strain shows only a single clone with an Eco RI site localized in the POL gene. The Sac I/Eco RI digestion also confirms the presence of two molecular clones in the bone marrow transplant recipient isolate; its major clone is similar to the LAV clone with only one Eco RI site, and its minor clone is different.

DISCUSSION

All isolates have shown degrees of heterogeneity as defined by restriction fragment polymorphisms. Dissimilarities in the restriction patterns of proviral DNA isolated from patient

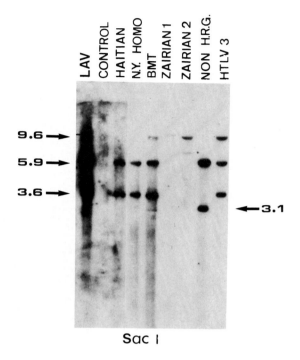

Sac I

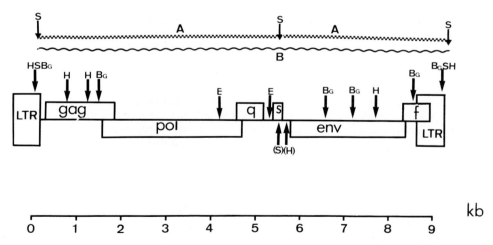

kb

Fig. 1. Sac I digestion of the proviral DNAs; 10 μg of DNA extracted from H9 cells infected with the various isolates was digested with 100 UI of Sac I (NE Biolabs). Restriction fragments were separated on a 0.8% agarose gel, and after blotting (Gene screen plus sheet) they were hybridized under stringent conditions with a p32 nick-translated pBT1 plasmid comprising 97% of the LAV1 genome. The restriction map of LAV/HTLV-III prototype is shown [7,8] in order to represent the different molecular clones A (checked line) and B (wavy line) that can be distinguished with the Sac I digestion. The restriction sites in parentheses are present only in certain clones and not in others. S, Sac I; H, Hind III; Bg, Bgl II; E, Eco R1.

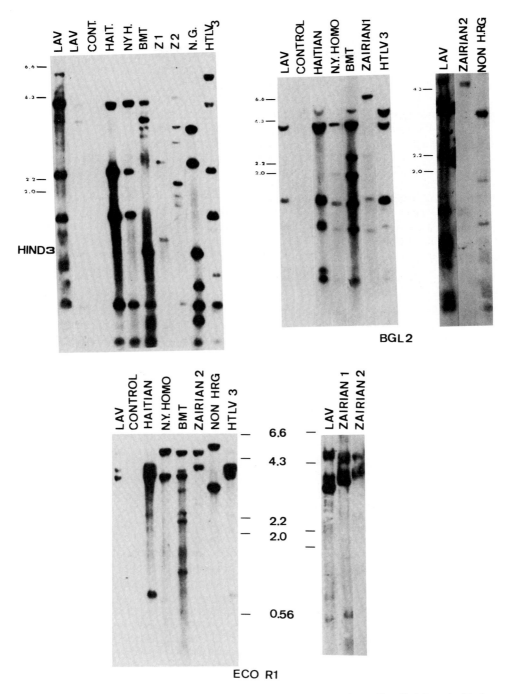

Fig. 2.   Genomic comparison of the isolates; 10 μg of DNA extracted from H9 cells infected with the various isolates (LAV, LAV-1 prototype; CONT, Control, uninfected H9; HAIT, Haitian isolate; NYH, New York homosexual isolate; BMT, Bone marrow transplant recipient isolate; Z1, first Zaïrian isolate; Z2, second Zaïrian isolate; N.G., N. HRG, nonhigh-risk-group isolate; HTLV III, HTLV III prototype) were digested with 100 UI of Sac I (NE Biolabs) and 100 UI of Hind III or Bgl II or Eco R1 (Amersham) as indicated. After electrophoresis and transfer, the restriction fragments were hybridized with the P32 nick-translated pBT1.

samples are a relatively quick and easy way to determine important differences between the proviral genomes. However, the disadvantage of this technique is that one cannot distinguish details, specific similarities or homologies. More time-consuming and expensive techniques of cloning and sequencing each provirus are necessary to characterize the genomes fully. Nonetheless, restriction digestion and Southern blotting remains a fast way to compare proviral DNA extracted from cells infected with patient isolates.

It has been possible to confirm Sac I and Hind III polymorphisms inside the LAV/HTLV-III-prototype, and such polymorphism at the Eco RI sites was also found. Only LAV and HTLV-III indicate the same restriction patterns; this is consistent with the 99% homology between the nucleotide sequences of LAV and HTLV-III [7,8]. The comparison of our isolates shows that all are different; however, some degree of variation can be detected. Clone A of LAV is rather similar to our Haitian isolate as well as to the early New York homosexual case isolate, which suggests a common origin for these viruses. Zaïrian strains and the isolate from a nonhigh-risk patient are more different. A bone marrow transplant recipient isolate seems to contain two rather different molecular clones; this suggests a double infection for this patient. Our technique did not enable us to build restriction maps, but some differences could be located in the ENV gene and also in more conserved regions. Core proteins as well as glycoproteins of our isolates are recognized by a reference anti-LAV-1 serum; however, it is interesting to note that comparison of glycoproteins of some isolates shows slight modifications of their apparent mobilities (unpublished observations).

On the way to comparing biological effects of these isolates, we found that one of the Zaïrian strains is highly cytopathic for normal T lymphocytes and for several continuous T lymphoblastoid cell lines. It will be of interest to characterize this virus further molecularly by cloning and sequencing in order to determine which genomic region is involved in the cytopathogenicity of this isolate.

All studies concerning variability of LAV, HTLV-III, and ARV indicate that these viruses are characterized by an important polymorphism [6,10,14]. This feature brings LAV/HTLV-III close to the lentivirus family. Lentiviruses give slow pathologies in animal and they all have a cytopathic effect in culture. Recently, the nucleotide sequence of the VISNA virus has shown a genomic organization similar to LAV [15]. However, this work supports the hypothesis that LAV has to be considered as the first human lentivirus.

ACKNOWLEDGMENTS

We thank Drs. W. Rozenbaum, E. Gluckman, A. Ellrodt, P. Rubinstein, J. Sonnet, and M. Lange for patient samples, Dr. S. Wain-Hobson for the gift of pBTl probe and Dr. R. Gallo for providing H9 and H9/HTLV-III cell lines. We thank Drs. M. Souyri and L. Montagnier for criticizing the manuscript and F. Kissian for helpful discussion. We thank H. Sinno for typing the manuscript. This work was supported by the French League Against Cancer, the Medical Research Foundation, the AIDS Medical Foundation (New York), the ARC (Association for Cancer Research), and the ADIP (Association pour le développement de l'Institut Pasteur).

REFERENCES

1. Barre-Sinoussi F, Chermann JC, Rey F, et al. Isolation of a T lymphotropic retrovirus from a patient at risk for acquired immune deficiency syndrome (AIDS). Science 1983; 220:868–71.
2. Gallo RC, Salahuddin SZ, Popovic M, et al. Frequent detection and isolation of cytopathic retrovirus (HTLV III) from patients with AIDS or at risk for AIDS and pre-AIDS. Science 1984; 224:500–2.
3. Levy JA, Hoffmann AD, Kramer SA, et al. Isolation of lymphocytopathic retrovirus from San Francisco patients with AIDS. Science 1984; 225:840–2.
4. Klatzmann D, Barre-Sinoussi F, Nugeyre MT, et al. Selective tropism of lymphadenopathy associated virus (LAV) for helper/inducer T lymphocytes. Science 1984; 225:59–62.
5. Alizon M, Sonigo P, Barre-Sinoussi F, et al. Molecular cloning of lymphadenopathy associated virus. Nature 1984; 312:757–60.

6. Luciw PA, Potter SJ, Steimer K, et al. Molecular cloning of AIDS associated retrovirus. Nature 1984; 312:760–3.
7. Wain-Hobson S, Sonigo P, Danos O, Coles S, Alizon M. Nucleotide sequence of the AIDS virus LAV. Cell 1985; 40:9–17.
8. Ratner L, Haseltine W, Patarca R, et al. Complete nucleotide sequence of the AIDS virus HTLV III. Nature 1985; 313:277–84.
9. Sanchez-Pescador R, Power MD, Barr PJ, et al. Nucleotide sequence and expression of an AIDS associated retrovirus (ARV-2). Science 1985; 227:484–92.
10. Shaw GM, Hahn BH, Arya SK, et al. Molecular characterization of human T cell leukemia (lymphotropic) virus type III in the acquired immune deficiency syndrome. Science 1984; 226:1165–71.
11. Ellrodt A, Barre-Sinoussi F, Lebras P, et al. Isolation of a T lymphotropic LAV retrovirus (LAV) from a Zaïrian married couple, one with AIDS, one with prodromes. Lancet 1984; i:1383–5.
12. Popovic M, Sarngadharan MG, Read E, et al. Detection, isolation and continuous production of cytopathic retroviruses (HTLV III) from patients with AIDS and pre-AIDS. Science 1984; 224:497–9.
13. Southern E. Detection of specific sequences among DNA fragments separated by gel electrophoresis. J Mol Biol 1975; 98:503–17.
14. Wong-Staal F, Shaw GM, Hahn BH, et al. Genomic diversity of human T lymphotropic virus type III (HTLV III). Science 1985; 229:563–6.
15. Sonigo P, Alizon M, Staskup K, et al. Nucleotide sequence of the visna lentivirus: Relationship to the AIDS virus. Cell 1985; 42:369–82.

Cancer Detection and Prevention Supplement 1:501–507 (1987)

Simian Models for AIDS

M.D. Daniel, DVM, PhD
R.C. Desrosiers, PhD
N.L. Letvin, MD
N.W. King, DVM

D.K. Schmidt, BS
P. Sehgal, DVM
R.D. Hunt, DVM

New England Regional Primate Research Center, Harvard Medical School, Southborough, MA

ABSTRACT The macaque immunodeficiency syndrome has many parallels to AIDS in humans. Affected monkeys develop profound, prolonged T lymphocyte dysfunction and die of lymphomas or opportunistic infections. We recently isolated a virus that we call SIV from four sick macaque monkeys. The morphology, growth characteristics, and antigenic properties of this virus indicate that it is related to the causative agent of human AIDS. The pathogenicity of this newly isolated virus was tested in macaque monkeys. Five of six died between 127 and 352 days following inoculation. The animals developed a wasting syndrome and died with adenovirus pancreatitis and/or pneumonia and primary retroviral encephalitis. Immunological abnormalities in these animals included a decrease in circulating $T4^+$ lymphocytes and depressed peripheral blood lymphocyte proliferative response to pokeweed mitogen. The SIV monkey model holds great promise for testing antiviral agents and for the development of vaccines against AIDS.

Key words: retrovirus, macaque monkeys, encephalitis

INTRODUCTION

The New England Regional Primate Research Center (NERPRC) houses over 1,300 animals; 864 of these are macaques of various species, and 436 are New World monkeys. In maintaining this large number of animals some deaths caused by bacterial, parasitic, and viral infections can be expected; however, the incidence of deaths in established colonies is usually low. During the years 1979 to 1983, deaths among macaques at the NERPRC increased, reaching 12 to 30% in some species [1]. The most affected species was *Macaca cyclopis* (the Taiwanese rock macaque), with losses caused by an unusual epidemic approaching two-thirds of our colony within 2 years. This increased mortality appeared to be largely the result of an immunodeficiency syndrome with deaths from cytomegalovirus (CMV), SV40, and adenovirus infections, necrotizing gingivitis (NOMA), and *Pneumocystis carinii* pneumonia [2]. In addition, some animals had systemic *Mycobacterium avium* complex, and a few had the flagellated protozoan *Hexamita* in the blood. In the preceeding 13 years, deaths with such opportunistic infections did not occur in any significant numbers.

Address reprint requests to Dr. M.D. Daniel, New England Regional Primate Research Center, Harvard Medical School, Southborough, MA 01772.

A systematic program for evaluating the nature of this unusual disease was initiated by looking at various parameters, including a study of necropsy reports of macaques that died during the period from 1979 to 1983 and a careful screening of affected animals for viral and other microbial agents and for immunological changes. The results of this evaluation revealed that some of these animals had lymphoproliferative disorders in addition to opportunistic infections and that immune functions were depressed [1].

Parallel experiments being performed at the same time with macaque lymphomas eventually converged with our studies on the immunodeficiency syndrome. Minced tissues from naturally occurring macaque lymphoma and filtrates of homogenated tumor tissue were inoculated into healthy macaques. Recipients developed lymphoma 14 to 26 months following inoculation [3,4]. Some of the inoculated animals, however, developed a fatal disease that bore a close resemblance to the naturally occurring immunodeficiency syndrome in macaques [1]. Since this fatal immunodeficiency syndrome was induced by filtered cell-free material, a viral etiology was suspected. Furthermore, epidemiological studies indicated that an infectious agent was the cause of the naturally occuring immunodeficiency syndrome.

In the search for possible etiologic viruses a variety of techniques were used, including organ cultures, explant cultures, and cocultivation with monolayer cells. The ubiquitous agents CMV, SV40, adenovirus, paramyxovirus, and foamy viruses were isolated; however, unusual viruses that might have been the cause were not observed. We reasoned that since the disease was one of immunosuppression, we might be able to isolate causative viruses using lymphoid cell cultures.

MATERIALS AND METHODS

For the isolation of lymphotropic viruses, established T, B, and Null cell lines were used as indicator cells instead of the usual monolayer cell lines for cocultivation with monkey lymphocytes. We mixed approximately equal numbers of each lymphoid cell line with macaque lymphocytes that had previously been separated by a standard Ficoll-Hypaque procedure. Of the 12 lymphoid cell lines tested, the human B cell line Raji exhibited formation of multinucleated giant cells following cocultivation with lymphocytes from macaques with immunodeficiency disease. This cytopathic effect developed in 9 days. Typical type D retroviral particles were demonstrated by electron microscopy, and reverse transcriptase activity was present in this supernatant [5]. Type D retrovirus was isolated from monkeys exhibiting fever, rash, diarrhea, and lymphadenopathy.

The prototype D retrovirus was first isolated by Chopra and Mason in 1970 [6] and termed *Mason-Pfizer monkey virus* (MPMV). It was isolated from a *Macaca mulatta* monkey with mammary carcinoma. In addition to the more recent isolates from the New England macaque colony, macaque type D retrovirus isolates have also been obtained at Regional Primate Research Centers in California [7,8] Washington [9], and Oregon [10]. MPMV and D retroviruses from New England and California are quite similar, sharing 90–92% sequence homology; however, these three are still easily distinguished [11–13]. In contrast, strain differences were not observed among D/New England isolates examined at over 30 restriction endonuclease sites [11]. Type D isolates from Washington and Oregon colonies are quite different from MPMV and the New England and California isolates, perhaps even of a different serotype [9,10].

Isolation of D retrovirus has been consistently associated with the immunodeficiency syndrome occurring sporadically among NERPRC macaques at the present time; D/New England has not been isolated from clinically healthy animals [11]. These results suggested that D/New England could be responsible for the immunodeficiency disease. This was supported by previous studies on the pathogenicity of MPMV. Inoculation of MPMV into infant rhesus monkeys resulted in deaths of 42 out of 68 animals with a wasting syndrome, opportunistic adenovirus, and cryptosporidia infections, thymic atrophy, profound neutropenia, anemia, and depletion of lymphocytes from lymph nodes [14]. Furthermore, experimental infection of juvenile macaques (10 to 30 months old) with SAIDS D retrovirus type 1 from California has induced death in 9 of 21 (43%) inoculated animals with generalized lymphodenopathy, splenomegaly, neutropenia, decreased lymphocyte mitogenic response, and opportunistic infections [8,15] (P. Marx, personal communication). Studies done at NERPRC demonstrated that juvenile macaques experimentally infected with D/New England developed lymphadenopathy without follicular hyperplasia, profound neutropenia, and a transient decrease in peripheral blood lymphocyte blastogenic responsiveness; this syndrome did differ, however, from the naturally occurring syndrome of macaques at the NERPRC [16].

RESULTS

The similar clinical features of the macaque immunodeficiency syndrome and human AIDS prompted us to look for HIV-like viruses that might contribute to spontaneous immunodeficiency disease in our macaque colony. Frozen lymphocytes from a macaque with lymphoma and immunodeficiency disease were retrieved from liquid nitrogen storage and cocultured with PHA-stimulated and IL-2–grown normal human peripheral blood lymphocytes (PBL) as had been described for HIV isolation [17,18]. On day 12 we detected reverse transcriptase activity, which increased in the subsequent days. When these cells were analyzed by electron microscopy, the presence of a lentivirus (Fig. 1) was confirmed [19]. In the succeeding days, other isolates were obtained from frozen sera from two other macaques which had died of the immunodeficiency disease and from PBL of a naturally infected macaque Mm 142-83 [19,20].

In cell culture the macaque virus had growth characteristics similar to those of HIV [17,18]. Moreover, the virus has been shown to be antigenically related to HIV [21]. The similar ultrastructural morphology and biological characteristics prompted the name SIV (simian T immunodeficiency virus). In cell cultures, SIV grew in macaque lymphocytes,

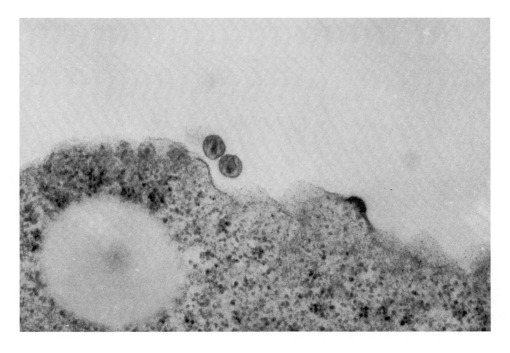

Fig. 1.   Electron micrograph showing one budding and two mature SIV virions. The manner of budding and cylindrical cores are characteristic of lentiviruses.

human lymphocytes, H-9, and Hut-78 cells. It did not grow in CEM cells, in EBV immortalized tumor cell lines, or in a variety of monolayer cell lines. Conversely, HIV did not grow in macaque T lymphocytes [22]. SIV induced a characteristic cytopathic effect in Hut-78 and H-9 cells but not in monkey or human PBL. Infected Hut-78 or H-9 cells became multinucleated and assumed a bizarre pleomorphic appearance; these giant cells were very prominent when viewed by light microscopy (Fig. 2). With an increase in the number of such cells, the reverse transcriptase activity in cell-free supernatant also increased and reached a peak between 2 to 4 weeks after low multiplicity infection. This high level of reverse transcriptase activity remained for several months, and after 8 to 9 months declined unless fresh uninfected cells were added periodically to the cultures.

Infection of susceptible cells was easily accomplished using cell-free virus, a feature similar to HIV but different from HTLV-I or II. SIV also grew preferentially in $T4^+$ cells and less efficiently in $T8^+$ cells [19,22]. The presence of viral antigens in infected cells could be demonstrated by indirect immunofluorescence. In freshly infected cells, antigenic expression was not readily detectable, but in older cultures a nuclear and cytoplasmic staining became discernible.

Thus, a virus with remarkable similarity to HIV was isolated at the New England Regional Primate Research Center from animals with immunodeficiency. To determine the pathogenicity of SIV, six *M. mulatta* monkeys between 6 and 18 months of age were inoculated intravenously with 1.7 ml of SIV propagated in PHA-stimulated, IL-2–grown human peripheral blood lymphocytes [23]. Four of the six died with immunodeficiency disease between 127 and 160 days and one at 352 days post-inoculation. All five developed rash, diarrhea, and weight loss. The number of $T4^+$ circulating lymphocytes was consistently depressed and there was a diminished blastogenic response of their PBL to pokeweed mitogen.

Pathologically, all five animals developed thymic atrophy, and their lymph nodes were depleted of lymphocytes. Three animals had necrotizing adenoviral pancreatitis, one animal had adenoviral pneumonia and cholangitis, and another had intestinal cryptosporidiosis. A striking finding in four of these five animals was the presence of multifocal granulomatous

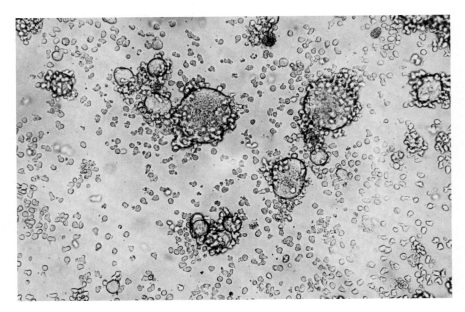

Fig. 2.   Photomicrograph of HUT-78 cells infected with SIV, showing large, multinucleated, bizzare-shaped cells.

encephalitis with syncytial giant cell formation (Fig. 3). Ultrastructural studies of the brain lesions revealed lentiviral particles within the macrophages, histiocytes, and syncytial cells in these granulomatous lesions. The brain lesions were indistinguishable from brain lesions called *microglial nodules* in human AIDS [24,25]. SIV was readily isolated from brain tissues of inoculated macaques following cocultivation of minced brain material with H-9 or Hut-78 cells. The presence of SIV in these cultures of brain material was confirmed by electron microscopy.

Antibody responses of the six inoculated animals were determined by radioimmunopre- cipitation and neutralization tests and quantitated by indirect immunofluorescence and ELISA assays. The strongest antibody response was seen in the animal that is still alive, while a moderate to strong response was observed in the animal that survived for 352 days. In contrast, the four animals that survived for less than 160 days had little or no antibody response. Thus, the ability of these infected animals to survive infection appeared to correlate directly with the strength of the antibody response.

SIV was regularly isolated from each of these animals beginning 2 weeks post-inocula- tion and up to the time of death. Virus is still being isolated from the one animal that is still alive 14 months after inoculation. In addition to virus recovery from lymphocytes, virus was also recovered from the brain, lymph nodes, spleen, and salivary gland.

DISCUSSION

Since the original isolation of SIV from captive macaques [19] other isolations of SIV have been reported from African green monkeys [26], sooty mangabeys [27,28], and pig-tailed macaques (R. Benveniste, personal communication). The precise relationship of these isolates to each other and to HIV is not yet determined; their potential pathogenicity is also not yet known. The antigenic relatedness of these SIV isolates to HIV has been demonstrated by radioimmune precipitation [21,26,27], by Western blotting [28], and by radioimmune compe- tition assay [29]. In the radioimmune competition assay SIV competed only partially in the homologous HIV P24 assay, indicating that core proteins of both viruses shared immunoreac-

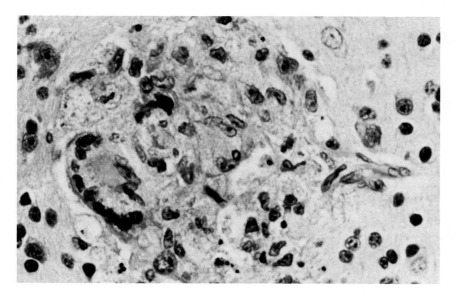

Fig. 3.   High power light micrograph of a granuloma composed of aggregates of foamy histiocytes and a single multinucleated syncytial giant cell present in the brain of an SIV–inoculated animal. These cells contained SIV particles by electron microscopy (not shown).

tive determinants, but differed immunologically because of the low level of competition. In the heterologous HIV P24 assay, common determinants on the major core proteins of the two viruses were demonstrated [28]. Radioimmune precipitation analysis of SIV–infected cell proteins using HIV–positive human sera has revealed cross-reactive specific proteins of approximately the same size as major envelope and core proteins of HIV [21,26,27,28].

The precise genetic relatedness of these various SIV isolates to HIV has not been established. The lack of a molecular clone has hampered progress in this direction. Analysis of molecular clones and sequence homologies will be needed to clarify these relationships. Preliminary evidence indicates less than 75% overall sequence homology between SIV and HIV [29].

More data will be needed to determine the extent to which HIV and type D retroviruses are causes of spontaneous immunodeficiency in monkeys. Of immediate importance is the identification of a virus from nonhuman primates with similarities to HIV and the experimental induction of an AIDS-like disease with this agent. This provides a unique, highly relevant animal model with which to study AIDS.

The increasing dissemination of AIDS in humans is alarming; the lack of a suitable animal model for drug evaluation and vaccine development is hampering progress toward the ultimate control of this deadly disease. Although HIV infection of chimpanzees will be important as an experimental model, chimpanzees are extremely limited in number and do not develop disease following HIV infections [30–33]. The similarity of the HIV macaque system to human AIDS provides hope that important research developments in this experimental model can be quickly extrapolated to human AIDS.

ACKNOWLEDGMENTS

The authors thank Ellen Hajema for bibliographical assistance and Joanne Newton for secretarial work. This work was supported by Public Health Service grants CA 38205, CA 34949, CA 40680, and AI 20729 from the National Institutes of Health and by grant RR00168 from the Division of Research Resources. Research was also sponsored, at least in part, by the National Cancer Institute, DHHS, under contract N01-CO-23910 with Program Resources, Incorporated. The contents of this publication do not necessarily reflect the views or policies of the DHHS, nor does mention of trade names, commercial products, or organizations imply endorsement by the U.S. Government.

REFERENCES

1. Letvin NL, Eaton KA, Aldrich WR, et al. Acquired immunodeficiency syndrome in a colony of macaque monkeys. Proc Natl Acad Sci USA 1983; 80:2718–22.
2. Letvin NL, King NW. Clinical and pathologic features of an acquired immune deficiency syndrome (AIDS) in macaque monkeys. Adv Vet Sci Comp Med 1984; 28:237–65.
3. Hunt RD, Blake BJ, Chalifoux LV, Sehgal PK, King NW, Letvin NL. Transmission of naturally occurring lymphoma in macaque monkeys. Proc Natl Acad Sci USA 1983; 80:5085–9.
4. Letvin NL, Aldrich WR, King NW, Blake BJ, Daniel MD, Hunt RD. Experimental transmission of macaque AIDS by means of inoculation of macaque lymphoma tissue. Lancet 1983; ii:599–602.
5. Daniel MD, King NW, Letvin NL, Hunt RD, Sehgal PK, Desrosiers RC. A new type D retrovirus isolated from macaques with an immunodeficiency syndrome. Science 1984; 223:602–5.
6. Chopra HC, Mason MM. A new virus in a spontaneous mammary tumor of a rhesus monkey. Cancer Res 1970; 30:2081–4.
7. Gravell M, London WT, Hamilton RS, et al. Transmission of simian AIDS with type D retrovirus isolates. Lancet 1984; i:334–5.
8. Marx, PA, Maul DM, Osborn KG, et al. Simian AIDS: Isolation of a type D retrovirus and transmission of the disease. Science 1984; 223:1083–6.
9. Stromberg K, Benveniste RE, Arthur LO, et al. Characterization of exogenous type D retrovirus from a fibroma of a macaque with simian AIDS and fibromatosis. Science 1984; 224:289–92.

10. Marx PA, Bryant ML, Osborn KG, et al. Isolation of a new serotype of simian acquired immune deficiency syndrome type D retrovirus from Celebes black macaques (*Macaca nigra*) with immune deficiency and retroperitoneal fibromatosis. J Virol 1985; 56:571–8.

11. Desrosiers RC, Daniel MD, Butler CV, et al. Retrovirus D/New England and its relation to Mason-Pfizer monkey virus. J Virol 1985; 54:552–60.

12. Power MD, Marx PA, Bryant ML, Gardner MB, Barr PJ, Luciw PA. Nucleotide sequence of SRV-1, a type D simian acquired immunodeficiency syndrome retrovirus. Science 1986; 231:1567–72.

13. Sonigo P, Barker C, Hunter E, Wain-Hobson S. Nucleotide sequence of Mason-Pfizer monkey virus: An immunosuppresive D-type retrovirus. Cell 1986; 45:375–85.

14. Fine DL, Landon JC, Pienta RJ, et al. Responses of infant rhesus monkeys to inoculation with Mason-Pfizer monkey virus materials. JNCI 1975; 54:651–8.

15. Maul DM, Lerche NW, Osborn KG, et al. Pathogenesis of simian AIDS in rhesus macaques inoculated with the SRV-1 strain of type D retrovirus. Am J Vet Res 1986; 47:863–8.

16. Letvin NL, Daniel MD, Sehgal PK, et al. Experimental infection of rhesus monkeys with type D retrovirus. J Virol 1984; 52:683–6.

17. Barre-Sinoussi F, Chermann JC, Rey F, et al. Isolation of a T-lymphotropic retrovirus from a patient at risk for acquired immune deficiency syndrome (AIDS). Science 1983; 220:868–71.

18. Popovic M, Sarngadharan MG, Read E, Gallo RC. Detection, isolation and continuous production of cytopathic retroviruses (HTLV-III) from patients with AIDS and pre-AIDS. Science 1984; 224:497–500.

19. Daniel MD, Letvin NL, King NW, et al. Isolation of T-cell tropic HTLV-III–like retrovirus from macaques. Science 1985; 228:1201–4.

20. Chalifoux LV, King NW, Daniel MD, et al. A lymphoproliferative syndrome in an immunodeficient rhesus monkey naturally infected with an HTLV-III–like virus (STLV-III). Lab Invest 1986; 55:43–50.

21. Kanki PJ, McLane MF, King NW, et al. Serologic identification and characaterization of a macaque T-lymphotropic retrovirus closely related to HTLV-III. Science 1985; 228:1199–201.

22. Kannagi M, Yetz JM, Letvin NL. In vitro growth characteristics of simian T lymphotropic virus type III. Proc Natl Acad Sci USA 1985; 82:7053–7.

23. Letvin NL, Daniel MD, Sehgal PK, et al. Induction of AIDS-like disease in macaque monkeys with T-cell tropic retrovirus STLV-III. Science 1985; 230:71–3.

24. Shaw GM, Harper ME, Hahn BH, et al. HTLV-III infections in brains of children and adults with AIDS encephalopathy. Science 1985; 227:177–82.

25. Sharer LR, Cho E-S, Epstein LG. Multinucleated giant cells and HTLV-III in AIDS encephalopathy. Hum Pathol 1985; 16:760.

26. Kanki PJ, Alroy J, Essex M. Isolation of T-lymphotropic retrovirus related to HTLV-III/LAV from wild-caught African Green monkeys. Science 1984; 230:951–4.

27. Fultz PN, McClure HM, Anderson DC, Swenson RB, Anand R, Srinivasan A. Isolation of a T-lymphotropic retrovirus from naturally infected sooty mangabey monkeys (*Cercocebus atys*). Proc Natl Acad Sci USA 1986; 83:5286–90.

28. Murphey-Corb M, Martin LN, Rangan SRS, et al. Isolation of an HTLV-III/LAV–related retrovirus from macaques with simian AIDS and its possible origin in asymptomatic mangabeys. Nature 1986; 321:435–7.

29. Desrosiers RC, Letvin NL, King NW, et al. Three retroviruses infecting macaques at the New England Regional Primate Research Center. In Gallo RC, Haseltine W, Klein G, zur Hausen H, eds: Viruses and human cancer. New York: A R Liss Inc., 1987; 451–66.

30. Alter JJ, Eichberg JW, Masur H, et al. Transmission of HTLV-III infection from human plasma to chimpanzees: An animal model for AIDS. Science 1984; 226:549–52.

31. Centers for Disease Control. Experimental infection of chimpanzees with lymphadenopathy-associated virus. Morbid Mortal Weekly Rep 1984; 33:442–4.

32. Gajdusek DC, Amyx HL, Gibbs CJ, et al. Transmission experiments with human T-lymphotropic retroviruses and human AIDS tissue. Lancet 1984; i:1415–6.

33. Fultz PN, McClure HM, Swenson RB, et al. Persistent infection of chimpanzees with human T-lymphotropic virus type III/lympadenopathy-associated virus: A potential model for acquired immunodeficiency syndrome. J Virol 1986; 58:116–24.

Cancer Detection and Prevention Supplement 1:509–514 (1987)

Extrathecal and Intrathecal IgG Response to the AIDS Virus LAV/HTLV-III in Experimental Infection of Chimpanzees

Jaap Goudsmit, MD
Clarence J. Gibbs Jr., PhD
David M.A. Asher, MD
D. Carleton Gajdusek, MD

Virology Department, Academic Medical Center of the University of Amsterdam, Amsterdam, The Netherlands (J.G.); Laboratory of Central Nervous System Studies, NINCDS, National Institutes of Health, Bethesda, MD (C.J.G., D.M.A.A., D.C.G.)

ABSTRACT Seven of seven chimpanzees inoculated with LAV/HTLV-III and three of three chimpanzee-to-chimpanzee passages seroconverted for LAV/HTLV-III as tested by ELISA and immunoblotting. Serum IgG reactivity to gag-gene products emerged between 3 and 6 weeks after inoculation, $p24^{gag}$ reactivity always reaching maximum titers first. Serum IgG antibodies to env-related proteins occurred 11–21 weeks after inoculation. Throughout the observation period (>36 weeks), IgG reactivity to gag, pol, and env gene products persisted. Matched serum and cerebrospinal fluid (CSF) from three LAV/HTLV-III-infected chimpanzees were available in the chronic phase of infection and titers of viral antibody and albumin and IgG content were determined. By calculation of antibody/albumin indices, evidence was obtained for intrathecal synthesis of IgG antibodies to LAV/HTLV-III in one animal.

Key words: serological HIV profiles, diagnostics, HIV vaccins

INTRODUCTION

Acquired immunodeficiency syndrome (AIDS) in humans is caused by lymphadenopathy-associated virus [1], also designated human T-lymphotropic retrovirus type III (LAV/HTLV-III) [2]. Immunoglobulin G (IgG) antibodies to LAV/HTLV-III are present in most, if not all, patients with AIDS or signs preceding AIDS [3–5], and LAV/HTLV-III can be isolated from the majority of these patients [6]. Person-to-person transmission of LAV/HTLV-III by blood transfusions and subsequent development of AIDS in the absence of infections by other viruses [7,8] contributes to the fulfillment of Koch's postulates. Persistent LAV/HTLV-III infection of chimpanzees has been accomplished by inoculation with tissues of AIDS patients as well as LAV/HTLV-III [9,10]. LAV/HTLV-III is both lymphotropic and neurotropic [10]. Viral infection of the central nervous system (CNS) may result in virus-specific antibody

---

Address reprint requests to Jaap Goudsmit, Virology Department, Academic Medical Center of the University of Amsterdam, 1105AZ Amsterdam, The Netherlands.

synthesis within the CNS. An increased antibody/albumin index [cerebrospinal fluid (CSF)/ serum levels of virus specific IgG divided by CSF/serum levels of albumin] reflects de novo rates of IgG synthesis in the CNS [11,12] and enables distinction between intrathecally produced antibody and CSF antibody derived from leakage of serum.

To study the time course of virus-specific IgG reactivity following LAV/HTLV-III infection, sequential serum samples of seven LAV/HTLV-III-inoculated chimpanzees and three chimpanzee-to-chimpanzee passages were tested by enzyme-linked immunosorbent assay (ELISA) and immunoblotting using purified HTLV-III as antigen. Matched serum and cerebro-spinal fluid was available from two HTLV-III infected chimpanzees and one chimpanzee-to-chimpanzee passage to titrate virus antibodies and determine albumin and IgG levels.

MATERIALS AND METHODS
Sera

Sequential serum samples were taken from five chimpanzees inoculated with superna-tants of HTLV-III producer cell lines (A3D, A3E, A86B, A251, and A275B) and two with supernatants from LAV producer cells (A22 and A286). One additional chimpanzee (A274B) was inoculated with whole blood from chimpanzee A3D taken 14 weeks after virus inoculation of A3D, and two chimpanzees (A3A and A243B) were inoculated with whole blood from chimpanzee A22 taken 8 weeks after virus inoculation of A22. Virus was isolated from each of these animals [10]. Matched serum and CSF were taken from chimpanzees A3D, A86B, and A274B more than 1 year after infection. The observation period reached until 36–45 weeks after inoculation. No clinical disease resulted from LAV/HTLV-III infection within the obser-vation period.

Enzyme-Linked Immunosorbent Assays (ELISA)
for IgG Antibodies to LAV/HTLV-III

Sera were tested for IgG antibodies to LAV/HTLV-III in serial twofold dilutions using ELISA (Vironostika, Organon, Oss, The Netherlands). Sucrose gradient-purified HTLV-III was used for coating polysterene microtiter strips. One hundred microliters of serum at twofold dilutions was added to each well and incubated for 30 min at 37°C. Subsequently 100 μl of goat antihuman IgG (Organon, Oss, The Netherlands) labeled with horseradish peroxidase was added after thorough washings. After another washing step, the reactivity was visualized using o-phenylene diamine as substrate. An IgG antibody titer was considered to be dilution of serum of which the ^{2}logarithm corresponded to an optical density at 450 nm of $[(OD_{maximum} + OD_{minimum})/2]$. The specificity for LAV/HTLV-III was confirmed by immunoblotting for all sera with an IgG titer of $>1:7$ in the ELISA.

Immunoblot Analysis of IgG Reactivity

Sucrose gradient-purified HTLV-III, inactivated by 1% Triton X-100 (final concentra-tion) and heat treatment (60 min at 56°C) was denatured by boiling for 2 min in 0.5 M Tris HCl (pH 6.8) containing 10% (w/v) SDS and 5% (v/v) β-mercaptoethanol. Viral proteins were separated on a 12% DSD polyacrylamide gel and transferred to nitrocellulose paper. After washing at room temperature, the paper was cut into strips and preincubated for 60 min at 37°C with normal goat serum. Subsequently strips were incubated at room temperature with a 1:100 (IgG) test serum dilution. After another washing, protein recognition patterns were visualised by incubation with biotinylated goat antihuman IgG (Vector Laboratories, CA), subsequent incubation with a complex of avidin and biotinylated horseradish peroxidase, and color development using 4-chloro-1-naphtol as substrate.

Albumin and IgG Assays

Total IgG and albumin in serum and CSF were determined with a Cobas Biocentrifugal Analyzer using procedures described by Hische et al [13]. Normal values for the albumin CSF/ serum ratio are below 7.8×10^{-3} and for the IgG index below 0.6.

RESULTS

IgG antibodies to LAV/HTLV-III occurred in all ten inoculated animals as tested by ELISA (Fig. 1). IgG reactivity to $p18^{gag}$, $p24^{gag}$, and $Pr55^{gag}$ emerged between 3 and 6 weeks after inoculation, $p24^{gag}$ reactivity always reaching maximum titers first (Fig. 2) [14]. IgG

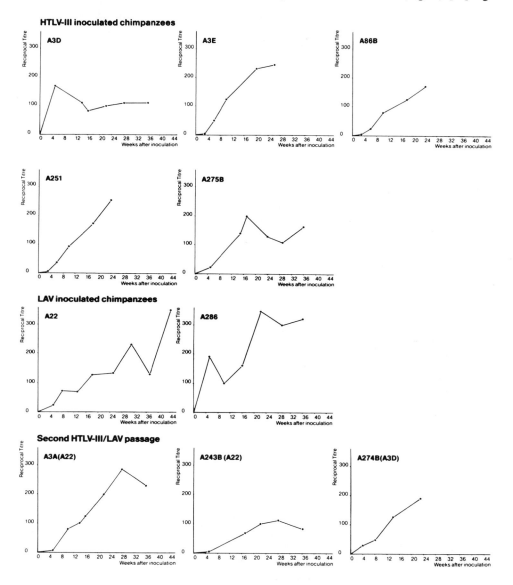

Fig. 1.   Evolution of IgG response to LAV/HTLV-III after experimental infection as tested by ELISA. Five chimpanzees were inoculated with supernatants from HTLV-III producer cell lines (A3D, A3E, A86B, A251, and A275B) and two with supernatants from LAV producer cells (A22 and A286). One additional chimpanzee (A274B) was inoculated with whole blood from chimpanzee A3D taken 14 weeks after virus inoculation of A3D, and two chimpanzees (A3A & A243B) were inoculated with whole blood from chimpanzee A22 taken 8 weeks after virus inoculation of A22. Virus was isolated from each of these animals.

LAV/HTLV-III inoculated chimpanzees

Second passage by whole blood

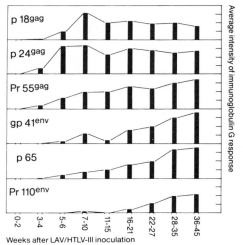
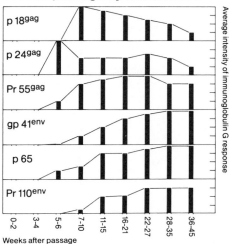

Fig. 2. LAV/HTLV-III protein recognition patterns of serum samples taken at various intervals after experimental infection as tested by immunoblotting. Virus-specific proteins were first detected at 3–6 weeks and subsequently throughout the observation period by sera from HTLV-III-inoculated and LAV-inoculated chimpanzees as well as by sera from chimpanzee-to-chimpanzee passages. Viral proteins and their assignment to the viral genome are indicated with their relative molecular masses.

TABLE I. IgG Antibody Titers to LAV/HTLV-III in Serum and CSF and Antibody Indices in Experimentally Infected Chimpanzees

| Chimpanzee No. | Inoculum | IgG antibody titer to LAV/HTLV-III in | | Antibody ALB/index* | Albumin CSF/serum ratio ($\times 10^{-3}$) | IgG index |
		Serum	CSF			
A3B	HTLV-III	46	0	0	11.7	0.6
A86B	HTLV-III	226	8	2.0	17.9	0.8
A274B	Second-passage HTLV-III (A3D)	80	10	4.6	26.9	0.6

*Upper normal limit is 2.0

antibodies to env gene products of M_r 41,000 (gp41^{env}) and M_r 65,000 (p65) occurred subsequently between 11 and 21 weeks after virus inoculation, and IgG reactivity to an env gene product of M_r 110,000 (Pr110^{env}) and a putative pol gene product of M_r 33,000 (p33^{pol}) occurred last between 22 and 27 weeks after inoculation. Throughout the observation period (>36 weeks) IgG reactivity to gag, pol, and env gene products persisted. A similar time-dependent protein recognition pattern was observed in the three chimpanzee-to-chimpanzee passages (Fig. 2). Table I shows IgG antibody titers to LAV/HTLV-III in serum and CSF and antibody indices of two virus inoculated chimpanzees and one chimpanzee-to-chimpanzee passage. In each of these animals, the albumin level in the CSF surpassed the upper normal limit for humans; the total IgG level in the CSF was proportional to albumin. The LAV/HTLV-III-specific antibody level in CSF was elevated in one animal (A274B) and borderline in another (A86B).

DISCUSSION

The IgG response to *gag* and *env* gene products after experimental LAV/HTLV-III infection follows characteristic patterns. Comparison of the titration curves in the ELISA (Fig. 1) and the immunoblot analysis indicates that the titers of ELISA IgG antibodies rise at least until recognition of all major *gag* and *env* gene products are established. Early responses are directed against *gag* gene products, recognizing $p24^{gag}$ first and $p18^{gag}$ and $Pr55^{gag}$ second. Late responses are directed against *env* and *pol* gene products, recognizing $gp41^{env}$ and p65 first and $Pr110^{env}$ and p33 second. The nature of p33 is still undetermined; however, Chang et al [15] have presented evidence that this protein is encoded by the 3' end of the LAV/HTLV-III *pol* gene and represents the RNase H of the virus.

These changes in LAV/HTLV-III protein recognition patterns as evaluated by immunoblotting allow us to relate an IgG response to the time-lapsed after infection. Acute LAV/HTLV-III infection is characterized by IgG antibodies to *gag* gene products in the absence of antibodies to *env* and *pol* gene products. Chronic LAV/HTLV-III infection is characterized by IgG antibodies to *gag*, *pol*, and *env* gene products. In the chronic phase of infection, IgG antibodies to LAV/HTLV-III were present in the CSF of two of three chimpanzees tested. Evidence was obtained that the titers of these antibodies were disproportional to both albumin and IgG in the CSF of one animal, indicating intrathecal synthesis of IgG antibodies to LAV/HTLV-III. These preliminary data suggest that LAV/HTLV-III can replicate in the brain without apparent symptoms of AIDS or AIDS encephalopathy, paralleling results obtained with visna virus in sheep [16].

Recent studies in humans [17] suggest that the human IgG response parellels the IgG respnose to LAV/HTLV-III in nonhuman primates and indicate that different phases of infection can be determined on the basis of protein recognition patterns. Further studies have to be initated to determine if replication of LAV/HTLV-III in the brain and concomitant intrathecal synthesis of LAV/HTLV-III specific antibodies occurs in asymptomatic phases of human LAV/HTLV-III infection and to predict development of neurological symptoms.

ACKNOWLEDGMENTS

We thank L. Montagnier and R.C. Gallo for providing LAV and HTLV-III. In addition, W. Greer and H.A. Amyx are thanked for taking care of the chimpanzees. E.A.H. Hische, J.A. Tutuarima, and H.J. van der Helm are acknowledged for determination of IgG and albumin levels in CSF and serum. This study was supported by a grant from the Netherlands Foundation for Preventive Medicine.

REFERENCES

1. Barré-Sinoussi F, Chermann JC, Rey F, et al. Isolation of a T-lymphotropic retrovirus from a patient at risk for acquired immune defiency syndrome (AIDS). Science 1983; 220:868–70.
2. Gallo RC, Salahuddin SZ, Popovic M, et al. Frequent detection and isolation of cytopathic retroviruses (HTLV-III) from patients with AIDS and at risk for AIDS. Science 1984; 224:500–3.
3. Safai B, Sarngadharan MG,Groopman et al. Seroepidemiological studies of human T-lymphotropic retrovirus type III in AIDS. Lancet 1984; i:1438–40.
4. Brun-Vezinet F, Rouzioux C, Barré-Sinoussi, et al. Detection of IgG antibodies to LAV by ELISA in patients with AIDS or LAS. Lancet 1984; i:1253–6.
5. Goedert J, Sarngadharan MG, Biggar RJ, et al. Determinants of retrovirus (HTLV-III) antibody and immunodeficiency conditions in homosexual men. Lancet 1984; ii:711–6.
6. Popovic J, Sarngadaharean MG, Read E, Gallo RC. Detection, isolation and continuous production of cytopathic retroviruses (HTLV-III) from patients with AIDS and pre-AIDS. Science 1984; 224:497–500.
7. Feorino P, Kalyanaraman VS, Haverkos HW, et al. Lymphadenopathy associated virus infection of a blood-donor-recipient pair with AIDS. Science 1984; 225:69–72.
8. Groopman J, et al. Virological studies in a case of transfusion associated AIDS. N Engl J Med 1984; 311:1419–22.

9. Alter H, Eichberg JW, Masin H. Transmission of HTLV-III infection from human plasma to chimpanzees: An animal model for AIDS. Science 1984; 226:549–52.

10. Gajdusek D, Gibbs Jr. CJ, Amyx HL, et al. Infection of chimpanzees by human T-lymphotropic retroviruses in brain and other tissues from AIDS patients. Lancet 1985; i:55–6.

11. Lefvert AK, Link H. IgG production within the central nervous system: A critical review of proposed formulae. Ann Neurol 1985; 17:13–20.

12. Tibbling CT, Link H, Öhman S. Principles of albumur and IgG analyses in neurological disorders. I. Establishment of reference values. Scand. J Clin Lab Invest 1977; 37:385–90.

13. Hische E.A.H. van Meegen MTA, van der Helm HJ. More precise determination of the cerebrospinal Fluid IgG index. Clin Chem 1985; 31:1417.

14. Muesing MA, et al. Nucleic acid structure and expression of the human AIDS lymphadenopathy retrovirus. Nature 1985; 313:450–8.

15. Chang NT, Huang J, Ghrayeb J, et al. An HTLV-III peptide produced by recombinat DNA is immunoreactive with sera from patients with AIDS. Nature 1985; 315:151–4.

16. Griffin DE, Narayan O, Bukowski JF, Adams RJ, Chohen SR. The cerebrospinal fluid in visna, a slow viral disease of sheep. Ann Neurol 1978; 4:212–8.

17. Schüpbach J, Haller O, Vogt M, et al. Antibodies to HTLV-III in Swiss patients with AIDS and pre-AIDS in gorups at risk for AIDS. N Engl J Med 1985; 312:265–70.

Cancer Detection and Prevention Supplement 1:515–523 (1987)

Human Lymphocyte Subpopulations: Analysis by Multiparameter Flow Cytometry and Monoclonal Antibodies

Noel L. Warner

Becton Dickinson Monoclonal Center, Inc, Mountain View, CA

Key words: monoclonal antibodies, immunophenotyping, flow cytometry

INTRODUCTION

The analysis of human lymphocyte differentiation has been greatly aided by the advent of many monoclonal antibodies (MAb) against human leukocyte cell surface structures, which at the same time has resulted in considerable confusion about the relationship of antibodies to each other and the various subsets one to the other. The number of such monoclonals is now counted in the hundreds, which has led to a major task of dissecting out those monoclonals that define distinct cell structures and that can be used to classify and characterize lymphocyte populations. A major step in this regard is the leukocyte workshop series [1, 2], and, when relevant, the CD system from this series will be used in this article.

The ultimate goal of immunophenotyping human lymphocyte populations is to define by the use of monoclonals against cell surface structures those specific and distinct lymphocyte subpopulations that mediate particular functions. Monitoring of such populations based on highly specific immunophenotypic patterns may detect changes in numbers of such distinct populations that are either causative or reflective of certain disease processes. This article reviews the current understanding of lymphocyte heterogeneity within the four major families of lymphocytes CD4-positive T cells, CD8-positive T cells, B cells, and NK cells, as revealed by an immunophenotypic analysis of these cells using multiple MAb in a multiparameter flow cytometry approach.

MULTIPARAMETER ANALYSIS

It is an essential premise in the approach to be described in this article that this goal of associating unique, functionally distinct lymphocyte subpopulations with a particular cell surface immunophenotype can *only* be achieved in a realistic and practical way using current monoclonal antileukocyte antibodies when they are combined together in a multiparameter approach. The majority of leukocyte antigens defined by MAb are *not* expressed uniquely on only one particular lymphocyte or leukocyte subpopulation. The first point to note is that a

---

Address reprint requests to Noel L. Warner, Becton Dickinson Monoclonal Center, Inc, 2375 Garcia Avenue, Mountain View, CA 94043.

particular antigen may be restricted in its expression within the lymphoid compartment to only one major subpopulation of lymphocytes and yet outside the lymphoid compartment, be expressed on other cell types. Three examples to illustrate this point are the following antigens: 1) CD4 (Leu-3): expressed uniquely at the cell surface level within the lymphoid compartment on only T lymphocytes of the CD4 subtype and yet also positive on virtually all peripheral blood monocytes at about one-tenth the cell surface density [3, 4] and contained intracytoplasmically in virtually all tissue macrophages [3, 5]; 2) CD16 (Leu-11): Fc receptor structure expressed by virtually all NK cells within the lymphoid compartment, and not expressed by other (Fc receptor-bearing) lymphoid cells [6], yet also expressed on the majority of neutrophils, 3) CD3 (Leu-4): expressed in association with the T cell receptor structure at the membrane level in virtually all mature T cells [7], and no other lymphoid cells, yet also expressed (at least as an epitope) in (or on) Purkinje cells of the cerebellum [8]. This example serves to illustrate the uncertainty that is frequently encountered in these situations of whether the same gene product is expressed in the "other" cell as in lymphocytes or whether this is simply an epitopic cross-reaction involving a different cellular component.

From the perspective of multiparameter analysis, the point that these illustrations demonstrate is that if one is studying a heterogeneous leukocyte population—such as in lysed whole blood—it will be essential to define first the leukocyte compartment containing the population of interest (eg, lymphocytes) and then identify within that compartment those cells that react with the particular antibody. In flow cytometry, this is achieved usually by the principle of biophysical measurements—low forward-angle light scatter, 90° light scatter, or cell volume, alone or in combination, to define the cellular population. Hence it is essential in multiparameter flow analysis first to make use of usually two biophysical parameters to set the leukocyte population windows and then proceed to use multiple fluorescence detectors to analyze the combination of staining given by different MAb tagged with different fluorescent dyes.

The second major point to note is that within lymphocyte populations, there are essentially two types of cell surface antigen expression: 1) lineage-associated and 2) restricted but cross-lineage. For example, anti-Leu-3 within lymphoid cells defines the CD4 T cell lineage compartment (type 1), and anti-Leu-8 defines an antigen that is restricted in expression to only some CD4-positive cells but also to some CD8-positive cells, most B cells, and some NK cells (type 2) [9]. The problems with single parameter analysis are thus that antibodies to type (1) lineage antigens react with *all* cells of the lineage and do not reveal the heterogeneity within the compartment and, second, that antibodies to type 2 restricted antigens may react with some cells of several different lineages, the sum of which has little meaning.

Multiparameter analysis, in which one antibody against a type (1) antigen is combined with another antibody against a type (2) antigen, permits their combined use both to identify the lineage set and see the specific subsets within it. In flow cytometry, the ability to "see" one antibody binding in the presence of the other, and to distinguish both together, is based on the use of different fluorescent dyes, each conjugated to the various MAbs and using appropriate light sources, filtering of emission spectra before detection, and dual compensation networks. Fluorochromes of primary choice are fluorescein isothyocyanate (FITC) and phycoerythrin (PE), together for two-color (two-antibody) analysis, and addition of either Texas red or allophycocyanin for three-color (three-antibody) analysis. All four together in a dual-dye laser configuration permit simultaneous four-antibody analysis. It is the essential premise of this approach that the majority of the functionally significant human lymphocyte compartments can be specifically identified only by such combined simultaneous two- (and even three-) MAb-immunophenotyping. Although this approach has been the province principally of research workers using complex instrumentation, and frequently indirect reagent staining procedures, the availability of direct FITC- and PE-conjugated antibodies and of relatively simple computer-based flow systems, has placed this multiparameter-based approach within routine clinical research programs for immunomonitoring leukocyte subpopulations in various disease states.

LEUKOCYTE DIFFERENTIATION

Leukocyte differentiation can be progressively subdivided into finer degrees of subsetting leukocyte compartments based on various criteria. The scheme depicted in Figure 1 illustrates a series of sequential subdivisions of leukocyte heterogeneity, which can be associated with expression of various MAb-defined cell surface antigens.

Hematopoietic cells. Distinction of the hematopoietic compartment from nonhematopoietic, most conveniently distinguished by the expression of the common (T200) leukocyte antigen on hematopoietic cells [10] and frequently intracellular cytokeratins in nonhematopoietic epithelial cells [11].

Leukocyte lineage. Major pathways of hematopoiesis, namely erythroid, myeloid, lymphoid, and megakaryocytic, usually distinguished either morphologically, by biophysical means, or histochemically. It is of interest to note that there are few (if any) monoclonals that are truly panlineage-specific at this level, for example, reacting with all lymphoid cells of all subtypes, and at all maturation stages, and not with any of the other lineages.

Differentiation sets and lymphocyte subsets. Restricting now to myeloid and lymphoid, these are subdivided, respectively, into the major monocytic and granulocytic pathways and into T and B, and non-T non-B lymphoid cells. Focusing only on lymphoid, these are in turn now divided into four major lymphocyte lineages, which can be defined by particular monoclonals (see discussion below and Tables I and II). This is the last level, however, where monoclonal antibodies as single reagents can define a compartment.

Functional subpopulations. Each of the four major lymphocyte lineages can be further subdivided into at least two and usually more subsets. At this level, distinct functional properties start to become associated with unique immunophenotypes. Thus T helper cells can be distinguished from certain T cells mediating induction functions and T cell suppression from certain types of T cell cytotoxicity.

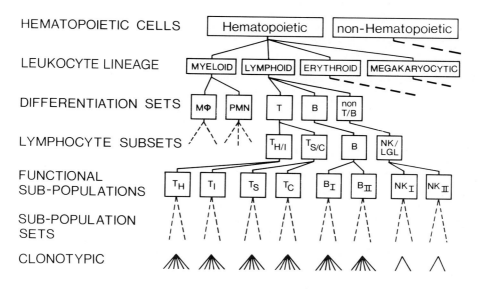

Fig. 1. Leukocyte differentiation.

Further subpopulations. As will be briefly summarized below, further heterogeneity is now becoming evident in some of these T cell compartments. Such subpopulation heterogeneity is, however, still short of the eventual clonotypic heterogeneity (line 7) based on T cell or B cell V gene-determined antigen receptor heterogeneity.

Association of the expression of MAb-defined antigens with the populations defined in lines 4 and 5 is summarized in Tables I and II, and several key points will be briefly explained as follows.

Major Myeloid and Lymphoid Lineages (Table I)

1. Common cell surface antigen (T200) refers to the differential quantitative levels of expression of the common leukocyte antigen being in highest density on lymphoid cells, medium density on monocytes, and lower density on granulocytes. This differential expression can provide a very convenient window to resolve these different compartments in heterogeneous cell populations. "Unique" cell surface antigens are those relatively restricted to only one or a few of the cell lineages within the context of the five compartments shown, whereas "restricted" antigens are expressed on only some subsets but in a cross-lineage fashion. In this article, specific antigens of myeloid cells will not be discussed.

2. Pan-T cell antigens: Of the potential pan-T cell lineage antigens that have been used to characterize *mature* T cells, the CD3 (Leu-4) antigen has become the single most specific and unique marker for this lineage. Points in favor of this notion include the following 1) CD3 (Leu-4) in cell membrane expression is tightly linked to T cell antigen receptor expression, itself the reflection of complete T cell α and β gene rearrangement, which is the essential definition of T cell lineage. 2) CD2 (Leu-5)—E rosette receptor is expressed on the majority of NK cells as well as on T cells. 3) CD5 (Leu-1)—although expressed on the majority of T cells, this is also expressed by a distinct B cell subset. 4) CD7 (Leu-9) is not expressed on all T cells; there is a small subpopulation of CD4 cells that lack CD7 in addition, CD7 is expressed on virtually all NK cells. 5) CD6 (T12), a small but significant subset of CD3-positive T cells, lacks expression of CD6.

3. Pan-NK antigens: Within the context of the five populations shown, there is *no* unique NK marker since most epitopes of the CD16 (Leu-11) antigen are also expressed on granulocytes, restricted to neutrophils (see next section).

4. Pan-B antigen: Three relatively unique non-MHC and non-Ig antigens have been defined as being expressed on virtually all normal mature B cells. These are the CD19 (Leu-12), CD20 (Leu-16), and CD22 (Leu-14) antigens. In view of the broader range of expression

TABLE I. Major Myeloid and Lymphoid Lineage-Associated Antigens

	Monocyte	PMN	LGL/NK	T	B
Common CSA					
T200	+ +	+	+ + +	+ + +	+ + +
"Unique" CSA					
LEU-M3	+	−	−	−	−
(PMN-associated)	−	+	(−)	−	−
CD3 (Leu-4)	−	−	−	+	−
CD19 (Leu-12)	−	−	−	−	+
CD22 (Leu-14)	−	−	−	−	+
Restricted CSA					
CD2 (Leu-5)	−	−	+ / −	+	−
CD7 (Leu-9)	−	−	+	+ / −	−
CD16 (Leu-11)	−	+	+	−	−
CD5 (Leu-1)	−	−	−	+	+ / −
CD4 (Leu-3)	+	−	−	+ / −	−

of the CD19 antigen, being very early in B cell maturation, this potentially serves the broadest value as a pan-B marker.

Major Lymphocyte Subsets

As is summarized in Table II, there are four major compartments of human lymphocytes, which were originally distinguished on the basis of T cell functions, B cells, and the NK/LGL family. Unfortunately, the immunophenotypic approach to lymphocyte differentiation does not exactly mesh with the earliest notions of subsets, and the so-called T helper-inducer versus T cytotoxic-suppressor compartments have frequently resulted in mistaken concepts of the association of certain cell surface antigens with T cell or NK cell functions. The so-called helper-suppressor ratio is an even more unfortunate name; in many clinical situations in which there is a striking change in the helper-suppressor ratio, it has absolutely nothing to do with helper or suppressor cells.

In considering this area of lymphocyte subsets in more detail, it might be of value first to state clearly several points that are frequently overlooked or misunderstood and then to consider these in the context of our current understanding. These points of emphasis are:

Not all CD8 (Leu-2) cells are T cells; some are NK cells.

Hence, the sum of percent CD4 cells and CD8 cells frequently exceeds the percent of CD3 cells but not of CD2 cells.

Not all LGL are NK cells, although most NK cells are LGL.

Leu-7 antigen-bearing cells are not all NK cells.

Not all NK cells express Leu-7.

There are CD4-bearing cytotoxic T cells.

CD11 (Leu-15, OKM1) is not a unique macrophage or macrophage and NK cell marker.

Non-MHC-restricted cytotoxicity is a property of both NK cells and a T cell subset.

With these and several other points in mind, the four main lymphocyte lineages might be minimally but specifically characterized as follows (referring specifically to mature cell stages).

CD4-positive T cells. Express cell surface CD3 and CD4, T cell $V\beta$ and $V\alpha$ gene rearrangement, primarily restricted to class II antigen-associated responses, primarily mediate helper or inducer functions but can also be cytotoxic cells.

CD8-positive T cells. Express cell surface CD3 and CD8 (the latter in high density), T cell $V\beta$ or $V\alpha$ gene rearrangement, primarily restricted to class I antigen associated responses, primarily mediate suppressor or cytotoxic functions.

TABLE II. Major Lymphocyte Subset-Associated Antigens

	T helper-inducer T class II-restricted	T-cytotoxic-suppressor T-class I-restricted	LGL/NK Nonrestricted	B
Common CSA				
None defined that is restricted to all of, but only these subsets				
"Unique" CSA				
CD4 (Leu-3)	+	−	−	−
CD8 (Leu-2)	−	+++	−(+)	−
CD16 (Leu-11)	−	−	+	−
CD19 (Leu-12)	−	−	−	+
Restricted CSA				
Leu-7	−/+	−/+	+/−	−
Leu-8	+/−	+/−	+/−	+/−
CD7 (Leu-9)	+/−	+	+	−
CD11 (Leu-15)	−/+	+/−	+	−

CD16-positive NK cells. Express cell surface CD16, do not rearrange T cell Vβ genes, are not MHC-restricted, primarily mediate cytotoxic functions, are large granular lymphocytes.

CD19-positive B cells. Express cell surface CD19, CD20, and CD22; rearrange Ig V genes in productive fashion; bear membrane immunoglobulin; are not MHC restricted.

Each of these four lymphocyte lineages is heterogeneous. Each contains both multiple functional properties, is heterogeneous in sensitivity to activation by various lymphokines, antigens, and other stimuli; and is heterogeneous in immunophenotype.

Considerable research effort has been focused on the goal of dissecting the heterogeneity within each of these compartments and attempting to *correlate* the variable parameters of phenotype, function, and susceptibility to activation, one with the other. The following section briefly summarizes some current results and interpretations in this area, using as a primary base the immunophenotypic dissection by two- (or three-) color multiparameter analysis.

NK Cell

The majority of NK cells are large granular lymphocytes that express CD16 (Leu-11), CD11 (Leu-15), and Leu-19 (NKH-1) as three primarily NK- associated antigens, and most NK cells also express CD2 (Leu-5) and CD7 (Leu-9). The major subdivision of NK cells is based on the pairing of anti-Leu-7 with anti-Leu-11 (CD16) [6]. This multiparameter analysis defines two populations of NK cells, Leu-7$^+$, 11$^+$ and Leu-7$^-$, 11$^+$. Functional distinctions between these two types of NK cells have been reviewed elsewhere [9], and a possible maturation scheme within the NK compartment has been proposed by Lanier and Phillips [13].

NK subpopulations can also be defined phenotypically on the basis of splitting CD16 (Leu-11)-positive (CD3-negative) cells with monoclonals against CD8, yielding two subpopulations of CD16 cells, one negative for CD8 and one expressing low-density CD8. These CD8 (Leu-2)-positive NK cells are not T cells and do not show significant differences in NK reactivity from other NK cells.

The major confusion about NK cells and phenotypic markers is not so much the disposition of markers within the NK lineage but rather that several markers considered initially as NK-specific are also found outside the NK compartment. Thus many Leu-7-positive cells are not NK cells but are T cells, and many NK cells do not possess Leu-7. Similarly, the Leu-19 (NKH-1) antigen, although present on virtually all NK cells, is also present on a subset of T cells (CD3-positive) that also mediate non-MHC restricted cytotoxicity [14]. The NK compartment has thus become reasonably well defined, and shows no clear differentiation relationship to the T cell lineage. Current research with this lineage is directed to an understanding of the maturation relationships of the presently defined subsets, with particular attention to the precursor stages.

B Cells

Several decades of studies of B cell maturation have led to a reasonable understanding of the pathways of differentiation of B cells following activation. However, recent immunophenotypic studies with cell surface markers that are not related to class II MHC antigens or Ig molecules have strongly indicated that there are distinct subsets of B cells.

Virtually all mature B cells express antigens CD19, CD20, and CD22, with CD19 being expressed very early in B cell maturation. Similarly, virtually all B cells express class II antigens HLA-DP, -DQ, and -DR; membrane immunoglobulin of μ and σ types; and CRII receptors. When any of these are paired with several other monoclonals, distinct B cell subsets can be found. This has been observed using anti-Leu-1 (CD5) and anti-Leu-17 (OKT10-like). In the former instance, two-color analysis using anti-Leu-1 paired with anti-Leu-4 shows a small subset of Leu-1$^+$ Leu-4$^-$ cells, in peripheral blood, which are of low-density CD5 and are the same cells as those CD5 that are B cells by other definitions. This Leu-1 B cell compartment in normal adult blood comprises 5–20% of the B cells, hence only about 1% of the total lymphocytes. Of particular interest is the possible association between murine Ly-1b cells and autoantibody production [15].

A second immunophenotypic split of tissue (tonsillar) B cells has recently been found by Ault et al [12], who showed that germinal center B cells express moderate CD20 cell surface density and no detectable Leu-17 antigen, whereas mantle B cells have high cell surface density of both Leu-17 and CD20 antigens. The possible functional significance of these subpopulations is under investigation.

CD4-Positive T Cells

The CD4 family of T cells can be subdivided into at least five major compartments based on a series of immunophenotypic studies and in some instances on correlated functional studies. This approach involves pairing anti-Leu-3 with several other antibodies, including anti-Leu-7, anti-Leu-9, anti-Leu-8, and anti-Leu-18. These studies can be summarized thus.

1. Leu-3,-7: A distinct subset of CD4$^+$, Leu-7$^+$ cells can be readily detected in germinal centers of lymphoid tissue and as a rare (usually <2%) subset of peripheral blood lymphocytes. Little is known of the function of these cells; however, they may be involved in B cell regulation [16].

2. Leu-3,-9: Anti-Leu-9 (CD7) reacts with virtually all CD8-positive T cells and most CD16-positive NK cells but not quite all of the CD4-positive T cells. The CD4$^+$ Leu-9$^-$ cells have not been associated with any unique function but are frequently found represented in *Mycosis fungoides* cases.

3. Leu-3,-8: The studies of Engleman and colleagues [9] have clearly established that the CD4$^+$, Leu-8$^-$ cells comprise only about 20% of the CD4 cells but contain virtually all T cell help function for immunoglobulin production. Conversely, the major population of CD4$^+$, Leu-8$^+$ cells contains suppressor inducer functional cells.

4. Leu-3,-18: Recent studies in our laboratories have shown that the Leu-18 antigen, a T200-like glycoprotein expressed on several T cell subsets, reacts in a similar fashion to the 2H4 antigen and reciprocally (mutually exclusively) within both CD4 and CD8 subsets to the 4B4 antigen. Thus Leu-3, CD4$^+$ cells that are 2H4$^+$ are Leu-18$^+$ but 4B4$^-$.

The function of T cell help and suppressor induction are associated respectively with the CD4$^+$, 4B4$^+$, ie, Leu-18$^-$ and CD4$^+$, 4B4$^-$, ie, Leu-18$^+$ subsets. These latter two groupings of monoclonals may be reconciled in the following manner. CD4$^+$ cells are divided into a minor CD4$^+$, Leu-8$^-$ set that has T cell help function and is also 4B4$^+$ or Leu-18$^-$ [17]. Since the 4B4 antigen is expressed on approximately twice as many CD4$^+$ cells as those that are Leu-8$^-$, Leu-18 or 4B4 must also split within the CD4$^+$, Leu-8$^+$ group. Hence the three major CD4 compartments based on these monoclonal antibodies are 1) CD4$^+$, Leu-8$^-$, Leu-18$^-$ (4B4$^+$)—T cell help for Ig secretion, 2) CD4$^+$, Leu-8$^+$, Leu-18$^+$ (4B4$^-$)—T cell suppressor-inducer function, and CD4$^+$, Leu-8$^+$, Leu-18$^-$(4B4$^+$)—unknown function.

The clearest pairing of monoclonal antibodies that defines these subsets are therefore: 1) T$_H$—CD4$^+$, Leu-8$^-$ and 2) T$_{SI}$—CD4$^+$, Leu-18$^+$. Studies are in progress to determine further possible functional association with these phenotypes.

CD8-Positive T Cells

Many studies have extensively documented the heterogeneity within this compartment that is revealed by pairing with anti-CD8 (Leu-2) the monoclonal antibodies against: Leu-7, Leu-8, Leu-15, and Leu-18. All four divisions of the CD8 compartment are clearly different, and the relationship between these subgroups have yet to be fully defined. The following brief comments pertain to this matter.

Cytotoxicity. Most cytotoxic T cells lack the CR3 receptor (CD11,Leu-15) and reciprocally express the 9.3 antigen [18]. In addition, it has been shown by Lanier et al (unpublished) that the Leu-2$^+$, 7$^+$cells can also be activated by anti-CD3 monoclonals to express cytotoxic functions. The phenotype of class I restricted cytotoxic T cells may therefore be CD8$^+$ (Leu-2$^+$), Leu-7$^+$, Leu-15$^-$. It is relevant to note that this is the population elevated in ARC, AIDS, and associated high-risk patients [19].

Suppression. Reciprocally, the CD8$^+$, -15$^+$ cells have been shown to mediate certain suppressor functions [20]. Since CD11 (Leu-15) is also expressed on most NK cells, some of which are CD8$^+$, it is essential to delineate between two distinct phenotypes (both Leu-2$^+$, -15$^+$), one T cell and one NK cell, which may both, in selected instances, mediate suppressor function. These populations are: Ts— CD3$^+$, CD8^{+++}, CD11$^+$, CD16$^-$ (ie, Leu-4$^+$, -2^{+++}, 15$^+$, 11$^-$) and NK cell subset—CD3$^-$, CD8$^+$, CD11$^+$, CD16$^+$ (ie, Leu-4$^-$, -2$^+$, -15$^+$, -11$^+$). Extensive analysis of the suppressor subset family by Engleman and associates has revealed several distinct phenotypic compartments (see Table III).

CONCLUSIONS

This brief, essentially highly summarized report on lymphocyte heterogeneity (summarized further in part in Table III) has tried to stress several key components in this quest for specific immunophenotypic definition of functionally relevant lymphocyte subsets. The goal is clearly attainable. Current two-, three-, and four-color simultaneous analysis will eventually clarify each of the interrelationships presently recognized and yield a final definition of the number of phenotypically *and* functionally distinct subsets of lymphocytes. It is already apparent that each of the four major lymphocyte families *is* heterogeneous and can be delineated, not by use of single monoclonals but by the multiparameter application of (at least) pairs of such monoclonals. This approach has now reached a routine level of utility in clinical research, and further studies of this type may reveal in more detail the selective changes in lymphocyte subpopulations that can occur in various immunologically induced or immunologically associated diseases.

TABLE III. Functional Lymphocyte Subpopulations

T cell	Help	Leu-3$^+$,-8^-
	Suppressor-inducer	Leu-3$^+$,-18^+
	Cytotoxic	Leu-2^+,-15^-
	Suppressor	Leu-2$^+$,-15^+
Suppression	Suppressor-inducer	Leu-3$^+$,-8^+
	Suppressor-amplifier	Leu-2$^+$,-8^+
	Suppressor-amplifier (act.)	Leu-2$^+$$-8^+$,$-DR^+$
	Suppressor-effector	Leu-2$^+$,8$^-$,-15^+
Cytoxicity	Class I-restricted	Leu-2$^+$,-7^+,-15^-
	Class II-restricted	Leu-3$^+$
	Non-MHC-restricted (NK)	Leu-7$^+$$-11^+$
		Leu-7$^-$,-11^+
		Leu-7$^-$,-11^+,$^-DR^+$
B cell populations subsets		Leu-12$^+$14$^+$$\kappa/\lambda^+DR^+$CRII$^+$
		Leu-12$^+$,1$^+$
		Leu-12$^+$,-1^-
		Leu-12$^+$,8$^+$
		Leu-12$^+$,8$^-$

REFERENCES

1. Bernard A, Boumsell L, Dausset J, Milstein C, Schlossman SF, eds. Leukocyte typing. New York: Springer Verlag, 1984.
2. Reinherz EL, Haynes BF, Nadler LM, Bernstein ID. Leukocyte typing II. New York: Springer Verlag, 1986.
3. Wood, GS, Warner NL, Warnke RA. Leu-3 antigen is expressed by cells of monocyte/macrophage and Langerhans lineage. J Immunol 1983; 131:212.
4. Warner NL, Kimura JY, Recktenwald DJ. Multiparameter flow cytometry analysis of normal and neoplastic human monocytes with Leu monoclonal antibodies. In: Monoclonal antibodies. Tom B, Allison J, eds. New York: Plenum Press, 1983.
5. Moscicki RA, Amento EP, Krane SM, Kurnick JT, Colvin RB. Modulation of surface antigens of a human monocyte cell line, U937, during incubation with T lymphocyte-conditioned medium: Detection of T4 antigen and its presence on normal blood monocytes. J Immunol 1983; 131:743.
6. Lanier LL, Le AM, Phillips JH, Warner NL, Babcock GF. Subpopulations of human natural killer cells defined by expression of the Leu-7 (HNK-1) and Leu-11 (NK-5) antigens. J Immunol, 1982; 131:1789.
7. Reinherz EL, Meuer SC, Fitgerald KA, Hussey RE, Hodgdon JC, Acuto O, Schlossman SF: Comparison of T3-associated 49- and 43- kilodalton cell surface molecules on individual human T-cell clones: evidence for peptide variability in the T cell receptor structures. Proc. Natl. Acad Sci (U.S.A.) 80:4104–4108 (1983).
8. Garson JA, Beverley PCL, Coakham HB, Harper EI. Monoclonal antibodies against human T lymphocytes label Purkinje neurones of many species. Nature 1982; 298:375.
9. Krensky AM, Lanier LL, Engleman EG. Lymphocyte subsets and surface molecules in man. Clin Immunol Rev 1985; 4:95.
10. Beverley PCL. Production and use of monoclonal antibodies in transplantation immunology. Transplant Clin Immunol 1980; 9:87–94.
11. Makin CA, Bobrow LG, Bodmer WF., Monoclonal antibody to cytokeratin for use in routine histopathology. J Clin Pathol 1984; 37:975.
12. Ault KA, and Gadol N. Unpublished observations.
13. Lanier LL, Phillips JH. A schema for the classification of cytotoxic lymphocytes based on T cell antigen receptor gene rearrangement and Fc receptor (CD16) or NKH-1/Leu 19 antigen expression. In: Proceedings of the International Symposium on Natural Immunity, RB Herberman, et al, eds. Krager, New York.
14. Lanier LL, Le AM, Civin CI, Loken MR, Phillips JH. "The relationship of CD16 (LEU 11) and Leu 19 (NKH-1) antigen expression on human peripheral blood NK cells and cytotoxic T lymphocytes. J Immunol 1986; 136:4480.
15. Hayakawa K, Hardy RR, Honda M, Herzenberg LA, Steinberg AD. Ly-1 B cells: Functionally distinct lymphocytes that secrete IgM autoantibodies. Proc Natl Acad Sci USA 1984; 81:2494.
16. Grossi, CE, Velardi A. Multiple marker analysis of human T-helper (Leu3$^+$) lymphocytes in blood and lymphoid tissues. Pinchera A, Doria G, Dammacco F, Bargellesi A, eds. Monoclonal antibodies '84: Biological and clinical applications. 1985, p129.
17. Morimoto C, Letvin N, Boyd A, Hagan M, Brown H, Kornacki M, Schlossman F. The isolation and characterization of the human helper inducer T cell subset. J Immunol 1985; 134:6.
18. Yamada H, Martin P, Bean M, Braun M, Beatty P, Sadamoto K, Hansen J. Monoclonal antibody 9.3 and anti-CD11 antibodies define reciprocal subsets of lymphocytes.1985; 15:1164–8.
19. Stites D, Casavant C, McHugh T, Moss A, Beal S, Ziegler J, Saunders A, Warner N. Flow cytometric analysis of lymphocyte phenotypes in AIDS using monoclonal antibodies and simultaneous dual immunofluorescence. Clin Immunol Immunopathol 1986; 38:161–77.
20. Landay A, Gartland L, and Clement LT. Characterization of a phenotypically distinct subpopulation of Leu·2$^+$ cells which suppresses T cell proliferative responses. J Immunol 1983; 131:2757.

Cancer Detection and Prevention Supplement 1:525–533 (1987)

AIDS and Lymphadenopathy Syndrome (LAS) Patients Display Similar Abnormal In Vitro Proliferation and Differentiation of T-Colony Forming Cells (T- CFC)

Yanto Lunardi Iskandar
Vassilis Georgoulias
Willy Rozenbaum
Daniel Vittecoq

Patrice Meyer
Marc Gentilini
Claude Jasmin

Unité d'Oncogénèse Appliquée (INSERM U-268) (Y.L.I., V.G., C.J.) and Institut de Cancérologie et d'Immunogénétique (ICIG) (P.M.) Hôpital Paul Brousse Villejuif, France; Département de Maladies infectieuses, Hôpital Saint-Louis, Service du Pr. Modai, France (D.V.); Département de Santé Publique et de Médecine Tropicale, Hôpital Pitié Salpêtrière, Paris, France (W.R., M.G.)

ABSTRACT   T-cell colonies were generated from the peripheral blood and bone marrow of 61 patients with acquired immunodeficiency syndrome (AIDS), 54 patients with persistent lymphadenopathy syndrome (LAS), 14 clinically normal male homosexuals, and 17 healthy heterosexuals. Mononuclear cells were cultured in methylcellulose in the presence of IL2-containing conditioned medium. The number of T-cell forming cells (T-CFC) from healthy male homosexuals and AIDS and LAS patients was significantly (P < 0.01) reduced compared to T-CFC from healthy heterosexuals. In AIDS patients, the low colony growth capacity of T-CFC was independent of the presence of either opportunistic infections or Kaposi sarcoma. Twelve LAS patients who subsequently developed AIDS showed the lowest capacity of peripheral blood and bone marrow T-CFC to proliferate. Pooled induced colonies from AIDS and LAS patients and normal homosexuals were composed of immature cells bearing the $T3^+$, $T4^+$, $T6^+$, and $T8^+$ surface phenotype, unlike colonies from normal heterosexuals, which displayed mature cells bearing the $T3^+$, $T4^+$, $T6^-$, and $T3^+$, $T8^+$, $T6^-$ surface phenotype. Moreover, most T-CFC from primary colonies had lost their self-renewal capacity. In some AIDS and LAS patients but not healthy homosexuals peripheral blood and bone marrow T-CFC were capable of generating colonies with recombinant IL2 (rIL2) without any other mitogenic stimulation. The rIL2-induced colony growth was abrogated by a monoclonal antibody against the IL2 receptor. These results suggest that early impairment of T-CFC plays a predominant role in the pathogenesis of AIDS.

Address reprint requests to Dr. Y. Lunardi-Iskandar, Unité d'Oncogénèse Appliquée (INSERM U-268), Hôpital Paul Brousse 14-16 Av Paul Vaillant Couturier, 94800 Villejuif, France.

Key words: T-cell colonies, lymphadenopathy syndrome

INTRODUCTION

A number of assays for the growth of T-cell colonies in semisolid media have been developed [1–5] that allow the detection and study of differentiation capacity of peripheral blood and bone marrow T-colony forming cells (T-CFC) in normal subjects [6–8] and in patients with a variety of pathological conditions [9–11]. The T-CFC of normal subjects have either an immature E^-T3^- (displaying neither receptors for sheep erythrocytes nor T3 molecule) or the presumably mature (E^+, $T3^+$) phenotype [7,8]. T-cell colony growth from peripheral blood and bone marrow T-CFC requires stimulation with phytohemagglutinin (PHA) and/or the addition of IL2-containing conditioned medium to the cultures [7,8]. Colonies are composed of mature T cells bearing mainly the $T3^+$ and $T4^+$ surface phenotypes [7,8], but some $T3^+$ and $T8^+$ cells have been also detected [12].

Patients with acquired immune deficiency syndrome (AIDS) have significant qualitative and quantitative T-lymphocyte modifications including (1) decreased absolute numbers of $T4^+$ cells resulting in the inversion of $T4^+/T8^+$ ratio [13], (2) reduction of T-cell proliferative responses to alloantigens and mitogens, (3) decreased IL-2 production [13], and (4) reduced proportion of circulating T lymphocyte expressing IL2 receptors after PHA stimulation. Finally, at advanced stages of the disease, a severe lymphopenia affecting all T-cell subsets is usually observed [13].

The lymphadenopathy syndrome (LAS) is defined as a syndrome of unexplained lymphadenopathy of more than 3 months duration at two or more extrainguinal sites [14–16] in high-risk patients. These patients present qualitative and quantitative T-lymphocyte modifications similar to those of AIDS patients, and prospective epidemiological studies suggest that about 10% of them will ultimately develop AIDS, opportunistic infections, or Kaposi sarcoma [13].

The qualitative and quantitative abnormalities in T lymphocytes and the evolution of the disease seem to indicate a primary involvement of T-cell precursors in the pathogenesis of AIDS. We therefore studied the proliferation and differentiation capacity of T-CFC in clinically normal male homosexuals and AIDS and LAS patients.

PATIENTS AND METHODS
Patients

Heparinized peripheral blood and bone marrow were obtained from 61 AIDS patients fulfilling the criteria defined by the Centers for Disease Control (CDC) [17, 18], 54 LAS patients, 14 clinically normal male homosexuals, and 17 healthy heterosexuals. All but two AIDS patients were male homosexuals. Both AIDS and LAS patients displayed serum antibodies against the lymphadenopathy-associated virus (LAV) as detected by ELISA and/or Western blot [19,20].

In LAS patients, cytological studies of lymph node biopsy sections revealed no evidence of malignant disease and were compatible with a diagnosis of LAS [15]. All patients were studied upon presentation before any treatment was applied.

Cell Separation

Peripheral blood (PBMC) and bone marrow (BMMC) mononuclear cells were obtained after Ficoll-Hypaque (Pharmacia Fine Chemicals, Uppsalla, Sweden) density centrifugation (d = 1.077). Interface cells were washed with Hanks balanced salt solution (HBSS) and resuspended in growth medium (α-MEM, Gibco, Grand Island, NY) at 10^6/ml.

T-Cell Colony Assay

Cells (5×10^5/ml; MNC or cell fractions) were seeded in 0.8% methylcellulose (Fluka, Bachs, Switzerland) in α-MEM supplemented with 20% (v/v) heat-inactivated fetal calf serum

(FCS; Gibco), 2 mM L glutamine, and antibiotics in the presence and the absence of 20% (v/v) PHA-leukocyte conditioned medium. This conditioned medium (PHA-LCM) was a 7 day supernatant from PHA (PHA-M 1%, v/v; Difco, Detroit, MI stimulated normal PBMC (10 cells/ml in α MEM supplemented with 10% FCS and 2 mM L-glutamine) and contained 0.2 U/ml of IL2 activity when tested on an IL2-dependent human T-cell line [21]. In addition, cells were seeded in the presence of 0.5 U/ml of recombinant IL2 (rIL2; a gift from Biogen, Switzerland). One-tenth milliliter of the methylcellulose-containing cell preparation was seeded per well in 96-well flat-bottomed microtest plates. Cultures were incubated for 5–7 days at 37°C in 5% CO_2 in air, and aggregates containing more than 50 cells were counted as colonies under an inverted microscope. In some experiments, 5×10^5 cells/ml were incubated for 45 min at 37°C with increasing concentrations (10^{-3}–10^{-7}) of anti-Tac monoclonal antibody, which recognizes the IL2 receptors (IL2-R; kindly provided by Dr. T.A. Waldmann, NIH). The cells were washed extensively and seeded in methylcellulose in the absence or presence of IL2 as above.

Self-Renewal Capacity

The clonogenic capacity of T-CFC was studied by two culture procedures. First, PBMC or BMMC (10^6 cells/ml) were incubated in growth medium supplemented with 10% FCS and 2 mM L-glutamine for 4 days at 37°C in 5% CO_2 in air. Washed viable cells (5×10^5/ml) were seeded in methylcellulose as described above (delayed plating). The second method was to pick individual, primary spontaneous colonies and pool and dissociate them by pipetting. After washing, 5×10^4 viable cells/ml were seeded as for primary colony growth in the absence or presence of PHA-LCM.

Phenotypic Characterization of PBMC, BMMC, and Colony Cells

Suspensions of PBMC and BMMC were phenotyped using a panel of monoclonal antibodies including the OKT series (Ortho, Ratiran, NJ), the T11 (Coultronics, Hialeah, FL), which recognizes SRBC receptors and fluoresceinated goat antimouse immunoglobulin (Cappel, Cochranville, PA) as a second reagent. Positive cells were counted using an Ortho Sepctrum III analyzer using a minimum sample size of 2,000 cells.

Colonies of the same size and morphology were individually picked, pooled, dissociated, and washed with HBSS. Colony cells were resuspended in phosphate-buffered saline supplemented with 0.01% sodium azide and 2% FCS and phenotyped by indirect immunofluorescence using the OKT series monoclonal antibodies. Nonspecific immunofluorescence was always less than 5%. At least 50–100 cells were evaluated for each determination. Slides were also prepared by cytocentrifugation and stained with May-Grunwald Giemsa for morphological examination.

Statistical Analysis

Statistical comparison of the mean values was made using Student's t test.

RESULTS
Peripheral Blood and Bone Marrow T-Cell Colony Formation From AIDS and LAS Patients

Healthy heterosexuals PBMC and BMMC generated a relatively high number of colonies in the presence of PHA-LCM (370 ± 179 and $248 \pm 86/5 \times 10^4$ cells, respectively; Table I). PHA-LCM-induced colony formation from AIDS patients' PBMC and BMMC was significantly decreased ($P < 0.001$). Indeed, in 43 of 61 patients, less than 50 colonies/5×10^4 PBMC were obtained, whereas in 16 of 30 patients BMMC did not generate colonies.

Peripheral blood and bone marrow T-CFC from LAS patients also demonstrated a very low colony growth capacity (61 ± 93 and 35 ± 53 colonies/5×10^4 cells, respectively; Table

TABLE I. T-Cell Colony Formation From AIDS and LAS Patients*

Group	PBMC†		BMMC‡	
	n	PHA-LCM	n	PHA-LCM
AIDS	61	108 ± 174§	30	76 ± 129
LAS	54	61 ± 93	19	35 ± 53
LAS-AIDS	12	17 ± 13	3	1 ± 2
Healthy male homosexuals	14	189 ± 52	7	185 ± 76
Healthy heterosexuals	17	370 ± 179	8	248 ± 86

*Cells (5 × 10^5/ml) were seeded in methylcellulose (0.8%, V/V) in growth medium supplemented with 20% FCS, 2 mM L-glutamine, and 20% (V/V) PHA-LCM. Cultures were incubated as described in Patients and Methods, and aggregates containing more than 50 cells were counted as colonies.
†Peripheral blood mononuclear cells.
‡Bone marrow mononuclear cells.
§Mean number of calories ± SD/5 × 10^4 cells.

TABLE II. T-Cell Colony Growth According to the Clinical Presentation of AIDS Patients

Clinical presentation	No. of colonies (mean ± SD)/5 × 10^4 cells	
	PBMC (n)	BMMC (n)
Kaposi sarcoma	129 ± 140 (13)	68 ± 85 (8)
Kaposi sarcoma + opportunistic infection	156 ± 240 (9)	99 ± 79 (12)
Opportunistic infection	79 ± 158 (40)	87 ± 169 (12)

I). PBMC from 22 of 54 patients and BMMC from ten of 21 patients did not give rise to colony formation at all.

It is interesting to note that LAS patients who subsequently developed AIDS during the 24 months of the study generated an extremely low number of colonies from both the PBMC and BMMC (Table I). Conversely, the colony growth capacity of PBMC and BMMC from clinically healthy male homosexuals, although lower than that of healthy heterosexuals (P < 0.01), was significantly higher than in LAS and AIDS patients (Table I).

Colony formation from BMMC does not seem to be significantly modified according to the clinical presentation of AIDS patients (Table II). Conversely, PBMC-derived colony formation was extremely decreased in patients presenting with opportunistic infections (79 ± 158 colonies/5 × 10^4 cells; Table II), whereas those who had Kaposi sarcoma with or without opportunistic infections displayed relatively higher numbers of colonies (Table II).

rIL2-Induced Colony Formation From PBMC and BMMC of AIDS and LAS Patients

PBMC from nine of 61 and five of 54 AIDS and LAS patients respectively, could be induced to generate colonies with rIL2 without any mitogenic stimulation (Table III). In 18 AIDS patients, 0–10% (mean ± SD 3 ± 6%) of the PBMC could be stained with the anti-Tac moAb. However, there was no correlation between the rIL2-induced colony formation and the percentage of Tac^+ cells, since patients with 10% Tac^+ PBMC failed to generate colonies. The same was observed in eight LAS patients. rIL2 could also induce the colony formation in five of 30 and three of 21 BMMC from AIDS and LAS patients, respectively (Table III). Again, in seven AIDS patients there was no correlation between the percentage of Tac^+ BMMC and the number of colonies, since Tac^- BMMC could be induced to proliferate in vitro with rIL2 (not shown).

Anti-Tac moAb was able to inhibit the rIL2-colony formation from either PBMC or BMMC of AIDS patients (Fig. 1). The same effect of anti-Tac has already been observed in rIL2-induced colony growth from T-CFC of LAS patients (manuscript submitted).

TABLE III. rIL2-Induced T Cell Colony Formation From LAS and AIDS Patients*

Group	PBMC†		BMMC‡	
	n	rIL2	n	rIL2
AIDS	61	53 ± 174§	30	61 ± 180
LAS	54	21 ± 81	19	12 ± 33
LAS-AIDS	12	0	3	0
Healthy male homosexuals	14	0	7	0
Healthy heterosexuals	17	0	8	0

*Cells (5×10^5/ml) were seeded in methylcellulose in the presence of 0.5 U/ml of rIL2 as described in Patients and Methods.
†Peripheral blood mononuclear cells.
‡Bone marrow mononuclear cells.
§Mean number of colonies ±SD/5×10^4 cells.

Phenotypic Characterization of Colony Cells

As is shown in Table IV, T-cell colonies from normal subjects were composed of mature lymphoblastoid cells bearing the $T3^+$, $T4^+$, or $T8^+$ phenotype. The percentage of $T6^+$ cell detected in the colonies was only 17% (Table IV). PBMC-derived induced colonies from AIDS and LAS patients were composed of significantly more $T4^+$ (50–80%, P < 0.01), $T6^+$ (44–87%, P < 0.01), and $T8^+$ (42–80%, P < 0.001) cells than colonies from normal subjects. Interestingly, PBMC-derived colonies from clinically normal homosexuals were also composed of significantly more $T6^+$ (50–77%, P < 0.01) and $T8^+$ (40–60%, P < 0.05) but not $T4^+$ cells (Table IV). rIL2-induced colonies from both AIDS and LAS patients were also composed of $T3^+$, $T6^+$, $T4^+$, and $T8^+$ cells, and the proportion of positive cells for each antigen was not significantly different from that of PHA-LCM-induced colonies (not shown).

Self-Renewal Capacity

Cells from pooled, primary spontaneous colonies were replated in methylcellulose in order to evaluate their self-renewal capacity in the absence and presence of added growth factors. In five AIDS and three LAS patients studied, no secondary colony growth could be obtained (data not shown). The proliferative capacity of peripheral blood T-CFC was also tested after a 4 day liquid culture of PBMC in the absence of added growth factors or/and mitogen. This delayed plating efficiency has been proposed as a measure of the proliferative capacity of the clonogenic cells [22]. In seven AIDS and three LAS patients and five control homosexuals, no delayed spontaneous colony growth could be obtained. Similarly, in six of seven AIDS patients and in all LAS and control homosexuals, delayed colony formation induced with PHA-LCM was significantly decreased (Table V). Conversely, in normal heterosexuals, the delayed plating yielded half of the observed immediate colony number (Table V).

DISCUSSION

The aim of these investigations was to study quantitatively and qualitatively the peripheral blood and bone marrow T-CFC of AIDS and LAS patients as well as of healthy male homosexuals. Indeed, patients showed an extremely low growth capacity, which was significantly decreased in those who subsequently developed AIDS. Similarly, we [23,24] and others [25,26] have shown impaired T-cell colony formation from PBMC of hemophiliacs with lymphadenopathy, AIDS, and other LAS patients.

In previous studies [25,26], T-cell colony formation was obtained by PHA stimulation of patients' PBMC without the addition of IL2; exogenous IL2 enhanced the colony growth, suggesting that the low plating efficiency observed in these studies is due to the impaired capacity of IL2 production by patients' PHA-stimulated T cells [27].

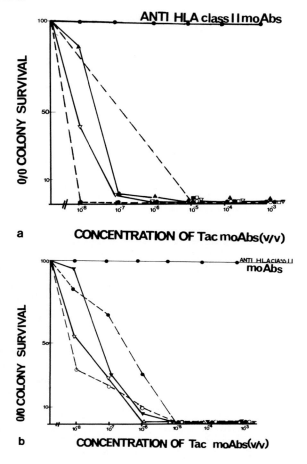

Fig. 1. a, Inhibition of IL2-induced T-cell colony formation with anti-Tac moAb. PBMC and/or BMMC (5×10^5 cells/ml) were incubated with increasing concentrations of either anti-Tac or a pool of three anti-HLA class II moAbs at 37°C for 1 hr. Extensively washed cells were seeded in methylcellulose in the presence of purified IL2 as described in Patients and Methods. Each sign represents a different patient: ▲, No. 1 (PBMC); ▽, No. 2 (PBMC); ●, No. 1 (BMMC); ○, No. 2 (BMMC); ■, No. 3 (BMMC); □, No. 4 (BMMC). b, Inhibition of spontaneous T-cell colony formation with anti-Tac moAb. PBMC and/or BMMC (5×10^5 cells/ml) were incubated with increasing concentrations of either anti-Tac or a pool of three anti-HLA class II moAbs at 37°C for 1 hr. Extensively washed cells were seeded in methylcellulose in the absence of added growth factors and mitogenic stimulation as described in Patients and Methods. Each sign represents a different patient: ▼, No. 1 (PBMC); △, No. 2 (PBMC); ●, No. 1 (BMMC); ○, No. 2 (BMMC).

In our experiments, colony formation was induced with crude conditioned medium containing both IL2 and very low amounts of PHA (0.001%). Contaminant PHA could not yield colony growth, whereas as little as 0.1 u/ml of IL2 is sufficient for normal T-cell colony formation [8]. Moreover, aggregates containing more than 50 cells were considered as colonies, whereas in the above-mentioned studies aggregates with as few as 25 cells counted as colonies. These methodological differences seem to indicate that the two different culture conditions recognize distinct T-CFC subsets and could explain our observation that IL2-containing conditioned medium did not enhance the plating efficiency.

TABLE IV. Phenotypic Characterization of Induced T-Cell Colonies From PBMC of AIDS and LAS Patients and Healthy Homosexuals and Healthy Heterosexuals*

Group	n	Mean ± SD percentage of positive cells			
		T3	T4	T6	T8
AIDS	12	67 ± 7	70 ± 8	73 ± 9	68 ± 4
LAS	7	64 ± 23	67 ± 30	74 ± 25	77 ± 24
Healthy male homosexuals	8	79 ± 9	60 ± 11	50 ± 14	48 ± 15
Healthy heterosexuals	7	75 ± 5	47 ± 13	17 ± 5	35 ± 4

*Individual colonies were pooled and washed colony cells were stained with various moAbs by indirect immunofluorescence.

TABLE V. Clonogenic Capacity of Peripheral Blood T-CFC From AIDS and LAS Patients

Group	n	Immediate plating (PHA-LCM)	Delayed plating*	
			MEM	PHA-LCM
AIDS	7	135 ± 180†	0	49 ± 100
LAS	3	189 ± 157	0	10 ± 10
Healthy homosexuals	5	203 ± 46	0	0
Healthy heterosexuals	7	370 ± 179	0	185 ± 86

*PBMC/(10^6 ml) were incubated for 3 days in culture medium in the absence of added growth factors or mitogens. Washed cells were subsequently seeded in methylcellulose in the presence and absence of PHA-LCM and the cultures incubated as described in Patients and Methods.
†Mean No. of colonies ± SD/5×10^4 cells.

An interesting observation in our study was that AIDS patients who had opportunistic infections had an extremely low number of colonies. Patients who presented with Kaposi sarcoma with/without opportunistic infection generated significantly more colonies than the previous group of patients, indicating that the low colony forming capacity of T-CFC from these patients is independent of the occurrence of opportunistic infections.

We have previously reported that PBMC from some AIDS [23] and LAS [24] patients as well as lymph node mononuclear cells from LAS patients [24] can generate colonies in the absence of added growth factor(s). In the present study, we demonstrated that rIL2 can also induce colony formation from T-CFC of some patients. Moreover, anti-Tac moAB could abrogate this rIL2-induced colony formation. Taken together, these observations strongly suggest that some patients' T-CFC are already activated cells bearing IL2 receptors [28,29]. The low proportion of Tac$^+$ cells detected is not contrary to this finding, since T-CFCs represent a very small subset of T cells (usually two or three clonogenic cells/10^3 PBMC [8]). A similar phenomenon has been observed in some human malignant T-cell lines [30] and in T-CFC from some patients with malignancies [9].

Patients' T-CFC displayed no self-renewal as well as a very low proliferating capacity. This observation, taken together with the fact that some T-CFC are already activated cells, seems to indicate that the majority of T-CFC are cycling and fully committed cells. This hypothesis is compatible with previous observations that mice inoculated with the myeloprolif-erative sarcoma virus (MPSV) develop CFU-GM that can proliferate in vitro but have lost their self-renewal capacity in the absence of colony-stimulating activity (CSA) [31].

In AIDS and LAS patients pooled T-cell colonies were composed of a high proportion of cells bearing the T4$^+$, T6$^+$, T8$^+$ surface phenotype. Conversely, colonies generated from normal subjects displayed less than 20% and 40% T6$^+$ and T8$^+$ cells, respectively [8]. Since a similar proportion of colony cells could be stained with the T4$^+$, T6$^+$, and T8$^+$ moAb, it can be assumed that most of them expressed, at the same time, all these antigenic determinants. However, double-staining studies are needed to verify this hypothesis. The increased expression of T6$^+$ antigen that characterizes immature lymphocytes [32] indicates a block of the in vitro differentiation of patients' T-CFC. This abnormal differentiation of T-CFC was also revealed in spontaneous colonies [23,24], indicating that this phenomenon is independent of added IL2. This observation strongly suggests that the observed reduced in vivo T4$^+$/T8$^+$ ratio in AIDS patients is not due to the impaired IL2 production by the patients' lymphocytes [13]. However, in that pooled colonies were used for phenotypic studies, it is unclear whether all colonies were composed of immature T cells or some of them of more differentiated cells.

Clinically normal male homosexuals present T-CFC abnormalities similar to those of AIDS and LAS patients although to a lesser degree. These findings might indicate that abnormalities of T-CFC represent early events in the establishment of an immunosuppressed status in male homosexuals [33].

In conclusion, our data indicate that T-cell lymphopenia observed in LAS and AIDS patients as well as in some male homosexuals might be the result of several mechanisms, such as impaired proliferative capacity, decreased number, and abnormal in vitro differentiation of T-CFC. In addition, the in vitro study of T-CFC could identify some LAS patients presenting a very low number of peripheral blood and lymph node T-CFC, whose risk of developing AIDS is extremely high. Longitudinal studies are needed to define exactly the prognostic value of this observation.

ACKNOWLEDGMENTS

We wish to thank Gerard Iglesia for technical assistance and Mrs. Nadiege Balliet for secretarial help. This study was supported by grants from the Association de la Recherche contre le Cancer (ARC).

REFERENCES

1. Fibach F, Gerasi E, Sachs L. Induction of colony formation in vitro by human lymphocytes. Nature 1976; 259:127.
2. Shen J, Wilson F, Shifrine M, Gershnin ME. Selective growth of human T lymphocytes in single phase semi-solid culture. Immunology 1977; 119:1299.
3. Riou N, Boizard G, Alcalay D, Goube De Laforest P, Tanzer J. In vitro growth of colonies from human peripheral blood lymphocytes by phytohemagglutin. Ann Immunol (Inst Pasteur) 1976; 127C:83.
4. Rozenszajn LA, Shohaw D, Kalecheman I. Clonal proliferation of PHA-stimulated human lymphocytes in soft agar culture. Immunology 1975; 29:1041.
5. Claesson MH, Rodger MB, Johnson GR, Wittingham S, Metcalf D. Colony formation by human lymphocytes in agar medium. Clin Exp Immunol 1977; 28:526.
6. Triebel F, Robinson WA, Hayward AR, Goube De Laforest P. Existence of a pool of lymphocyte colony forming cells (T-CFC) in human bone marrow and their place in the differentiation of the T lymphocyte lineage. Blood 1981; 58:911.
7. Triebel F, Robinson WA, Hayward AR, Goube De Laforest P. Characterization of the T lymphocyte colony forming cells and evidence for the acquisition of T markers in the absence of thymic microenvironment in man. J Immunol 1981; 126:2020.
8. Georgoulias V, Marion S, Consolini R, Jasmin C. Characterization of normal peripheral blood T- and B-cell colony forming cells: Growth factor(s) and accessory cell requirements for their in vitro proliferation. Cell Immunol 1985; 90:1.
9. Georgoulias V, Auclair H, Jasmin C. Heterogeneity of peripheral blood T-cell colony forming cells in patients with T-cell malignancies. Leuk Res 1984; 8:1025.
10. Sutherland DC, Dalton G, Wilson JD. T lymphocyte colonies in malignant diseases. Lancet 1976; ii:1113.
11. Bernstein ML, Winkelstein A, Dobson SA. Depressed T cell colony growth in systematic lupus erythematosus. Arthritis Rheum 1980; 23:385.

12. Claesson MH, Petersen J, Sonderstup-Hansen G, Rozke C, Sorensen T. Colony formation by subpopulations of human T lymphocytes III. Antigenic phenotype and function of colony-forming cells, colony cells and their expanded progeny. Cell Immunol 1983; 81:526.

13. Seligmann M, Chess L, Fahey JL, Fauci AS, Lachmann PJ, et al. AIDS—An immunologic reevaluation. N Engl J Med 1984; 311:1287.

14. Miller B, Stansfilld SK, Zack MM, Curran JW, Kaplan JE, Schonberger LB, Falk H, Spira TJ, Mildvan D. The syndrome of unexplained generalized lymphadenopathy in young men in New York City. JAMA 1984; 151:242.

15. Ioachim HL, Lerner CW, Tapper ML. Lymphadenopathies in homosexual men. Relationship with the acquired immune deficiency syndrome. JAMA 1983; 250:1306.

16. Metroka CE, Cunningham Rundles S, Pollack MS. Generalized lymphadenopathy in homosexual men. Ann Intern Med 1983; 99:505.

17. Centers for Diseases Task Force: Morbid Mortal Weekly Rep 1982; 31:365..

18. Centers for Diseases Task Force: Morbid Mortal Weekly Rep 1982; 31:644.

19. Brun Vesinet F, Rouzioux C, Barre-Sinoussi F, Klatzmann D, Saimot AG, Rozenbaum W, Christol D, Gluckman JC, Montaigner L, Cherman JC. Detection of Ig G antibodies to lymphadenopathy associated virus in patients with AIDS or lymphadenopathy syndrome. Lancet 1984; 1:1253.

20. Montagnier L, Calvel F, Krust B, Chamaret S, Rey F, Barre-Sinoussi F, Chermann JC. Identification and antigenicity of major envelope glycoprotein of lymphadenopathy associated virus (LAV). J Virol 1985; 144:283.

21. Bertoglia NA, Boison N, Bonnet MC, Chatenoud L, et al. First workshop on standardization of human IL2. A joint report. Lymphokine Res 1984; 1:121.

22. Nicola NA, Metcalf D, Von Melcher H, Burgess AW. Isolation of murine fetal hematopoietic progenitor cells and selective fractionation of various erythroid precursors. Blood 1981; 58:376.

23. Lunardi-Iskandar Y, Georgoulias V, Allouche M, Rozenbaum W, Klatzmann D, Cavaille-Coll M, Meyer P, Gluckman JC, Gentilini M, Jasmin C. Abnormal in vitro proliferation and differentiation of T colony forming cells in AIDS patients and clinically normal male homosexuals. J Clin Exp Immunol 1985; 60:285.

24. Lunardi-Iskandar Y, Georgoulias V, Rozenbaum W, Klatzmann D, Cavaille-Coll M, Meyer P, Gentilini M, Gluckman JC, Jasmin C. Abnormal in vitro proliferation and differentiation of T colony-forming cells in patients with lymphadenopathy syndrome (LAS). Blood 1986; 67:1063.

25. Winkelstein A, Klein RS, Evans TL, Dixon BW, Holder WL, Weaver LD. Defective in vitro T cell colony formation in the acquired immunodeficiency syndrome. J Immunol 1985; 134:151.

26. Gluckman JC, Klatzmann D, Cavaille-Coll M, Brisson E, Messiah A, Lachiver D, Rozenbaum W. Is there correlation of T cell proliferative functions and surface marker phenotypes in patients with acquired immunedeficiency syndrome or lymphadenopathy syndrome? Clin Exp Immunol 1985; 60:8.

27. Robb RJ, Greene WC, Rusk CM, Low and high affinity cellular receptors for interleukin 2. Implications for the level of Tac antigen. J Exp Med 1984; 160:1126.

28. Talle MA, Alleger N, Makowski M, Goldstein G. Distinct classes of human T-cell activation antigens. Cell Immunol 1984; 84:185.

29. Gootenberg JE, Ruscetti FW, Mier JM, Gazdar A, Gallo RC. Human cutaneous T-cell lymphoma and leucemie cell lines produce and respond to T-cell growth factor. J Exp Med 1981; 154:1403.

30. Klein B, Le Bousse Kerdiles C, Smadja Joffe F, Pragnall IA, Ostertag W, Jasmin C. A study of added GM-CSF independent granulocyte and macrophage precursors in mouse spleen infected with myeloproliferative sarcoma virus (MPSV). J Exp Hematol 1982; 10:373.

31. Reinherz EL, Schlossman SF. The differentiation and function of human T cell lymphocytes. Cell 1980; 19:821.

32. Pinching AJ, McManus JJ, Jeffries DJ, Moshtael O, Perkin JM, Munday PE, Harris JRW. Studies of cellular immunity in male homosexuals in London. Lancet 1983; ii:126.

Cancer Detection and Prevention Supplement 1:535–541 (1987)

Immune Status of Drug Abusers

D. Fuchs, PhD
A. Hausen, PhD
G. Reibnegger, DSc
D. Schönitzer, MD
B. Unterweger, MD

H.G. Blecha, MD
P. Hengster, MD
H. Rössler, MD
T. Schulz, MD
E.R. Werner, DSc

M.P. Dierich, MD
H. Hinterhuber, MD
K. Schauenstein, MD
K. Traill, MD
H. Wachter, PhD

Institute of Medical Chemistry and Biochemistry (D.F., A.H., G.R., E.R.W., H.W.), Clinic of Psychiatry (H.G.B., H.H., H.R., B.U.), Institute of Hygiene (M.P.D., P.H., T.S.), Institute of Experimental Pathology (K.S., K.T.), Institute for Blood Transfusion and Immunology (D.S.), and Ludwig Boltzmann Institute for AIDS Research, University of Innsbruck, Innsbruck, Austria

ABSTRACT This study followed 184 drug abusers. Examined in all of them were urinary neopterin levels, HBV, SGOT, and Luestest. Seventy-three percent of IV drug addicts showed elevated neopterin levels reflecting activated cellular immunity. Statistically, no correlation of neopterin levels with, eg, excessive alcohol consumption, duration of drug abuse, or studied laboratory parameters was found. Individuals using cocaine revealed higher neopterin levels than those not doing so. Twenty-one of twenty-two patients with no parenteral drug use had normal neopterin excretion. In 34 drug detoxification patients, we examined in addition: T-lymphocyte subsets (T_4/T_8 ratio) and serum neopterin levels. Thirty-eight of ninety-four parenteral drug addicts presented with anti-LAV/HTLV-III* antibodies (ELISA + Western blot + IFT). Our data demonstrate an activated cellular immune status in parenteral drug addicts that cannot be attributed to LAV/HTLV-III infection in all cases. The development of AIDS seems to depend not only on the exposure to LAV/HTLV-III but also on activated cellular immunity, which is easily assessed by neopterin measurement.

Key words: drug addicts, LAV/HTLV-III, neopterin, T_4/T_8 ratio, activated cellular immunity

INTRODUCTION

The acquired immunodeficiency syndrome (AIDS) is a new epidemic form of immunodeficiency that was first recognized in 1981 [1]. Spread of disease is almost exclusively limited to such "at-risk" groups as homosexually active men, parenteral drug abusers, and recipients of blood products [2]. AIDS is clinically characterized by opportunistic infections and/or

---

*According to the Internal Committee on Taxonomy of Viruses now termed HIV (human immunodeficiency virus).

Address reprint requests to Dr. D. Fuchs, Institute of Medical Chemistry and Biochemistry, University of Innsbruck, A-6020 Innsbruck, Austria.

malignant disease in patients without known cause for immunodeficiency [3]. It is a distinctive disease of the cellular immune system with persistent quantitative and functional depression within the T_4-lymphocyte subset, and it is caused by a cytopathogenic lymphotropic human retrovirus [4,5] designed as lymphadenopathy-associated virus (LAV) or human T-cell lymphotropic virus III (HTLV-III).

It has been mentioned that, besides confrontation with LAV/HTLV-III, the special immunologic situation in AIDS risk groups might contribute to progressive infection and to development of AIDS [6–8]. Immunological abnormalities have also been demonstrated in homosexuals [9,10] and hemophilia patients [11] not seropositive for LAV/HTLV-III antibodies.

We studied the immunologic situation of heterosexual parenteral drug abusers to see if alterations similar to those observed in other risk groups are relevant in this group, too. Further, we investigated the presence of antibodies to LAV/HTLV-III and the relationship between antibody status and the immunologic findings. Finally, the relevance of neopterin levels besides anti-LAV/HTLV-III testing in AIDS risk groups should be examined. Neopterin is a sensitive marker for AIDS and AIDS-related complex (ARC) reflecting cellular immune activation [12–14].

PATIENTS AND METHODS

The present study comprises 188 imprisoned drug abusers (34 female and 154 male) investigated during the last 20 months. Twenty-two of them were nonparenteral drug abusers; 166 were parenteral addicts. We examined urinary neopterin levels by HPLC as described previously [15,16]. In addition, hepatitis A and B serology, SGOT test, and cardiolipin test were performed. Anamnesis concerning alcohol consumption (no, moderate, excessive), duration of drug abuse (1–12 years), duration of detoxification (1 week–1 year), previous hepatitis infections, and travel activities in the past few years was elaborated. As tests for antibodies against LAV/HTLV-III became available, we screened 94 parenteral drug abusers by ELISA (Organon). Positive results were confirmed by Western blot and immunofluorescence test. In 31 individuals of this group, T_4/T_8 ratios were determined by a fluorescence-activated cell sorter, and, in addition, serum neopterin levels were measured by radioimmunoassay (RiAcid; Fa. Henning, Berlin, Federal Republic of Germany).

RESULTS

Figure 1 shows urinary neopterin levels of the first 94 drug abusers investigated in 1983. A clear separation (P < 0.0001, Fisher exact test) between nonparenteral and parenteral drug abusers is expressed: Only 5% of 22 nonparenteral addicts but 68% of 72 parenteral addicts showed elevated neopterin levels reflecting activated cellular immune status. Statistical comparison of neopterin levels within the parenteral drug addicts (Table I) revealed no association between increased neopterin levels and duration of drug abuse, duration of detoxification, alcohol consumption, previous hepatitis infections, HB antigen/antibody status, SGPT values, or cardiolipin test. A difference concerning neopterin levels was found in addicts using cocaine compared to those not doing so (P = 0.017, Wilcoxon test). As testing for antibodies against LAV/HTLV-III became available, a group of 34 parenteral drug abusers was evaluated additionally concerning seroconversion (Organon-ELISA, Western blot, immunofluorescence test) T_4/T_8 ratio, and neopterin serum levels (Fig. 2). Fifteen of thirty-four (44%) were found to be seropositive [17]. Statistical comparison of the seronegative group with the seropositive one showed that urinary neopterin discriminates better (P = 0.0002, Wilcoxon test) than serum neopterin (P = 0.0113). Difference in T_4/T_8 ratios is only marginally significant (P = 0.0483). It is important to recognize that abnormal immunologic parameters such as T_4/T_8 ratio <1 and neopterin above normal are demonstrated also in healthy seronegative drug addicts.

In Figure 3, antibody testing in parenteral drug addicts is extended to 94 individuals. All of 36 sera with positive ELISA tests were confirmed by Western blotting and IFT, which

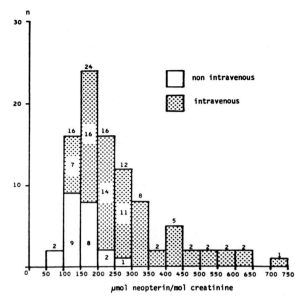

Fig. 1.   Urinary neopterin levels of 72 parenteral and 22 nonparenteral drug abusers.

TABLE I. Influence of Various Parameters on Neopterin Excretion of Parenteral Drug Abusers

Variable	P (Wilcoxon test)
LAV/HTLV-III antibody status	0.001
Opiate versus opiate + cocaine users	0.017
Previous hepatitis	NS*
Hepatitis antigen-antibody status	NS
Cardiolipin test	NS
Alcohol consumption	NS

Variable	P (Student's t test of linear correlation coefficient)
Age	NS
Sex	NS
Duration of drug consumption	NS
Duration of detoxification	NS
SGPT	NS

*NS, not significant.

indicates 40% seropositives among parenteral drug abusers in the Austrian Tyrol. There were no clinical signs of AIDS or an AIDS-related disease apparent in the drug addicts examined. No difference in seropositivity rate was observed between male and female addicts. Most of the 14 seropositive female addicts admitted prostitution. All but one of the seropositives showed partially highly increased urinary neopterin levels (97%). Fifty percent of the seronegative addicts had elevated neopterin levels as well. There exists a clear shift in neopterin levels when seronegative individuals are compared with seropositives ($P < 0.001$, Wilcoxon test).

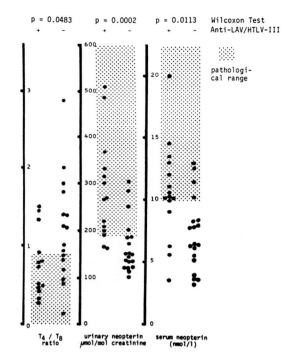

Fig. 2. T_4/T_8 ratio and urine and serum neopterin levels correlated to anti-LAV/HTLV-III antibody status of 34 drug abusers.

DISCUSSION

This study provides further evidence that in parenteral drug addicts immunological abnormalities are detectable to a similar extent as in other groups at risk for AIDS. In agreement with the clinical picture, an immunocompromised situation is expressed in most of the patenteral drug addicts examined as indicated by a reduced T_4/T_8 ratio. Additionally, neopterin levels reflect a persistent activation of cell-mediated immunity in a high percentage. This observation is in agreement with findings in other populations at risk for AIDS as in homosexuals and in hemophiliacs ([6,18]. It should be emphasized that immunologic abnormalities are not restricted to anti-LAV/HTLV-III seropositives.

Surprisingly, a very high rate (40%) of anti-LAV/HTLV-III seropositivity is observed in the Tyrol [17]. It is comparable to the Swiss [19], Italian [20], and Scottish [21] results. In contrast, English drug addicts showed only a 6% seropositivity for LAV/HTLV-III antibodies [19]. The question remains open as to whether giving syringes to drug addicts could reduce the spread of the virus in the near future [22] in countries where syringes have been limited for drug addicts in the past. In this respect, education programs for drug addicts would be necessary. Furthermore, drug addicts have to be sure of not being suspicious for police when caught with syringes.

Increased neopterin excretion in seropositive individuals could be due to immunologic activation caused by acute infection with LAV/HTLV-III, since progressive infection is accompanied by a further increase of neopterin levels [14]. The elevated levels found in seronegative drug addicts are not easily explained. Previous infections had no significant influence on neopterin levels. Nevertheless, most of the addicts have had previous hepatitis infections. The influence of parenteral administration of drugs or common diluents that might be immunogenic warrants further investigation. Probably, repeated injection of diluents can lead to persistently activated immune status. Increased neopterin levels were observed also during drug-detoxifi-

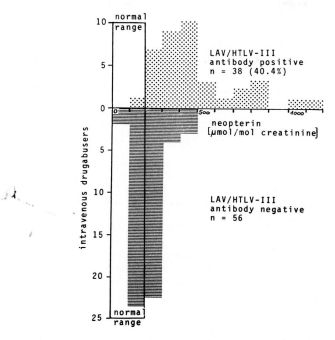

Fig. 3.   Distribution of urinary neopterin levels of 94 drug abusers with respect to anti-LAV/HTLV-III antibody status.

cation periods in seronegatives, only slightly decreasing during the first few weeks. As in homosexuals and in hemophiliacs [6] this situation of persistent activated cellular immunity is demonstrable in parenteral drug addicts. Therefore, we suggest that activated T-cells might be the most relevant predisposition for development of AIDS subsequent to infection with LAV/HTLV-III. Such an activated T-lymphocyte system is also a prerequisite for cultivation of LAV/HTLV-III in vitro.

Elevated urinary neopterin excretion was found to be present in almost all drug addicts seropositive for LAV/HTLV-III. Besides its high sensitivity, neopterin seems to allow a quantification of the progression of the disease. All these drug addicts were free of any clinical symptom associated with AIDS or ARC. There are several hints from studies on patients with AIDS and ARC that development of AIDS is associated with a continuous increase of neopterin levels [12–14]. Therefore, neopterin represents not only a very sensitive parameter in recognizing seropositives for anti-LAV/HTLV-III but also an easily assessable parameter quantifying the susceptibility for developing progressive infection in seropositives [8]. The one addict seropositive for anti-LAV/HTLV-III and with normal neopterin levels who is also still quite healthy and finished his drug career half a year ago in this respect would have the very best prognosis of not developing ARC and AIDS in the near future. He may even be free from any viral promotion now. The situation of the neopterin positives but anti-LAV/HTLV-III seronegatives is not quite clear at the moment. As mentioned above, one aspect will be the immunologic challenge initiated by administration of drugs and diluents, which might lead to a persistently activated immune status. On the other hand, minor chronic infections by, eg, HBV could be the cause. Both possibilities are independent of the onset of the AIDS epidemic in the latter 1970s, since the immunocompromised situation of parenteral heroin or cocaine addicts has been well established for more than 10 years [23,24]. Even generalized lymphadenitis in drug addicts was published long before AIDS was considered to exist [25]. The third possibility is that at least some of the neopterin positives but anti-LAV/HTLV-III negatives are carriers of the virus as well. These subjects possibly will develop measurable antibody titers in the near future. They are considered to be in the lack phase concerning antibody development [26], since it is well known that measurable antibodies will occur 6–8 weeks after contact with the virus at earliest. On the other hand neopterin is established to be increased during the acute phase of viral infections and is even elevated in children after vaccination [27]. Both cases demonstrate neopterin elevation before measurable antibody titers exist. Thus using neopterin in the screening of blood donors might lower the false-negative rate concerning potential carriers of LAV/HTLV-III.

REFERENCES

1. Gottlieb MS, Schroff R, Schanker HM, et al. Pneumocystis carinii pneumonia and mucosal candidiasis in previously healthy homosexual men: evidence of a new acquired cellular immunodeficiency. N Engl J Med 1981; 305:1425–31.
2. Seligmann, Chess L, Fahey JL, et al. AIDS—An immunologic reevaluation. N Engl J Med 1984; 311:1286–92.
3. Centers for Disease Control. Update on acquired immunodeficiency syndrome (AIDS). United States. Morbid Mortal Weekly Rep 1982; 3:507–14.
4. Barré-Sinoussi F, Cherman JC, Rey F, et al. Isolation of a T lymphotropic retrovirus from a patient at risk for acquired immune deficiency syndrome (AIDS). Science 1983; 220:868–71.
5. Popovic M, Sarngadharan MG, Read E, Gallo RC. Detection, isolation and continous production of cytopathic retrovirus (HTLV-III) from patients with AIDS and pre-AIDS. Science 1984; 224:497–500.
6. Fuchs D, Hausen A, Reibnegger G, et al. Urinary neopterin evaluation in risk groups for the acquired immunodeficiency syndrome (AIDS). In Pfleiderer W, Curtius HC, Wachter H, eds: Biochemical and clinical aspects of pteridines. Berlin: Walter de Gruyter, 1984; Vol 3, 457–67.
7. Levy JA, Ziegler JL. Acquired immunodeficiency syndrome is an opportunistic infection and Kaposi's sarcoma results from secondary immune stimulation. Lancet 1983; ii:78–81.
8. Fuchs D, Dierich MP, Hausen A, et al. Are homosexuals less at risk of AIDS than intravenous drug abusers and haemophiliacs? Lancet 1985; ii:1130.
9. Mavligitt GM, Talpaz M, Hsia FT, et al. Chronic immune stimulation by sperm alloantigens: Support for the hypothesis that spermatozoa induce immune dysregulation in homosexual males. JAMA 1984; 251:237–41.
10. Detels R, Schwartz K, Visscher BR, Fahey JL, Greene RS, Gottlieb MS. Relation between sexual practices and T-cell subsets in homosexually active men. Lancet 1983; ii:609–11.
11. Ludlam CA, Steel CM, Cheingsong-Popov R, et al. Human T-lymphotropic virus Type III (HTLV-III) infection in seronegative haemophiliacs after transfusion of factor VIII. Lancet 1985; ii:233–6.
12. Wachter H, Fuchs D, Hausen A, et al. Elevated urinary neopterin levels in patients with the acquired immune deficiency syndrome (AIDS). Hoppe Seyler Z Physiol Chem 1983; 364:1345–6.
13. Fuchs D, Hausen A, Reibnegger G, et al. Urinary neopterin in the diagnosis of acquired immune deficiency syndrome. Eur J Clin Microbiol 1984; 3:70–1.
14. Abita JP, Cost H, Milstien S, Kaufman S, Saimont G. Urinary neopterin and biopterin levels in patients with AIDS and AIDS-related complex. Lancet 1985; ii:51.
15. Hausen A, Fuchs D, Koenig K, Wachter H. Determination of neopterin in human urine by reversed phase high performance liquid chromatography. J. Chromatogr 1982; 227:61–70.
16. Fuchs D, Hausen A, Reibnegger G, Wachter H. Automatized routine estimation of neopterin in human urine by HPLC on reversed phase. In Wachter H, Curtius HC, Pfleiderer W, eds: Biochemical and clinical aspects of pteridines. Berlin: Walter de Gruyter, 1982; Vol 1, 67–79.
17. Fuchs D, Blecha HG, Deinhardt F, et al. High Frequency of HTLV-III antibodies among heterosexual intravenous drug abusers in the Austrian Tyrol. Lancet 1985, i:1506.
18. Buimovici-Klein E, Lange M, Klein RJ, Cooper LZ, Grieco MH. Is the presence of interferon predictive for AIDS? Lancet 1983; ii:344.
19. Mortimer PP, Vandervelde EM, Jesson EM, Pereira MS, Burkhardt F. HTLV-III antibody in Swiss and English intravenous drug abusers. Lancet 1985; 11:449–50.
20. Ferroni P, Geroldi D, Galli C, Zanetti AR, Cargnel A. HTLV-III antibody among Italian drug addicts. Lancet 1985; ii:52.

21. Peutherer JF, Edmond E, Simmonds P, Dickson JD, Bath GE. HTLV-III antibody in Edinburgh drug addicts. Lancet 1985; ii:1129–30.
22. Andreyew HJN. Selling syringes to drug addicts. Lancet 1985; ii:1192–3.
23. Elliott JH, O'Day DM, Gutow GS, Podgorski SF, Akrabawi P. Mycotic endophthalmitis in drug abusers. Am J Ophthalmol 1979; 88:66–72.
24. Marugg D, Martenet AC, Morell B, Oelz O. Candida-Endophthalmitis: Diagnostik, Verlauf und Therapie bei 8 Patienten. Schweiz Med Wochenschr 1985; 115:132–4.
25. Geller SA, Stimmel B. Diagnostic confusion from lymphatic lesions in heroin addicts. Ann Intern Med 1973; 78:703–5.
26. Salahuddin SZ, Groopman JF, Markham PD, et al. HTLV-III in symptom-free seronegative persons. Lancet 1984; ii:1416–20.
27. Reibnegger G, Fuchs D, Grubauer G, Hausen A, Wachter H. Neopterin excretion during incubation period, clinical manifestation and reconvalescence of viral infection. In Pfleiderer W, Wachter H, Curtius HCh, eds: Biochemical and clinical aspects of pteridines. Berlin: Walter de Gruyter, 1984: Vol 3, 433–47.

Cancer Detection and Prevention Supplement 1:543–548 (1987)

B-Cell Reactivity in Homosexuals With Persistent Generalized Lymphadenopathy (PGL)

J. Kekow, MD
P. Kern, MD
H. Schmitz, MD
W.L. Gross, MD

*Department of Internal Medicine, Christian Albrecht University,
Kiel (J.K., W.L.G.), and Clinical Department (P.K.) and Department of Virology
(H.S.), Bernhard-Nocht-Institut, Hamburg, Federal Republic of Germany*

ABSTRACT   In addition to the well known T-cell dysfunctions in AIDS, hypergammaglobulinaemia and autoimmune phenomena indicate an involvement of the B cell as well. Reports of HTLV-III/LAV-infected B cells suggest T-cell-independent B-cell abnormalities. To look for early B-cell dysfunctions, we examined a high-risk group of AIDS consisting of six homosexuals with PGL and HTLV-III/LAV antibodies, comparing these data to those of patients with AIDS/ARC and a normal control. In vitro studies included the B-cell proliferation response (^{3}H-thymidine uptake) to *Staphylococcus aureus* Cowan I and the differentiation response (Ig secretion into culture supernatants) to T-cell-dependent/-independent polyclonal B-cell activators (PBAs). Profound alterations were found in both the proliferation and the differentiation responses. The weak response even to T-cell-independent PBAs indicates a B-cell dysfunction that is not due only to a T-cell defect in patients with PGL, similar to that observed in AIDS.

Key words: AIDS, risk groups for AIDS, HTLV-III/LAV, B-cell function

INTRODUCTION

The acquired immunodeficiency syndrome (AIDS) is a new clinical entity associated with pronounced immunologic abnormalities [for review, see 1]. Investigations of full-blown AIDS to assess the immunodeficiency in detail have revealed a broad scope of abnormalities, which are not restricted to T lymphocytes. Looking at the B-cell system, Lane et al [2] reported a defect in the proliferation response to *Staphylococcus aureus* Cowan I (SAC) and, in addition, a separate B-cell differentiation defect. This was shown in a pokeweed mitogen (PWM)-driven allogenetic coculture experiment. Although this observation was questioned by Gottlieb and Benveniste [3], recently another group presented evidence of a T-cell-independent B-cell dysfunction in hemophiliacs, a risk group for AIDS [4].

Address reprint requests to Dr. W.L. Gross, I. Medizinische Klinik, Klinikum der CAU, Schittenhelmstrasse 12, D-2300 Kiel, Federal Republic of Germany.

We attempted to evaluate B-cell alterations by using a previously reported model of human B-cell activation via T-cell-independent polyclonal B-cell activators (PBAs). In contrast to PWM, crude preparations of gram-negative bacteria can trigger highly purified B cells to undergo terminal differentiation without prior proliferation [5,6]. With mice, Mosier et al [7] recently demonstrated that T-cell-independent PBAs are a useful tool for elaborating B-cell functions after infection with a retrovirus. We were particularly interested in determining with this model the extent of possible B-cell dysfunction in patients with a history of homosexual practice and persistent generalized lymph node enlargement (PGL), a group thought to be particularly likely to develop AIDS or an AIDS-related complex, recognized as an AIDS prodrome [8]. In parallel studies, these patients were examined for their proliferation response after stimulation with SAC. Our results on B-cell function using PBAs coincide closely with findings in a PWM-driven allogenetic coculture system and demonstrate that a dysfunction of both the proliferative and the differentiation response has to be considered for homosexuals, who are particularly likely to develop AIDS. Particularly, B-cell proliferation is affected at an early stage, while T-cell proliferation can still be detected.

MATERIALS AND METHODS
Patients

Twelve homosexuals from the Clinical Department of the Bernhard-Nocht-Institut, Hamburg, were studied. Six homosexuals were categorized as having AIDS or ARC [for definition, see 8, p 70]. The six others showed persistent generalized lymph node enlargement. Table I contains further information on clinical and laboratory findings from these patients. All homosexuals investigated were seropositive for HTLV-III antibodies. The control group consisted of healthy heterosexual men paired by age. Lymphocyte tests were done in the form of parallel in vitro culture studies, testing AIDS/ARC patients, patients with PGL, and healthy heterosexual men.

Cell Preparation and Culture Conditions

Mononuclear cells (MNC) were separated by density centrifugation as described elsewhere [11] and cultivated in microtiter plates (2×10^5 MNC in 200 μl per well) at 37°C in a 5% CO_2-95% air humidified atmosphere. For stimulation, SAC (Calbiochem, Frankfurt/Main, Federal Republic of Germany), PWM (Difco, Detroit, MI), concanavalin A (Con A) (Difco), or a membrane preparation of A-*Streptococcus* (AScM) [for details, see 11] was added. For T-cell-independent B-cell differentiation, *Klebsiella* and *Salmonella* membrane preparations (Klebs M, Salm) were employed [for detailed methods, refer to 6]. All cultures were carried out in triplicate.

Lymphocyte Proliferation Assay

DNA synthesis was determined by measuring the incorporation of ^{3}H-thymidine by proliferating cells. The culture period of 3 days was terminated with a 4 hr pulse with 0.5 μCi/well. The trichloroacetic acid-insoluble ^{3}H-thymidine in the cells was collected on Millipore filters, and the radioactivity was counted in a liquid scintillation counter.

Lymphocyte Differentiation Assay

Secreted immunoglobulins (IgM and IgG) in culture supernatants were assessed by ELISA [12]. After a 6 day culture period, the culture supernatants were transferred into microtiter plates, precoated with anti-IgM or anti-IgG, and incubated overnight. Following extensive washing, anti-IgM or anti-IgG peroxidase conjugates were added. Two hours later, the plates were washed and Orthophenylendiamindihydrochloride was added as substrate. Then, extinction was measured at 492 nm.

TABLE I. Main Clinical Characteristics and Laboratory Findings in the Homosexuals

Patients		Age (years)	Clinical features	Serum immunoglobulins*			Delayed hyper-sensitivity†	Lymphocyte marker‡ Ratio OKT4/OKT8	HTLV III§ (IgG AB)
				IgA	IgG	IgM (mg/dl)			
Homosexuals presenting with PGL	1	23		101	1,070	145	2/1	0.7	+
	2	26	Persistent generalized	558	1,430	130	12/2	0.5	+
	3	34		190	2,380	261	4/2	0.6	+
	4	44	Lymph node enlargement only	263	1,560	192	NL.‖	0.8	+
	5	51		139	1,740	252	14/3	1.0	+
	6	62		198	1,740	192	NL.‖	0.6	+
Homosexuals presenting with ARC/AIDS	1	34	*Salmonella* sepsis	181	2,260	168	5/2	0.6	+
	2	40	Kaposi sarcoma	386	1,442	186	0/0	0.3	+
	3	42	PGL, weight loss	242	1,165	138	20/4	0.6	+
	4	43	Kaposi sarcoma	395	3,663	192	0/0	0.4	+
	5	43	PGL, weight loss, diarrhea	395	3,219	317	8/3	0.8	+
	6	44	PGL, weight loss, interst. pneumonia	82	2,059	252	5/1	0.8	+

*Normal values: IgA 90–450, IgG 800–1,800, IgM 69–280 mg/dl.
†Composed scores of Multitest Mérieux, France [10].
‡Detected by indirect immunoflourescence and monoclonal AB's from Ortho (Heidelberg, Federal Republic of Germany). Values of the control group: x̄ = 2.0 (1.6–2.4).
§AB to HTLV-III were sought by means of indirect immunoflourescence [9].
‖NL., not listed because different skin tests were used.

Statistics

The results from the different groups were compared, and the significance was analyzed with Wilcoxon's rank sum test. Data are expressed as arithmetic mean $\pm$ SEM as appropriate.

RESULTS

Table II gives details of the proliferation studies. Stimulation with Con A (a T-cell mitogen) and AScM (a microbial antigen for T-cell stimulation) showed significantly less ^{3}H-thymidine incorporation in all homosexuals than in the heterosexual control group. In each group, Con A led to a significant proliferative response (stimulation index >3 [13]). Using SAC, a pure T-cell-independent B-cell mitogen [14], no significant proliferative response could be obtained in any of the patients, including the homosexuals with PGL. The stimulation results of the AIDS/ARC group did not differ from the initial levels, which were obtained by omitting the stimulants.

The Ig levels in the culture supernatants were determined by ELISA. High spontaneous IgG levels were seen in all homosexuals. In patients with PGL, IgG was increased by a factor of four and in AIDS/ARC patients by a factor of ten. In contrast, only slightly elevated spontaneous IgM levels were seen in AIDS/ARC. None of the homosexuals responded with an increase in IgG in their culture supernatants when PWM and AScM, two T-cell-dependent B-cell activators, were used for stimulation. The same was true for stimulation with Klebs M and Salm, two T-cell-independent polyclonal B-cell activators. The spontaneous IgG levels even ranged above the values obtained after lymphocyte stimulation.

Examination of the IgM isotype in culture supernatants of stimulated MNCs revealed results similar to those obtained for IgG in patients with AIDS/ARC. In patients with PGL, the IgM levels in the culture supernatants were four to six times above the initial levels when Klebs M and Salm were employed. The results were compiled in Table III.

To allow conclusions from the observed abnormalities and from the clinical and laboratory findings, we investigated three other healthy homosexually active men who were HTLV-III antibody-negative. Identical in vitro experiments performed in this "control group" showed no evidence of a lack in proliferation response or defects in their differentiation capacities. Specifically, ^{3}H-thymidine uptake after SAC stimulation revealed a more than threefold increase, and Klebs M induced an increase in IgM to 788 ng/ml and in IgG to 546 ng/ml. The spontaneous Ig levels did not differ from the normal controls.

DISCUSSION

This study on B-cell reactivity, using previously characterized T-cell-independent PBAs and a T-cell-independent B-cell mitogen, shows an abnormal B-cell response in AIDS/ARC patients and in homosexuals who are particularly likely to develop AIDS/ARC. First, there was no significant increase in proliferation of MNC from AIDS/ARC patients after stimulation with SAC. This was also true for a group of homosexuals presenting clinically with PGL and having HTLV-III antibodies. This contrasts with the significant MNC response to T-cell stimulators in this group. Second, the last step in the B-cell maturation process induced by PBAs was also affected: In addition to elevated spontaneous IgG production by MNC, we

TABLE II. Proliferative Response (^{3}H-Thymidine Uptake:cpm) of MNC From the Homosexuals

Stimulant	Dose	Heterosexual control group	Homosexuals presenting with PGL	Homosexuals presenting with ARC/AIDS
None (day 3)		568 $\pm$ 98	642 $\pm$ 100	450 $\pm$ 44
SAC	1:5,000 v/v	2,898 $\pm$ 221	1,253 $\pm$ 303†	477 $\pm$ 81*
Con A	20.0 μg/ml	20,067 $\pm$ 8,192	5,198 $\pm$ 1,589*	5,057 $\pm$ 744*

Significance in comparison with the control group: *P $\leqslant$ 0.01, †P $\leqslant$ 0.05.

TABLE III. Differentiation Response (Ig Secretion, ng/ml) of MNC From the Homosexuals

Stimulant	Dose	Heterosexual control group	Homosexuals presenting with PGL	Homosexuals presenting with ARC/AIDS
A. IgG secretion				
None		126 ± 49	586 ± 134[*]	1,220 ± 386[*]
PWM	1.5 μl/ml	969 ± 243	508 ± 121	375 ± 113[†]
AScM	100.0 μg/ml	369 ± 31	167 ± 46	410 ± 127
Klebs M	100.0 μg/ml	1,032 ± 192	362 ± 102[†]	496 ± 95[†]
Salm	100.0 μg/ml	1,193 ± 173	624 ± 145	562 ± 165[†]
B. IgM secretion				
None		199 ± 46	152 ± 61	325 ± 168
PWM	1.5 μl/ml	1,113 ± 190	384 ± 125[†]	284 ± 102[*]
AScM	100.0 μg/ml	1,457 ± 279	207 ± 94[*]	232 ± 139[*]
Klebs M	100.0 μg/ml	4,182 ± 491	634 ± 240[*]	322 ± 155[*]
Salm	100.0 μg/ml	5,140 ± 898	983 ± 472[†]	311 ± 119[*]

Significance in comparison with the control group: [*]P ≤ 0.01, [†]P ≤ 0.05.

found an impaired B-cell differentiation response to both T-cell-dependent (as described by Lane et al [2]) and T-cell-independent PBAs. B cells from patients with AIDS/ARC or PGL appeared to be refractory to the stimulation signal given by Klebs M and Salm. These two B-cell activators obviously bypass the network of B-cell-triggering T cells that is necessary, for instance, in a PWM-driven T-cell-dependent system of B-cell activation. The only noteworthy difference was seen when the ELISA results for IgM were compared. Here, Klebs M and Salm were able to induce an increase in the spontaneous IgM production in the patients with PGL. All B-cell activators employed failed to induce further IgM production in patients with AIDS/ARC. In addition, high spontaneous IgG levels were reduced under stimulatory conditions, a phenomenon that needs further assessment. Therefore, this study extends the first observations on this subject by Lane et al [2], who investigated total IgA/M/G levels. Our data on different isotypes show elevated spontaneous IgG levels. They also show that patients with PGL were still able to respond to stimulation by enhancing their IgM release into culture supernatants. The detection of HTLV-III antibodies has enabled a more convincing definition of certain at risk groups previously determined only by epidemiologic criteria, so we were able to choose a group that is particularly likely to develop AIDS or ARC. Positive HTLV-III antibody results indicated contact with the retrovirus responsible for the disease.

The hyporesponsiveness of B cells is thought to be due to B-cell activation in vivo [2], as is possible in recurrent infectious diseases. This explanation is also supported by the appearance of elevated serum Ig levels (mainly IgG) and autoimmune phenomena [15]. Recently, B-cell infection by HTLV-III/LAV has been documented in addition to the well known trophism of HTLV-III/LAV to T4-positive cells [16,17]; thus B cells can serve as a target for the retrovirus themselves. From this observation, it can be concluded that HTLV-III causes a direct B-cell dysfunction. The evidence of changes in B-cell function early in the disease supports the hypothesis that some of the reported T-cell abnormalities could even be secondary to B-cell abnormalities [18]. This pathogenetic concept is well known from studies in animals [19,20]. For instance, the treatment of rodents with anti-μ results in functional T-cell defects similar to AIDS, and bursectomy in chickens initiates an increase of T8-positive cells. Thus the evaluation of immunodeficiency in ARC/AIDS patients and in patients at risk for AIDS should include functional studies on B cells. A follow-up is necessary to elucidate the particular significance of B-cell dysfunction in patients and to develop diagnostic programs.

ACKNOWLEDGMENTS
This work was supported by the BMFT "Forschungsförderung AIDS."

REFERENCES

1. Bowen DL, Lane HC, Fauci AS. Cellular immunity. In Ebbesen P, Biggar RJ, Melbye M, eds: AIDS. Copenhagen: Munksgaard, 1984; 135–73.
2. Lane HC, Masur H, Edgar LC, Whalen G, Rook AH, Fauci AS. Abnormalities of B-cell activation and immunoregulation in patients with the acquired immunodeficiency syndrome. N Engl J Med 1983; 309:453–8.
3. Gottlieb MS, Benveniste E. B-cell abnormalities in AIDS. N Engl J Med 1984; 310:258.
4. Brieva JA, Sequi J, Zabay JM, Pardo A, Campos A, Luz de la Sen M, Bootello A. Abnormal B cell function in haemophiliacs and their relationship with factor concentrates administration. Clin Exp Immunol 1985; 59:491–8.
5. Chen WY, Fudenberg HH. Polyclonal activation of human peripheral blood B-lymphocytes. III. Cellular interaction and immunoregulation of immunoglobulin-secreting cells induced by formaldehyde-fixed Salmonella paratyphy B. Clin Immunol Immunpathol 1982; 22:279–90.
6. Gross WL, Rucks A. Klebsiella pneumoniae stimulate highly purified human blood B cells to mature into plaque forming cells without prior proliferation. Clin Exp Immunol 1983; 52:372–80.
7. Mosier DE, Yetter RA, Morse HC. Retroviral induction of acute lymphoproliferative disease and profound immunosuppression in adult C57B1/6 mice. J Exp Med 1985; 161:766–84.
8. Quinn TC. Early symptoms and signs of AIDS and the AIDS-related complex. In Ebbesen P, Biggar RJ, Melbye M, eds: AIDS. Copenhagen: Munksgaard, 1984; 69–83.
9. Popovic M, Sarngadharan MG, Read E, Gallo RC. Detection, isolation, and continuous production of cytopathic retroviruses (HTLV-III) from patients with AIDS and pre-AIDS. Science 1984; 224:497–500.
10. Knicker WT, Anderson CT, Roumiantzeff M. The multitest system: A standardized approach to evaluation of delayed hypersensitivity and cell mediated immunity. Ann Allerg 1983; 43:73–9.
11. Gross WL. Lymphocytenantwort auf humanpathogene Streptokokken. Zelluläre Immunphänomene, ausgelöst durch somatische Streptokokkenantigenpräparationen. Stuttgart: Thieme, 1982.
12. Voller A, Bartlett A, Bidwell D. Enzyme immunoassays with special reference to ELISA techniques. J Clin Pathol 1978; 31:507–20.
13. Ling NR, Kay JE. Lymphocyte stimulation. New York: American Elsevier, 1975; 179.
14. Schuurman RKB, Gelfand EW, Dosch HM. Polyclonal activation of human lymphocytes in vitro. I. Characterisation of the lymphocyte response to a T-cell-independent B-cell mitogen. J Immunol 1980; 125:820–6.
15. Sonnabend JA, Witkin SS, Purtilo DT. Acquired immune deficiency syndrome—An explanation for its occurence among homosexual men. In Ma P, Armstrong D, eds: The acquired immune dificiency syndrome and infections of the homosexual men. New York: Yorke Medical Books, 1984; 409–25.
16. Montagnier L, Gruest J, Charmaret S, Dauguet C, Axler C, Guétard D, Nugeyre MT, Barré-Sinoussi F, Chermann JC, Brunet JB, Klatzmann D, Gluckman JC. Adaptation of lymphadenopathy associated virus (LAV) to replication in EBV-transformed B lymphoblastoid cell lines. Science 1984; 225:63–66.
17. Volsky DJ, Sinangil F, Sonnabend J, Casareale D. Isolation of HTLV-III and EBV-positive B lymphoblastoid cell lines from peripheral blood lymphocytes of AIDS patients. Ann Intern Med (in press).
18. Zolla-Pazner S. B cells in the pathogenesis of AIDS. Immunol Today 1984; 5:289–91.
19. Gray D. B cells and the development of the T-cell repertoire. Immunol Today 1984; 5:316–7.
20. Seligman M, Chess L, Fahey JL, Fauci AS, Lachmann PJ, L'Age-Stehr J, NGU J, Pinching AJ, Rosen FS, Spira TJ, Wybran J. AIDS—An immunologic reevaluation. N Engl J Med 1984; 311:1286–97.

Cancer Detection and Prevention Supplement 1:549–552 (1987)

Imbalance of the Epstein-Barr Virus–Host Relationship in AIDS-Related Complex Patients

Giuseppe Ragona, PhD
Maria Caterina Sirianni, MD

Department of Experimental Medicine (G.R.) and Department of Allergology and Clinical Immunology (M.C.S.), University of Rome "La Sapienza," Rome, Italy

ABSTRACT Patients affected by AIDS related-complex (ARC) showed several immunological abnormalities that could lead to a disregulation of immunosurveillance against viral latent infections. We report Epstein-Barr virus (EBV) reactivation was found in seven of eight ARC patients and in two of seven affected by persistent generalized lymphoadenopathy. These patients showed either elevated levels of circulating EBV-positive transformed cells and/or depressed EBV-specific T cell cytotoxicity as assessed by the regression assay. Natural killer cell activity was found to be decreased and correlated with evidence of circulating EBV-infected cells and with impaired EBV-specific immune control. Our data demonstrate that loss of control of EBV latency in the infected host by specific immune mechanisms increases the risk for EBV reactivation and emergence of clones with unlimited growth potential. A role of EBV as a cofactor in the development of ARC is suggested.

Key words: EBV, generalized lymphadenopathy, T cell cytotoxicity

INTRODUCTION

Since its discovery in 1964, Epstein-Barr virus (EBV) appeared to have a role, at least as a cofactor, in the development of several different pathological entities. This role is linked to its powerful ability to "immortalize" cells, mainly B lymphocytes, and to affect a large human population, establishing a persistent infection. When EBV infects target cells, they acquire the property to proliferate indefinitely, giving origin in vitro to polyclonal lymphoblastoid cell lines that maintain for a long period a euploid diploid karyotype. However, the immortalized cell is only partly transformed since it has not acquired a neoplastic phenotype. EBV-immortalized B cells are normally controlled in vivo by an efficient immune system. In the EBV-positive Burkitt lymphoma (BL) all tumor cells are not only infected-immortalized by EBV, but they also carry a specific translocation of the long arm of chromosome 8, involving the activation of a human myc oncogene [1].

EBV was confirmed to be the cause of infectious mononucleosis (IM) and has been etiologically associated to BL, nasopharyngeal carcinoma, thymic carcinoma, CNS primary

Address reprint requests to Giuseppe Ragona, Department of Experimental Medicine, University of Rome "La Sapienza," 00185 Rome, Italy.

lymphoma, and to polyclonal lymphoproliferations in a variety of immunodeficiency states such as Duncan syndrome, acquired immunodeficiency syndrome (AIDS), and patients undergoing organ or bone marrow transplantation. In AIDS, several cases of BL have been documented [2].

A heterogeneous reactive population of lymphoid cells containing several functional components is operative in the protection against the EBV-induced lymphoproliferation: They include an active suppressor T cell, which appears during the acute phase of IM, perhaps as a response to the EBV-induced increased immunoglobulin synthesis [3], and a cytotoxic component detected in assays involving EBV-positive cell lines, consisting of both EBV-specific T killer cells and HLA nonrestricted natural killer (NK) cells. In addition, all healthy individuals previously infected by EBV possess circulating virus-specific memory T cells, whose cytotoxic potential can be reactivated in vitro by an appropriate challenge with autologous virus-infected B cells. This cytotoxic response can be assayed in cultures of experimentally infected blood mononuclear cells through its capacity to cause regression of outgrowth of the emerging virus-transformed B cell line. Prospective studies using this regression assay revealed the remarkable stability of EB virus-specific memory T cell levels in individual donors over periods of up to 5 years [4].

METHOD OF STUDY

How can the EBV-related B cell proliferative disturbances arise in spite of the complex immune mechanisms devoted to EBV control? In an attempt to answer this question, we investigated a group of patients at risk for AIDS who were suffering from AIDS-related complex (ARC). The choice of this group of patients was based on the hypothesis that an impairment of the immune system in a previously infected person could be followed by EBV reactivation from the latent carrier state. Such reactivation can be monitored by the appearance of EBV-infected cells in the peripheral blood. This event is usually found solely during the acute phase of primary EBV infection, before an adequate specific immune response has developed [5].

Experiments were performed for detection and quantiation of antibodies to different EBV-related antigens and of EBV-infected circulating lymphocytes and EBV-specific cytotoxic T cells. An analysis of T cell subsets and of the NK activity of peripheral blood lymphocytes was also performed.

Blood was collected from eight patients with ARC and from seven patients with a persistent generalized lymphoadenopathy (PGL) but without any other clinical signs of ARC. The great majority of both ARC and PGL patients had antibodies to HTLV-III. A number of controls have been subjected to the investigation, including five apparently healthy individuals, one boy with Bruton agammaglobulinemia, and one patient with non-Hodgkin lymphoma. None of the controls had antibodies to HTLV-III.

RESULTS

High levels (> 1:320) of antibodies to EBV-viral capsid antigen (VCA) were present in five of eight ARC patients, one of seven PGL patients, and none of the healthy controls [6]. Unexpectedly elevated levels of circulating EBV-infected cells were found in six of seven ARC patients. Their values were derived from the minimal concentration of total mononuclear cells, which in culture provided the spontaneous outgrowth of EBV-positive transformed cells, and were integrated as a direct index of the in vivo burden of infected cells in each individual tested [5]. This proliferation index provided values ranging from 50,000 to more than 600,000 mononuclear cells per well. Only two patients suffering from PGL showed significantly elevated levels of virus-infected cells. Proliferation indexes were negative (more than 600,000 mononuclear cell per well) in all controls.

Abnormalities in the cytotoxic T cell memory response to EBV as expressed by the regression index were found in all ARC cases harboring proliferating EBV-infected cells in the peripheral blood. Regression indexes are given in terms of the minimal concentration per well of T cells (OKT3 positive) required to cause regression of transformation in 50% of replicate cultures [4]. In the ARC patient group, values ranged from 167,500 to more than 350,000 (absence of regression). Among PGL and controls, only two subjects were found devoid of regression activity: a PGL patient with an elevated proliferation index and an individual who never acquired EBV infection. The proliferation and regression indexes are highly correlated ($r = 0.74$, $P < 0.001$).

NK activity was significantly decreased ($P < 0.005$) in patients with impaired EBV-specific cytotoxicity and elevated numbers of circulating EBV-positive lymphocytes. Proliferation and regression indexes and data on NK activity are presented in Table I. Data referring to the percentages of frequency of total T cells, T cell subpopulations with helper and suppressor/cytotoxic phenotype, and NK activities of PBL showed slightly abnormal values for all parameters in ARC and PGL patients (data not shown) [7].

DISCUSSION

The presence of EBV-positive lymphoid cells in ARC suggests a marked proliferation of EBV-infected cell clones in the peripheral blood of these patients. The specific cytotoxic

TABLE I. Proliferation, Regression, and Natural Killer Activity

Cases	Proliferation index*	Regression index[†]	NK activity[‡]
ARC			
1.	250,000	>350,000	ND
2.	250,000	325,000	ND
3.	80,000	ND	24.3
4.	>600,000	167,500	31.3
5.	ND	>350,000	33.4
6.	180,000	ND	34.4
7.	60,000	>350,000	40.2
8.	180,000	>350,000	30.4
PGL			
9.	>600,000	160,000	77.3
10.	>600,000	112,000	ND
11.	>600,000	58,750	48.4
12.	>600,000	176,000	49.2
13.	ND	45,000	31.2
14.	50,000	68,000	5.1
15.	50,000	>350,000	32.1
Control			
16.	>600,000	126,000	68.3
17.	>600,000	204,000	70.1
18.	>600,000	>350,000	61.0
19.	>600,000	86,400	ND
20.	>600,000	35,000	63.0
21.	>600,000	42,000	ND
22.	>600,000	21,000	70.0
23.	>600,000	27,000	72.0

*The lowest number of total mononuclear cells giving outgrowth of EBV-positive lymphoblasts in 50% of replicate microcultures is reported. When " > " is indicated, no proliferation at all is observed at the reported concentration, which corresponds to the highest number of cells seeded per well.
[†]The lowest number of T lymphocytes at which regression of proliferation of in vitro EBV-infected autologous lymphocytes has been observed in 50% of replicate microcultures is reported. When " > " is indicated, no regression at all is observed at the reported concentration, which corresponds to the highest number of cells seeded per well.
[‡]Percentage of specific lysis at the effector:target ratio of 100:1.

response was also found to be impaired. According to our findings, replication and spreading of EBV-immortalized lymphoblasts in the peripheral blood of patients with ARC and in some cases of PGL could be reasonably caused by a decreased EBV-specific immune control.

NK activity was also found to be depressed in our patients who had EBV-related lymphoproliferation. It was recently demonstrated that NK cells participate in the early phase of the cytotoxic response to autologous EBV-immortalized cells [8]. Characterization of lymphocyte subpopulations by monoclonal antibodies showed a slight increase in OKT8-positive cells in patients with ARC and PGL but did not result in higher cytotoxic activity toward circulating EBV-infected cells. The evidence of circulating EBV-positive cells is of interest because of their possible relationship to the EBV-induced B cell proliferations in immunodeficient patients. Its striking correlation with the reduced or absent EBV-specific cytotoxic T cell response, assayed by the regression test, is also noteworthy. Analysis of the cause and effect relationship between the appearance of EBV-infected cells and the inability of control by the immune system, suggests that the cause is most likely an impairment of the specific immune response rather than an overall aspecific dysfunction of the immune system. Additional studies are needed to evaluate the contribution of the EBV-specific T memory cells in the control of the EBV-related B cell proliferation.

Finally, with regard to the appearance of infected cells in the blood based on serological data such as the absence of class M antibodies to VCA, the presence of antibodies to Epstein-Barr nuclear antigen at increased levels supports the evidence for an EBV reactivation rather than for a primary infection (data not shown). Such reactivation may have a role in the pathogenesis of ARC or, at least, in the onset of those clinical manifestations, such as lymphoadenopathy, known to be associated with the clinical response to EBV infection.

REFERENCES

1. Klein G, Klein E. Evolution of tumors and the impact of molecular oncology. Nature 1985; 315:190–5.
2. Rosen FS. The acquired immunodeficiency syndrome (AIDS). J Clin Invest 1985; 75:1–3.
3. Tosato G, Magrath I, Koski I, Dooley N, Blease M. Activation of suppressor T cells during Epstein-Barr virus induced infectious mononucleosis. N Engl J Med 1979; 301:1133–7.
4. Rickinson AB, Moss DJ, Pope JH, Ahlberg N. Long-term T-cell-mediated immunity to Epstein-Barr virus in man. IV. Development of T-cell memory in convalescent infectious mononucleosis patients. Int J Cancer 1980; 25:59–65.
5. Rocchi G, De Felici A, Ragona G, Heinz A. Quantitative evaluation of Epstein-Barr virus-infected peripheral blood leukocytes in infectious mononucleosis. N Engl J Med 1977; 296:132–4.
6. Henle W, Henle G: Epstein Barr virus-specific serology in immunologically compromised individuals. Cancer Res 1981; 41:4222–5.
7. Sirianni MC, Rossi P, Scarpati B, et al. Immunological and virological investigation in patients with lymphoadenopathy syndrome and in a population at risk for AIDS with particular focus on the detection of antibodies to lymphotropic retroviruses (HTLV-III). J Clin Immunol 1985; 5:261–8.
8. Masucci MG, Bejarano MT, Masucci G, Klein E. Large granular lymphocytes inhibit the in vitro growth of autologous Epstein-Barr virus infected B cells. Cell Immunol 1983; 76:311–21.

Cancer Detection and Prevention Supplement 1:553–556 (1987)

Distribution of P24 HTLV3 Major Core Protein in Lymph Nodes of LAS Patients

Carlo D. Baroni, MD
Francesco Pezzella, MD

2nd Chair of Pathological Anatomy, Section of Immunopathology, Department of Biopathology, University "La Sapienza," Roma, Italy

ABSTRACT   Lymph nodes of patients with lymphadenopathy syndrome (LAS) are characterized by two main histological patterns: hyperplastic reactive (H) and regressive (R). In both conditions, the paracortex (PC) is markedly activated with presence of selectively Ia-1$^+$ high endothelial venules. Using a monoclonal antibody for p24, the major core protein of HTLV3, we have immunohistochemically determined the distribution of p24$^+$ cells in lymph nodes from 23 LAS patients' HTLV3-ab serologically positive. p24$^+$ cells were demonstrated in 11 cases. Control nodes were negative. p24$^+$ cells included high endothelial cells of PC postcapillary venules, large perivenular cells, large mono- or binucleated cells in PC and in GC, and few lymphocytelike cells. Our preliminary observations indicate that the majority of p24$^+$ cells are high endothelial and accessory cells that may act either as virus reservoir or as antigen-presenting cells to T4 lymphocytes and to GC B cells. In addition, the positivity of high endothelial cells for p24 might help to explain their selective Ia-1$^+$.

Key words: LAS, p24$^+$ cells, distribution, lymph node, HTLV3

INTRODUCTION

Lymph nodes of patients affected by the lymphadenopathy syndrome (LAS) are characterized by distinctive histological features. We have recently described in these lymph nodes two histological patterns: 1) hyperplastic reactive (H) and 2) regressive (R), indicating that LAS may eventually turn into AIDS, progressing from a hyperplastic reactive to a regressive-involuting phase [1]. The regressive phase, when very pronounced, may be considered as a morphological marker of a disease turning into AIDS.

The complete nucleotide sequence of the HTLV3 virus has recently been published [2]. In the core of the virus is expressed a gag product, protein p24, which is the major viral core protein. A mouse monoclonal antibody has been produced against protein p24 [3].

In the present paper, we describe the results of a study in which we have determined, using immunohistochemical methods, the distribution of cells positive for the HLA-DR-related OK Ia-1 monoclonal antibody and for the p24 monoclonal antibody in hyperplastic and regressive nodes of patients serologically HTLV3 positive affected by LAS.

Address reprint requests to Dr. Carlo D. Baroni, 2nd Chair of Pathological Anatomy, Viale Regina Elena 324, 00161 Roma, Italy.

MATERIALS AND METHODS

Lymph nodes were obtained from 23 patients of either sex affected by LAS; control nodes were removed from ten patients not at risk for AIDS (Table I). Briefly, 6 μm acetone fixed cryostat sections were incubated for 30 min with anti-p24 (1:200; kindly provided by Dr. R.C. Gallo) and with OK Ia-1 (Ortho Pharmaceutical Corporation, Raritan, NJ) mouse monoclonal antibodies. The sections were then washed and reincubated using the indirect biotin avidin complex method (ABC Kit, mouse IgG PK-4002, Vectastain; Vector Laboratories, Burlingame, NJ); the reaction product was developed using 0.06% 3-3'-diaminobenzidine (Sigma Chemical Co., St. Louis, Missouri). In negative controls, the primary antibody was substituted by a nonreactive mouse monoclonal antibody (anti-Cytokeratin PKK1; Labsystems

TABLE I. Immunohistochemical Demonstration of p24$^+$ Cells: Listing of Cases

Case	Age (years)	Sex	Risk*	Histology†	Serology‡	p24$^+$ cells GC§	p24$^+$ cells PC‖	Ia$^+$ vessels GC	Ia$^+$ vessels PC
LAS patients									
1	38	M	hom.	H	+	+	+	−	+
2	21	F	d.a.	H	+	+	+	−	+
3	43	M	he.	H	+	−	+	−	+
4	25	M	d.a.	H	+	+	−	−	+
5	34	F	d.a.	H	+	+	−	−	+
6	2	F	child of d.a.	H	+	+	−	−	+
7	24	M	hom.	H	+	+	−	−	+
8	31	M	d.a.	H	+	+	−	−	+
9	28	M	hom.	H	+	+	−	−	+
10	27	M	n.d.	H	+	+	−	−	+
11	19	M	d.a.	H	n.d.	−	−	−	+
12	26	M	d.a.	H	n.d.	−	−	−	n.d.
13	31	M	nos	H	n.d.	−	−	−	+
14	21	M	hom.	H	+	−	−	−	+
15	30	M	hom.	H	n.d.	−	−	−	n.d.
16	23	F	d.a.	H	+	−	−	−	+
17	21	M	he.	H	+	−	−	−	+
18	23	M	d.a.	R	+	+	−	−	+
19	30	F	d.a.	R	+	−	−	−	+
20	25	F	d.a.	R	+	−	−	−	+
21	24	F	d.a.	R	n.d.	−	−	−	+
22	21	F	d.a.	R	n.d.	−	−	−	+
23	31	M	hom.	R	+	−	−	−	+
Control patients									
1	17	M	−	FL	n.d.	−	−	−	−
2	20	M	−	FL	n.d.	−	−	−	−
3	45	F	−	FL	n.d.	−	−	−	−
4	8	M	−	FL	n.d.	−	−	−	−
5	7	M	−	FL	n.d.	−	−	−	−
6	24	F	−	FL	n.d.	−	−	−	−
7	12	M	−	FL	n.d.	−	−	−	−
8	50	M	−	FL	n.d.	−	−	−	−
9	25	F	−	HD	n.d.	−	−	−	−
10	53	F	−	HD	n.d.	−	−	−	−

*d.a., drug abuser; hom., homosexual; he., hemophiliac; nos, not otherwise specified.
†H, hyperplastic reactive; R, regressive; FL, follicular lymphadenitis; HD, Hodgkin disease.
‡Anti-HTLV-III antibodies.
§Germinal center.
‖Paracortical areas.

Oy, Helsinki, Finland). H9 T-cell culture lines, infected by the HTLV3 virus, were used as positive controls.

RESULTS

In both histological patterns we have always observed in paracortical areas a prominent postcapillary venule proliferation. Immunohistology has clearly demonstrated that the high endothelial postcapillary venules were activated, being strongly positive for the HLA-DR-related Ia-1 antibody. Furthermore, germinal centers were strongly positive for the OKT9 monoclonal antibody, a marker for activated lymphoid cells, and contained scattered T4$^+$ lymphocytes and T8$^+$ cells mainly located in perivascular position. All LAS cases were subgrouped according to their histological patterns (Table I). In both groups, prominent high endothelium postcapillary venules were constantly observed in paracortical areas.

When cryostat sections were treated with the OK Ia-1 monoclonal antibody, which primarily detects HLA-DR-related antigens and thus identifies activated cells, it was found that, besides positive cells present in germinal centers and in paracortex, high endothelial cells of postcapillary venules were also strongly Ia-1 positive. Immunohistology revealed the presence of p24 positive cells in ten hyperplastic nodes and in one regressive node. All these cases were HTLV3 serologically positive. p24 positivity was never observed in control nodes.

p24$^+$ cells, characterized by intracytoplasmic granular pattern, were observed in ten instances in germinal centers and in three instances in paracortical area. In two cases, positive cells were present both in germinal centers and in paracortical areas.

The distribution of p24 positive cells among the various cell types is summarized in Table II. In germinal centers, small lymphocytelike cells were found positive in all but one case: in three instances, they were observed in perivenular position. Other cells expressing p24 in germinal centers included few large mono- and binucleated cells, which in one instance were detected in strict contact with a small blood vessel. Large and small mononucleated p24$^+$ cells were noticed in paracortical areas, where they were occasionally in strict contact with postcapillary venules. High endothelial cells of postcapillary venules were found to be p24$^+$ in two cases. It must be pointed out that p24 endothelial positivity was strictly confined to postcapillary venules of paracortical areas.

DISCUSSION

The present observations indicate that in nodes of LAS patients there are cells immuno-stained by a monoclonal antibody specific for p24 protein. It is perhaps worth noting that in most cases p24$^+$ cells were observed in hyperplastic nodes, whereas in only one instance they were present in a regressive node. This observation suggests, on morphological grounds, that viral expression and replication require and/or promote initial proliferation of lymphocytes,

TABLE II. Nature and Distribution of p24$^+$ Cells in Germinal Centers and Paracortical Areas of Lymph Nodes From LAS Patients

	Germinal centers	Paracortical areas
Endothelial	−	−
High endothelial	−	+ 2 cases
Large mononucleated PV*	+ 1 case	+ 1 case
non-PV†	+ 2 cases	+ 1 case
Large binucleated PV	−	−
non-PV	+ 3 cases	−
Lymphocytelike PV	+ 3 cases	−
non-PV	+ 9 cases	+ 2 cases

*perivascular.
†Nonperivascular.

which is indicated by the germinal centers hyperplasia and activation, both observed at histological and immunohistochemical levels.

In addition, if we compare the number of p24$^+$ cells in germinal centers and in paracortex, we see that in most cases positive cells are present in germinal centers. It has been reported [4] that follicular dendritic cells of germinal centers represent antigen-trapping cells containing viruslike particles in AIDS-related lymphadenopathy. The presence of virions trapped in germinal centers might help to explain their marked activation. In paracortical areas, fewer p24$^+$ cells were observed, thus confirming the prominent role played by the germinal centers in the early phase of the disease.

Finally, it is interesting to note that high endothelial cells of postcapillary venules were found to be positive for the p24 monoclonal antibody in two instances. This last finding might help to explain the selective HLA-DR Ia-1 positivity of paracortical venules and may also be related to the recent evidence implicating endothelial cells in antigen presentation to T lymphocytes [5]. Our observation of some p24$^+$ cells in perivascular position is also in line with this interpretation.

The role played by endothelial and histiocyticlike accessory cells in relation to the development of LAS and AIDS has not been fully investigated until now. The only conclusions we can draw now, on the basis of these results, are that both endothelial and accessory cells may act as a reservoir of the LAV/HTLV3 virus and/or as antigen-presenting cells.

ACKNOWLEDGMENTS

This study was supported by grants from CNR, Progetto Finalizzato "Oncologia," No. 84.00440.44.

REFERENCES

1. Baroni CD, Pezzella F, Stoppacciaro A, et al. Systemic lymphadenopathy (LAS) in intravenous drug abusers. Histology, immunohistochemistry and electron microscopy: Pathogenetic correlations. Histopathology 1985; 9:1275–93.
2. Ratner L, Haseltine W, Patarca L, et al. Complete nucleotide sequence of the AIDS virus. HTLV-III. Nature 1985; 313:277–84.
3. di Marzo-Veronese F, Sarngadharan MG, Raman R, et al. Monoclonal antibodies specific for P24, the major core protein for HTLV-III. Proc Natl Acad Sci USA 1985; 82:5199–202.
4. Armstrong JA, Horne R. (1984) Follicular dendritic cells and viruslike particles in AIDS-related lymphadenopathy. Lancet 1984; ii:370–2.
5. Hirschberg H, Bergh OJ, Thorsby E. Antigen-presenting properties of human vascular endothelial cells. J Exp Med 1980; 152:249s–55s.

Cancer Detection and Prevention Supplement 1:557–565 (1987)

Lymphomas Associated With the Acquired Immune Deficiency Syndrome (AIDS): A Study of 35 Cases

Harry L. Ioachim, MD
Marvin C. Cooper, MD
Gerard C. Hellman, MD

Departments of Pathology (H.L.I.) and Medicine (M.C.C., G.C.H.), Lenox Hill Hospital, New York, NY

ABSTRACT   An increased incidence of lymphoid neoplasias is associated with the states of immune deficiency both congenital and acquired. Thirty-five cases of lymphoma in males at high risk for AIDS were diagnosed in one community hospital in New York City within the past 2 years. The mean age of these patients was 39.6 years; 34 were homosexual, and one was an intravenous drug abuser. There were four Hodgkin and 31 non-Hodgkin lymphomas of various histologic types but almost all of high-grade categories. The proportion of extranodal lymphomas, the involvement of the gastrointestinal tract, central nervous system, bone marrow, and myocardium were significantly higher than in the lymphomas of the general population. The phenotypes were B-cell and non-B-non-T-cell types without any T-cell lymphomas. All patients had reversed helper-suppressor T-cell ratios, and all those tested had circulating HTLV-III and antilymphocyte antibodies. Nine patients have had previous lymph node biopsies showing the lesions of AIDS-related lymphadenopathies that were often directly associated with lymphoma. A variety of severe opportunistic infections and Kaposi sarcoma affected these patients. All lymphomas associated with immune deficiency were highly aggressive, involved multiple organs, and responded poorly to treatment resulting in early deaths.

Key words: non-Hodgkin lymphoma, Hodgkin lymphoma, lymphomas in homosexuals, lymphadenopathies in AIDS, Kaposi sarcoma in AIDS

INTRODUCTION

In 1982, only 1 year after issuing the account on the first cases of AIDS [1] the Centers for Disease Control reported the occurrence of 4 cases of non-Hodgkin lymphomas among homosexual males [2]. During the past 2 years, additional cases of lymphoma in the population of homosexual males at risk for AIDS were reported [3–9], and the picture of a distinctive type of neoplasia began to emerge. The current clinical experience with AIDS-related lymphomas was summarized in a recent review of 90 cases of non-Hodgkin lymphomas in homosexual men collected from six major national medical centers by a large group of contributing physicians [9].

Address reprint requests to Dr. Harry L. Ioachim, Department of Pathology, Lenox Hill Hospital, New York, NY 10021.

In Lenox Hill Hospital in New York City, 21 cases of lymphomas in patients at risk for AIDS had been diagnosed by January, 1985, when a study on this subject was submitted for publication [10]. Presently, (September, 1985), we have seen in our hospital a total of 35 cases of lymphomas in homosexual males who also manifested clinical or immunologic symptoms of AIDS. They were similar to those already reported in the literature and as a group resembled in all respects the lymphomas associated with various types of genetic and induced immune deficiencies [11,12].

MATERIALS AND METHODS

All cases of lymphoid malignancy first diagnosed between February 1982 and September 1985 in Lenox Hill Hospital were reviewed to identify those occurring in males at high risk for AIDS. In 35 cases, lymphomas of Hodgkin and non-Hodgkin type occurred in males homosexuals, bisexuals, and drug abusers. Some of the patients had been previously diagnosed, biopsied, treated, and followed-up for opportunistic infections, Kaposi sarcoma, or AIDS-related lymphadenopathy; others were seen for the first time with lymphoma.

The clinical and laboratory records of all patients were reviewed for age, previous history, prodromes, presence and location of principal and additional neoplasms, and hematological and immunological status. Treatment, response to treatment, recurrence, and death or survival until September 1985 were recorded.

Immunologic evaluation was conducted in most cases and included protein electrophoresis and immunoelectrophoresis, determination of total lymphocyte amount, B- and T-cell counts, helper and suppressor T-cell ratio, and in some cases, lymphocyte function and skin testing for various antigens. Serum HTLV-III antibodies were determined by an ELISA assay using purified whole virus extract. The presence of antilymphocyte antibodies was estimated according to a method previously published [13]. Tissues from biopsy or autopsy were processed routinely for light and electron microscopy. For immunohistochemical examination, unfixed tissues were stained with fluorescein-isothiocyanate (FITC)-labeled monospecific antisera to IgM, IgG, IgD, Kappa, and λ immunoglobulins for the identification of B-cells and with monoclonal OKT3, OKT4, OKT6, and OKT11 antibodies and the peroxidase-antiperoxidase reagents for the identification of T-cells. Bouin-fixed tissues were also stained for heavy- and light-chain immunoglobulins by the peroxidase antiperoxidase (PAP) technique.

Complete autopsies were performed on the 18 patients who died in the hospital. Tissues of all organs were examined microscopically and in selected cases also by electron microscopy and immunohistochemistry. The lymphoma classifications of Rappaport, Lukes-Collins, and the Working Formulation [14] were used.

RESULTS

From February 1982 to September 1985, 35 cases of lymphoma in males at high risk for AIDS were diagnosed at Lenox Hill Hospital. Thirty-four patients were homosexual or bisexual and one patient was an IV drug abuser. Their ages ranged from 26 to 55 years, with a mean age of 39.6 years. There were four cases of Hodgkin lymphomas and 31 cases on non-Hodgkin lymphomas. The four patients with Hodgkin disease were 34, 35, 38, and 52 years old. Two had their initial diagnosis made on the basis of a bone marrow biopsy (Fig. 1). The oldest patient with Hodgkin disease had a rapid downhill course, having presented with stage IV B disease and bone marrow involvement. Inguinal lymph node and bone marrow lesions were classified as mixed cellularity type. He was treated with MOPP-ABVD chemotherapy and expired of rapidly progressive disease including massive liver involvement. Two of the younger patients had lesions classified as nodular sclerosis in axillary lymph nodes and the third mixed cellularity in submaxillary lymph nodes. These patients had helper/suppressor T-cell ratios between 0.6 and 0.9. Two patients had positive tests for antibodies to HTLV-III. Of the 31 patients with non-Hodgkin lymphoma, 15 had fever from several days to 4 months prior to diagnosis and 11 had moderate weight loss. Eight patients had noneoplastic lymphadeno-

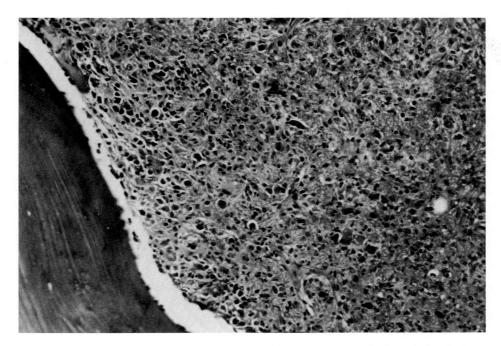

Fig. 1. Hodgkin lymphoma, mixed cellularity type of bone marrow completely replacing the hemopoetic and adipose tissues. Multiple Reed-Sternberg cells and fibrosis. Original magnification × 100.

TABLE I. Principal Location of Lymphoma at Diagnosis in 35 Patients

| | Nodal | | Extranodal | |
	Location	n	Location	n
Non-Hodgkin (n = 31)	Cervical	3	Bone marrow	2
	Axillary	5	Stomach	2
	Inguinal	2	Duodenum, ileum	4
	Mediastinal	1	Colon	3
	Retroperitoneal	5	Brain	2
	Total	16	Palate, tonsil	2
			Total	15
Hodgkin (n = 4)	Cervical	1	Bone marrow	1
	Inguinal	1	Total	1
	Axillary	1		
	Total	3		

pathies biopsied at the same time or before the diagnosis of lymphoma was made. Of these, three had the acute lymphadenitis histologic pattern characterized by marked follicular hyperplasia, and five had the chronic histologic pattern, with lymphocyte depletion, effacement of lymphoid follicles, and extensive vascular proliferation as previously described [15,16]. The principal location of non-Hodgkin lymphoma at diagnosis involved lymph nodes in 16 cases and extranodal organs in 15 cases. The lymph node groups biopsied are indicated in Table I. The extranodal lymphomas had the principal location in bone marrow (2) and gastrointestinal tract (9), of which two were in the stomach, four in the small intestine, and three in the colon

(Table I, Fig. 2). In addition, the central nervous system was involved and clinically symptomatic in four cases. Massive involvement of the pericardium and myocardium was found at autopsy in two cases (Fig. 3).

Clinically, most of the patients had extensive disease and rapid progression of lesions. The intestinal involvement present in six patients was considerable, including a constricting ileocecal tumor in one case requiring urgent laparotomy. Lymphoma of the CNS evolved as a space-occupying parietal lesion in one case, extension to the base of the brain of a tumor initially in the cervical lymph nodes in one case, and leptomeningitis in two cases. Lymphoma localized in two cases in the parotid and submaxillary lymph nodes presented as salivary gland tumors and were originally seen by ENT specialists [17]. One patient after 1 year of chemotherapy for nodal lymphoma had an exploratory laparotomy for persistent splenomegaly. There was congestive splenomegaly with no evidence of residual lymphoma; however, six months later he developed skin lesions on his face and lower extremities that on biopsy were diagnosed as cutaneous lymphoma.

Hematologic evaluation revealed great variation of peripheral white blood cell count. At the time of presentation, counts ranged from 3,200 to 13,500 wbc/mm^3 excluding a patient with Burkitt lymphoma/leukemia who had 19,8000 wbc/mm^3. The mean wbc was 7,400 per mm^3. Absolute lymphocyte counts varied from 50 to 8,000/m^3 with a mean of 2,014/mm^3. Hemoglobins ranged from 7.5 to 16.9 g% with a mean of 12.2 g%, and platelets ranged from 19,000 to 450,000/mm^3, with a mean of 224,000/mm^3. The patients with the lowest hemoglobin concentrations tended to be lymphopenic. Immunoglobulin levels were determined in 14 patients. IgG levels ranged from 75 to 1,900 mg% (mean 1,127 mg%), IgA from 71 to 700 mg% (mean 198 mg%), and IgM from 44 to 320 mg% (mean 159 mg%). IgD was measurable in four of the 14 patients, two within normal range and one with a polyclonal IgD of 210 mg%. The helper/suppressor T-cell ratio (h/s) was below 1 in 14 of 18 patients for whom it was determined. Ten of ten patients tested had circulating HTLV-III antibodies, whereas none of 30 patients with disease unrelated to AIDS had positive tests. Eleven of 14 patients evaluated

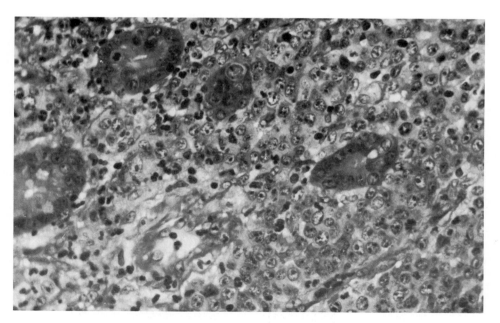

Fig. 2.   Intestinal non-Hodgkin lymphoma, diffuse, large, noncleaved cell type. Residual colonic crypts in a mass of lymphoma cells. Original magnification ×250.

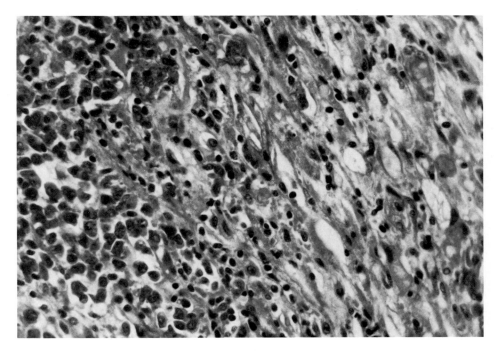

Fig. 3. Non-Hodgkin lymphoma, diffuse, large, cleaved cell type invading myocardium. Original magnification ×250.

TABLE II. Histopathological Diagnosis of Lymphoma in 35 Patients

Lymphoma	No. of patients
Non-Hodgkin	31
Nodular, small cell, cleaved	1
Diffuse, small cell, cleaved	1
Diffuse, large cell, cleaved	13
Diffuse, large cell, noncleaved	7
Diffuse, large cell, plasmacytoid	3
Undifferentiated Burkitt type	2
Undifferentiated non-Burkitt type	4
Hodgkin	4
Nodular sclerosis	1
Mixed cellularity	3

for antilymphocyte antibodies had positive tests expressed as a significant increase in the number of surface immunoglobulin-positive lymphocytes occurring after incubation with patients' sera [13]. The histopathology diagnoses listed in Table II show that with one exception all non-Hodgkin lymphomas were classified in the intermediate- and high-grade categories of the Working Formulation (Fig. 4). In several cases, focal areas of lymphoma were observed within lymph nodes that displayed the typical lesions of lymphadenopathy. Aggregates of lymphoma cells were present within the markedly hyperplastic germinal centers of AIDS-associated lymphadenopathy, where they appeared to originate. In one patient, lymphoma in the small intestine co-existed with Kaposi sarcoma.

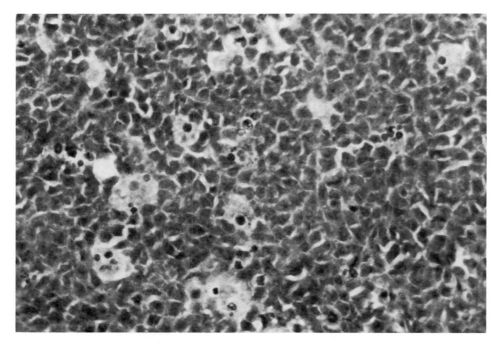

Fig. 4.   Non-Hodgkin lymphoma, diffuse, undifferentiated, non-Burkitt type. Characteristic starry-sky pattern resulting from scattered macropages containing nuclear debris as a result of widespread cell necrosis. Original magnification ×250.

Electron microscopic examination of seven cases of non-Hodgkin lymphoma showed the characteristic features of the various lymphoma types, confirming their histologic classification [14]. Immunohistochemistry performed on 12 non-Hodgkin lymphoma patients showed monoclonal light- and heavy-chain immunoglobulin staining in eight cases and no staining for either T or B markers in four cases (Fig. 5).

All patients were treated with multidrug chemotherapy CHOP, M-BACOD, or BACOD. CNS radiotherapy with or without intrathecal methotrexate was instituted at the time of CNS involvement. Complete or partial responses to these therapeutic regimens were noted in most cases, with the longest partial remissions of 15 and 28 months after diagnosis. These responses, however, represent only 30% of patients, which is significantly inferior to the 70% rates of response to similar chemotherapy combinations reported in the literature [18]. The incidence of opportunistic infections was impressive, with 1 case each of nocardiosis, aspergillus fungus ball, CMV esophagitis, and mycobacteriosis. There were also five cases of pneumocystis pneumonia and six cases of oral candidiasis. One of these patients developed pneumocystis pneumonia one year after he had been off all chemotherapy. Kaposi sarcoma was present in three patients. This considerable amount of opportunistic infections is not commonly seen in association with lymphomas and must be attributed to the underlying immune deficiency of AIDS. Twenty of 31 patients with non-Hodgkin lymphoma died of their disease 1 week to 28 months after diagnosis. The autopsies performed in 18 cases showed that systemic lymphoma was the prevalent cause of death, although opportunistic infections frequently were contributing factors. The patients that are alive had histologic diagnoses with the most favorable prognostic implications. These survivors are also the most recently diagnosed, with only 2–6 months of follow-up for the patients with non-Hodgkin lymphoma and 1–4 months for the patients with Hodgkin lymphoma.

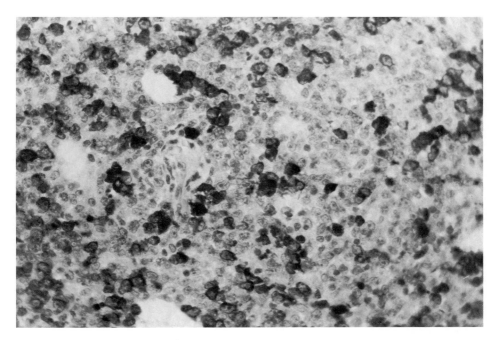

Fig. 5. Non-Hodgkin lymphoma invading omentum. B-cell phenotype demonstrated by uniform cell staining with anti-κ light-chain antibody using immunoperoxidase techinque. Original magnification ×250.

DISCUSSION

The existence of a relationship between immune deficiency and neoplasia had been recognized more than a decade before the present epidemic of AIDS [11,12]. The risk of developing a malignant tumor is 4% in patients with genetic immune deficiencies, which represents an incidence of over 10,000 times that recorded in the general age-matched population [12,19]. In immunosuppressed renal transplant recipients, the occurrence of neoplasia is 6%, with a total of 1,767 tumors that have developed in 1,661 patients as of May, 1983, according to the transplantation register [19,20]. Of all the tumors developing in immundeficient individuals, by far the most common are those of the lymphoid system. Non-Hodgkin lymphomas represent 3–4% of all the tumors in the general population but constitute 26% of the tumors arising in recipients of renal transplants and 71% in recipients of cardiac transplants [20]. In the course of Kaposi sarcoma, a tumor clearly associated with the status of immune deficiency, additional neoplasms may develop in as many as 37% of patients, and, of these, lymphoid tumors are 20 times more common than other tumors [21]. These and other statistics strongly indicate that lymphoid tumors more than any other malignancies are related to the various states of immune deficiency.

The lymphomas in immunodeficient patients are not only more common but also different from those in immunocompetent patients in relation to their location, histology, natural history, and response to treatment. In the present study, all patients were males with an age distribution predominantly in the late thirties. Of the 35 cases of lymphoma, only four were of Hodgkin type. Among the previously published cases, only one report mentions cases of Hodgkin lymphoma related to AIDS [22]. Thus a reversal of the ratio between the incidence of Hodgkin and non-Hodgkin lymphomas in this patient population is noted. Whereas in the general population in young adults the first is more common, in homosexual males the incidence of non-Hodgkin disease is significantly higher. Similarly altered is the ratio of nodal vs extranodal location of non-Hodgkin lymphomas, which in the population at large is heavily weighted toward the lymph nodes as the primary site of tumors. In our series, only 16 lymphomas originated in lymph nodes, whereas 15 occurred in other locations, again similar to the other cases published, in which extranodal location of lymphomas was more common than usual [2,4,9]. Involvement of the CNS appears to be another characteristic feature of lymphomas in AIDS. Whereas no more than 2% of non-Hodgkin lymphomas involve the brain primarily (and, not too often, secondarily) in the general population, there was 42% involvement of the CNS in the series of Ziegler et al [9] and 18% in the present series. The lymphomas in AIDS patients studied by us and by others were highly aggressive and uniformly involved multiple organs. In the 18 autopsies performed in this study, extensive tumor involvement was present, and massive invasion of organs not commonly affected such as myocardium, stomach, kidney, testis, urinary bladder and skin were noted. In contrast to the first reports of lymphomas in AIDS, in which all cases were recorded as being Burkitt-like type [2,3,7], the non-Hodgkin lymphomas in the present series as well as those in the two other more recently published series [4,9] were heterogeneous. However, 30 of 31 were of diffuse pattern and of large-cell or undifferentiated cytology, thus of generally high-grade histologic types indicative of poor response to treatment and short survival. The phenotype determined in 12 non-Hodgkin lymphomas in this study was of monoclonal B-cell type in 8 and of non-B- non-T-cell type in four. The only lymphoma in which the skin was involved belonged to this second group. No lymphoma of T-cell phenotype has yet been reported to have occurred in AIDS-related patients. The relationship with the acquired immune deficiency and the previous viral infection was obvious. Eight of eight of the non-Hodgkin and two of two of the Hodgkin lymphoma patients tested had circulating HTLV-III antibodies, which were not present in any of the controls. Fourteen of eighteen patients tested had reversed helper/suppressor T-cell ratios with markedly depressed amounts of helper T-cells, and 11 of 14 patients evaluated for the presence of antilymphocyte antibodies had positive tests. Nonneoplastic lymphadenopathies preceded the lymphomas in most patients and showed the characteristic AIDS-related morphologic changes in the seven cases of non-Hodgkin and one case of Hodgkin lymphoma in whom they were biopsied. In four of the first and one of the second, the lymph node alterations were those generally associated with an involuted phase, showing hypervascularity and atrophic lymphoid follicles [16]. Similar lymph node lesions have been noted in other patients to precede or coexist with Kaposi sarcoma of lymph nodes. The observation in this study of focal areas of lymphoma or Kaposi sarcoma coexistent in lymph nodes with lesions of AIDS-related lymphadenopathy clearly establishes the sequence between the inflammatory and neoplastic lesions. The potential of reactive lymph nodes in individuals at high risk for AIDS to develop neoplasia justifies the biopsy and, if persistent, the rebiopsy of enlarged lymph nodes. The course of lymphomas in AIDS-related patients has been highly malignant, reflecting the immature tumor cell types and the defective immune response. The mortality, both in non-Hodgkin lymphoma (20 of 31) and Hodgkins lymphoma (one of four), with most of the survivors among the patients more recently diagnosed, is far greater than in lymphomas diagnosed and treated in the general population. Despite a variety of chemotherapy regimens applied and a generally positive initial response, almost all patients have relapsed. The poor results obtained in the treatment of AIDS-related lymphomas represent another feature that distinguishes them from the corresponding lymphomas in the general population. The morphologic, biologic, and clinical characteristics mentioned above indicate that the AIDS-related lymphomas are a distinct clinicopathologic entity. We suggest that they therefore be considered as a separate group and not be included in general clinical or chemotherapy studies. In the absence of this distinction, the poor prognosis of AIDS-associated lymphomas may obscure the advances obtained in the therapy of lymphomas unrelated to AIDS.

REFERENCES

1. Centers for Disease Control. Kaposi's sarcoma and pneumocystis pneumonia among homosexual men—New York City and California. Morbid Mortal Weekly Rep 1982; 31:249.

2. Centers for Disease Control. Diffuse, undifferentiated non-Hodgkin's lymphoma among homosexual males—United States. Morbid Mortal Weekly Rep 1982; 31:277.

3. Ziegler JL, Miner RC, Rosenbaum ET, et al. Outbreak of Burkitt's like lymphoma in homosexual men. Lancet 1982; 2:631.

4. Levine AM, Meyer PR, Begandy MK, et al. Development of B-cell lymphoma in homosexual men. Ann Intern Med 1984; 100:7–13.

5. Ioachim HL, Lerner CW, Tapper ML. Lymphadenopathies and lymphoma in immunocompromised homosexual men (abstract). Lab Invest 1983; 48:39A.

6. Snider WD, Simpson DM, Aronyk KE, Nielsen SL. Primary lymphoma of the nervous system associated with acquired immune-deficiency syndrome. N Engl J Med 1983; 308:45.

7. Doll DC, List AF. Burkitt's lymphoma in a homosexual. Lancet 1982; 2:1026–7.

8. Ciobanu N, Andreef M, Safai B, Koziner B, Mertelsmann R. Lymphoblastic neoplasia in a homosexual patient with Kaposi's sarcoma. Ann Intern Med 1983; 98:151–5.

9. Ziegler JL, et al. Non-Hodgkin's lymphoma in 90 homosexual men: Relationship to generalized lymphadenopathy and acquired immunodeficiency syndrome (AIDS). N Engl J Med 1984; 311:565–71.

10. Ioachim HL, Cooper MC, Hellman GC. Lymphomas in males at high risk for the acquired immune deficiency syndrome (AIDS): A study of 21 cases. Cancer 1985; 56:2831–2842.

11. Penn I, Hammond A, Brett Scheider L, Starzl TE. Malignant lymphomas in transplantation patients. Transplant Proc 1969; 1:106.

12. Gatti RA, Good RA. Occurrence of malignancy in immunodeficiency diseases. A literature review. Cancer 1971; 28:89–98.

13. Dorsett B, Cronin W, Chuma V, Ioachim HL. Anti-lymphocyte antibodies in patients with the acquired immune deficiency syndrome. Am J Med 1985; 78:621–5.

14. Ioachim HL. Lymph node biopsy. Philadelphia: J.B. Lippincott Co. Publ., 1982.

15. Ioachim HL, Lerner CW, Tapper ML. Lymphadenopathies in homosexual men: Relationships with the acquired immune deficiency syndrome. JAMA 1983; 250:1306–9.

16. Ioachim HL, Lerner CW, Tapper ML. The lympoid lesions associated with the acquired immunodeficiency syndrome. Am J Surg Pathol 1983; 7:543–53.

17. Ryan JR, Ioachim HL, Marmer J, Loubeau JM. Acquired immune deficiency syndrome-related lymphadenopathies presenting in the salivary gland lymph nodes. Arch Otolaryngol 1985; 111:554–56.

18. Skarin AT, Canellos GP, Rosenthal DS, et al. Improved prognosis of diffuse histiocytic and undifferentiated lymphoma by use of high dose methotrexate alternating with standard agents (M-BACOD). J Clin Oncol 1983; 1:91–8.

19. Hanto WH, Frizzera G, Purtillo DT, et al. Clinical spectrum of lymphoproliferative disorders in renal transplant recipients and evidence for the role of Epstein-Barr virus. Cancer Res 1981; 4253–61.

20. Penn I: Lymphomas complicating transplantation patients. Transplant Proc 1983; 15:2790–7.

21. Safai B, Mike V, Giraldo G, Beth E, Good G. Association of Kaposi's sarcoma with second primary malignancies. Possible etiopathogenic implications. Cancer 1980; 45:1472–9.

22. Schoeppel SL, Hoppe RT, Dorfman RF. Hodgkin's disease in homosexual men with generalized lymphadenopathy. Ann Intern Med 1985; 102:68–70.

Cancer Detection and Prevention Supplement 1:567–570 (1987)

Exposure to Hair Dyes and Polychlorinated Dibenzo-p-Dioxins in AIDS Patients With Kaposi Sarcoma:
An Epidemiological Investigation

Lennart Hardell, MD
Andrew Moss, PhD
Dennis Osmond, PhD
Paul Volberding, MD

School of Public Health, University of California (L.H.), Berkeley, CA 94720; Departments of Epidemiology and International Health (A.M., D.O.) and of Medical Oncology (P.V.), University of California, San Francisco General Hospital, San Francisco, CA 94110

ABSTRACT Fifty male AIDS patients with Kaposi sarcoma and 50 matched controls were interviewed about occupation, exposure to pesticides, Vietnam service, smoking habits, etc. No difference in use of pesticides was seen. One case but no control had served in Vietnam and was thereby exposed to agent orange. Dioxins are known to be immunosuppressive in animals. No significant difference in exposure to dioxin-containing products was found between cases and controls, however. Of interest was the fact that four cases but no control were occupationally exposed to hair dyes, some of which have been reported to be carcinogenic.

Key words: pesticide exposure, agent orange, hair dyes, Kaposi sarcoma, AIDS

INTRODUCTION

It has recently been suggested that exposure to agent orange might constitute a risk factor in AIDS (Bergh D, personal communication, 1984). Agent orange consisted of the two phenoxy acids 2,4-dichlorophenoxyacetic acid (2,4-D) and 2,4,5-trichlorophenoxyacetic acid (2,4,5-T); which have been used widely as weed killers. These phenoxy acids are contaminated with dioxins. The highest level of 2,3,7,8-tetrachlorodibenzo-p-dioxin (TCDD) reported in agent orange was 47 ppm [1]. Dioxins have also been reported as contaminants in chlorophenols, which are used as wood preservatives in tanneries, in cutting oils, etc.

In all studied animals species, TCDD exposure causes thymic atrophy with cortical thymic depletion [2]. The lymphocytes in T-dependant regions of peripheral lymphoid tissue

---

Dr. Lennart Hardell is now at the Department of Oncology, University Hospital, S-901 85 Umeå, Sweden. Address reprint requests there.

are also depleted [3]. Studies of cellular immunity have shown suppression of T-cell functions. These changes have been observed in both acute and chronic TCDD-exposed animals and are most pronounced in neonatal animals [2]. Studies on immunological effects of TCDD exposure in humans are more scarce. One investigation on the immune capability of workers previously exposed to 2,3,7,8,-TCDD suggested that persons in the highest exposed group were relatively deficient in primary immune capability and in T-cell and B-cell cooperation [Ward AM. Investigation of the immune capability of workers previously exposed to 2,3,7,8-tetrachloro-dibenzo-para-dioxin (TCDD). Unpublished observations]. A medical health survey of Missouri residents exposed to TCDD-contaminated soil in the Times Beach area suggested a greater percentage of individuals with a T4/T8 ratio < 1.0 in the high-risk group compared to the low-risk group (15% vs 6%), although this was not significant [4]. Exposure to dioxins might cause immunosuppression and decrease the host resistance to subsequent infection.

It was thus of interest to test if exposure to dioxins is a cofactor in the development of AIDS. Initially, 53 male AIDS patients were interviewed about Vietnam service and exposure to agent orange. Four of them (7.5%) had served in Vietnam, but none stated exposure to agent orange. Several of the cases reported exposure to pesticides during their leisure time, however. The hypothesis that dioxin exposure is a risk factor was then further tested in a case-control study.

MATERIAL AND METHODS

The present investigation consisted of 50 male AIDS patients with Kaposi sarcoma (KS). Only AIDS patients with KS were used since this is a well defined entity. Fifty male homosexual persons were used as controls. They were matched by age to each case. The cases were interviewed at the outpatient clinic and the controls over the phone about their job, occupational exposure to pesticides, service in Vietnam and exposure to agent orange, home use of pesticides, smoking habits, etc.

RESULTS

No case or control refused to participate. The median age of the cases and controls was 35 years (ranges 23–52 and 25–53 years for cases and controls, respectively). Twelve of the controls were lymphadenopathy-associated virus-positive (LAV+), and 29 were LAV−; nine controls were not tested.

Exposure to various agents is given in Table I. No difference in overall exposure to pesticides was seen in cases and controls. Most of the exposures were occasionally in their own gardens; eg, only two cases and two controls were occupationally exposed. All of these four subjects were exposed to phenoxy acids. Furthermore, one case was exposed to agent orange during his service in Vietnam in 1967–1968. No other case or control had served in Vietnam.

If a minimum total exposure time of 30 days was applied, four cases and three controls were exposed to pesticides. All were exposed to weed killers for more than 30 days in total. Three of these cases and two controls were exposed to dioxin containing phenoxy acids.

Exposure to wood preservatives was reported by ten cases and two controls. Two cases and both of the controls reported the preservative to be creosote. Only one subject, a case, was occupationally exposed to wood preservatives. He was exposed to pentachlorophenol for 8 years. The rest of the cases did not know the type of wood preservative.

One case was occupationally exposed to cutting oils for 4 years. He did not know if chlorophenols had been added to the cutting oils.

One control was exposed to leather dust from hides for two years, and another control was occasionally exposed to PCB in his work as an electrician for 10 years. PCBs are known to be contaminated by dibenzofurans, which are related to dioxins in their toxic effects.

Two cases and two controls had lived in sawmill areas but were never occupied in such industry. One case had for 5 years worked in a sawmill that used wood preservatives, although he never participated in such work.

TABLE I. Frequency of Exposure (%) to Different
Agents in 50 Cases and 50 Controls

Agents	Exposure frequency (%)	
	Cases	Controls
Asbestos*	4	2
Cutting oils	2	0
Hair dyes	8	0
Leather dust	0	2
Organic solvents*	12	6
PCB	0	2
Pesticides		
Total	44	50
Weed killers	20	22
2,4-D,2,4,5-T	12	6
Other	2	8
Unknown	6	8
Pesticides (30 days)		
Total	8	6
Weed-killers	8	6
2,4-D,2,4,5-T	6	4
Smoking	32	36
Wood preservatives	20	4
Creosote	4	4
Pentachlorophenol	2	0
Unknown	14	0

*Self reported exposure, eg, not included in the
questionnaire.

Exposure for more than 30 days to dioxin- or furan-contaminated products was thus stated by four cases and three controls, eg, three cases and two controls exposed to phenoxy acids, one case exposed to pentachlorophenol, and one control exposed to PCB. In addition, potential exposure was reported by two cases and one control.

Of the 12 LAV+ controls, six were exposed to pesticides (50%) vs 14 of the 29 LAV− controls (48%).

Regarding other exposures, interestingly, four cases had worked as hairdressers for 6, 6, 7, and 26 years. All of them reported exposure to hair dyes on a regular basis. Some of the hair dyes have been reported to be carcinogenic [5]. No control reported work as hairdresser or exposure to hair dyes. Smoking habits did not differ between cases and controls.

DISCUSSION

This investigation did not show any significant difference in exposure to dioxin-containing products in AIDS patients with KS vs controls. The study suggests that such exposure could not be a major cofactor in the development of AIDS as defined by KS lesions. To detect any difference of significance, a larger epidemiological study would be necessary. The difference in the use of wood preservatives in cases and controls could be caused by observational bias, since the cases were interviewed at the clinic and the controls over the phone. Further studies should especially evaluate use of hair dyes in these patients. It would also be of interest to analyze for dioxins and dibenzofurans in adipose tissue of AIDS patients to find out if the levels differ from the general population.

REFERENCES

1. Rappe C, Buser HR, Bosshardt HP. Dioxins, dibenzofurans, and other polyhalogenated aromatics production, use, formation and destruction. Ann NY Acad Sci 1979; 320:1–18.

2. McConnell EE. Acute and chronic toxicity, carcinogenesis, reproduction teratogenesis and mutagenesis in animals. In: Kimbrough RD, ed. Halogenated biphenyls, terphenyls, naphthalenes, dibenzodioxins and related products. Amsterdam: Elsevier/North-Holland, 1980; 109–50.
3. Vos JG, Faith RE, Luster MI. Immune alternations. In: Kimbrough RD, ed. Halogenated biphenyls, terphenyls, naphthalenes, dibenzodioxins and related products. Amsterdam: Elsevier/North-Holland, 1980; 241–66.
4. Knutsen AP. Immunologic effects of TCDD exposure in humans. Bull Environ Contam Toxicol 1984; 33:673–81.
5. Some aromatic amines and related nitro compounds–hair dyes, colouring agents and miscellaneous industrial chemicals. IARC Monogr Carcinog Risk Chem Hum 1978; 16; 25–42.

Cancer Detection and Prevention Supplement 1:571–576 (1987)

Lymphocyte Subsets, Natural Killer Cytotoxicity, and Perioperative Blood Transfusion for Elective Colorectal Cancer Surgery

Paul Ian Tartter, MD, FACS
Giorgio Martinelli, PhD

Department of Surgery, The Mount Sinai Medical Center, New York, NY

ABSTRACT Blood transfusions are associated with phenomena attributable to immune suppression. Since perioperative blood transfusion is associated with early cancer recurrence in patients with malignancies, we prospectively studied T-cell subsets and natural killer cytotoxicity in patients undergoing potentially curative surgery for colorectal cancer. Preoperative total peripheral lymphocyte number was significantly ($P = 0.0191$) depressed in patients who were subsequently transfused, but returned to normal by follow-up 1 to 3 months after surgery. Natural killer cytotoxicity declined significantly ($P < 0.05$) at follow-up in patients who were not transfused. These results do not explain the association of blood transfusion with cancer recurrence observed in colorectal cancer patients. Blood transfusion in this study was followed by increased numbers of peripheral lymphocytes and higher natural killer cytotoxicity.

Key words: immunology, oncology, hematology

INTRODUCTION

Numerous clinical studies have linked perioperative blood transfusion to tumor recurrence. Retrospective studies of sarcomas [1] and breast [2], colon [3–5], and lung [6,7] cancers have found that transfused patients undergoing potentially curative surgery have higher recurrence rates, lower disease-free survival, and poorer overall survival than patients who are not transfused.

The precise mechanism of the association between blood transfusion and cancer recurrence is elusive despite numerous hypotheses. Since pretransplant blood transfusion is associated with immunosuppression and prolonged survival of subsequently transplanted kidney allografts [8], and tumor growth is associated with immune suppression, these hypotheses have focused on immunologic mechanisms. Blood transfusion of dialysis patients is followed by inversion of the helper-suppressor T-cell ratio [9], the appearance of plasma lymphocyte suppressive factors [10], and marked suppression of lymphoctye response to mitogens and antigens [11]. Blood transfusions are also immune modulating in other clinical situations. Chronic transfusion therapy for sickle cell disease, hemophilia, thalessemia, and pyruvate

Address reprint requests to Dr. Paul Ian Tartter, Department of Surgery, Mount Sinai Medical Center, Gustave L. Levy Place, New York, NY 10029.

kinase deficiency is associated with depressed helper-suppressor T-cell ratios and depressed natural killer cytotoxicity [12,13]. Neonatal exchange transfusion is followed by measureable suppression of lymphocyte response to mitogens and allogeneic lymphocytes even 20 years after transfusion [14]. Perioperative blood transfusion in general surgical patients is associated with postoperative depression of lymphocyte proliferative responses [15], and transfusion for surgery of inflammatory bowel disease is followed by continued depression of peripheral lymphocyte number [16]. Since depressed natural killer cell number and cytotoxicity have been observed following transfusion in dialysis and other patients and are associated with tumor progression in cancer patients, we studied T-cell subsets and natural killer cytotoxicity in transfused and untransfused colorectal cancer patients.

MATERIALS AND METHODS
Patients

The study population consisted of 64 consecutive patients scheduled for elective colorectal cancer surgery between February 1, 1984 and October 31, 1984, without preoperative evidence of liver or other metastases.

Disease Staging

Staging was by a modification of Dukes' staging: A, limited to mucosa and submucosa; B1, infiltration of muscularis, nodes uninvolved; C1, one to three involved nodes; C2, more than three involved nodes; D, liver or other metastases. No patients received chemotherapy or radiotherapy during the study. Blood for T-cell subset determinations was drawn directly into heparinized tubes between 8 and 10 AM to eliminate diurnal variability.

Peripheral Blood Mononuclear Cell Isolation

Peripheral blood mononuclear cells were isolated using standard Ficoll-Hypaque density gradients. Cells were then resuspended in RPMI 1640 medium supplemented with 10% heat-inactivated fetal calf serum, penicillin (100 IU/ml), and streptomycin (100 μg/ml). Peripheral blood mononuclear cells were reacted with saturated amounts of monoclonal antibody (Ortho Pharmaceutical, Rahway, NJ) for 30 min at 4°C. The monoclonal antibodies used in the study were Leu-1 (reactive with T lymphocytes), Leu-2 (reactive with T lymphocytes of the suppressor phenotype), Leu-3 (reactive with lymphocytes of the helper phenotype), and Leu-7 (reactive with lymphocytes of the natural killer phenotype). Samples were then stained with flouresceinated goat antimouse immunoglobulin (Tago, Burlingame, CA) and analyzed with a flourescence-activated cell sorter (FACS IV, Becton Dickinson & Co., Sunnyvale, CA).

Natural Killer Cell Activity Assay

Natural killer cytotoxicity in peripheral blood mononuclear cells isolated as described above was assayed using labeled K562 tumor cells as targets. The assay was carried out as follows: 50,000 peripheral blood mononuclear cells were mixed in triplicate with 10,000, 20,000, 30,000, and 50,000 ^{51}Cr-labeled K562 cells in a final volume of 0.150 nl in round-bottomed trays. Following a brief spin to pack the cells lightly, trays were incubated for 4 hr in a humidified carbon dioxide incubator. The microtiter trays were then centrifuged at 150g for 5 min, and the radioactivity in a 100 μl aliquot of supernatant was measured in a γ-counter. The percentage of lysis was calculated according to the following formula: 100 $\times$ [cpm (experimental release) − cpm (spontaneous release)]/[cpm (total release) − cpm (spontaneous release)]. Spontaneous release of ^{51}Cr from the target cells determined in the presence of medium alone was always less than 10% of total release. Total release was determined by adding 1% NP40 to the cultures. Natural killer activity was assayed for each subject at effector: target ratios of 50:1, 25:1, 17:1, and 10:1 by varying the number of target cells.

Data Analysis

The data were analyzed by comparing the preoperative and follow-up T-cell subset numbers and natural killer cytotoxicity for transfused and untransfused patients. The preoperative values for each patient were compared to the follow-up values for each patient using a paired t test. Transfused and untransfused group means were compared using Student's unpaired t test. Multivariate anlaysis with stage, admission hematocrit, duration of surgery, estimated blood loss, and blood transfusion as dependent variables was performed on an IBM 370 computer system using the BMDP statistical package [17].

RESULTS

Preoperative depression of peripheral lymphocytes was significantly associated with subsequent blood transfusion (P = 0.0191; Table I). Both absolute numbers of lymphocytes (1,812 vs 2,231) and lymphocytes as percentage of white blood cells (21.9 vs 28.5) were depressed preoperatively in patients subsequently transfused.

Since patients with low admission hematocrit were significantly more likely to be transfused than patients with normal hematocrits (P = 0.0014), the association of low lymphocytes with subsequent transfusion may be a reflection of low hematocrits. To examine this posssiblity, we compared the lymphocyte numbers and percentages of patients with admission hematocrits above and below the mean of 38.7. There was no association between lymphocyte number (2,171 vs 2,134) and percentage (26.1 vs 26.9) with admission hematocrit.

Preoperative white blood count, subset numbers and percentages, and natural killer cytotoxicity were generally lower in patients who were subsequently transfused, but none of these differences were significant. There was no apparent relationship between preoperative cell numbers or cytotoxicity and stage of disease.

Patients returned for follow-up testing between 1 and 3 months after surgery. By this time there were no differences in peripheral cell numbers or T-cell subsets between the transfused and untransfused patients (Table II). The number of natural killer cells had increased significantly at follow-up in both transfused and untransfused patients who had potentially curative surgery (P = 0.0219, after eliminating stage D). Peripheral lymphocytes of transfused patients had increased and approximated the values for untransfused patients.

Natural killer cytotoxicity had declined significantly (P < 0.05) for all effector to target ratios in untransfused patients at the time of follow-up despite a slight increase in natural killer cell number. Cytotoxicity of natural killer cells from transfused patients had increased slightly from preoperative values. These differences in cytotoxicity could not be attributed to natural killer cell number or percentages since both of these values had increased at follow-up in both transfused and untransfused patients.

Multivariate analysis revealed no significant relationships between lymphocyte or subset numbers or cytotoxicity and admission hematocrit, duration of procedure, stage, size of tumor, number of involved nodes, location of tumor, or estimated operative blood loss.

TABLE I. Preoperative Lymphocyte Evaluation

	Untransfused		Transfused		
	No./mm^3	%	No./mm^3	%	P
White blood count	7,820		8,279		0.4762
Lymphocytes	2,231	28.5	1,812	21.9	0.0191
T cells (Leu 1$^+$)	1,263	56.6	1,107	61.1	0.2841
Helper cells (Leu 3$^+$)	785	35.2	690	38.1	0.3112
Suppressor cells (Leu 2$^+$)	466	21.9	390	21.5	0.7850
NK cells (Leu 7$^+$)	296	13.3	236	13.0	0.9136
Cytotoxicity (%)	68.6		65.0		
N	45		19		

TABLE II. Follow-Up Lymphocyte Evaluation

	Untransfused		Transfused		
	No./mm^3	%	No./mm^3	%	P
White blood count	7,341		7,728		0.6403
Lymphocytes	2,092	28.5	2,063	26.7*	0.5141
T cells (Leu 1$^+$)	1,109	53.0	1,118	54.2	0.8141
Helper cells (Leu 3$^+$)	674	32.2	747	36.2	0.2497
Suppressor cells (Leu 2$^+$)	441	21.1	398	19.3	0.4997
NK cells (Leu 7$^+$)	318	15.2	314	15.2	0.9765
Cytotoxicity (%)	60.8*		68.7		
N	45		19		

*$P < 0.05$ compared to preoperative value.

The statistically significant findings are that depressed preoperative lymphocyte levels were associated with subsequent blood transfusion and lymphocyte levels of transfused patients had increased at the time of follow-up. Natural killer cytotoxicity had decreased at follow-up in untransfused patients, and this could not be attributed to changes in natural killer cell number.

DISCUSSION

Two significant findings of the study are the association of low preoperative lymphocyte levels with blood transfusion and the subsequent normalization of peripheral lymphocyte number at follow-up. The former suggests that lymphocytes vary with some other variable associated with the need for transfusion, such as stage, admission hematocrit, duration of surgery, or estimated blood loss. Indeed, lymphocyte number has been reported to correlate with stage of colorectal cancer [18]. However, we did not find a relationship between lymphocyte number and stage, size of tumor, nodal staus, operative time, estimated blood loss, or admission hematocrit. A second potential explanation for the observed association of low preoperative lymphocytes with transfusion may be that low lymphocytes are associated with coagulopathy leading to excess intraoperative bleeding and transfusion. However, lymphocytes were not related to estimated operative blood loss, and all of these patients had normal platelet counts and prothrombin times prior to surgery. This does not rule out an association of lymphocytes with some unmeasured coagulation factor or with a circulating tumor-associated anticoagulant. A final possible explanation for the data comes from the observation that iron deficiency is associated with diminished numbers of peripheral lymphocytes in man [19]. Patients with low preoperative lymphocytes may be iron deficient, although not yet anemic, and the operative losses would have to be made up with transfused blood since the patient has inadequate iron stores.

The second significant finding of the study is the recovery of lymphocyte number in transfused patients. Recovery of lymphocyte number and function is associated with tumor excision in experimental animals [20], and normal peripheral lymphocyte numbers are restored by curative colorectal cancer surgery in man [21]. The recovery of normal lymphocyte number may merely reflect the excision of tumor, or it may reflect stimulation by allogeneic antigens present in transfused blood that continue to circulate in the recipient.

Natural killer cytotoxicity declined significantly at follow-up in patients who were not transfused despite a slight increase in natural killer cell number in these patients. This indicates that changes in natural killer cytotoxicity are not simply a reflection of natural killer cell number. The decline may refect the removal of tumor, which normally stimulates cytotoxicity. The continued high level of cytotoxicity noted at follow-up in transfused patients may reflect stimulation by transfused allogeneic antigens, as noted above, present in transfused blood that have continued to circulate in the recipient.

These results do not provide an explanation for the observed association of blood transfusion with immune suppression and tumor growth. The increase in natural killer cell number and cytotoxicity observed in transfused patients is not in agreement with hypotheses linking blood transfusion to immune suppression.

The increase in natural killer cell number following surgery has been previously reported by us [21] and others [22]. Peripheral lymphocytes decline in number following surgery [23, 24] with proportionate decreases in helper and suppressor cells and return to normal levels by 48 hr. Since the depression is transient and closely follows the peak of serum cortisol, it is probably due to a redistribution of lymphocytes from the blood to the tissues [24]. Blood transfusion does not seem to correlate with changes in the postoperative suppressor/helper ratio [23]. Our studies of helper and suppressor subsets are in complete agreement.

Postoperative lymphocyte function appears to be relatively independent of the observed depression in numbers. For example, Hamid et al [24] note that the proportion of activated lymphocytes as measured by the incorporation of tritiated thymidine in vitro without added mitogen is substantially increased 5 to 8 days after surgery or blood transfusion with the greatest number found after operation combined with blood transfusion. Indeed, enhanced natural killer cytotoxicity has been noted during surgery for benign disease and localized primary tumors, but this has been attributed to increased natural killer cell number [22]. The effect of surgery on natural killer cell number and cytotoxicity may be independent. We noted a significant cell increase in numbers of natural killer cells at 30 to 90 days of follow-up, suggesting that the effect of surgery on natural killer cell number may be prolonged. However, cytotoxicity declined significantly in the absence of blood transfusion despite increased natural killer cell number. This supports the observations of Vose and Moudgil [25] and Uchida et al [26], who noted that cytotoxicity was depressed following surgery for breast cancer. Uchida et al attributed their observation to increased suppressor activity.

The role of natural killer cells and natural killer cytotoxicity in the host's defenses against tumors as well as the effects of surgery and blood transfusion on host defenses are ill-defined at present. The results of cytotoxicity studies may be profoundly affected by the target cell line used [27]. In addition, the peripheral blood cells responsible for in vitro cytotoxicity may not be the same T cells as those isolated from tumors that kill cells in vivo [28]. This empirically attractive in vitro assay of tumor cell killing by patients' lymphocytes may not reflect in vivo events. Studies of natural killer cytotoxicity with simultaneous determinations of natural killer cell number are needed to refine the role of these cells in patients with malignancies.

ACKNOWLEDGMENTS

This work was supported by the Frieda and George Zinberg Foundation and by NCI-NIH grant 1 RO1-CA-35558-01.

REFERENCES

1. Rosenburg SA, Seipp CA, White DE, Wesley R. Perioperative blood transfusions are associated with increased rates of recurrence and decreased survival in patients with high-grade soft-tissue sarcomas of the extremities. J Clin Oncol 1985; 3:698–709.
2. Tartter PI, Burrows L, Papatestas AE, Lesnick G, Aufses AH Jr. Perioperative blood transfusion has prognostic significance for breast cancer. Surgery 1985; 97:225–9.
3. Blumberg N, Agarwal MM, Chuang C. Relation between recurrence of cancer of the colon and blood transfusion. Br Med J 1985; 290:1037–39.
4. Foster RS Jr, Costanza MC, Foster JC, Wammer MC, Foster CB. Adverse relationship between blood transfusions and survival after colectomy for colon cancer. Cancer 1985; 55:1195–1201.
5. Burrows L, Tartter P. Effect of blood transfusions on colonic malignancy recurrence rates. Lancet 1982; ii:661.
6. Hyman NH, Foster RS, DeMueles JE, Costanza MC. Blood transfusions and survival after lung cancer resection. Am J Surg 1985; 149:502–7.

7. Tartter PI, Burrows L, Kirschner P. Perioperative blood transfusions adversely affect survival after resection of stage I (subset NO) non-oat cell lung cancer. J Thorac Cardiovasc Surg 1984; 88:659–62.

8. Opelz G, Terasaki PI. Improvement of kidney-graft survival with increased numbers of blood transfusions. N Engl J Med 1978; 299:799–803.

9. Kerman RM, VanBuren CT, Payne W. Influence of blood transfusions on immune responsiveness. Transplant Proc 1982; 14:335–7.

10. Shenton BK, Proud G, Smith BM, Taylor RMR. Identification of immunosuppressive factors in plasma following multiple blood transfusions. Transplant Proc 1979; 11:171–4.

11. Fischer E, Lenhard V, Seifert P, Kluge A, Johannsen R. Blood transfusion-induced suppression of cellular immunity in man. Human Immunol 1980; 3:187–94.

12. Kaplan J, Sarnaik S, Gitlin J, Lusher J. Diminished helper/suppressor lymphocyte ratios and natural killer activity in recipients of repeated blood transfusions. Blood 1984; 64:308–10.

13. Gascon P, Zoumbos NC, Young NS. Immunologic abnormalities in patients receiving multiple blood transfusions. Ann Intern Med 1984; 100:173–7.

14. Beck I, Scott JS, Pepper M, Speck EH. The effect of neonatal exchange and later blood transfusion on lymphocyte cultures. Am J Reprod Immunol 1981; 1:224–5.

15. Roth JA, Golub SH, Grimm EA, Eilber FR, Morton DL. Effects of operation on immune response in cancer patients: Sequential evaluation of in vitro lymphocyte function. Surgery 1976; 79:46–51.

16. Tartter PI, Heimann TM, Aufses AH Jr. Blood transfusion, skin test reactivity and lymphocytes in inflammatory bowel disease. Am J Surg 1986; 151:358–61.

17. Engelman L. Stepwise logistic regression. In Dixon WJ, ed: *BMDP statistical software* c. Berkeley: University of California Press, 1981.

18. Slater G, Kim U, Papatestas AE, Aufses AH Jr. Peripheral lymphocytes in carcinoma of the colon and rectum. Surg Gynecol Obstet 1979; 149:719–21.

19. Flether J, Mather J, Lewis MJ, Whiting G. Mouth lesions in iron-deficient anemia: Relationship to candida albicans in saliva and to impairment of lymphocyte transformation. J Infect Dis 1975, 131:44–50.

20. Whitney RB, Levy JG, Smith AG. Influence of tumor size and surgical resection on cell-mediated immunity in mice. JNCI 1974; 53:111–6.

21. Tartter PI, Martinelli G, Steinberg B, Barron D. Changes in peripheral T cell subsets and natural killer cytotoxicity in relation to colorectal cancer surgery. Can Det and Prev 1986; 9:347–52.

22. Griffith CD, Rees RC, Platts A, Jermy A, Peel J, Rogers D. The nature of enhanced natural killer cytotoxicity during anesthesia and surgery in patients with benign disease and cancer. Ann Surg 1984; 200:753–8.

23. Hole A, Bakke O. T-lymphocytes and subpopulations of T-helper and T-suppressor cells measured by monoclonal antibodies (T11, T4, and T8) in relation to surgery under epidural and general anesthesia. Acta Anaesthesiol Scand 1984; 28:296–300.

24. Hamid J, Bancewicz J, Brown R, Ward C, Irving MH, Ford WL. The significance of changes in blood lymphocyte populations following surgical operations. Clin Exp Immunol 1984; 56:49–57.

25. Vose BM, Moudgil GC. Effect of surgery on tumor-directed leukocyte responses. Br Med J 1975; 1:56–8.

26. Uchida A, Kolb R, Micksche M. Generation of suppressor cells for natural killer activity in cancer patients after surgery. JNCI 1982; 68:735–41.

27. Takasugi M, Ramseyer A, Takasugi J. Decline of natural nonselective cell-mediated cytotoxicity with tumor progression. Ca Res 1977; 37:413–18.

28. Hutchinson GH, Symes MO, Williamson RCN. Cytotoxicity of lymphocytes from blood, tumour and regional lymph nodes against K562 cells and autoplastic colorectal tumour cells. Br J Cancer 1982; 46:682–6.

Cancer Detection and Prevention Supplement 1:577–582 (1987)

Immunohistochemical Studies of Lymph Nodes From LAS and AIDS Patients

H. Müller, MD
S. Falk, MD
H.J. Stutte, MD

Zentrum der Pathologie, J.W. Goethe Universität, Frankfurt, Federal Republic of Germany

ABSTRACT Lymph nodes from eight LAS and six AIDS patients were studied by routine histology, immunohistochemistry, and ultraimmunohistochemistry. LAS lymph nodes show a peculiar follicular hyperplasia with a characteristic increase of proliferating dendritic and interdigitating reticulum cells. In AIDS, these cells are reduced and the expression of proliferation-associated antigens is diminished. The immunohistochemical analysis of dendritic and interdigitating reticulum cells and of proliferation-associated antigens in lymph nodes thus allows a clear distinction between LAS and AIDS and may have important prognostic implications.

Key words: reticulum cells, proliferation-associated antigen, HIV, ultraimmunohistochemistry

INTRODUCTION

About 40% of all AIDS patients experience a phase of generalized lymphadenopathy that is of variable duration and may be associated with constitutional symptoms [1,2]. This clinical picture has been designated lymphadenopathy syndrome (LAS) and possibly constitutes either a benign form of AIDS or a prodromic phase [1,3,4]. The clinical distinction of LAS from AIDS in the setting of persistent generalized lymphadenopathy and seropositivity for HIV is based on the absence of opportunistic infections and unusual neoplasms as defined by the Centers for Disease Control surveillance criteria [5]. The histologic patterns encountered in lymph nodes from LAS and AIDS patients are variable [1–3,6,7] and in many instances do not permit a clear-cut distinction between LAS and AIDS. In the present study, immunohistochemical and ultraimmunohistochemical techniques were used to develop additional criteria for the morphologic evaluation of lymph nodes from patients with HIV-induced immunodeficiency.

MATERIALS AND METHODS

Lymph nodes from eight LAS and six AIDS patients were studied by routine histology. In addition, fresh-frozen sections were stained by a panel of monoclonal antibodies including

Address reprint requests to H.J. Stutte, MD, Zentrum der Pathologie, J.W. Goethe Universität, Theodor-Stern-Kai 7, D-6000 Frankfurt, Federal Republic of Germany.

TABLE I. Distribution of Dendritic Reticulum Cells (KiM4), Proliferation-Associated Antigen (Ki67), Interdigitating Reticulum Cells (S-100), and Natural Killer Cells (Leu7, Leu11b)*

No.	KiM4[†]		Ki67[‡]		S-100[‡]		Leu7[§]		Leu11b[§]	
	T	B	T	B	T	B	T	B	T	B
Lymphadenopathy syndrome (LAS)										
1	−	+ + + +	(+)	+ + + +	+ +	(+)	(+)	(+)	+	+
2	−	+ + + +	+	+ + +	+ + +	(+)	−	−	(+)	(+)
3	−	+ + + +	+	+ + + +	+ +	(+)	(+)	+	+	(+)
4	−	+ +	+	+ +	+ + +	+	−	−	−	−
5	−	+ + + +	+	+ + +	+ + +	(+)	(+)	−	−	(+)
6	−	+ + +	(+)	+ +	+ +	+	−	+	(+)	−
7	−	+ + +	+	+ + +	+ +	(+)	−	−	−	−
8	−	+ +	+	+ +	+ +	(+)	−	(+)	(+)	−
Acquired immunodeficiency syndrome (AIDS)										
1	−	−	−	−	−	−	−	−	−	−
2	−	+ + +	−	(+)	(+)	−	(+)	−	(+)	−
3	−	+	−	(+)	+	−	−	−	−	−
4	−	+ +	−	(+)	+	−	(+)	−	−	(+)
5	−	+	−	(+)	+	−	(+)	−	−	(+)
6	−	+ +	(+)	+	+ +	(+)	(+)	−	(+)	−

*Compared to LAS, lymph nodes in AIDS show a characteristic reduction of dendritic and interdigitating reticulum cells as well as of proliferating cells.
†Behring (Marburg, Federal Republic of Germany).
‡Dako (Hamburg, Federal Republic of Germany).
§Becton Dickinson (Heidelberg, Federal Republic of Germany).

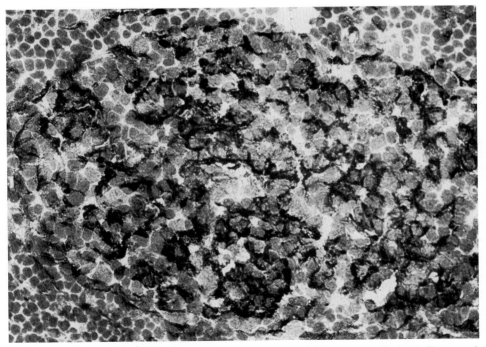

Fig. 1.   In comparison to AIDS, a marked increase of KiM4-positive dendritic reticulum cells occurs in germinal centers of lymph nodes from LAS patients. APAAP, hematoxilin counterstain; original magnification ×300.

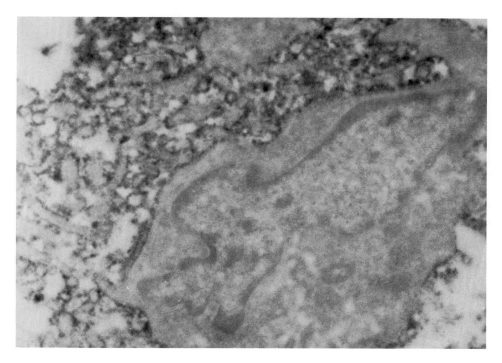

Fig. 2. Ultraimmunohistochemical demonstration of the KiM4 antibody as granular densities on the cell membrane of a dendritic reticulum cell from an LAS lymph node. Preembedding indirect immuno-peroxidase method without uranyl acetate and lead citrate stain; original magnification ×18,000.

those shown in Table I. Tissue fixed in a mixture of paraformaldehyde and glutaraldehyde and incubated with monoclonal antibodies was processed for electron microscopy. All patients were serologically positive for HIV as determined by an ELISA test and confirmed by a Western blotting technique, whereas six controls gave negative results.

RESULTS

All patients exhibited an inversion of the T4:T8 ratio in the peripheral blood as well as in the lymph nodes. In AIDS, T4:T8 ratios in lymph nodes correlated closely with values obtained in the peripheral blood; in LAS, obvious discrepancies were noted. In three LAS patients T4:T8 ratios in lymph nodes exceeded peripheral blood values, whereas in the five remaining LAS patients T4:T8 ratios were significantly lower in lymph nodes than in the peripheral blood. In two cases this discrepancy can be explained by the fact that 39% and 46% of all lymphocytes in these lymph nodes expressed neither T4 nor T8 antigens but were positive for the common T-cell antigen only. Lymph nodes from LAS patients histologically show a peculiar follicular hyperplasia that is expecially evident after staining with the common B-cell marker anti-Leu12 (Becton Dickinson, Heidelberg, Federal Republic of Germany).

Within the germinal centers, however, the number of dendritic reticulum cells (DRC) stained by the monoclonal antibody KiM4 (Behring, Marburg, Federal Republic of Germany) is substantially increased (Fig. 1). The KiM4 antibody may also be demonstrated by the ultraimmunohistochemical indirect immunoperoxidase method. The antibody is localized on the cell membrane of DRC as electron-dense granular material (Fig. 2).

Numerous cells within the germinal centers express a proliferation-associated antigen reacting with the monoclonal antibody Ki67 (Dako, Hamburg, Federal Republic of Germany). As evidenced by double staining with KiM4 and Ki67, the majority of these cells are DRC

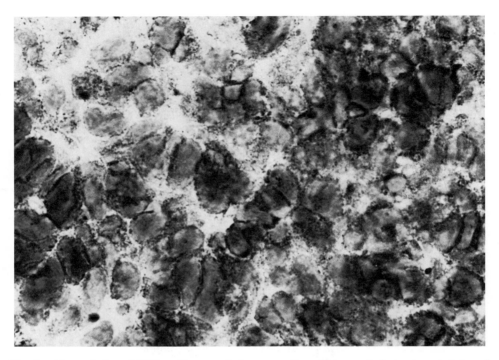

Fig. 3.   The majority of Ki67-positive germinal center cells exhibit morphologic characteristics of dendritic reticulum cells. APAAP, hematoxilin counterstain; original magnification ×800.

(Fig. 3). Ultraimmunohistochemically, the proliferation-associated antigen is situated on the nuclear membrane, within the cytoplasm, and on the cell membrane of the DRC.

In the T regions of LAS lymph nodes, the number of interdigitating reticulum cells (IDRC) that are positive for S-100 protein is markedly increased (Fig. 4). Staining with antibody Ki67 shows that this species of reticulum cells in LAS also expresses a proliferation-associated antigen (Fig. 5).

In AIDS lymph nodes, however, the number of DRC and IDRC is substantially reduced. Moreover, the expression of proliferation-associated antigens is markedly reduced and in some cases virtually absent. In comparison to HIV negative controls the number of natural killer cells is reduced in LAS as well as in AIDS. The results are summarized in Table I.

DISCUSSION

An increase of cells staining with the monoclonal antibodies KiM4, Ki67 and with antibodies against S-100 protein, ie proliferating DRC and IDRC, is highly typical of lymph nodes from LAS patients. In full-blown AIDS, however, the number of DRC and IDRC is conspicuously reduced and the expression of proliferation-associated antigens markedly diminished. In some AIDS cases, proliferation-associated antigens eventually are no longer detectable. These observations once more underscore the importance of the so-called accessory cells with respect to the HIV-induced immunodeficiency [8–11]. Like Jothy et al [12] but unlike Wood et al [11] we observed a diminished number of natural killer cells in lymph nodes from LAS and AIDS patients. Therefore we regard a reduction and not an increase of natural killer cells in lymph nodes as an indicator of a functional impairment of the immune system in HIV infection. Since the number of natural killer cells is reduced in both LAS and AIDS this parameter does not allow a distinction between these two stages of HIV-induced immunodeficiency.

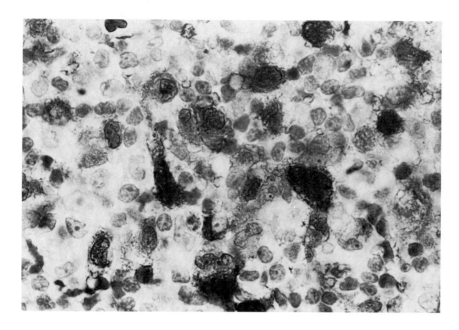

Fig. 4. In comparison to controls and to AIDS patients, increased numbers of protein S-100-positive interdigitating reticulum cells are scattered throughout the T regions of LAS lymph nodes. APAAP, hematoxilin counterstain; original magnification ×800.

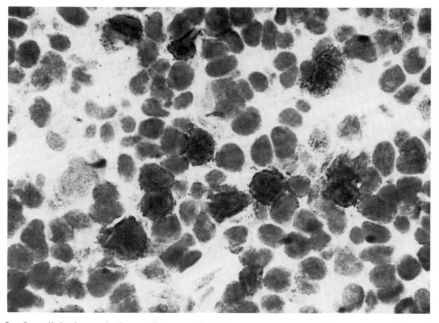

Fig. 5. Interdigitating reticulum cells expressing a proliferation-associated antigen reacting with the monoclonal antibody Ki67. APAAP, hematoxilin counterstain; original magnification ×800.

Immunohistochemical studies of DRC and IDRC as well as of proliferation-associated antigens clearly distinguish between LAS and AIDS. The somewhat arbitrary staging of the HIV infection on clinical grounds may thus be substantiated by objective morphologic criteria. The clinical significance and prognostic implications of the expression of proliferation-associated antigens on reticulum cells and on lymphatic cells have yet to be determined.

REFERENCES

1. Guarda LA, Butler JJ, Mansell P, et al. Lymphadenopathy in homosexual men: Morbid anatomy with clinical and immunological correlations. Am J Clin Pathol 1983; 79:559–68.
2. Mathur-Wagh U, Spigland J, Sachs H, et al. Longitudinal study of persistent generalized lymphadenopathy in homosexual men: Relation to acquired immunodeficiency syndrome. Lancet 1984; i:1033–8.
3. Fernandez R, Mourdian J, Metroka C, Davis J. The prognostic value of histopathology in persistent generalized lymphadenopathy in homosexual men. N Engl J Med 1983; 309:185–6.
4. Metroka CE, Cunningham-Rundles S, Pollack MS, et al. Generalized lymphadenopathy in homosexual men. Ann Intern Med 1982; 96:700–4.
5. Centers for Disease Control. Acquired immunodeficiency syndrome (AIDS)—United States. Morbid Mortal Weekly Rep 1983; 32:389–91.
6. Ioachim HL, Lerner CW, Tapper ML. Lymphadenopathies in homosexual men. JAMA 1983; 250:1306–9.
7. Burns BF, Wood GS, Dorfman RF. The varied histopathology of lymphadenopathy in the homosexual male. Am J Surg Pathol 1985; 9:287–97.
8. Armstrong JA, Dawkins RL, Horne R. Retroviral infection of accessory cells and the immunological paradox in AIDS. Immunol Today 1985; 6:121–2.
9. Müller H, Falk S, Stutte HJ. Lymph nodes, accessory cells and the staging of AIDS. Immunol Today 1985; 6:257.
10. Müller H, Falk S, Schmidts HL, Stutte HJ. Lymphknotenveränderungen beim Lymphadenopathie-Syndrom (LAS) und beim erworbenen Immun-defekt-Syndrom (AIDS). Verh Dtsch Ges Pathol 1985; 69:643.
11. Wood GS, Burns BF, Dorfman RF, Warnke RA. The immunohistology of non-T cells in the acquired immunodeficiency syndrome. Am J Pathol 1985; 120:371–9.
12. Jothy S, Gilmore N, El'Gabalawy H, Prchal G. Decreased population of Leu 7 + natural killer cells in lymph nodes of homosexual men with AIDS-related persistent generalized lymphadenopathy. Can Med Ass J 1985; 132:141–5.

Cancer Detection and Prevention Supplement 1:583–587 (1987)

Activated T Cells in Addition to LAV/HTLV-III[†] Infection:
A Necessary Precondition for Development of AIDS

D. Fuchs, PhD
A. Hausen, PhD
E. Hoefler, MD
D. Schönitzer, MD
E.R. Werner, DSc

M.P. Dierich, MD
P. Hengster, MD
G. Reibnegger, DSc
T. Schulz, MD
H. Wachter, PhD

Institutes for Medical Chemistry and Biochemistry (D.F., A.H., G.R., E.R.W., H.W.), for Hygiene (M.P.D., P.H., T.S.), Blood Transfusion and for Immunology (E.H., D.S.), and Ludwig Boltzmann Institute for AIDS Research, University of Innsbruck, Innsbruck, Austria

ABSTRACT Urinary neopterin levels are raised with a high incidence in all risk groups for AIDS. Neopterin elevations reflect activated cellular immunity in risk group members, in some cases independently of LAV/HTLV-III infection. Moreover, we are able to show that in patients receiving multiple blood transfusions at least a transient challenge of cell-mediated immunity occurs, which is indicated in part by increasing neopterin levels. We conclude that neopterin levels are a reliable index for assessment of susceptibility for AIDS when infection with LAV/HTLV-III occurs. Activated status of cell-mediated immunity might predispose infected persons to an overwhelming infection and secondary spreading of LAV/HTLV-III, thus leading to the development of full-blown AIDS or ARC. As a consequence of these observations, T-cell-stimulatory actions and agents should intentionally be avoided. Treatment of AIDS patients with immunosuppressants should be examined. The success of therapeutic regimens should be monitored by measurement of neopterin levels.

Key words: cellular immune system, neopterin, susceptibility for AIDS, blood transfusion, parenteral drug abusers

INTRODUCTION

The pathogenic role of LAV/HTLV-III in the acquired immunodeficiency syndrome (AIDS) is well established [1,2]. However, it has been suggested that other factors, eg, antigen overload and/or repeated exposure to other viral pathogens (CMV, EBV, HBV), contribute to the development of clinical AIDS or AIDS-related complex (ARC) in the risk groups [3–5].

---

†According to the International Committee on Taxonomy of Viruses now termed HIV (human immunodeficiency virus).

Address reprint requests to Dr. D. Fuchs, Institute for Medical Chemistry and Biochemistry, University of Innsbruck, A-6010 Innsbruck, Austria.

Particularly, an already compromised immune system has been considered to predispose individuals to progressive LAV/HTLV-III infection. According to that view, AIDS is an opportunistic infection [5].

Our investigations on neopterin excretion in members of AIDS risk groups do not exclude the proposed impact of such a preexisting immune deficiency for susceptibility but suggest that conditions linked with T-cell stimulation are more important for progressive LAV/HTLV-III infection. Similarly, the in vitro cultivation data of LAV/HTLV-III does not support the view of AIDS as an opportunistic infection: As virus production by infected cells is dependent on their proliferation [6], phytohemagglutinin and interleukin-2 have to be present. In vivo, the proliferative response of T4 cells is induced by antigenic stimulation via the lymphokine cascade [7].

Neopterin levels represent a reliable and easily measurable parameter for assessment of the activation of a cell-mediated immune system in vivo. Neopterin is produced by monocytes/macrophages upon stimulation with interferon-γ (IFN-γ) in a dose-dependent manner [8]. IFN-γ release is a function of the activation state of T cells. Therefore, high serum and urinary neopterin levels indicate stimulated T cells and an initiated lymphokine cascade in vivo. Increased neopterin levels are observed in approximately 100% of AIDS and ARC patients [9–11].

Activation of the cellular immune system is reported in AIDS risk groups: homosexuals [12], hemophiliacs [12], and parenteral drug abusers [13]. The activation of the immune system might be caused by alloreactions against sperm in homosexuals [14] and by protein load through substitution therapy in hemophiliacs [15]. The reasons for T-cell stimulation in parenteral drug abusers and possible activations in recipients of blood transfusions are examined in this report.

PATIENTS AND METHODS

Urinary samples from 20 patients were collected daily for 10 days following implantation of an artificial hip. These patients received 2–4 units of whole blood on the first day and five patients further 2 or 3 units on the third day subsequent to surgery. Urine samples were chromatographed by high-pressure liquid chromatography (HPLC) as described previously [16,17], with slight updating modifications: 100 μl urine diluted with 1,000 μl of Sorensen potassium phosphate buffer (pH 6.4, 0.015 mol/liter). Ten microliters were injected on the column (125 mm/4 mm, LiChroCart-rp-18; Fa. Merck, Darmstadt, Federal Republic of Germany). A guard column (125 mm/4 mm, LiChroCart-rp-18; Fa. Merck) was used and renewed after each 100 samples. In this way, at least 1,500 urinary samples can be evaluated with one main column. The effluent is monitored for pteridines with a fluorescence spectrophotometer (Shimadzu RF 530, Kyoto, Japan) with excitation set at 353 nm and emission at 438 nm. Simultaneously, urinary creatinine is quantified using its absorption at a 235 nm wavelength (UV 100; Fa. Varian, Palo Alto, CA). Pteridine levels were expressed as μmol/mol creatinine, taking physiologically varying urine concentration into account. Antibodies against milk powder as one commonly used diluent for drugs were tested with standard ELISA procedures. Sera of 34 drug abusers and of 30 controls were diluted 1:40, 1:80, 1:160, 1:320, and 1:640. Peroxidase-marked antibodies and 2,2′-azino-di-3-ethylbenzthiazoline sulfonate [6] as substrate were used.

RESULTS

Twenty patients who had received 1–7 units of whole blood during implantation of an artificial hip because of severe coxarthrosis showed increased urinary neopterin levels at 1–6 days posttransfusion. The daily neopterin excretion of a patient who received 6 units of whole blood is shown in Figure 1 as an example. The second set of transfusions revealed, similar to the example, in each case a more pronounced rise of urinary neopterin levels. This had led to the study of whether a booster effect produced by the minor mismatches of the second units

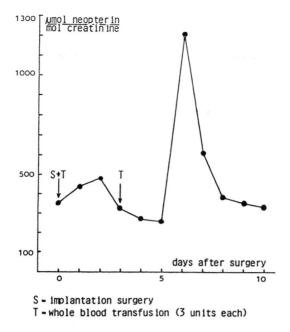

S = Implantation surgery
T = whole blood transfusion (3 units each)

Fig. 1.   Serial urinary neopterin levels (μmol/mol creatinine) of a patient, after artificial hip implantation surgery because of severe Cox arthrosis, receiving repeated whole blood transfusions.

with respect to blood groups Kell, Duffy, Kidd, and Lewis and the M, S, and P1 antigens is responsible for this increase. This possible explanation was refuted in that none of the patients developed antibodies against these blood group antigens as examined 3 months after surgery. Some of the patients presented at that time with antileukocyte antibodies. The possible HLA mismatches as cause of the observed immune stimulation remain to be examined.

Since persistently elevated neopterin levels have been observed in parenteral drug addicts and no correlation was found with previous infections we examined the immunogeneity of common diluents for opioids. Nine sera from 34 addicts as well as eight from 30 controls contained IgG antibodies to milk powder. Therefore, at least one commonly used diluent for drugs can induce antibody formation. Repeated intravenous injection of diluents might lead to immune complex formation, to activation, and thus to proliferation of T cells in parenteral drug addicts.

DISCUSSION

Our studies show that activations of T cells can be observed also in recipients of blood transfusions as a risk group among whom such a condition was so far unknown. Furthermore, milk powder, often used as a diluent for opioids, was found to be able to stimulate the cellular immune system. Therefore, the activation of the cellular immune system appears to represent an important feature in all risk groups. Since in vitro also the replication of LAV/HTLV-III in cultured T lymphocytes requires antigenic stimulation [18], we conclude that a repeatedly or permanently stimulated cellular immune system influences the clinical outcome of risk group members besides the LAV/HTLV-III infection. A scheme describing the situation proposed for the pathogenesis of AIDS is shown in Figure 2. As can be concluded from our results, immunologic activation of T-helper cells is a prerequisite for viral propagation as a second event in addition to infection with LAV/HTLV-III. This activation is achievable by alloreaction against sperm after receptive anal intercourse or immunogenicity of parenterally administered drugs and diluents. Blood transfusions also activate the cellular immune response. In addition,

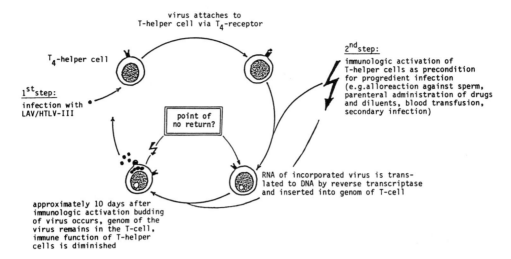

Fig. 2.   Proposal for the pathogenesis of AIDS.

activation of T lymphocytes because of secondary infection has to be considered. In advanced LAV/HTLV-III disease states, a self-sustaining activation of T-helper cells by recognition of virally transformed cells might be relevant. This situation is indicated in Figure 2 as "point of no return."

The proposed scheme appears to be supported by the following consideration. The magnitude of the elevations in the neopterin levels in risk group members reflects the susceptibility for development of AIDS [19]. We have observed a lower percentage of elevated neopterin levels and a lesser mean in homosexuals than in parenteral drug abusers [20]. In fact, the incidence of AIDS cases per number of individuals at risk among homosexuals represents only one-fourth compared to the other groups. Furthermore, Kaposi sarcoma represents a clinical manifestation of AIDS seen almost exclusively in homosexuals [21]. It should be noted that patients with Kaposi's sarcoma have the best prognosis among AIDS cases [22] and that immunologic abnormalities are less pronounced.

This influence of the T-cell activation associated with T-cell proliferation is in contradiction to the established treatment of AIDS patients: T-cell-stimulatory actions and agents should be avoided. AIDS and ARC patients should be kept free from secondary infections. The effect of hospitalization should be considered. Clinical trials using immunosuppressants possibly combined with inhibitors of reverse transcriptase and/or immunomodulatory agents that induce maturation of T cells without mitogenic activity should be established.

The success of such therapeutic regimens can be assessed by measurement of neopterin levels. Since treatment with immunostimulatory agents leads to rising and with immunosuppressants to decreasing neopterin levels, they represent a convenient and unique means of monitoring therapy in AIDS patients.

REFERENCES

1. Barré-Sinoussi F, Cherman JC, Rey F, et al. Isolation of a T-lymphotropic retrovirus from a patient at risk for acquired immune deficiency syndrome (AIDS). Science 1983; 220:868–71.
2. Popovic M, Sarngadharan MG, Read E, Gallo RC. Detection, isolation and continuous production of cytopathic retroviruses (HTLV-III) from patients with AIDS and pre-AIDS. Science 1984; 224:497–500.

3. Cavaille-Coll M, Messiah A, Klatzmann D, et al. Critical analysis of T cell subset and function evaluation in patients with persistent lymphadenopathy in groups at risk for AIDS. Clin Exp Immunol 1984; 57:511–9.

4. Kaplan J, Sarnaik S, Levy J. Transfusion-induced immunologic abnormalities not related to AIDS virus. N Engl J Med 1985; 313:1226–7.

5. Levy J, Ziegler JL. Acquired immunodeficiency syndrome is an opportunistic infection and Kaposi's sarcoma results from secondary immune stimulation. Lancet 1983; ii:78–80.

6. Klatzmann D, Barré-Sinoussi F, Nugeyre MT. Selective tropism of lymphadenopathy associated virus (LAV) for helper-inducer T-lymphocytes. Science 1984; 225:59–63.

7. Ettinghausen SE, Lipford EH, Mule JJ, Rosenberg SA. Systemic administration of recombinant interleukin 2 stimulated in vivo lymphoid cell proliferation in tissues. J Immunol 1985; 135:1488–97.

8. Huber C, Batchelor JR, Fuchs D, et al. Immune response associated production of neopterin, release from macrophages primarily under control of interferon-gamma. J Exp Med 1984; 160:310–6.

9. Wachter H, Fuchs D, Hausen A, et al. Elevated urinary neopterin levels in patients with the acquired immunodeficiency syndrome (AIDS). Hoppe-Seyler Z Physiol Chem 1983; 364:1345–6.

10. Abita JP, Cost H, Milstien S, Kaufman S, Saimot G. Urinary neopterin and biopterin levels in patients with AIDS and AIDS-related complex. Lancet 1985; ii:51–2.

11. Perna M, Nitsch F, Santelli G, et al. Urinary neopterin, a useful marker for AIDS? Lancet 1985; i:1098.

12. Fuchs D, Hausen A, Reibnegger G, et al. Urinary neopterin evaluation in risk groups for the acquired immunodeficiency syndrome (AIDS). In Pfleiderer W, Wachter H, Curtius HCh, eds: Biochemical and clinical aspects of pteridines. Berlin: Walter de Gruyter, 1984; 1613; 457–67.

13. Fuchs D, Blecha HG, Deinhardt F, et al. High frequency of HTLV-III antibodies among heterosexual intravenous drug abusers in the Austrian Tyrol. Lancet 1985; i:1506.

14. Mavligitt GM, Talpaz M, Hsia FT, et al. Chronic immune stimulation by sperm alloantigens. JAMA 1984; 251:237–41.

15. Landay A, Poon MC, Abo T, Stagno O, Lutie A, Cooper MD. Immunologic studies in asymptomatic hemophilia patients. J Clin Invest 1983; 71:1500–4.

16. Hausen A, Fuchs D, König K, Wachter H. Determination of neopterin human urine by reversed-phase high-performance liquid chromatography. J Chrom 1982; 227:61–70.

17. Fuchs D, Hausen A, Reibnegger G, Wachter H. Automatized routine estimation of neopterin in human urine by HPLC on reversed phase. In Wachter H, Curtius HC, Pfleiderer W, eds: Biochemical and clinical aspects of pteridines. Berlin: Walter de Gruyter, 1982; Vol 1; 67–79.

18. Montagnier L, Chermann JC, Barré-Sinoussi F, et al. A new human T-lymphotropic retrovirus: Characterization and possible role in lymphadenopathy and acquired immune deficiency syndromes. In Gallo RC, Essex ME, Gross L, eds: Human T-cell leukemia/lymphoma virus. Cold Spring Harbor, New York: Cold Spring Harbor Laboratory, 1984; 363–79.

19. Wachter H, Fuchs D, Hausen A, et al. Are conditions linked with T-cell stimulation necessary for progressive HTLV-III infection? Lancet 1986; i:97.

20. Fuchs D, Dierich MP, Hausen A, et al. Are homosexuals less at risk for AIDS than intravenous drug abusers and haemophiliacs? Lancet 1985; ii:1130.

21. Haverkos HW, Drotman DP, Morgan M. Prevalence of Kaposi's sarcoma among patients with AIDS. N Engl J Med 1985;6:1518.

22. Pinching AJ. The acquired immune deficiency syndrome. Clin Exp Immunol 1984; 56:1–13.

Cancer Detection and Prevention Supplement 1:589–596 (1987)

Modified Nucleosides in Patients With Acquired Immune Deficiency Syndrome (AIDS) and Individuals at High Risk of AIDS: Correlations With Lymphadenomegaly and Immunological Parameters

Alf Fischbein, MD
J. George Bekesi, PhD
Stephen Solomon, PhD
Ernest Borek, PhD
Opendra K. Sharma, PhD

Environmental Sciences Laboratory (A.F.) and Department of Neoplastic Diseases (J.G.B., S.S.), Mount Sinai School of Medicine, The City University of New York, New York, NY 10029; Department of Molecular Biology, AMC Cancer Research Center (E.B., O.K.S.), Denver, CO 80214

ABSTRACT   Patients with certain malignant diseases excrete in their urine elevated levels of modified nucleosides originating predominantly from the breakdown of transfer RNA (tRNA). Acquired immune deficiency syndrome (AIDS), often associated with rapidly progressing Kaposi's sarcoma (KS), is currently occurring in many countries. Male homosexuals are considered to be at highest risk of developing these disorders. We have previously reported that patients with AIDS excrete elevated levels of modified nucleosides. In this communication, we report on modified nucleoside levels measured in 77 male homosexuals without clinical manifestations of AIDS at the time of examination. A high frequency of abnormal nucleoside levels was found in this high-risk group. There was a trend towards higher levels in individuals with lymphadenomegaly, considered a prodrome of AIDS. Statistically significant correlations were found between some of the nucleosides (pseudouridine and dimethylguanosine) and degree of lymphadenomegaly. Pseudouridine, 1-methyladenosine and dimethylguanosine were inversely related to percentages of total T-lymphocytes (T_{11}), suppressor T-lymphocytes (T_8), and number of natural killer cells (Leu-7). These findings suggest that determination of urinary nucleoside levels may help identify individuals at high risk of developing AIDS.

Key words: Kaposi's sarcoma, homosexual males, tumor markers, tRNA, neoplastic risk, modified nucleosides

INTRODUCTION

Transfer RNA (tRNA) is a biomacromolecule with complex structure and function. Normally, tRNA undergoes modifications, the most important being methylation. It has been

Address reprint requests to Dr. Alf Fischbein, Environmental Sciences Laboratory, Mount Sinai School of Medicine, City University of New York, New York, NY 10029.

demonstrated that tRNA methylating enzymes are aberrantly hyperactive in malignant tumor tissue and that the turnover rate of tRNA is higher [1]. A clinical manifestation of these biochemical events is the observation that cancer patients excrete higher levels of modified nucleosides in their urine than healthy individuals [2]. Several investigations have demonstrated the usefulness of urinary nucleosides as diagnostic tumor markers in patients with cancer or as a means of evaluating the effectiveness of chemotherapy, ie, nucleoside excretion approaches normal levels in patients who have undergone successful treatment [3]. We have also reported that patients with asbestos-related malignant mesothelioma excrete high levels of nucleosides; moreover, we have found a high occurrence of elevated nucleoside levels in asbestos insulation workers with long-term exposure to asbestos and thus at high risk of developing cancer [4,5]. These investigations suggested the extended use of modified nucleosides as a means of identifying individuals at high neoplastic risk. This would be in addition to their previously mentioned function as tumor markers and as a monitoring tool for cancer treatment. A well defined high-risk group, without evidence of clinical disease, would be a suitable study group in which to explore modified nucleosides as potential preclinical indicators of future disease. We have attempted to address this matter in an investigation of a population at high risk for acquired immune deficiency syndrome (AIDS).

AIDS constitutes a severe public health problem in the United States [6]. The first reports of this disease appeared in 1981 [7–9]. AIDS is characterized by a wide spectrum of immunological alterations associated with an aggressive form of Kaposi's sarcoma's or by a wide spectrum of opportunistic infections [10,11], particularly *Pneumocystis carinii* pneumonia. Although a variety of therapeutic approaches are currently being evaluated, the disease has been quite resistant to treatment and has a poor prognosis.

Although approximately 75% of the recorded cases of AIDS in the United States have occurred in homosexual men, the disease has also been observed in intravenous drug users [12,13] as well as in male and female sexual partners of men with acquired immune deficiency [14]. In addition, AIDS has been reported in hemophiliacs receiving factor VIII concentrate [15]. Though the exact cause for AIDS is not yet known, the epidemiological picture suggests an agent, or agents, transmissible both sexually and percutaneously [16,17].

Recently, several investigations have linked lymphotropic retrovirus (HTLV-III/LAV) with AIDS and have proposed HTLV-III/LAV as the primary etiologic agent [18–21]. However, a predictive marker for the development of AIDS has not yet been identified, although a broad spectrum of possible "prodromal" clinical signs and symptoms have been described in male homosexuals. These include lymphadenomegaly, weight loss, fever, and fatigue.[22]. Generalized lymphadenopathy has also been related to serologic evidence of HTLV-III/LAV [23]. In the absence of any specific predictive marker for AIDS, it seems to be an important public health matter to attempt to detect individuals at high risk of developing AIDS. This could facilitate control of the current epidemic.

We have previously reported on urinary nucleoside levels in male homosexuals not suffering from clinically evident AIDS at the time of the examination [24]. In this communication, we have extended the initial investigation to a study of the relationship between urinary nucleosides, lymphadenomegaly, and immunological parameters.

MATERIALS AND METHODS

A clinical survey of 100 male homosexual volunteers without AIDS was undertaken. Subjects were recruited to participate in the examination through contacts with community organizations and the local press. Adequate quantities of urine were obtained from 77 individuals. Detailed questionnaires were administered in order to characterize demographic information, past medical and occupational histories, drug and alcohol use, and sexual practices. Each subject underwent a physical examination. Venous blood samples were obtained for a wide spectrum of laboratory tests, which included routine blood count, clinical biochemistry analyses, and detailed immunological evaluation.

Forty-five healthy male hospital employee volunteers served as a comparison group for the nucleoside studies. They had been recruited as laboratory controls and were unaware of the nature of the study.

Collection of Urine Samples, and Laboratory Techniques

Special requirements as to medications or diet were not imposed on the study subjects. All urine samples were collected in plastic containers and maintained at $-20°C$ to $-15°C$ without any preservatives. The samples were packed in dry ice and shipped to the AMC Cancer Research Center, Denver, where the samples were stored at $-80°C$ until analysis. The compounds measured were pseudouridine (ψ), 1-methyladenosine (m'A), 2-pyridone-5-carboxamide-N'-ribofuranoside (PCNR), 1-methylinosine (m'I), N^2-methylguanosine (m^2G), N^2-N^2-dimethylguanosine (m_2^2G), and β-aminoisobutyric acid (BAIB). The analytical methods utilizing high-performance liquid chromatography (HPLC), for the quantitation of modified nucleosides, and for BAIB, have been described in detail [25,26]. Urinary nucleosides and total BAIB (free and conjugated) were determined in duplicate aliquots of urine. Analyses of those samples with more than 5% variation were repeated and average values recorded. Creatinine was measured in three different dilutions of the urine by a creatinine analyzer (Beckmann Instruments). The rate of reaction was measured 25.6 sec after sample introduction to minimize interference resulting from the presence of nonspecific chromogens.

Immunodiagnostic Methods: Lymphocyte Separation, Surface Markers, and NK Assay

Peripheral blood (50 ml) was taken by venipuncture in a plastic syringe containing 15 U/ml preservative-free heparin. Separation of peripheral blood lymphocytes (PBL) was achieved by Ficoll-Hypaque gradient centrifugation. Briefly, 50 ml of blood was diluted with an equal volume of saline, overlaid onto a $25-ml$ Ficoll-Hypaque gradient, and centrifuged at 850g and 20°C for 45 min. The lymphocytes in the buffy-coat interphase were washed twice in saline and resuspended in RPMI-1640 supplemented with 20% heat-inactivated autologous plasma.

Mononuclear cells were analyzed for cell surface phenotypes by indirect immunofluorescence. Monoclonal antibodies directed against E receptors of human T lymphocytes (T11), helper T lymphocytes (T4), suppressor/cytotoxic T lymphocytes (T8), and B lymphocytes (B1) were obtained from Coulter Immunological (Hialeah, FL). Leu-7 against granulated lymphocytes associated with NK-cell activity was purchased from Becton-Dickinson (Mountain View, CA).

The standard NK cytotoxicity target K562 cells, a myelogenous leukemia cell line, were kindly supplied by E.C. Borden, University of Wisconsin. The cells were maintained in optimal growth and passed twice weekly in RPMI-1640, pH 7.3, fortified with 10% heat-inactivated pooled human serum (GIBCO, Grand Island, NY), 100 $\mu g/ml$ gentamicin (Wyeth Laboratories, Philadelphia, PA) and 25 mM Hepes (Sigma Chemical Company, St. Louis, MO). Detailed description of the immunodiagnostic methods has been published elsewhere [27,28].

Statistical Methods

The univariate statistics and the nature of the underlying distributions were determined for each nucleoside. For any given subject, a nucleoside value in the study group was considered to be elevated if it exceeded the 95th percentile level observed in the comparison group. An index of nucleoside abnormality, therefore, was defined as the cumulative frequency of elevated values for each particular subject. Since the nature of this latter variable is categorical, nonparametric techniques or distribution-free statistics (viz, Spearman ρ correlation coefficient) were applied in order to explore interrelationships with specific immunological parameters.

An important objective of the data analysis was to determine the accuracy of a linear multiregression model in discriminating between the control subjects and the homosexual men based exclusively on their nucleoside profiles. The actual computations were performed using the packages provided by the Statistical Analysis System [29]. Inasmuch as this higher-order correlational technique requires multiple measurements on each subject, only individuals with complete nucleoside profiles could be considered for developing any particular discriminant function, explaining reductions in sample sizes from the study populations described above. The rationale of discriminant analysis is to develop a classification algorithm that ascribes group membership predicated on a set of discriminator variables, ie, nucleoside level in this study. Increasing the number of unique relevant discriminator variables should greatly improve the efficiency (ie, predictability) of the discriminant function.

RESULTS

The age distribution of the examined populations is shown in Tables I and II. No significant differences were found in age between the high-risk and comparison groups. With respect to ethnic background, 71 (92%) of the 77 homosexual males without AIDS were white. Sixty-one (79%) described themselves as strictly homosexual, 14 (18%) as predominantly homosexual, and two (3%) as bisexual.

Figure 1 shows the number of subjects in the two examined groups with elevated nucleoside levels and provides a comparison with nucleoside levels of patients with confirmed AIDS [24]. In the homosexual group, nucleoside level failed to correlate with either the number of reported infectious diseases or with a cumulative index of the frequency of sexually transmitted diseases. Lymphadenomegaly has been a frequent observation in male homosexuals, and it has been suggested that this may be an important prodromal sign of AIDS. The extent of lymphadenomegaly was defined with respect to the number of sites at which lymph

TABLE I. Age Distribution of 77 Individuals at Risk of Developing AIDS and 45 Comparison Subjects

Age (years)	High-risk subjects		Comparison subjects	
	No.	%	No.	%
≤ 30	19	25	14	31
31–40	34	44	13	29
41–50	16	21	9	20
> 50	8	10	9	20
Total	77	100	45	100

TABLE II. Spearman Correlation Coefficients* Between Psuedouridine (ψ), Dimethylguanosine (m_2^2G) Levels and Palpable Lymph Nodes on Physical Examination of 77 Homosexual Men

Nucleoside	Palpable nodes No. of sites		No. of sites (inguinal excluded)		No. of sites (inguinal and submandibular excluded)	
	R	P	R	P	R	P
ψ	0.32	0.005	0.34	0.003	0.34	0.003
m_2^2G	0.37	0.001	0.38	0.0006	0.40	0.0003
Total number of elevated nucleosides	0.25	0.03	0.32	0.004	0.32	0.005

*Correlations with P < 0.05 are italicized.

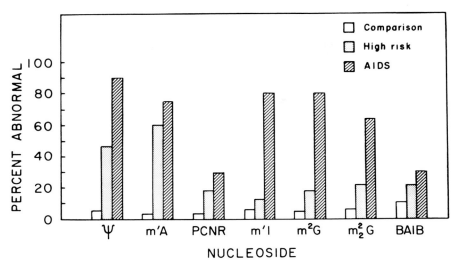

Figure 1.   Percent of patients with confirmed AIDS and male homosexuals showing elevated levels on each nucleoside in relation to the control subjects.

nodes were palpable on physical examination; it was found that pseudouridine and m_2^2G were significantly related to the degree of lymphadenomegaly (Table II). The magnitude of the relationship was unaffected by excluding either inguinal and/or submandibular lymph nodes from the computations. Moreover, the index of nucleoside abnormality, defined as the total number of elevated nucleosides, was significantly correlated with the extent of lymphadenomegaly.

The correlation coefficients between nucleoside levels and immunological parameters are presented in Table III. ψ, m'A, and m_2^2G were inversely related to T_{11}, T_4, T_8, and Leu-7. It has been suggested that especially ψ and perhaps m'A are crucial biochemical markers in identifying patients with confirmed malignant lymphoma [30]. Table IV presents the results of the discriminant model using only these two nucleosides. A 94% "hit rate" was observed for the normal controls (ie, 17 correct out of 18) and 82% of the homosexual men were correctly identified by the model, or an 18% "miss rate," on the basis of ψ and m'A levels alone (see the footnotes to Table IV for explanations of "hits" and "misses"). Subsequent inclusion of m'I, m_2G, m_2^2G, and PCNR improved prediction of both the control subjects and the homosexual men. The results of this discriminant function are shown in Table V. The need to monitor a broader range of biochemical markers may reflect the existence of an underlying biological gradient that requires more information in order to increase the accuracy of a multivariate prediction model.

DISCUSSION

Since 1981, when AIDS was first recognized as a serious disease in the United States, it has also become a serious public health problem in many countries. Just as the etiology for AIDS is unknown, the development of effective therapy has not yet been achieved. Viral etiology of AIDS has been suggested [18–21], and serologic tests are currently being evaluated as an attempt to identify individuals at high risk for developing AIDS; the successful use of such tests would be invaluable in meeting the challenge posed by this disease. We have attempted to approach this issue by evaluating the urinary excretion of biochemical products, ie, modified nucleosides, thought to be related to the carcinogenic process [1].

A pilot investigation was therefore undertaken to study the urinary excretion patterns of modified nucleosides in a group of AIDS patients and in one of the groups at high risk, ie,

TABLE III. Spearman Correlation Coefficients (P < 0.005) Between Pseudouridine (ψ), 1-Methyladenosine (m′A), Dimethylguanosine (m$_2^2$G), and Selected Immunological Parameters in 77 Homosexual Males

Immunological parameter	Pseudouridine	1-Methyladenosine	Dimethylguanosine
Percent T_{11} (T-lymphocytes)	−0.30	−0.32	−0.45
Percent T_4 (helper T-lymphocytes)	−0.24	NS*	−0.28
Percent T_8 (suppressor T-lymphocytes)	−0.24	−0.25	−0.34
Number of Leu-7 (natural killer cells)	−0.35	−0.26	−0.33

*Not statistically significant.

TABLE IV. Classification of Homosexual Men and Healthy Male Controls on the Basis of ψ and m′A Levels

Actual group	Predicted group	
	Controls	Homosexuals
Controls	17*	1†
	94%	6%
Homosexuals	14†	63*
	18%	82%

*Individuals correctly classified, "hit."
†Individuals misclassified, "miss."

TABLE V. Classification of Homosexual Men and Controls on the Basis of ψ, m′A, m^{2}G, m$_2^2$G, and PCNR Levels

Actual group	Predicted group	
	Controls	Homosexuals
Controls	17*	0†
	100%	0%
Homosexuals	19†	64*
	13%	87%

*Individuals correctly classified, "hit."
† Individuals misclassified, "miss."

male homosexuals without AIDS. Our results indicate that patients with AIDS excrete elevated levels of nucleosides; of added interest, however, is the observation that, within the group of disease-free (but at-risk) homosexuals, a high prevalence of abnormal nucleoside patterns was likewise found [24]. The study, therefore, raises the possibility that these biochemical markers can be used to identify persons at high risk of developing AIDS and that the presence of an abnormal nucleoside pattern among high-risk individuals may represent a prodromal stage prior to clinically manifest AIDS.

Recently, in another male homosexual population, we have observed that asymptomatic adult male homosexuals excreted elevated amounts of several modified nucleosides as compared to asymptomatic adult male controls. This aberrant excretion was more pronounced in asymptomatic adult male homosexuals with antibodies to HTLV-III/LAV [31].

The observed association between nucleoside abnormalities, lymphadenomegaly and immunological parameters is of interest and gives credence to the possibility that these are pathogenically related. It also suggests that there are manifestations of AIDS that will require a broader definition for epidemiologic surveillance [32–33].

Studies to investigate whether a specific nucleoside profile is characteristic for high-risk individuals are currently in progress. The predictive value of the initial findings presented here is also being investigated by prospective observation of the study group.

ACKNOWLEDGMENTS

We are grateful to Mr. Frank Buschman for performing analyses of modified nucleosides. We thank The City University of New York Computer Center for support in computer operations. Thanks are due to Mr. Mohammed Zanjani and Ms. Ratchanee Songsakphisarn for their excellent immunological work. This study was supported in part by T.J. Martell Foundation for Cancer and Leukemia Research (J.G.B., S.S.). We are grateful to Mr. Sidney Sibel for skillful typing of our manuscript.

REFERENCES

1. Borek E, Baliga BS, Gehrke CW, et al. High turnover rate of transfer RNA in tumor tissue. Cancer Res 1977; 37:3362–6.
2. Spear J, Gehrke CW, Kuo KC, Waalkes TP, Borek E. tRNA breakdown products as markers for cancer. Cancer 1979; 44:2120–3.
3. Gehrke CW, Kuo KC, Waalkes TP, Borek E. Patterns of urinary excretion of modified nucleosides. Cancer Res 1978; 39:1150–3.
4. Fischbein A., Sharma OK, Selikoff IJ, Borek E. Urinary excretion of modified nucleosides in patients with malignant mesothelioma. Cancer Res 1983; 43:2971–4.
5. Fischbein A, Sharma OK, Solomon S, et al. Transfer RNA breakdown products in the urine of asbestos workers. Cancer Detect Prevent 1984; 7:247–52.
6. Centers for Disease Control. Update: Acquired immunodeficiency syndrome (AIDS)—U.S. Morbid Mortal Weekly Rep 1983; 32:465–7.
7. Centers for Disease Control. Pneumocystis pneumonia–L.A. Morbid Mortal Weekly Rep 1981; 30:250–2.
8. Gottlieb MS, Schroff R, Schanker HM, et al. Pneumocystis carinii pneumonia and mucosal cardidiasis in previously healthy homosexual men. N Engl J. Med 1981; 305:1425–31.
9. Siegal FP, Lopez C, Hamner GS, et al. Severe acquired immunodeficiency in male homosexuals, manifested by chronic perianal ulcerative herpes simplex lesions. N Engl J Med 1981; 305:1439–44.
10. Gottlieb MS, Groopman JE, Weinstein WN, Fahey JL, Detels R. The acquired immunodeficiency syndrome. Ann Intern Med 1983; 99:208–20.
11. Sonnabend J, Witkin SS, Purtilo DT. Acquired immunodeficiency syndrome, opportunistic infections and malignancies in male homosexuals. JAMA 1983; 249:17:2370–4.
12. Masur H, Michelis MA, Greene JB, et al. An outbreak of community acquired pneumocystis carinii pneumonia. N Engl J Med 1981; 305:1431–8.
13. Masur H, Michelis MA, Wormser GP, et al. Opportunistic infection in previously healthy women. Ann Intern Med 1982; 97:533–9.
14. Harris C, Small CB, Klein RS, et al. Immunodeficiency in female sexual partners of men with acquired immunodeficiency syndrome. N Engl J Med 1983; 308:1181–4.
15. Centers for Disease Control. Update on acquired immune deficiency syndrome (AIDS) among patients with hemophilia A. Morbid Mortal Weekly Rep 1982; 31:644–6, 652.
16. Centers for Disease Control. Acquired immunodeficiency syndrome (AIDS): Precautions for health care workers and allied professionals. Morbid Mortal Weekly Rep 1983; 32:450–1.
17. Mildvan D, Mathur U, Enlow RW, et al. Opportunistic infections and immune deficiency in homosexual men. Ann Intern Med 1982; 97:700–4.
18. Essex M, McLane MF, Lee TH, Falk L, Howe CWS, Mullins JI. Antibodies to cell membrane antigens associated with human T-cell leukemia virus in patients with AIDS. Science 1983; 220:859–62.
19. Barré-Sinoussi F, Chermann C, Rey F, et al. Isolation of a T-lymphotropic retrovirus from a patient at risk for acquired immune deficiency syndrome (AIDS). Science 1983; 220:868–71.
20. Popovic M, Samagadharan MG, Read E, Gallo RC. Detection, isolation and continuous production of cytopathic retroviruses (HTLV-III) from patients with AIDS and pre-AIDS. Science 1984; 224:497–500.

21. Broder S, Gallo RC. A pathogenic retrovirus (HTLV-III) linked to AIDS. N Engl J Med 1984; 311:1292–1297.
22. Centers for Disease Control. Persistent, generalized lymphadenopathy among homosexual males. Morbid Mortal Weekly Rep 1982; 31:249–51.
23. Laurence J, Brun-Vezinet F, Schutzer SE, et al. Lymphadenopathy-associated viral antibody in AIDS. N Engl J Med 1984; 311:1269–73.
24. Fischbein A, Sharma OK, Valciukas JA, et al. Urinary excretion of modified nucleosides in patients with acquired immune deficiency syndrome and individuals at high risk of developing these diseases. Cancer Detect Prevent 1985; 8:271–7.
25. Gehrke CW, Kuo KC, Davis GE, Suits RP, Waalkes TP, Borek E. Quantitative high performance liquid chromatography of nucleosides in biological materials. J Chromatogr 1978; 150:455–76.
26. Kuo KC, Cole BF, Gehrke CW, Waalkes TP, Borek E. Dual column cation exchange for chromatographic method for BAIB and beta-alanine in biological samples. Clin Chem 1978; 24:1373–80.
27. Lew F, Tsang P, Solomon S, Selikoff IJ, Bekesi JG. Natural killer cell function and modulation by α-IFN and IL$_2$ in AIDS patients and prodromal subjects. J Clin Lab Immunol 1984; 14:115–21.
28. Tsang P, Tangnavarad K, Solomon S, Bekesi JG. Modulation of T and B-lymphocyte functions by Isoprinosine in homosexual subjects with prodromata and patients with acquired immune deficiency syndrome (AIDS) J Clin Immunol 1984; 4:469–78.
29. SAS User's Guide: Basics. SAS Institute Inc, 1982; Cary, NC: 27511.
30. Rasmuson T, Björk GR, Damber L, et al. Evaluation of carcinogenic antigen, tissue polypeptide antigen, placental alkaline phosphatase, and modified nucleosides as biological markers in malignant lymphomas. Rec Results Cancer Res 1983; 84:332–43.
31. Borek E, Sharma OK, Buschman FL, Cohn DL, Penley KA, Judson FN, Dobozin BS, Horsburgh Jr CR, Kirkpatrick CH. Altered excretion of modified nucleosides and β-aminoisobutyric acid in subjects with acquired immunodeficiency syndrome or at risk for acquired immunodeficiency syndrome. Cancer Research 1986; 46:2557–2561.
32. Centers for Disease Control. Update: Acquired immunodeficiency syndrome (AIDS)–U.S. Morbid Mortal Weekly Rep 1983; 32:389–91.
33. Centers for Disease Control. Revision of the case definition of acquired immunodeficiency syndrome for national reporting–United States. Morbid Mortal Weekly Rep 1985; 34:373–5.

Cancer Detection and Prevention Supplement 1:597–609 (1987)

Isoprinosine (Inosine Pranobex BAN, INPX) in the Treatment of AIDS and Other Acquired Immunodeficiencies of Clinical Importance

Alvin J. Glasky, PhD
Judy F. Gordon, DVM

Newport Institute for Medical Research, Newport Beach, CA

ABSTRACT   The immunopharmacologic effects of Isoprinosine (INPX) have been associated with clinical benefit to the patient in a number of conditions characterized by immunodeficiency of diverse etiology. Immunodepressed homosexuals at risk of developing acquired immunodeficiency syndrome (AIDS) treated with placebo or INPX experienced an increase in the function and number of immunocompetent cells associated with clinical improvement. A multicenter trial designed to confirm these results has demonstrated that INPX produced an increase in natural killer (NK)-cell activity, total T cells, and T-helper cells, with certain effects persisting for months after completion of the 28-day treatment period. INPX-treated patients also experienced clinical improvement and decreased incidence of progression to AIDS. The administration of INPX for longer periods to patients with frank AIDS under a compassionate-use protocol has also proved useful. Clinical benefit associated with INPX treatment has been demonstrated in other patients with a depressed immune response, such as aged patients, cancer patients, severely burned patients, ill patients, and surgery patients. This program of clinical trials supports the therapeutic use of INPX in the treatment of AIDS and other acquired immunodeficiencies of clinical importance.

Key words: AIDS-related complex, persistent generalized lymphadenopathy, cancer, aging, surgery, burns

INTRODUCTION

The use of immunomodulators in the treatment of diverse clinical conditions characterized by an underlying cellular immune defect is a therapeutic concept that has gained recent attention with the emergence of acquired immunodeficiency syndrome (AIDS) and the related conditions, including AIDS-related complex (ARC) and persistent generalized lymphadenopathy (PGL) Clinical application of immunotherapy, such as the use of interferon in the treatment of Kaposi sarcoma, has yielded mixed results [1,2] in this patient population, and trials evaluating other immunomodulators are still in early stages [3,4].

Isoprinosine (inosine pranobex, INPX) is an immunopharmacologically active agent that has been evaluated in numerous clinical trials for the treatment of viral diseases and immunodeficiency conditions. The efficacy of INPX treatment has been demonstrated in double-blind trials in herpes simplex virus infections [5–7], viral hepatitis [8], influenza [9], and rhinovirus infection [10], as well as in subacute sclerosing panencephalitis (SSPE), a disease of the central nervous system associated with measles infection [11–14].

Most recently, the therapeutic efficacy of INPX has been demonstrated in a series of clinical trials that establishes the usefulness of an immunomodulator in patients with acquired immunodeficiency associated with HTLV-III/LAV infection, ie, ARC and PGL patients. Additional trials conducted in patients with immunodeficiency of diverse etiology, including severely burned patients, cancer patients undergoing chemotherapy and/or radiation therapy, surgery patients, aged patients suffering recurrent infections, and other seriously ill patients, further established the clinical application of the immunopharmacological properties of INPX. This report will discuss those studies that demonstrate the ability of INPX to restore the immune response in patients with a range of clinical conditions all characterized by an underlying immune defect.

CLINICAL EXPERIENCE IN AIDS AND RELATED CONDITIONS

A number of in vitro studies [15–22] demonstrating the significant effects of INPX in enhancing lymphocyte function, interleukin-1 (IL-1) production and absorption, and production of and receptors for interleukin-2 (IL-2) provided a rationale for the design and implementation of clinical studies to evaluate the in vivo effects of the drug in this patient population. An early pilot study involving both AIDS and ARC patients indicated that INPX (4 g/day for 28 days) enhanced lymphocyte proliferative responses in patients with ARC but not in patients with frank AIDS [23]. This was the first indication that 28 days of treatment with INPX in patients with frank AIDS was not sufficient to trigger the chain of events that results in immunorestoration. Mansell and colleagues [24] also observed that only 28 days of treatment and observation of patient conditions was not sufficient in patients with AIDS. The lack of response seen particularly in patients with the profuse and persistent diarrhea typical of AIDS may have been associated with problems of drug absorption.

A double-blind placebo-controlled clinical study was then undertaken to evaluate the effect of INPX in a group of immunodepressed male homosexuals, all at risk of developing AIDS [25,26]. Patients were treated with placebo or INPX for 28 days and were followed clincially and immunologically for 1 year. Treatment with INPX at 3 g/day had a significant enhancing effect on several immune parameters. By day 7 of treatment, natural killer (NK) activity had increased by 60% relative to the initial baseline value. Total T cells showed an increase at day 28, and T-helper cells were increased at day 90. All three of these immunologic parameters remained elevated at day 180, 5 months after termination of drug treatment. NK-cell activity remained significantly elevated at Day 360, 11 months after completion of the treatment period, whereas T cells and T-helper cells had returned to baseline levels (Table I).

INPX was also of clinical benefit to this patient population. Based on cumulative clinical improvement scores, INPX-treated patients showed a substantially better clinical response than the placebo-treated patients at all time intervals examined (Fig. 1). By day 180, 52% of the drug group experienced clinical improvement compared to only 15% of the placebo group (P<.01).

These findings have been confirmed in two multicenter trials conducted under similar protocols. A total of 157 immunodepressed male homosexual patients at risk of developing AIDS have been treated with either INPX (3 g/day) or placebo for 28 days. As is shown in Figure 2, treatment with INPX resulted in substantial and sustained improvement in NK-cell activity, total T lymphocytes, and T-helper lymphocytes, whereas the placebo controls have shown little or no change. The most striking drug effect was the substantial increase in NK-cell activity. In patients followed for 90 days, NK-cell activity remained increased at day 90, 2 months after cessation of treatment. Drug effects on total and T-helper lymphocytes, although of lesser magnitude and duration, serve to support the concept that INPX promotes normal

TABLE I. Effect of INPX (3 g/day) on Immune Cell Activity in Pre-AIDS Patients

Day	Total T_{11} lymphocytes		Total T_4 helper cells		NK-cell activity	
	Placebo	INPX	Placebo	INPX	Placebo	INPX
0	1,251	1,209	606	515	11.5	11.9
7	1,049	1,141	527	478	14.4	19.3
14	1,047	1,186	529	508	13.4	26.6***
28	1,213	1,390	582	563	16.3	22.8
90	1,311	1,562**	646	686*	18.2	25.0*
180	1,298	1,365	570	572	14.3	22.3**
360	1,157	1,025	479	488	12.4	21.0

*P < .05.
** < .025.
***P < .01.
Reprinted from Wallace and Bekesi [25], with permission

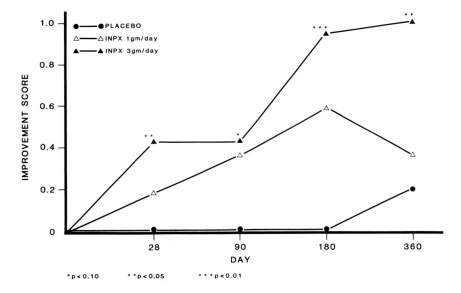

Fig. 1.   Effect of two doses of INPX on cumulative clinical improvement scores. Clinical improvement was scored as improved, 2; slightly improved, 1; unchanged, 0; slightly worse, −1; worse, 0. *P < .10, **P < .05, ***P < .01 significantly different from placebo: two sided Mann-Whitney u test. Reprinted from Wallace and Bekesi [25], with permission

stem cell production and differentiation, as manifested by increased NK cytotoxicity and greater numbers of cells phenotypically identifiable as thymus-derived.

The effect of treatment with INPX on the progression to AIDS in the total study population is shown in Figure 3. Patients treated with placebo had a higher probability of developing AIDS than patients treated with INPX. By day 210, six placebo-treated patients had progressed to AIDS, as compared to only three INPX-treated patients. Life table analysis indicates that, by day 210, 6% of the drug-treated patients would be expected to progress to AIDS as compared to 17% of the placebo patients. This constitutes a 65% reduction in the progression to the more serious forms of disease.

It is apparent from these data that INPX administered at a dose of 3 g/day had a profound and lasting effect on a number of cellular immunologic parameters as evaluated in this group

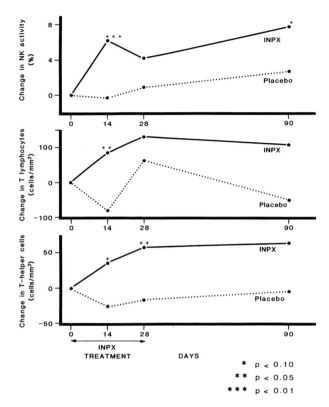

Fig. 2. Change in Nk-cell activity, total T lymphocytes, and T-helper cells following treatment with INPX or placebo. *P < .10, **P < .05, ***P < .01.

of immunodepressed homosexuals. The time course of this immune potentiation suggests that the drug induces the production of undifferentiated stem cells that can then naturally acquire the differentiated characteristics of one or more cell types, including cell phenotypically identifiable as thymus-derived. This is manifested by the rapid increase in NK cells, an early product of stem-cell differentiation. It is possible that undifferentiated stem cells whose production the drug has enhanced could differentiate along normal pathways to generate other phenotypically recognizable cell populations, such as T cells. Consistent with the duration of time required for thymic development, total T lymphocytes were increased at 1 month, and T-helper cells, a later stage of phenotypic development, were increased at 3 months. This lasting immunoenhancing effect was mirrored in the significantly improved clinical status of the patients 11 months after completion of treatment.

Interim results from an ongoing study of INPX in the treatment of frank AIDS, conducted under a compassionate-use protocol, suggest that the drug is useful in patients with more serious disease when administered for longer periods of time. Out of a total of 48 patients who have received INPX at a dose of 3 g/day for at least 60 days, 40 patients (84%) had improved or remained stable, and only eight patients (16%) had deteriorated clinically when evaluated at day 60.

SUPPORTIVE STUDIES IN IMMUNORESTORATION

Data from supportive controlled studies in other immunodepressed clinical states involved burn patients, cancer patients, aging patients, patients undergoing surgery, and other

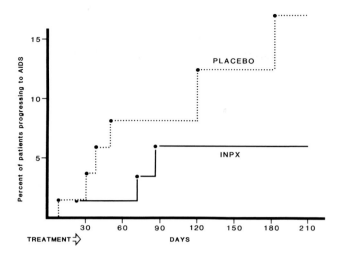

Fig. 3.   Kaplan-Meier life table estimate of the proportion of patients developing AIDS in the INPX- and placebo-treated groups.

seriously ill patients serve to establish further the usefulness of INPX in the management of various clinically distinct immunodeficiencies (Table II).

Cancer

In a series of studies, INPX was administered to cancer patients undergoing radiotherapy and/or chemotherapy [27–29]. Patients were evaluated immunologically both prior to and following treatment with INPX. Immunological parameters measured included E, EA, and EAC rosettes, mitogen-induced lymphoproliferative response, lymphocyte count, and skin test response (delayed-type hypersensitivity; DTH). INPX-treated patients experienced an immunorestorative effect, whereas placebo-treated patients remained immunodepressed. Among patients receiving pelvic radiation for genital cancer, 54% of the INPX-treated patients experienced immunorestoration following 3 months of treatment compared to only 13% of the placebo controls [27]. In another group of patients with mammary cancer, this difference persisted to the fifth month of the study, with 40% of the treated patients showing an immunorestorative effect as compared to only 6% of the controls.

This more rapid restoration of the immune response following cancer therapy was also seen in a group of 106 solid tumor patients (46 patients with breast cancer, 31 with cancer of the mouth and neck, and 20 with uterine cancer) treated with INPX or placebo in a double-blind study [30]. Patients were evaluated immunologically prior to radiotherapy, immediately thereafter, and after 1, 3, and 5 months of treatment by measuring mitogen response and percentage of E and EA rosettes and by performing lymphocyte counts and skin testing with a variety of antigens. After 3 months of treatment, 64% of the INPX-treated patients had a normal immune response as compared to 23% of the placebo-treated patients (Fig. 4). This effect was even more significant when evaluating breast cancer patients as a subgroup; 71% of the INPX-treated patients experienced normalization of the immune response as compared to 23% of the controls.

In a comparative study [31], the immunorestorative effects of INPX were compared to total parenteral nutrition (TPN) in a group of patients undergoing chemotherapy and/or radiation therapy after surgery for advanced esophageal and gastric cancer. TPN treatment was initiated 5 days before surgery and continued for 20 days; INPX treatment was initiated 14 days after surgery and continued for 28 days. A control group consisted of patients receiving only electrolyte-replacement fluids. INPX-treated patients experienced a significant improve-

TABLE II.

Investigator	Indication	No. of Patients	Dosage	Duration of Treatment	Comments
Benedetti et al [30]	Esophageal and gastric cancer	40	4 g/day	4 weeks	INPX patients had increased skin test response and EA rosette-forming T lymphocytes
Catania et al [3,35]	Surgery for malignant neoplasias	32	4 g/day	7 days	INPX patients had increased E rosettes and T lymphocytes
Cirulli and Roxas [38]	Surgery patients	96	4 g/day	14 days	INPX increased skin test response and decreased incidence of infection and mortality
Delogu et al [40]	Intensive care unit patients	57	8 g/day	14 days	INPX restored the immune response and decreased the incidence of mortality and infection
De Simone et al [29]	Solid tumors (Radiotherapy and/or chemotherapy)	30	4 g/day	28 days	INPX restored immune response as measured by skin test response and E, EA, and EAC rosettes
Donati et al [44]	Severe burns	20	70–100 mg/kg	8 days	INPX enhanced functional activity of neutrophils and reduced mortality and infections
Fenton [27]	Cancer patients (pelvic radiotherapy)	—	—	—	INPX accelerated return to normal of immune response following radiotherapy
Fridman et al [30]	Solid tumors (radiotherapy)	106	3 g/day	28 days, then 4 days/wk for 4 months	INPX accelerated normalization of immune response following radiotherapy
Gui et al [36]	Anergic surgical patients	62	4 g/day	10 days	81% of INPX patients had an increased skin test response compared to 16% of controls
Meroni et al [43]	Aged patients	50	4 g/day	90 days	INPX decreased the frequency and duration of episodes of respiratory tract and urinary tract infections
Midiri et al [25]	Gastric or colorectal adenocarcinoma	40	4 g/day	4 weeks	INPX patients had increase in skin test response and active E rosettes
Nanni et al [39]	Surgery patients	46	4 g/day	14 days	INPX patients had significantly fewer infections and less mortality
Ronconi et al [37]	Surgery patients	37	4 g/day	14 days	INPX decreased incidence of infection and mortality

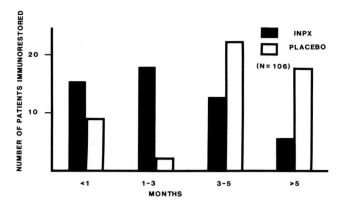

Fig. 4.   Number of cancer patients experiencing immunorestoration (as defined by lymphocyte/mono-cyte count, surface E and EA rosettes, lymphoblast transformation response to PHA, PWM, and PPD, and skin test response to candida at various intervals) during a 5 month course of treatment with INPX or placebo. There were 53 patients in each group Reprinted from Fridman et al [30], with permission.

ment in skin test response following a decrease from day 0 to day 14, ie, before treatment was initiated. EA rosette-forming T lymphocytes were also increased following treatment with INPX. TPN had a similar effect on skin test response but no effect on the number of EA rosette-forming T lymphocytes. Control patients experienced a decreased skin test response.

INPX also demonstrated efficacy in treating viral infections in patients with malignant hematologic disorders and in preventing opportunistic infections in a group of high-risk leukemia patients [32,33]. Although viral infections are generally severe in this patient population, 19 of 25 patients with a variety of viral infections (cytomegalovirus, varicella-zoster, herpes zoster, perpes genitalis) recovered completely following treatment with INPX. In leukemia patients treatment prophylactically with INPX, no viral infections were noted.

Surgery

INPX has been evaluated in controlled studies involving a substantial number of surgical patients [34–40]. Catania et al [34,35] found that the immune response was more rapidly restored to normal levels in INPX-treated patients undergoing surgery for malignant neoplasias than in the controls. The number of T lymphocytes and E rosettes had returned to presurgical levels within 7 days in the INPX-treated patients as compared to 15 days in the control patients. Control patients also experienced a depression of the lymphoproliferative response to PHA mitogen, which persisted until day 10 following surgery, whereas INPX-treated patients showed no surgery-associated depression of PHA response.

A group of investigators [36–38] evaluated the immunorestorative effect of INPX in surgical patients by identifying immunodeficient individuals through skin testing and then randomizing these patients to receive either INPX or placebo. Skin testing was then repeated at intervals following surgery and treatment. Gui et al [36] found that 81% of the INPX-treated patients experienced an increased skin test response as compared to only 16% of the placebo patients, and 56% of the drug-treated patients had a complete restoration of normal skin test reactivity as compared to 3% of the placebo patients.

In addition to evaluating skin test response, Ronconi et al [37] and Cirulli and Roxas [38] studied the incidence of local and systemic infections as well as postoperative mortality in two double-blind placebo-controlled studies in surgical patients. Following the same protocol, these investigators identified immunodeficient patients through the use of skin testing, random-ized these patients into INPX and placebo groups, and then repeated the skin testing following the treatment period. Patients treated with INPX experienced a significantly lower incidence of local sepsis, systemic sepsis, and postoperative mortality. These differences between the drug and placebo patients were directly related to the significant increase in the number of INPX-treated patients who experienced immunorestoration ie, became normoergic (Table III.)

These findings were confirmed by Nanni et al [39] in a study of the incidence of infection in patients treated with INPX or placebo for 14 days prior to surgery. Post surgical infections were experienced by only 13% of the INPX-treated patients as compared to 39% of the placebo-treated patients.

The results of these studies lead to the conclusion that the immunorestorative properties of INPX can be applied to lower the incidence of complications in surgical patients. Similar results were seen in critically ill patients admitted to the intensive care unit (ICU) of a hospital [40]. Patients treated with INPX experienced immunorestoration and, associated with this improvement in the immune response, a lower incidence of mortality and infection: 34.7% mortality in the treated patients as compared to 61.7% mortality in the controls and 52.5% incidence of infection as compared to 76.8% in the control patients.

Aging

The effects of INPX on the immune responses of aged humans have been evaluated in several clinical trials [41–43]. Moulias et al [41] studied the immunorestorative effect of INPX in a group of individuals with a mean age of 83 years. Although those immunological parameters that were initially normal were not affected by treatment, INPX normalized deficient immunological parameters in this population. In another study [42], 20 women between 68 and 95 years of age were divided into four groups and treated with INPX (3 g/day) or placebo for 2, 5, or 10 days. OKT3+, OKT4+, and OKT8+ cells were measured on days 0, 4, 8, 10, and 12. As in the earlier study, INPX had no effect on individuals whose cells were at normal levels at the initiation of treatment, although abnormally low levels of OKT8+ cells were increased in the 5 day treatment group and the 10 day treatment reduced the excess of OKT8+ cells present in that patient group. Thus, INPX corrected varied immune abnormalities present in aged individuals.

These effects were associated with significant clinical benefit in a group of elderly patients suffering from recurrent upper respiratory tract (URI) or urinary tract infections (UTI) [43]. Patients were treated with either INPX (4 g/day) or placebo, for 90 days, and were evaluated for the number of duration of respiratory tract and urinary tract infections during the trial period. INPX was effective in decreasing both the number and duration of infections in these patients. A significant decrease in the mean number of infectious episodes was seen following 60 days of treatment, and a significant decrease in the duration of these infections was noted after 30 days of treatment (Fig. 5). Simultaneously, treated patients showed an increased skin response to candida antigen.

Burns

Patients with severe burns represent another population with a depressed immune response and high risk and incidence of infection. Following treatment with INPX, a group of severely burned patients experienced marked improvement in their immune response characterized by increased functional activity of polymorphonuclear leukocytes as demonstrated by increased phagocytosis and increased killing [44] (Fig. 6). These immunological effects were

TABLE III. Effects of INPX on Incidence of Complications in Surgical Patients

	Normal skin test response (%)		Infection (%)		Mortality (%)
	Day 0	Day 14	Local	Generalized	
INPX	54.2	87.5	14.6	6.25	2.08
Placebo	58.4	60.5	25.0	18.70	12.50

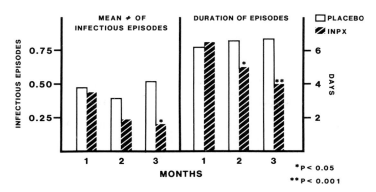

Fig. 5.   Mean number and duration of urinary and respiratory infections in elderly subjects treated for 3 months with INPX (N = 25) or placebo (N = 25). *P < .05, **P < .001. Reprinted from Meroni et al [43], with permission.

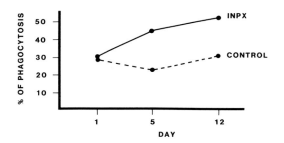

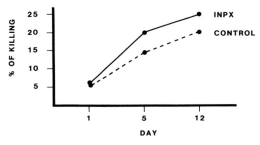

Fig. 6.   Immunorestoration in severely burned patients treated for 8 days with INPX (N = 10) or untreated controls (N = 10). Upper panel, percent phagocytosis of candida by polymorphonuclear cell, lower panel, percent killings of candida by polymorphonuclear cells. Reprinted from Donati et al [44], with permission.

associated with a reduction of mortality to 10% as compred to 30% in the untreated control group and a reduction of septic complications to 40% as compared to 90% in the controls.

DISCUSSION

The efficacy of INPX as an immunomodulating agent has been evaluated in a series of clinical trials involving patients with various acquired immunodeficiencies associated with diverse clinical presentations ranging from pre-AIDS to severe burns, cancer, surgery, and recurrent infections. The ability of INPX to restore the deficient immune response in this large and varied patient population is not surprising, based on the immunopharmacological activity of INPX as demonstrated in numerous in vitro and in vivo systems. In vitro studies have shown that INPX induces significant enhancement of NK-cell activity [45–47] and production of interferon [48] and interleukin-2 (IL-2) [17,18]. In animal models, INPX has been shown to produce increased NK-cell cytotoxicity [49], restoration of IL-2 production and receptors [50], and augmentation of the antitumor effect of interferon [51]. INPX restored depressed immune responses in human osteosarcoma-bearing hamsters [52], in animals immunosuppressed with cyclophosphamide [53], and in influenza virus (INFV)-infected mice [54]. In humans, INPX enhances lymphocyte proliferative responses to mitogens [55] and antigens [56] and increases production of lymphotoxin [55] and interferon [57].

Recently, the immunopotentiating effects of INPX have been studied in AIDS and related conditions, eg, ARC and PGL. Incubation of INPX with human peripheral blood monocytes (HPBMC) from patients with AIDS and ARC resulted in significant increases, and in some cases normalization, of mitogen-induced lymphocyte proliferative responses, with the greatest increases seen in cells from ARC patients [15,16,58]. It has also been reported that incubation of INPX with HPBMC from ARC patients resulted in a significant increase in both the percentage and absolute number of T-helper lymphocytes [59].

Although the precise biochemical mechanism through which INPX modulates immunologic functions is not entirely understood, data indicate that HPBMC from patients with AIDS respond to in vitro INPX with increased production of IL-1 and IL-2. Tsang et al [20] demonstrated that INPX potentiates IL-1 production by monocytes from both normal subjects and AIDS patients. These observations have been amplified by showing that Leu 3 + T lymphocytes (helper/inducer) from both controls and AIDS patients absorbed more IL-1 and produced significantly greater quantities of IL-2 in the presence of INPX [22]. In addition, Leu 2 + cells (suppressor/cytotoxic T lymphocytes) responded to in vitro INPX with increased expression of Tac antigen, the putative IL-2 receptor on this T-cell subset, thereby increasing the utilization of IL-2 in AIDS patients. Pompidou et al [60] have demonstrated the direct antiviral activity of INPX against HTLV-III/LAV, the etiologic agents of AIDS, further suggesting an effect of INPX on lymphocyte surface receptors. Cells infected with HTLV-III/LAV exhibited a 48% decrease in reverse transcriptase activity in peripheral blood lymphocytes (PBL) when virus and cells were coincubated with INPX at a concentration of 200 μg/ml [60]. Pompidou et al concluded that INPX is active against HTLV-III/LAV during the first steps of viral infection of T-helper cells, at the stage of viral transduction through the cell membrane, or in preventing incorporation of DNA in the nucleus. It is possible that the effects of INPX on lymphocyte surface receptors are responsible for triggering the molecular events that lead to the enhanced immune function seen in patients treated with INPX.

The results of human clinical trials in immunodepressed male homosexuals reported herein serve to establish the therapeutic application of this enhanced immune function in patients at risk of developing AIDS, ie, patients with AIDS syndrome, PGL, and ARC. INPX had a profound and lasting effect on both the immunological and clinical status of these patients. Treatment with INPX at 3 g/day for 28 days resulted in significant increases in NK-cell activity, total T lymphocytes, and T-helper cells. In patients followed for 1 year, NK-cell activity remained elevated 11 months following the completion of the 28-day treatment period. These immunological effects were associated with clinical benefit to the patients, with fewer treated patients going on to develop AIDS than placebo patients and significantly greater numbers of INPX-treated patients experiencing clinical improvement than placebo-treated patients.

A pattern of clinical improvement and lowered incidence of complications following treatment with INPX was also seen in studies dealing with a number of clinical states characterized by some degree of immunodeficiency, ie, surgery, cancer, burns, etc. The parallel results in each of these studies correlating the level of immune competence with the clinical response to treatment has established a link between enhancement of immunologic status and clinical improvement in conditions of apparently diverse clinical presentation. Collectively, these data suggest that numerous, seemingly unrelated conditions share a common immunologic defect that can be correlated by INPX. More specifically, the data support the use of the immunopharmacologic agent INPX as an effective means of restoring immunity and controlling infection in a broad range of clinical indications, including AIDS and AIDS-related conditions.

REFERENCES

1. Kriegel RL, Odajynk CM, Laubenstein LJ, et al. Therapeutic trial of interferon for patients with epidemic kaposi's sarcoma. J Biol Response Modif 1985; 4:358–64.
2. Krown SE, Real FX, Cunningham-Rundles S, et al. Preliminary observations on the effect of recombinant leukocyte a interferon in homosexual men with kaposi's sarcoma. N Eng J Med 1983; 308:1071–6.
3. Lifsdon JD, Mark DF, Benike CJ, Koths K, Engleman EG. Human recombinant interleukin-2 partly reconstitutes deficient in vitro immune responses of lymphocytes from patients with AIDS. Lancet 1984; ii:698–702.
4. Clumeck N, Van De Perre D, Mascart-Lemone F, Cran S, Bolla K. Preliminary results on clinical and immunological effects of thymopentin and AIDS. Int J Clin Pharmocal Res 1984; 6:459–63.
5. Salo O, Lassus A. Treatment of recurrent genital herpes with Isoprinosine. Eur J Sex Transm Dis 1983; 1:101–5.
6. Bouffaut P, Saurat J. Isoprinosine as a therapeutic agent in recurrent mucocutaneous infections due to herpes virus. Int J Immunopharmacol 1980; 2:193.
7. Bradshaw L, Summer H. In vitro studies on cell-mediated immunity in patients treated with inosiplex for herpes virus infection. Ann NY Acad Sci 1977; 284:190–6.
8. Scasso A, Paladini A, Della Santa M. Methisoprinol in the treatment of acute B viral hepatitis: Controlled clinical study. Curr Ther Res 1983; 34:423–35.
9. Betts R, Douglas R, George S, Rinehart C. Isoprinosine in experimental influenza a infection in volunteers. Paper presented at the 78th Annual Meeting of American Society for Microbiology, Las Vegas, Nevada, 1978.
10. Waldman R, Ganguly R. Therapeutic efficacy of inosiplex in rhinovirus infection. Ann NY Acad Sci 1978; 84:153–60.
11. Jones C, Dyken P, Huttenlocher P, Jabbour J, Maxwell K. Inosiplex therapy in subacute sclerosing panencephalitis. Lancet 1982; ii:1034–7.
12. Huttenlocher PR, Mattson RH. Isoprinosine in subacute sclerosing panencephalitis. Neurology 1979; 29:763–71.
13. Mattson RH, Lott T, Fink AJ. Treatment of SSPE with inosiplex. Arch Neurol 1975; 32:503.
14. Durant RH, Dyken PR. The effect of inosiplex on the survival of subacute sclerosing panencephalitis. Neurology 1983; 33:1053–55.
15. Tsang P, Lew F, O'Brien G, Selikoff IJ, Bekesi GJ. Immunopotentiation of impaired lymphocyte functions in vitro by Isoprinosine in prodromal subjects and AIDS patients. Int J Immunol 1985; 7:511–4.
16. Tsang P, Tangnavard K, Solomon S, Bekesi G. Modulation of T- and B-lymphocyte functions by Isoprinosine in homosexual subjects with prodromata and in patients with acquired immune deficiency syndrome (AIDS). J Clin Immunol 1984; 4:469–78.
17. Nakamura T, Miyasaka N, Pope RM, Talal N, Russell IJ. Immunomodulation by Isoprinosine: effects on in vitro immune functions of lymphocytes from humans with autoimmune diseases. Clin Exp Immunol 1983; 52:67–74.
18. Tsang KY, Pan JF, Swanger DL, Fudenberg HH. In vitro restoration of immune responses in aging humans by Isoprinosine. Int J Immunopharmacol 1985; 7:199–206.
19. Hersey P, Bindon C, Bradely M, Hasic E. Effect of Isoprinosine on interleukin 1 and 2 production and on suppressor cell activity in pokeweed mitogen stimulated cultures of B and T cells. Int J Immunopharmacol 1984; 6:321–8.
20. Tsang KY, Donnely RP, Galbraith GMP, Fudenberg HH. Isoprinosine effects on interleukin-1 production in Acquired Immune Deficiency Syndrome (AIDS). Int J Immunopharm (in press).
21. Tsang KY, Boutin B, Pathak S, et al. Effect of Isoprinosine on the sialylation of interleukin-2. Int J Immunopharm (in press).

22. Tsang KY, Fudenberg HH, Galbraith GMP, et al. Partial restoration of impaired interleukin-2 production and Tac antigen (putative interleukin-2 receptor) expression in AIDS patients by Isoprinosine treatment in vitro. J Clin Invest 1985; 75:1538–44.

23. Grieco M, Reddy M, Manvar D, Ahuja K, Moriarty M. In vitro immunomodulation by Isoprinosine in patients with Acquired Immunodeficiency Syndrome (AIDS) and related complexes. Ann Intern Med 1984; 101:206–7.

24. Mansell P, Reuben J, Odem M, Rios A, Hersh E. The use of Isoprinosine in an attempt to improve immune function in AIDS and AIDS related complex. Paper presented at the International Conference on Acquired Immunodeficiency Syndrome (AIDS), Atlanta, Georgia, 1985.

25. Wallace J, Bekesi G. A double-blind clinical trial of the effects of inosine pranobex in immunodepressed patients with prolonged generalized lymphadenopathy. Clin Immunol Immunopathol (in press).

26. Tsang P, Warner N, Bekesi JG. Impaired B and T-lymphocyte subsets and function restored by Isoprinosine in prodromal homosexuals and AIDS patients. Cancer Detect Prevent 1985; 8:580.

27. Fenton J. Double-blind study of the effect of Isoprinosine upon immunity tests in patients with pelvic radiation. Bull Cancer 1981; 68:200.

28. Midiri G, De Simone C. Meli D, et al. Studi preliminari sull 'effetto del methisoprinolo nei soggetti affetti de cancro dell' apparato digerente. Prog Med 1981; 37:1–7.

29. De Simone C, Midiri G, Meli D, Del Buono S, Di Paola M. Methisoprinol as an immunomodulating agent in G.I. cancer patients, preliminary report. Paper presented at the 4th International Congress of Immunology, Paris, France. 1980.

30. Fridman H, Calle R, Morin A. Double-blind study of Isoprinosine influence on immune parameters in solid tumor-bearing patients treated by radiotherapy. Int J Immunopharmacol 1980; 2:194.

31. Benedetti M, Amanti C, Midiri G. Comparative evaluation between total parenteral nutrition and methisoprinol as immunomodulating agent in cancer patients. Drug Exp Clin Res 1984; 10:471–8.

32. Schaison G, Gluckman E, Souillet JF, Turc JM. Isoprinosine curative and prophylactic treatment of viral infections in patients with malignant hemotologic disorders. Paper presented at the 4th International Congress of Immunology, Paris, France, 1980.

33. Souillet G, Schaison G, Gluckman E, Turc JM. Essai de l'Isoprinosine dans le traitement d'affections virales intercurrentes en hematologie. Paper presented at the 7th International Congress of Pharmacology, Paris, Frnce, 1978.

34. Catania G, Basile F, Cardi F, et al. Effect of methisoprinol on post-surgical immunodepression in subjects suffering from malignant neoplasias. Min Med 1981; 72:569–73.

35. Catania G, Cardi F, Basile F, Azzarello G, Chiavaro I, Giovineto A. Role of Ievamisole and methisoprinol in the treatment of immunodepression in patients undergoing surgery for malignant neoplasias. Policlin Chir 1981; 8:448–54.

36. Gui D, Borgogone A, Pittiruti M, Ronconi P. Immunostimulation of the anergic surgical patient with methisoprinol. Clin Eur 1982; 21:3–8.

37. Ronconi P, Bellantone R, Pittiruti M. Treatment of anergy in the surgical patients using methisoprinol. Chir Patol Sper 1982; 24:20–33.

38. Cirulli G, Roxas MA. Clinical evaluation of skin test responses in surgical patients treated with methisoprinol. Riv Gen Ital Chir 1980; 31:553–64.

39. Nanni G, Picari M, Chiodine A, Pepoli R, Koverech A. Studio clinico preliminare sull' uso del methisoprinolo nella profilassi e nel tratamento delle infezioni di interesse chirurgico. Riv Gen Ital Chir 1982; 23:127–38.

40. Delogu C, Lozzi A, Campanelli A, et al. Cell-mediated immunity and immunomodulatory drugs in critically ill patients. Acta Anes Ital 1982; 33:619–25.

41. Moulias I, Proust MR, Marescot M, Piette A, Devillechabrolle A. Action of Isoprinosine (inosiplex) on the immunological parameters of aged people. Paper presented at the 7th International Congress of Pharmacology Paris, France, 1978.

42. Renoux G, Renoux M, Froge E, Colombat PH. Influence of Isoprinosine on the T-cell phenotypes in elderly females. Int J Immunother (in press).

43. Meroni P, Palmieri R, Palmieri G, Froldi M, Zanussi C. Effetto di un trattamento con methisoprinolo sulia frequenza e durata di episodi infettivi delle vie ed urinarie in soggetti in eta' avanzata. Rec Prog Med 1984; 75:2–8.

44. Donati L, Lazzarin A, Signorini M, Candiani P, Klinger M, Moroni M. Preliminary clinical experiences with the use of immunomodulators in burns. J Trauma 1983; 23:816–31.

45. Balestrino C, Montesoro E, Nocera A, Ferrarini M, Hoffman T. Augmentation of human peripheral blood natural killer activity by methisoprinol. J Biol Response Modif 1983; 2:577–85.

46. Tsang KY, Fudenberg HH, Pan JF, Gnagy MJ, Bristow CB. An in vitro study on the effects of Isoprinosine on the immune responses in cancer patients. Int J Immunopharmacol 1983; 5:481–90.

47. Welch W, Duong L. Isoprinosine enhances human natural killer cell activity. Paper presented at the 2nd International Conference on Immunopharmacology, Washington 1982.

48. Tsang K, Fudenberg HH. In vitro modulation of virus susceptibility by Isoprinosine and NPT 15392. Clin Res 1982; 30:564.

49. Tsang KY, Fudenberg HH, Gnagy MJ. Restoration of immune responses of aging hamsters by treatment with Isoprinosine. J Clin Invest 1983; 71:1750–5.

50. Fischbach M, Talal N. Restoration of Interleukin-2 production and immune function in autoimmune mice. Clin Exp Immunol 1985; 61:242–7.

51. Cerutti I, Chany C, Schlumberger J. Isoprinosine increases the antitumor action of interferon. Cancer Treat Rep 1978; 62:1971–4.

52. Tsang KY, Fudenberg HH. Isoprinosine as an immunopotentiator in an animal model of human osteosarcoma. Int J Immunopharmacol 1982; 3:383–9.

53. Binderup L. Effects of Isoprinosine on animal models depressed T-cell function. Int J Immunopharmacol 1985; 7:93–101.

54. Ohnishi H, Kosuzume H, Inaba H, et al. Mechanism of host defense suppression induced by viral infection: Mode of action of inosiplex as an antiviral agent. Infect Immun 1982; 38:243–50.

55. Bradshaw L, Sumner H. In vitro studies are cell-mediated immunity in patients treated with inosiplex for herpes virus infection. Ann NY Acad Sci 1977; 284:190–6.

56. Corey L, Chiang W, Reeves W, Stamm W, Brewer L, Holmes L. Effect of Isoprinosine on the cellular immune response in initial genital herpes virus infection. Clin Res 1979; 27:41.

57. Kott E, Gadoth N, Levin S, et al. Stimulation of the interferon system by Isoprinosine (inosiplex) in subacute sclerosing panencephalitis (SSPE). Paper presented at the 13th Symposium of the Israeli Immunological Society, 1982.

58. Manvar D, Ahuja K, Reddy M, Moriarty M, Grieco MH. Immunomodulation with Isoprinosine in AIDS. J Allerg Immunol 1983;71:133.

59. Pompidou A, Delsaux MC, Telvi L, et al. Isoprinosine and imuthiol, two potentially active compounds in patients with AIDS-related complex symptoms. Cancer Res 1985; 45:4671–3.

60. Pompidou A, Zagury D, Gallo R, Sun D, Thorton A, Sarin P. In vitro inhibition of LAV/HTLV-III infected lymphocytes by dithiocarb and inosine pranobex. Lancet 1985; ii;1423.

Cancer Detection and Prevention Supplement 1:611–618 (1987)

Normalization of Immunoregulatory T-Helper T-Suppressor Sublineages and Cell-Mediated Immunity by Isoprinosine In Vitro in the Early Stages of AIDS

Peter Tsang
J. George Bekesi

Department of Neoplastic Diseases, Mount Sinai School of Medicine and Hospital, New York, NY

ABSTRACT Applying flow cytometric analysis and a panel of monoclonal antibodies that define functional subsets and stages of lymphocyte differentiation, we found both inducer and suppressor regulating subsets of helper T cells to be depressed with concurrent increase in the functionally active effector suppressor T cells in prodromal homosexuals and patients with AIDS. Concomitantly a broad spectrum of aberrations in all stages of B cell developments were observed. Failure of isolated peripheral blood lymphocytes from these subjects to respond to formalin-fixed *Staphylococcus aureus* cowan 1 (SAC) indicated intrinsic defects in their resting B cells, while impairment in pokeweed mitogen (PWM)-induced blastogenesis coupled with increased levels of Ig secretion signified regulatory defects in their mature B cells, which may be related to helper-suppressor dysfunctions. Based on these findings, a multifactorial immunodysfunction in AIDS was proposed. The antiviral biological modulator drug isoprinosine was shown to enhance PWM-induced, T-cell dependent, B-cell blastogenesis and normalize the spontaneous secretion of Ig while showing no modulative effects on SAC-induced (resting B-cell) transformations. It also modified, in a selective fashion, the phenotypic coexpression of both HLA-DR and Leu8 antigen on helper and suppressor T cells. Among prodromal subjects at risk to develop AIDS, isoprinosine augmented the expression of both helper T-cell subsets while reducing the number of suppressor effector cells and activated suppressor cells. These interferences with the helper-suppressor regulatory loop may explain the therapeutic efficacy of this drug in the early stages of AIDS.

Key words: monoclonal antibodies, flow cytometry, Ig secretion

INTRODUCTION

Previous studies have shown phenotypic and functional abnormalities in both homosexual males and AIDS patients but in different degrees [1–10]. Responses to T cell-dependent, B-cell mitogens were severely impaired in the homosexual subjects and more so in the AIDS patients [1–4]. Decrease in B-cell function was closely associated with a significant decrease

Address reprint requests to Dr. J. George Bekesi, Clinical Immunology—Cancer Center, Mount Sinai School of Medicine and Hospital, Basic Sciences Building, 10 East 102nd Street, New York, NY 10029.

in the number of T lymphocytes and in the ratio of helper/suppressor ($Leu3^+$/$Leu2^+$) cells [2,3]. Application of dual-color flow cytometry and monoclonal antibodies that define functional subsets (Leu8, Leu15, HLA-DR) within the T-helper and T-suppressor lymphocyte populations allowed us to demonstrate a possible defect in the feedback suppressor loop, which regulates both the helper and suppressor T-cell systems as well as B-cell functions in AIDS and prodromal subjects [2,3]. A variety of biological and chemical substances are being examined for their capacity to normalize regulatory pathways and to augment the depressed lymphocyte functions of these individuals [5,11–13]. Our preliminary findings suggest that the antiviral drug isoprinosine may be effective as a modulator of immune function in the prodromal stage of AIDS [4,5]. In a double blind randomized clinical trial in homosexual males at risk to develop AIDS, isoprinosine promoted clinical and immunological improvements [14]. In the work to be reported, the cellular mechanism of isoprinosine regulatory actions on the peripheral blood lymphocytes (PBL) derived from prodromal homosexual males and AIDS patients was examined in detail.

MATERIALS AND METHODS

Comprehensive clinical and immunological testing was performed in the following groups of subjects: 1) 72 homosexual males at risk of developing AIDS (average age 38.4 $\pm$ 8 years with a mean leukocyte count of 5,137 $\pm$ 1,122 mm^3) showing symptoms such as fever lasting more than a week, weight loss (>10 lb), diarrhea, venereal and herpes infection, anogenital lesions, lymphadenopathy at multiple sites, and antibody against HTLV-III/LAV, all of which have been associated with acquired immune deficiency syndrome [1-10]; 2) ten patients clinically diagnosed with AIDS (average age 37.5 $\pm$ 7 years with a mean leukocyte count of 3,850 $\pm$ 1,050; eight had Kaposi sarcoma and two had opportunistic infections; and 3) a control group of 19 healthy heterosexual males (average age 41.4 $\pm$ 7 years with a mean leukocyte count of 6,800 $\pm$ 700). The functional integrity of peripheral blood lymphocytes of the study groups was assessed by means of lymphoblastogenesis induced by highly purified phytohemagglutinin (PHA; Wellcome, Dartford, England) for T-lymphocyte functions, pokeweed mitogen (PWM; Wellcome, Dartford, England) for T cell-dependent B-lymphocyte function, and formalin-fixed *Staphylococcus aureus* cowan strain 1 (SAC) (BRL, Bethesda, MD) for resting B cells. B-cell activation and regulation of immunoglobulin synthesis were quantitated by measurement of spontaneous secretion of IgG and by staining of intracytoplasmic antibodies. Levels of IgG secreted during the 4 day incubation were measured in harvested culture supernatants by nephelometric technique as reported previously [2].

Enumeration of Cytoplasmic Antibody

The cultured mononuclear cells were fixed in ice-cold PBS containing 2% paraformaldehyde with 0.25% saponin, stained with an FITC-conjugated goat antihuman IgG antiserum, and analyzed with single parameter flow cytometry.

Determination of Surface Phenotypes

Mononuclear cells from the various patient and control groups were studied with dual-color direct immunofluorescence method as reported previously [1]. Monoclonal antibodies directed against T-helper ($Leu3^+$) antigen and T-suppressor ($Leu2^+$) antigen were conjugated with fluorescein, (FITC), while Leu8 and HLA-DR (Ia) monoclonal antibodies were conjugated with phycoerythrin (PE). Stained lymphocytes were analyzed for fluorescence in a Becton Dickinson FACS Analyzer. Two parameter data (x-axis = log FITC fluorescence and Y-axis = PE fluorescence) were displayed as contour maps indicating increasing numbers of cells in a defined area of display. Areas within the contour maps were integrated to determine the percentages of positive and negative cells [1].

Statistical Analysis

All data were encoded and entered into an IBM 370 computer and cataloged. The Statistical Analysis System (SAS) and Biomedical Programs P-series (BMDP) statistical packages were used in the data analysis. The data were characterized by parametric and nonparametric tests as the nature of the distributions demanded. The values obtained from the control male subjects served as our normative standard. Student t tests were computed between the control samples and all other groups on all clinical and immunological variables. The normal range of each variable was defined as either the 5th or 95th percentile of the control group. The values from each of the other groups were compared to these standards, the frequency of cases that exceeded the range tabulated, and the tendency for related multivariable involvement assessed.

RESULTS
Functional Studies of AIDS and Prodromal Subjects

Results in Figure 1A–C show marked deficiency among both homosexuals at risk and AIDS patients in their SAC-induced (T cell-independent B-cell) lymphocyte function and a less striking but still significant reduction in the PBL responses to PWM (T cell-dependent B-lymphocyte) and to PHA (T cell). The degree of dysfunction was consistent with a prodromal state among the homosexual males, leading to the more severe immunodepressive stage in the AIDS patients. Incorporation of ^{3}H-TdR as an index for DNA synthesis for SAC-induced responses (cpm) were $2.1 \pm 1.1 \times 10^3$ for the prodromal homosexual males and $0.8 \pm 0.2 \times 10^3$ for AIDS patients compared to $11.3 \pm 3.1 \times 10^3$ for the heterosexual controls. For PWM-induced blastogenesis the mean cpm were 91.9 ± 18.2, 38.8 ± 9.5, and $1.5 \pm 0.3 \times 10^3$ for the controls, prodromal homosexuals, and AIDS patients, respectively. The PHA-induced responses of the same study groups were 99.6 ± 17.3, 43.0 ± 11.0, and $8.8 \pm 2.4 \times 10^3$, respectively.

Despite the poor blastogenesis responses of lymphocytes from AIDS and prodromal subjects to various mitogens, heightened spontaneous immunoglobulin secretion by the unstimulated PBL was observed. Specifically, the value of IgG synthesized by unstimulated PBL over a 4 day culture was 55 μg per 10^6 cells for heterosexual controls, 127 μg for homosexual subjects, and 323 μg for the AIDS patients. Similarly, there was a marked increase in intracytoplasmic antibody-containing (clg$^+$) cells in both the AIDS and prodromal subjects. The relative number of cells reactive to goat antihuman immunoglobulin preparations was less than 3% in heterosexual controls, 16.3% in homosexuals, and 33.3% in AIDS patients.

Phenotypic Studies in AIDS and Prodromal Subjects

The decrease in PWM- and PHA-induced responses can be explained partially by a depression of T-helper (Leu3$^+$) cell-associated functions or by the increased activity of T-suppressor cell activity. The results in Figure 2 may support this hypothesis. An examination of T-helper (Leu3$^+$) and T-suppressor (Leu2$^+$) phenotypes demonstrated significant reductions in the number and percentage of Leu3$^+$ cells in the homosexual population and even more so in patients with AIDS, while the value of Leu2$^+$ cells was concurrently increased compared to the T-helper cell population

Among Leu3$^+$ cells, dual-color analysis following PWM stimulation demonstrated significant decreases in both regulator-helper (Leu3$^+$, Leu8$^+$) subset and inducer-helper (Leu3$^+$ Leu^8) subset. The numbers of activated helper T cells (Leu3$^+$ HLA-DR$^+$) were not significantly affected in the PBL of homosexuals at risk and the AIDS patients. Among the T-suppressor (Leu2$^+$) subset of lymphocytes (see Fig. 3) we observed an increase in the effector Ts (Leu2$^+$ Leu8$^-$) and the activated Ts (Leu2$^+$ HLA-DR$^+$) subsets for both homosexuals and AIDS patients, while Ts precursor (Leu2$^+$ for Leu8$^+$) cells were within the normal range.

Effects of Isoprinosine on Lymphocyte Functions

Coincubation with isoprinosine promoted various degrees of increase in the PWM (25.4%)-, PHA (29.3%)-, and in the SAC (10.6%)-induced lymphoblastogenesis of lymphocytes derived from heterosexual control subjects. In its application to the PBL of AIDS and

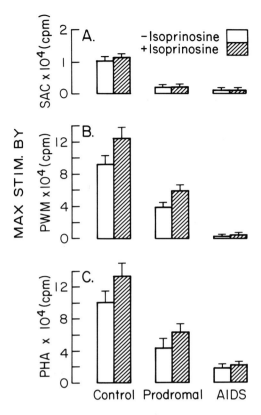

Fig. 1. Modulative effects of isoprinosine on T-, B, and pre-B-cell functions among prodromal homosexual males and patients with AIDS.

prodromal subjects, isoprinosine did not modulate SAC-induced lymphocyte responses but significantly increased and in many cases normalized both T- and B-lymphocyte functions (Fig. 1A–C).

To elucidate the mechanism of isoprinosine's modulative action on lymphocyte function, PBL from prodromal and AIDS subjects were analyzed with dual-color flow cytometry following PWM-induced blastogenesis. Prodromal subjects' lymphocytes coincubated with isoprinosine produced near normalization of both T_h-inducer (Leu3$^+$ Leu8$^-$) and T_h-regulator (Leu3$^+$ Leu8$^+$) subsets with concurrent elevation of their activated T-helper (Leu3$^+$ HLA-DR$^+$) cells. As for the T-suppressor subsets of prodromal subjects, coincubation with isoprinosine significantly reduced their effector Ts (Leu2$^+$ Leu8$^-$) and activated T-suppressor (Leu2$^+$ HLA-DR$^+$) subsets to levels comparable with heterosexual controls while the reciprocal subsets of precursor Ts (Leu2$^+$ Leu8$^+$) cells were not affected by such treatment. Similar coincubation of lymphocytes from AIDS patients with isoprinosine did not induce significant changes in the surface expression of T-helper and T-suppressor lymphocyte subsets (see Figs. 2, 3).

DISCUSSION

It is now well established that infections with the retroviruses T-lymphotropic virus type III (HTLV-III) or lymphadenopathy-associated virus (LAC) precede the onset of immunodysfunctions in AIDS [15–20]. T cells with the helper-inducer (T-4$^+$) phenotype have been shown

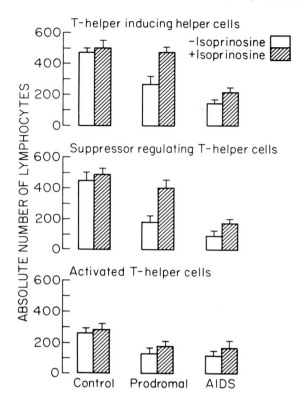

Fig. 2.   Phenotypic coexpressions of T-helper lymphocyte subsets selectively modified by isoprinosine in prodromal homosexual males and in patients with AIDS.

to be specifically susceptible to viral attack. Klatzmann et al [21] and Popovic [22] interrupted in vitro viral replication of HTLV-III in purified human lymphocytes by pretreating these cells with monoclonal antibodies to the T-4 antigen. More recently, McDougal et al [23] showed that the T-4 molecule itself was the surface receptor to the virus when they coprecipitated radiolabeled membrane particles from T helper/inducer cells with an isolated viral glycoprotein (GP110) from HTLV-III. Our report of a close association between depressed lymphocyte functions and a profound depression in circulating T-helper cell numbers among both prodromal and AIDS subjects [4,5] further supports the hypothesis that quantitative and functional aberrations in helper T cells are instrumental in the immunoregulatory imbalance in AIDS patients and prodromal homosexuals.

The lack of correlation between altered lymphocyte functions and the number of T-suppressor cells does not rule out the possibility that a subset of Ts cells may still be abnormally activated. Applying dual-color flow cytometric analyses and a panel of monoclonal antibodies that define functional subsets and stages of lymphocyte differentiation (Leu8, Leu 15, and HLA-DR), we have demonstrated that while both subsets of helper T cells (inducer-helper and regulator-helper) were indeed depressed in these subjects, there was also a concurrent increase in the functionally active suppressor T cells (Leu2$^+$ Leu15$^+$, Leu2$^+$ Leu8$^+$, Leu2$^+$ HLA-DR$^+$) while the reciprocal cytotoxic Ts cells (Leu2$^+$ Leu15$^-$ and Leu2$^+$ HLA-DR$^+$) were unchanged [2,3,]. Besides these abnormalities in helper and suppressor T-cell subsets, the results presented here illustrate a broad spectrum of impairments in all stages of B-cell developments as well. Failure of PBL from both prodromal subjects and AIDS patients to

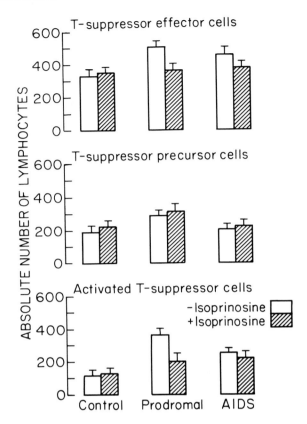

Fig. 3. Normalization of Ts-effector, Ts-precursor, and activated Ts-lymphocytic subsets in high risk homosexuals and in AIDS patients with isoprinosine.

respond to SAC indicated intrinsic defects in their resting B cells, while impairments in PWM blastogenesis together with increased levels of plasma cells and Ig secretion signified regulatory defects in T cell-regulated mature B-lymphocyte functions [24,25]. In an earlier study [5], we found both numerical and functional deficiencies in circulating NK cells and a general lack of response to endogenous interferon among both prodromal and AIDS subjects. Based on this information, we conclude that the cellular dysfunction in AIDS is multifactorial in mechanism and may involve defects in the feedback regulatory loop that modulates both helper and suppressor T-cell systems as well as B-cell and NK-cell functions.

Among helper cell subsets, the inducing helper cells (Leu3$^+$ Leu8$^-$) provide the majority of helper functions for B-lymphocyte activities while the reciprocal Leu3$^+$ Leu8$^+$ cells have been shown to regulate suppressor cell differentiation and activation [26–29]. Defects in the former may be responsible for the depressed T cell-dependent B-lymphocyte functions (PWM-inducted blastogenesis and Ig secretion) in AIDS. Quantitative deficiencies in the latter subset, on the other hand, may lead to abnormally high numbers of T-suppressor effector cells (Leu2$^+$ Leu8$^-$) and activated Ts cells (Leu2$^+$ HLA-DR$^+$). The elevated activities of these two suppressor subsets in turn affect both helper T cells and suppressor T cells as well as B- and NK-cell functions [30,31].

Recognition of these phenotypical and functional deficiencies provides information relating to immunomodulative management of both prodromal and AIDS subjects. Isoprinosine did not affect SAC-induced blastogenesis and therefore appears to have no modulative effects on the resting B-cell population. It effectively restored PWM-induced transformation and normalized the spontaneous secretion of Ig, suggesting that this agent may exert its regulative influence through its interference with the helper and suppressor regulatory pathways. Direct support for this view was provided by experiments with dual-color flow cytometric analyses. Isoprinosine modified the phenotypic coexpression of both HLA-DR and Leu8 antigen on helper and suppressor T cells in a selective fashion. Among prodromal homosexuals with mild symptoms, in vitro treatment with isoprinosine was able to augment the expression of both the inducer cells for helper function (Leu3$^+$ Leu8$^-$ subset) and suppressor regulating helper T cell function (Leu3$^+$ Leu8$^+$ subset) while reducing the number of suppressor effector lymphocytes (Leu2$^+$ Leu8$^-$) and activated suppressor (Leu2$^+$ HLA-DR$^+$) cells. Among AIDS patients with severe symptoms, coincubating their lymphocytes with isoprinosine reduced the number of the elevated subset of Leu2$^+$ Leu8$^-$ lymphocytes but exerted no modulative effects on the differentiation and activities of any other lymphocyte subsets. These selective interferences with the defective helper-suppressor regulatory loop may explain the therapeutic efficacies of this drug in restoring at least partially the depressed cell-mediated immunity associated with the early stages of AIDS.

ACKNOWLEDGMENTS

This work was supported in part by the T.J. Martell Foundation for Cancer and Leukemia Research, Newport Pharmaceuticals International, and NIH-NIAID-No1-A1-52572. The authors acknowledge the excellent technical assistance of Pat Mason, Ratchanee Songsakphisarn, and Sophie Kurdziel and the secretarial assistance of Ms. Diane Andujar.

REFERENCES

 1. Tsang PH, Warner N, Bekesi JG. Phenotypic and functional correlations in circulating lymphocytes of prodromal homosexuals and patients with AIDS. J Clin Lab Immunol 1985; 17:7.
 2. Bekesi JG, Tsang P, Roboz JP. The mechanism and modulation of immune dysfunction in AIDS associated syndromes. In Gupta S, ed: AIDS-associated syndromes. New York: Plenum, 1985.
 3. Bekesi JG, Tsang P, Lew F, Roboz JP, Teirstein A, Selikoff IJ. Functional integrity of T, B, and natural killer cells in homosexual subjects with prodromata and in patients with AIDS. Ann NY Acad Sci. 1984; 437-28.
 4. Tsang P, Lew F, O'Brien G, Selikoff IJ, Bekesi JG. Immunopotentiation of impaired lymphocyte functions in vitro by isoprinosine in prodromal subjects and AIDS patients. Int J Immunopharmacol, 1985; 7:511.
 5. Lew F, Tsang P, Solomon S, Selikoff IJ, Bekesi JG. Natural killer cell function and modulation by IFN and IL2 in patients and prodromal subjects. J Clin Lab Immunol 1984; 14:115.
 6. Tsang PH, Tangnavarad K, Solomon S, Bekesi JG. Modulation of T- and B-lymphocytes functions by isoprinosine in homosexual subjects with prodromata and in patients with acquired immune deficiency syndrome (AIDS). J Clin Immunol 1984; 4:469.
 7. Sonnbend J, Witkin SS, Purtilo DT. Acquired immunodeficiency syndrome, opportunistic infections, and malignancies in male homosexuals: A hypothesis of etiologic factors in pathogenesis. JAMA 1983; 249:2370.
 8. Reuben JM, Hersh EM, Mansell PW, et al. Immunological characterization of homosexual males. Cancer Res 1983; 43:897.
 9. Stahl RE, Friedman-Kien A, Dubin R, Marmor M, Zolla-Pazner S. Immunologic abnormalities in homosexual men: Relationship to Kaposi's sarcoma. Am J Med 1982; 73:171.
10. Rasmussen EO, Cooper KD, Kang K, White CR Jr, Regan DH, Hanifin JM. Immunosuppression in a homosexual man with Kaposi's sarcoma. J Am Acad Dermatol 1982; 6:870.
11. Krown SD, Real FX, Cunningham-Rundles S, et al. Preliminary observations of the effect of recombinant leukocyte A interferon in homosexual men with Kaposi's sarcoma. N Engl J Med 1983; 308:1071.
12. Rook AH, Masur H, Lane HC, et al. Interleukin-2 enhances the depressed natural killer and cytomegalovirus-specific cytoxic activities of lymphocytes from patients with the acquired immune deficiency syndrome. Clin Invest 1983; 72:398.

13. Coutinho RA, Lelie N, Albrecht-Van-Lent P, et al. Efficacy of a heat inactivated hepatitis B vaccine in male homosexuals: Outcome of a placebo controlled double blind trial. Br Med J Clin Res 1983; 286:1305.

14. Wallace JI, Bekesi JG. A double blind clinical trial of the effects of inosiplex in immunodepressed patients at risk of developing AIDS. Clin Immuno and Immunopath 1986; 39:179–86.

15. Vilmer E, Rouzioux C, Fischer A, et al. Isolation of new lymphotropic retrovirus from two siblings with haemophilia B, one with AIDS. Lancet 1984; 1:753–6.

16. Essex M, McLean MF, Lee TH, et al. Antibodies to cell membrane antigens associated with human T-cell leukemia virus in patients with AIDS. Science 1983; 220:859.

17. Barre-Sinoussi F, Chermann JC, Rey F, et al. Isolation of a T-lymphotropic retrovirus from a patient at risk for acquired immune deficiency syndrome (AIDS). Science 1983; 220:868.

18. Gelmann EP, Popovic M, Blayney D, et al. Proviral DNA of a retrovirus, human T-cell leukemia virus in two patients with AIDS. Science 1983; 220:862.

19. Montagnier I, Chermann JC, Barre-Sinoussi F. A new human T-lymphotropic retrovirus: Characterization and possible role in lymphadenopathy and acquired immune deficiency syndrome. In Levin AJ (ed): The cancer cell 3. Cold Spring Harbor NY: Cold Spring Harbor Laboratory, 1983.

20. Zolla-Pazner S, Leibowitch J, Popovic M. Isolation of human T-cell leukemia virus in acquired immune deficiency syndrome (AIDS). Science 1983; 220:865.

21. Klazmann D, Champagne E, Chamaret S, et al. T-lymphocyte T4 molecule behaves as the receptor for human retrovirus LAV. Nature, 1985; 312:767.

22. Popovic M, Read-Connole E, Gallo RC. T4 positive human neoplastic cell lines susceptible to and permissive for HTLV III. Lancet 1984; ii: 1472.

23. McDougal JS, Kennedy MS, Sligh JM, Cort SP, Mawle A, Nicholson JKA. Binding of HTLV III/LAV to T4[+] T cells by a complex of the 110 K viral protein and the T4 molecule. Science 1985; 231:382.

24. Lane HC, Massur H, Edgar LC, et al. Abnormalities of B-cell activation and immunogeneration in patients with the acquired immunodeficiency syndrome. N Engl J Med 1983; 309:453.

25. Howard M, Paul WE. Regulation of B-cell growth and differentiation by soluble factors. Annu Rev Immunol 1983; 1:307.

26. Gatenby PA, Kansas GS, Xian CY, Evans RL. Dissection of immunoregulatory subpopulations of T-lymphocytes within the helper and suppressor sublineages in man. J Immunol 1982; 129:1997.

27. Nicholson JKA, McDougal JS, Spira TJ, Cross GD, Jones BM, Reinherz EL. Immunoregulatory subsets of the T helper and T suppressor cell populations in homosexual men with chronic unexplained lymphadenopathy. J Clin Invest 1984; 73:191.

28. Landay A, Gartland GL, Clement LT. Characterization of a phenotypically distinct subpopulation of Leu2[+] cells that suppressor T cell proliferative responses. J Immunol 1983; 131:2757.

29. Reinherz EL, Morimoti C, Pinta AC, Schlossman SF. Subpopulations of the T4[+] inducer T cell subset in man evidence for an amplifier population preferentially expressing Ia antigen upon activation. J Immunol 1981; 126:67.

30. Yachie A, Miyawaki T, Yokoi T, Nagaoki T, Taniguchi N. Ia-positive cells generated by PWM-stimulation within OKT4[+] subset interact with OKT8[+] cells for inducing active suppression on B cell differentiation in vitro. J Immunol 1983; 129:103.

31. Damle NK, Mohagheghpour N, Englamen EG. Soluble antigen primed inducer T cells activate antigen-specific suppressor T cells in the absence of antigen-pulsed accessory cells: Phenotypic definition of suppressor-inducer and suppressor-effector cells. J Immunol 1984; 132:644.

Cancer Detection and Prevention Supplement 1:619–626 (1987)

Immunological Studies in Acquired Immunodeficiency Syndrome: Effect of TCGF and Indomethacine on the In Vitro Lymphocyte Response

Bo Hofmann, MD
Lars Fugger, MD
Lars P. Ryder, MSc
Johannes Gaub, MD

Niels Ødum, MD
Per Platz, MD
Jan Gerstoft, MD
Arne Svejgaard, MD, DSci

Tissue Typing Laboratory of the Department of Clinical Immunology (B.H., N.Ø., L.F., P.P., L.P.R., A.S.) and University Clinic for Infectious Diseases (J.Ga.), University Hospital (Rigshospitalet) and State Serum Institute, Department of Rubella, (J.Ge.) Copenhagen, Denmark

ABSTRACT   We studied the effects of exogenous T cell growth factor (TCGF) (= interleukin-2) and indomethacine on the lymphocyte transformation response in vitro to allogeneic cells, mitogens, and antigens in AIDS patients, those with AIDS-related complex (ARC), and in healthy controls. While low amounts of TCGF reduced the response of peripheral blood mononuclear cells (PBMC) to allogeneic cells in both healthy controls and AIDS patients, large amounts of TCGF augmented the response in both groups, although the response of the patients' cells were still subnormal. By depleting the PBMC for either CD4-positive or CD8-positive cells, the effect of TCGF on suboptimally mitogen-stimulated PBMC from controls was shown to be due to an increased response in both the CD4-positive and the CD8-positive cells. In contrast, with patient cells, TCGF only increased the response of the CD4-positive cells, while that of the CD8-positive cells was largely unchanged. Thus, the lack of normalization of the mitogen response of patient cells upon addition of TCGF may be largely due to unresponsiveness of CD8-positive cells to TCGF. This observation further supports the idea that CD8-positive cells are abnormal.

To investigate the role of the inhibitor of TCGF production, PGE2, in AIDS, indomethacine was added to cultures of mitogen-stimulated PBMC from controls and patients. No differences were found between the three groups: the responses to PHA were slightly increased and those to Con A were unchanged.

Key words: PGE2, ARC, CD4, CD8, IL2

INTRODUCTION

T cell growth factor (TCGF) (= interleukin-2) plays a crucial role in normal T lymphocyte-dependent immune responses. It has been repeatedly observed that patients with

Address reprint requests to Dr. Bo Hofmann, Tissue Typing Laboratory, 7631, University Hospital (Rigshospitalet), Tagensvej 18-20, Copenhagen, Denmark.

acquired immune dificiency syndrome (AIDS) and AIDS-related complex (ARC) have a reduced or even an extinct response in lymphocyte transformation [1,2], and we as well as others [3–5] have previously suggested an underlying defect in the capacity to produce TCGF.

The addition of irradiated HLA-DR identical peripheral blood mononuclear cells (PBMC) from healthy controls as well as supernatants from mitogen-stimulated cultures of PBMC from these controls and exogeneous TCGF increase the responses to mitogens of PBMC from patients with AIDS, suggesting that the production of TCGF in these patients is impaired [3]. Part of this decreased production is undoubtedly caused by a decreased number of circulating CD4-positive cells [6], since a subset of these CD4-positive cells are believed to be the main producers of TCGF [7] upon interleukin 1 stimulation. However, even when the number of CD4-positive cells was adjusted to a normal number, the transformation responses were still subnormal [2]. Moreover, CD8-positive cells are also capable of producing TCGF [7], and PBMC from controls, when depleted for CD4-positive cells, retain about 50% of their original responding capacity to mitogens, while AIDS PBMC depleted for CD4-positive cells did not respond at all [2].

This finding is enigmatic, since the human T cell lymphotropic virus-III lymphadenopathy virus (HTLV-III/LAV), believed to be the cause of AIDS, infects the CD4-positive helper cells and some monocytes but not the circulating CD8-positive cells. Prostaglandin E2 (PGE2) inhibits the production of TCGF, the expression of transferrin receptors, and the Ia antigen expression on macrophages [8–12]. Only macrophages expressing HLA-DR antigen can present antigen, but we previously found a normal mitogen and antigen "presentation" including interleukin 1 production by AIDS PBMC [3]. Our previous conclusion was that TCGF could restore the decreased response in AIDS PBMC to a subnormal level. However, whether TCGF can restore the response in both CD4-positive and CD8-positive cells is unknown as is the relationship between TCGF concentration and the transformation responses in PBMC from patients with AIDS and from healthy controls. The aim of the present study was to explore these problems by comparing the effect of TCGF (in AIDS patients and in controls by the lymphocyte transformation test.)

MATERIALS AND METHODS
Patients

All patients included in the study were men admitted to the University Clinic for Infectious Diseases in Copenhagen. The patients were male homosexuals between 24 and 52 years of age at the time of investigation. All patients with AIDS fulfilled the criteria for AIDS given by the Centers for Disease Control (CDC; Atlanta GA), and all patients were known to be positive for antibodies to HTLV-III/LAV [13].

Three patients with AIDS and three patients with ARC were included in the experiments with CD4- or CD8-depleted cells [see Table I (for details, see 2)]. One of the AIDS patients had Kaposi sarcoma, and two had pneumonia caused by *pneumocystis carinii*. The ARC patients were selected for the present study on the basis of a persistently decreased CD4:CD8 ratio of less than 0.5 and a decreased transformation response to mitogens and antigens accompanied by clinical symptoms. The number of experiments were limited by the large number of PBMC needed for the depletion experiments.

Four patients with AIDS and four patients with ARC were included in the mixed lymphocyte culture (MLC) experiments with TCGF (see Fig. 1). Besides the three patients with AIDS described above, an additional patient with generalized cytomegalovirus infection were included. The four ARC patients were selected by the same criteria as described above.

In the indomethacine experiments (see Fig. 2), ten patients with AIDS and six patients with ARC were included. Among the additional six patients with AIDS, four had pneumonia caused by *P. carinii* and two had Kaposi sarcoma. The six patients with ARC all had a CD4:CD8 ratio less than 0.9. In three of the patients, severely decreased responses to mitogens and antigens were found ie, less than 50% mitogen response compared to that of two

TABLE I. The Effect of TCGF (interleukin-2) on the Transformation Responses in Different Lymphocyte Subsets in AIDS/ARC Patients and in Healthy Controls

| | Responder cells | | | | | | | |
| | PBMC | | CD4-depleted | | CD8-depleted | | CD4-adjusted† | |
	None	TCGF	None	TCGF	None	TCGF	None	TCGF
PHA								
Controls								
1.	27*	53	0	29	38	42	39	49
2.	27	75	13	14	45	48	85	107
3.	138	118	64	103	79	88	19	55
4.	26	55	7	26	23	40	28	57
5.	9	43	9	46	56	63	50	55
6.	8	48	11	33	35	64	30	115
Median	27	54	10	31	42	56	35	56
AIDS/ARC								
1.	0	6	0	2	1	4	2	8
2.	2	21	2	8	1	11	5	18
3.	5	16	5	11	4	11	10	27
4.	8	30	2	5	49	50	44	48
5.	1	0	3	6	2	3	7	5
6.	1	24	3	1	12	22	12	22
Median	2	19	3	6	3	11	9	20
Con A								
Normal controls								
1.	63	70	0	24	51	25	76	67
2.	94	101	10	9	50	46	120	124
3.	102	120	38	44	65	73	115	102
4.	41	23	10	18	31	30	60	43
5.	21	15	11	7	28	13	38	19
6.	54	30	16	9	63	18	77	31
Median	59	50	11	14	51	28	77	55
AIDS/ARC								
1.	3	5	0	3	4	16	41	51
2.	4	23	1	7	13	17	14	20
3.	15	1	12	2	9	0	75	0
4.	2	12	3	5	14	17	16	20
5.	3	0	2	3	3	1	14	1
6.	1	7	29	0	42	51	42	51
Median	3	6	3	3	11	17	29	20

*Entries are increment cpm $\times 10^{-3}$. Median and range of values for unstimulated cultures of PBMC with TCGF added: Normal controls 6×10^3 cpm (range 3–20); AIDS/ARC 1×10^3 cpm (range 0–1).
†CD8-depleted cells adjusted to contain 20,000 CD4-positive cells per well.

simultaneously investigated controls for at least two of the three mitogens: phytohemagglutinin (PHA), concanavalin A (Con A), and pokeweek mitogen (PWM). Five of the six patients fulfilled the proposed criteria for ARC given by CDC, and one had abnormal immunological parameters and clinical symptoms compatible with acute HTLV-III/LAV infection.

Controls

Seventy-six volunteer donors or members of the medical staff served as normal controls.

Isolation of Lymphocytes

Isolation of lymphocytes has been described in detail [2]. Briefly, PBMC were isolated by lymphoprep (Nyegaard and Co., Oslo, Norway) density gradient centrifugation. Monocyte-enriched cells were prepared with the AET-rosetting technique. A mixture of 2 ml 10% 2-aminoethylisothiouronum bromide hydrobromide (AET)-treated sheep erythrocytes, 5×10^6 PBMC, 2 ml medium (RPMI 1640, Gibco, Grand Island, NY), and 1 ml fetal calf serum was centrifuged at 500 rpm for 10 min and incubated for 30 min at 4°C. After incubation, the pellet was gently resuspended, and the nonrosetting (monocyte-enriched) cells were separated by lymphoprep density gradient centrifugation. All monocyte-enriched cells were irradiated with 2,100 rad (γ cell, Risø, Denmark). Before use, all monocyte-enriched cells were washed twice. Initial experiments showed that 20,000 irradiated normal monocyte-enriched cells were able fully to reconstitute the lymphocyte transformation response of nylon wool-separated control T lymphocytes, and, accordingly, this amount was used in subsequent experiments.

T Cell Subset Depletion

PBMC were diluted to 10^7/ml of medium (RPMI with 10% pooled human serum [HS]), and monoclonal antibodies (OKT4 or OKT8; Ortho-mune, Raritan, NJ) were added (10 μl antibody/10^6 cells to be removed). The cell depletion was checked on a fluorescence-activated cell analyzer (Becton Dickinson, Mountain View, CA) with biotin-conjugated monoclonal antibodies (Leu-1, Leu-2, and Leu-3 from Becton Dickinson) and fluorescein isothiocyanate (FITC)-conjugated avidin (Vector, Burlingame, CA).

Culture Techniques

Cultures were prepared in triplicates in 0.35 ml round-bottomed plastic microtiter plates (Grainer, Nurtingen, FRG). Each culture contained 50,000 responder cells. For the mixed lymphocyte culture (MLC), 50,000 irradiated stimulator cells from a pool of more than five blood donors were added. In the lymphocyte transformation test, 20,000 irradiated monocyte-enriched autologous cells were added to all cultures except those with PBMC, since the macrophage function is damaged by subset depletion. The total volume of medium was 170 μl per well (RPMI supplemented with antibiotics, heparin, L-glutamine, and 15% HS). The amounts of mitogen and antigen per well were 2 μg for PHA (DIFCO, Detroit, MI), 10 μg for Con A (Pharmacia, Uppsala, Sweden), and 2 μg for purified protein derivate (PPD; State Serum Institute, Copenhagen, Denmark). The stock solution of TCGF (Lymphocult-TLF, Biotest, Dreiich, FRG), was diluted to 1:4 and used in amounts of 5, 10, 20, 30, 40, 50, and 100 μl per well. The PHA concentration in this dilution was 3.7 ng ml, which even in the highest concentration used is about 1:1,000 of the normal concentration used in PHA-stimulated cultures and much below the amount needed to cause stimulation. Indomethacine (Dumex, Copenhagen, Denmark) was used in an amount of 10 μg per well (this concentration was shown in initial experiments to have maximal effect without being toxic). One microcurie of ^{3}H-labeled thymidine was added to cultures stimulated with mitogens after 72 hr and to cultures stimulated with antigens after 120 hr. After a further 24 hr the cells were collected on glass fiber filters with an automatic harvesting machine (SKATRON, Lierbyen, Norway), and the incorporated radioactivity was measured in a liquid scintillation counter (Beckman LS 1800) after the addition of 1.5 ml scintillation fluid. The results are given as medians of the triplicate determinations.

Statistical Methods

The sign test and The Wilcoxon matched-pairs signed-ranks test were used.

RESULTS

The correlation between the MLC responses and the amount of TCGF added to PBMC from healthy controls and from patients with AIDS/ARC is shown in Figure 1. A decreased

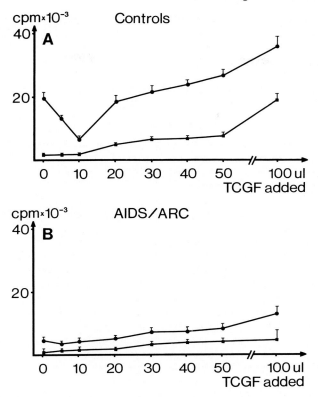

Fig. 1.   The transformation responses of PBMC from healthy controls (N = 11) (A) and from patients with AIDS/ARC (N = 8) (B) unstimulated (■) or stimulated with a pool of irradiated allogeneic cells (●) and with addition of variable amounts of TCGF. Mean values of the crude responses in CPM are connected with a line. Standard errors of the mean are given.

MLC response was found after addition of 5–10 μl of TCGF to PBMC in nine of 11 controls (P < 0.05, sign test), and a slightly decreased MLC response was found in seven of eight AIDS/ARC patients (P < 0.05). Addition of larger amounts of TCGF increased the responses of PBMC from both control and patients, but the maximal response of the patient PBMC was only one third of the response found in PBMC from normal controls. TCGF in larger amounts also increased the thymidine uptake in unstimulated PBMC from both controls and patients.

The effects of 50 μl TCGF on the response of crude PBMC, PBMC depleted for CD4-positive cells, and PBMC depleted for CD8-positive cells from controls and from AIDS/ARC patients are shown in Table I. CD8-depleted PBMC from controls and from patients, however, did not contain the same number of CD4-positive cells as control suspensions, and, accordingly, the numbers were adjusted to 20,000, shown in Table I as "CD4-adjusted." All suspensions contained a variable number of Null cells (CD4- and CD8-negative). In controls, the responses of both the CD4- and the CD8-positive PBMC increased in the presence of TCGF when stimulated with suboptimal doses of PHA (six of six experiments, P < 0.05, sign test). In contrast, in AIDS/ARC patients, only the responses of the CD4-positive (CD4-adjusted) PBMC were increased (five of six experiments), while the responses of the CD8-positive PBMC were unchanged. When similar experiments were performed with optimally Con A-stimulated cells, the responses could not be increased further by the addition of TCGF of either normal cells or patient cells. If the cell subsets were stimulated with the antigen PPD, the responses of normal cells were not changed by TCGF and patient cells did not respond to the antigen at all (data not shown). Even with TCGF added, all responses of AIDS/ARC cells were lower than the responses of cells from normal controls (P < 0.001, Wilcoxon matched-pairs signed-ranks test).

The effects of indomethacine on the responses of PHA-stimulated PBMC from controls, patients with ARC, and AIDS patients are shown in Figure 2. Addition of indomethacine seems to increase slightly the responses of PBMC from all three different groups, but the responses of patient cells were not normalized.

DISCUSSION

The above experiments aimed at clarifying the mechanisms behind the low responses of AIDS and ARC PBMC to mitogens and antigens in the in vitro lymphocyte transformation test by studying 1) the effects of exogenously added TCGF in various concentrations on the in vitro responses of PBMC to allogeneic cells, 2) the effects of TCGF on the mitogen and antigen responses of either CD4-positive or CD8-positive cells by depleting for the complementary subset, and 3) the effects on the mitogen response of inhibiting the TCGF-regulating PGE2 by indomethacine.

To evaluate the effect of TCGF on the lymphocyte transformation response, increasing amounts of TCGF were added to cultures of PBMC from controls and patients stimulated with allogeneic cells (MLC) (Fig. 1). An MLC response was chosen because it is believed to be largely independent of the responder's accessory cells. We found that addition of small amounts of TCGF inhibited the response in cells from both controls and patients, while addition of larger amounts of TCGF almost linearly increased the response, but the maximal responses of AIDS/ARC PBMC were significantly lower than the responses of PBMC from normal controls. The decreased responses seen when small amounts of TCGF were added might be due to an interference with the normal regulation of TCGF production, ie, reflect a feedback inhibition of TCGF production. The inhibition might be a direct inhibition on the producer cells connected with the high and low density Tac receptors or an indirect inhibition effectuated by, for example, the PGE2 regulatory system. Others have reported the same kind of inhibition

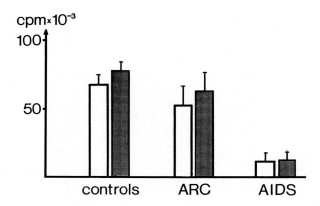

Fig. 2.   The transformation responses of suboptimally PHA-stimulated PBMC from controls (N = 75), patients with ARC (N = 6), and patients with AIDS (N = 10) without (□) and with (■) addition of indomethacine.

of the response to allogeneic cells without TCGF added when stimulator cells were added in small numbers [14]. The responses of PBMC to the mitogens PHA and Con A can also be inhibited by certain concentrations of TCGF (N. Ødum, unpublished observations). Larger amounts of TCGF also increased the response of unstimulated PBMC, indicating that TCGF exerts a direct blastogenic effect on PBMC.

The effects of TCGF on the CD4- and the CD8-positive T cell subsets were investigated by depleting PBMC from healthy controls and from patients for the complementary CD8- or for the CD4-positive cells (Table I). The patient suspensions were adjusted to 20,000 CD4-positive cells (CD4-adjusted), ie, the same number as control suspensions. In controls TCGF increased the responses of suboptimally PHA-stimulated PBMC by an increase of the response of both the CD4-positive and CD8-positive cells. In PBMC from AIDS/ARC patients, the increased response was mainly due to an increase in the responses of the CD4-positive cells, and the responses of the CD8-positive cells were largely unchanged. When the same experiment was performed with an optimal concentration of Con A, the responses of PBMC from controls could not be further increased and only small increases in the responses were observed in patient cells. For the antigen PPD, the responses were not changed in either group. Our data show that the deficient response of the CD4-positive cells from AIDS/ARC patients can be largely normalized by TCGF, suggesting that, apart from the decreased production of TCGF, the CD4-positive cells have a largely normal responding capacity despite being infected with HTLV-III/LAV. Furthermore, our data show that the CD8-positive cells from AIDS/ARC patients are defective even when supplied with sufficient amounts of TCGF. These CD8-positive cells should not be LAV/HTLV-III infected, and the lacking response to TCGF supports the suggestion that these cells may be immature.

PGE2 inhibits the production of TCGF, the proliferation of TCGF-treated cell lines, the expression of the transferrin receptor, and the Ia expression on macrophages. To investigate whether an overproduction of PGE2 is involved in the decreased responses of AIDS PBMC, indomethacine was added to mitogen-stimulated PBMC from healthy controls and from patients (Fig. 2). Indomethacine seems to augment slightly the responses to a suboptimal concentration of PHA in all groups, but the increases were only small, and the responses to an optimal concentration of Con A were largely unaffected. These findings indicated that the decreased production of TCGF in AIDS cells is not due to an increased production of the regulatory PGE2.

In conclusion, our experiments suggest that a reduction in the mitogen-induced production of TCGF in PBMC from patients with AIDS is not the only reason for the severely decreased response in the lymphocyte transformation test. The responses of the CD4-positive cells were increased when the cell numbers were adjusted to normal and TCGF was added, but the responses were still subnormal. Moreover, the responses of the CD8-positive cells could not be increased substantially by TCGF. Bearing in mind that CD8-positive cells from controls respond to mitogens with about 50% of the response of PBMC [2], the decreased responses of the AIDS CD8-positive cells indicate that these supposedly uninfected cells might be immature and that the lacking response of these CD8-positive cells contribute significantly to the reduction in the response of AIDS lymphocytes found in routine testing.

ACKNOWLEDGMENTS

This work was supported by the Danish Cancer Society (86-073) and the Danish Medical Research Council.

REFERENCES

1. Schroff TW, Gottlieb MS, Prince HE, Chai LL, Fahey JL. Immunological studies of homosexual men with immunodeficiency and Kaposi's sarcoma. Clin Immunol Immunopathol 1983; 27:300–5.
2. Hofmann B, Ødum N, Platz P, Ryder LP, Svejgaard A, Nielsen JO. Immunological studies in acquired immunodeficiency syndrome; Functional studies of lymphocyte subpopulations. Scand J Immunol 1985; 21:235–43.

3. Hofmann B, Ødum N, Jakobsen BK, et al. Immunological studies in AIDS II; Active suppression or intrinsic defect investigated by mixing AIDS cells with HLA-DR identical normal cells. Scand J Immunol 1986; 23:669–78.

4. Ciobanu N, Welter K, Kryger G, et al. Defective T-cell response to PHA and mitogenic monoclonal antibodies in male homosexuals with acquired immunodeficiency syndrome and its in vitro correction by interleukin 2. J Clin Immunol 1983; 3:332–9.

5. Murray HW, Rubin BY, Mazur H, Roberts RB. Impaired production of lymphokines and immune gamma interferon in the acquired immunodeficiency syndrome. N Engl J Med 1984; 310:883–9.

6. Gerstoft J, Malchow-Møller A, Bygbjerg I, et al. Severe acquired immunodeficiency in European homosexual men. Br Med J 1982; 285:17–9.

7. Luger TA, Smolen JS, Chused TM, Steinberg AD, Oppenheim JJ. Human Lymphocytes with either the OKT4 or OKT8 phenotype produce interleukin-2 culture. J Clin Invest 1982; 70:470–3.

8. Chouaib S, Welte K, Mertelsmann R, Dupont B. Prostaglandin E2 acts at two distinct pathways of T lymphocyte activation: Inhibition of interleukin 2 production and down regulation of transferrin receptor expression. J Immunol 1985; 135:1172–9.

9. Snyder DS, Beller DI, Unanue ER. Prostaglandins modulate macrophage Ia expression. Nature 1982; 299:163–5.

10. Maca RD. The effects of prostaglandins on the proliferation of cultured human T lymphocytes. Immunopharmacology 1983; 6:267–77.

11. Steeg PS, Moore RN, Johnson HM, Oppenheim JJ. Regulation of murine macrophage Ia antigen expression by a lymphokine with immune interferon activity. J Exp Med 1982; 156:1780–93.

12. Goodwin JS, Ceuppens J. Regulation of the immune response by prostaglandins. J Clin Immunol 1983; 3:295–315.

13. Hofmann B, Platz P, Ødum N, et al. Occurrence of anti-HTLV-III antibodies in Danish high risk homosexuals in 1982–83—Seroconversion rate and risk of AIDS. AIDS Res 1986; 2:1–3.

14. Rosenkrantz K, Dupont B, Flomenberg N. Generation and regulation of autocytotoxicity in mixed lymphocyte cultures: Evidence for active suppression of autocytotoxic cells. Proc Natl Acad Sci USA 1985; 82:4508–12.

Subject Index and List of References Cited

A-Sepharose, 74
Ab complexes, 2
Abortions, unexplained recurrent, 41
Acetone, 237
N-Acetylgalactosamine, 74–75
N-Acetyllactosamine, 82
Acetylcholine, 449
Acevedo, H.F., 478
Acheson, E.D., 378
Acidosis, lactic, 160
ACTH, 62, 378, 450
Acute phase transport protein-inducing factor, 433, 435
Acyclovir, 160, 169
Acyltransferases, 362
ADCC, 402
Addicts, immune status of, 535–540
Adenitis, 446
Adenocarcinoma, 145, 207, 212, 450
    colorectal, 91–93, 95, 602
    gastric, 603
    lung, 294
    mammary, 183, 477–484
    M alveolar, 317, 321–322, 326
    pleural effusion, 293
    vaginal, 98
Adenoma, lung, 301–302, 304–307
Adenovirus, 160, 501–502
    mouse, 292
    pancreatitis, 501
    type 12, 430–431
Adrenal glands, 293
Adriamycin, 400–401
Africa, AIDS and, 487–489, 495, 497–498
Ag/Ab, 66, 68–70
Agarose, avidine, 77
Aging, 419, 449, 600, 602, 605
    relevance of cancer-related research on, 97–100
AIDS, 43, 46–47, 99, 150, 162, 409–411, 419, 438, 457, 459, 493–496, 509, 525–532, 543–544, 546–547, 550, 553–556, 577–582, 589–595, 597–607, 611–617, 619–625
    Agent orange and, 567–569
    drug abuse and, 535–540
    enteropathic, 488
    hair dyes and, 567–569
    heterosexual spread of, 487, 489
    homosexual spread of, 487–489
    lymphomas associated with, 557–564

pathogenesis of, 586
pesticide exposure and, 567–569
pre-AIDS, 599, 605
preconditions for, 583–586
predictive markers for, 590
risk groups for, 543–547, 557, 563, 584, 586, 589–595, 597–598, 600, 606, 612–613
simian models for, 501–506
in Subsaharan Africa, 487–489
AIDS-related complex (ARC), 46–47, 409–411, 457–459, 461–462, 546–547, 583–584, 586, 597–598, 606, 621–625
    drug abuse and, 536, 539
    EBV imbalance and, 549–552
    risk groups for, 544–547
Alberts, D., 284
Alcohol, 3, 5, 61, 535
Alexanian, R., 282
Alkaline phosphatase, 363–364, 367–368, 446
    monoclonal antialkaline phosphatase complex, 264, 266
1-S-Alkyllysophosphocholine, 362, 370
Alkyllysophospholipids, 361–362, 367, 369–370
Allen, L.H., 3
Alloantigens, 526; see also Antigens
Allophycocyanin, 516
Alopecia, 18, 30
Amano, K., 412
Amanti, C., 602
Amico Roxas, M., 331
Amiel, J.L., 283
Amino acids. See specific amino acids
Aminoethylcarbazol, 237
2-Aminoethylisothiouronum bromide hydrobrom- ide (AET), 622
β-Aminoisobutyric acid (BAIB), 591, 593–594
Aminopeptidase, 450–451
Aminopeptides, 445
Aminopterin, 270
Amphotericin B, 165, 167, 169, 171
Amputation, 364, 366
Amyloidosis, 100
An-Ab complexes, 2
Analgesics. See specific agents
Anaplasia, cervical, 203
Anderson, C.F., 4
Andersson, B., 282
Andersson, L., 451
Andujar, D., 36
Anemia, 502

Anergy, 7–8, 331, 602
Ankylosing spondylitis, 99
Anorexia, 7, 23, 30, 166
Antibiotics. *See specific drugs*
Antibodies
    791T/36, 249–261
    AE1, 81–83, 85–87
    antisialo GMI, 22, 323
    antitumor, 111–120
    AP-antialpha-chain, 209
    AP-antigamma, 209
    AP-anti-my, 209
    CA1, 243
    CEA, 93–94, 243, 250, 261
    D, 118
    diphtheria toxoid, 482
    F11348, 212–214
    FH6, 128, 132
    G6146, 212–213
    generation of, stress and, 58
    H-2, 113–117
    H-2D/K, 118–119
    H-2K, 118
    H17, 189, 192, 195–203
    HB, 536
    hCG, 477, 479–481, 484
    hepatitis, 537
    HISL-19, 263–266, 268
    HLA, 351–353, 357–358, 530
    HLA-DR, 553–556, 613
    HMFG-1, 243
    HMFG-2, 241, 243–244
    HNK-1, 463–464, 466, 470–471, 473
    HSV neutralizing, 53
    HTLV-III, 46–47, 554, 558, 560, 564
    HTLV-III/LAV, 537, 538–539
    I-113, 249
    Ia-1, 555–556
    In-111, 249
    induced modulation of, 65–70
    IXF9, 183–186
    J5, 226–228, 279–281
    Ki-1, 134
    Ki67, 579–580
    KiM4, 579
    Leu1, 572
    Leu2, 572
    Leu3, 572
    Leu7, 91, 94, 572
    Leu8, 613
    Leu15, 613
    LeuM1, 132–134
    M8, 243
    M18, 243
    monoclonal, 73–74, 76–78, 82–83, 103–109,
        128, 133, 137, 145–148, 150, 173–180,
        183–187, 189–203, 207–214, 226, 231–

    239, 241–245, 250–257, 259–261, 270–
    277, 279–286, 463–464, 471, 473, 515–
    522, 530–531, 545, 553–555, 572, 577,
    579, 611–617
    islet, 263–268
    mononuclear, 466, 470
    monospecific, 160
    natural, 21
    OK Ia-1, 553–554
    OKT3, 558
    OKT4, 558
    OKT6, 558
    OKT9, 555
    OKT11, 558
    polyclonal, 231–234
    T3, 93–94
    T12, 226
    Tac, 137–139, 530–531
    t-PA, 269, 271, 273–276
    u-PA, 272, 275–276
    VE7, 183–186
    VIG3, 183–186
    VILAI, 280–281
    see also Antigens; Autoantibodies; B cell; Cell
        lines; T cell
Antibody-drug conjugates, 249–261
Anticarcinogens, 301–307
Antigen/antibody complexes. *See* Ag/Ab
Antigenicity sharing, 91–95
Antigens
    ABO blood group, 82
    AScM, 546–547
    B, 82, 84
    B-1, 168
    cancer-associated, 231–234
    Candida, 604–605
    carcinoembryonic, 231–234
    CD2, 518–520
    CD3, 518, 519, 522
    CD4, 518–519, 521
    CD5, 518, 521
    CD6, 518
    CD7, 518, 519–520
    CD8, 519, 521–522
    CD11, 519, 522
    CD12, 518
    CD16, 518–522
    CD19, 518, 519–520
    CD20, 518, 520–521
    CD22, 518, 520
    CEA, 91, 250
    common ALL, 225–229, 272
    cytoplasmic, 207
    D113, 119
    D4123, 211–212, 214
    differentiation, 211, 280
    EBV, 218–221, 550, 552

4B4, 521
gp69/71, 112, 117
H, 81–87
H-2, 119
H-2D, 112–113
H-2K, 112–113, 119
H-2Kb, 68–70
H-2Kd, 118
H17, 194
HB, 536
hepatitis, 537
HISL-19, 265–267
HLA-DP, 520
HLA-DQ, 520
HLA-DR, 520, 611–617
HMFG-2, 244
HMy-2, 211
HSVII, 189–197, 200–201, 203
Klebs M, 547
Leu1, 518, 520–521
Leu2, 519, 522
Leu3, 516, 521, 612–614, 616–617
Leu4, 518, 520, 522
Leu5, 518, 520
Leu7, 519, 521–522
Leu8, 516, 519, 521, 613–617
Leu9, 518–521
Leu11, 516, 519–520
Leu12, 518–519
Leu14, 518
Leu15, 519–522
Leu16, 518
Leu17, 520–521
Leu18, 521
Leu19, 520
Lewis, 145–148
M, 585
M1, 276
melanoma-associated, 350
NKH-1, 520
OKM1, 519
OKT10, 520
P1, 585
pan-NK, 518
pan-T cell, 518
PPD, 625
proliferation-associated, 577–582
recall, 374, 378
S, 585
Salm, 547T-3, 95
T-4, 579, 615
T-8, 579
T-11, 168
T-200, 517–519
Tac, 137–142
Thomsen-Friedenreich, 237
tissue-polypeptide, 232–234

tumor-associated, 74, 117, 214, 235–239, 241–
    245, 285–286, 400
viral capsid, 218–219, 221
    see also Alloantigens; Antibodies; B cell; Cell
    lines; T cell
Antimetastatics. *See specific drugs*
Antineoplastics. *See specific drugs*
Antiserum. *See specific sera*
Aoyagi, T., 450
Aparisi, T., 283
Arachidonic acid, 61–62
Arachis hypogaea, 132
Arginine, 445
Arlacel A, 478–479
Arnetz, D.B., 59–60
Arthropathy, psoriatic, 154
Asbestos, 590
Asparaginase, 166–168
Aspergillus fungus, 562
Assay
    Clq-binding, 351, 353, 356, 358
    antibody-dependent cellular cytotoxicity, 221
    conglutinin-binding, 351, 353, 358
    EBV-related, 217–221
    HIV P24, 505–506
    immunodot, 235–239
    Komuro-Boyce, 413, 416
    leukocyte migration, 221
    Limulus lysate, 386
    NK, 591
    Staphylococcus protein A, 351–353, 356–357
Ataxia telangiectasia, 123
Athymic
    humans, 417–418
    nude mice, 51, 95, 133, 175–176, 251–252,
        257–260, 412, 418, 432–433, 435
    metastasis models for human tumors in,
        291–298
Augmentation, of NK cell activity, 316–326
Auquier, A., 282
Autoantibodies, 410; *see also* Antibodies
Autofluorescence, 68
Autonomic nervous system, 62
Avidin, 128
    peroxidase, 134
Avidin phycoerythrin, 104
5-Azacytidine (5-Aza), 311–314, 316
8-Azaguanine, 208
Azathioprine, 150, 154, 159–161, 378
Azimexone, 386, 390–391, 411
Azzarello, G., 602, 604

Bagshawe, K.D., 482
Baley, A.C., 99
Balliet, N., 532
Bancewicz, J., 575
Barot-Ciorbaru, R., 43, 47
Bartrop, R.W., 59

Basidiomycetes, 423
Basile, F., 602, 604
Basophils, 62
B cell
    function, 3, 5, 9, 23, 29, 32–34, 36, 40, 47,
            127, 152, 162, 164–165, 185, 187, 225,
            273, 275, 385, 410–411, 515–522, 550,
            553, 557, 611–613, 615–617
    lymphadenopathy and, 543–547
    oligoclonal proliferation of, 160, 163
    polyclonal activators, 44, 46–47, 544
    response of in hemophiliacs, 43–47
    see also B lymphocytes; Cell lines
BCG282–285, 399, 432, 464
Beattie, E.J., 214
Bekesi, J.G., 284, 599
Bellantone, R., 331, 602
Benedetti, M., 602
Benveniste, E., 533
Benveniste, R., 505
Benzo(a)pyrene, 300–306
Bergh, D., 567
Bernardini, A., 478
Bernstein, I.D., 279
Bestatin, 283–285, 445–446, 450–451
Biological response modifiers, 15–16, 23–24,
        385–395, 399, 402–404, 445, 447–451
Biphenyls
    polybrominated, 29–36
    polychlorinated, 30
Bird, A.G., 121
Bjorkholm, M., 283
Black, S., 59
Blastogenesis, 58, 138–139, 374, 450, 613–614,
        616–617, 625
Blindness, 167
Blomgren, H., 284, 450
Blood group types, correlative studies on antigen-
        icity of pancreatic cancer and, 145–148
B lymphocytes, 33–34, 36, 40, 160–161, 183–187,
        210–211, 611–614
    see also B cell; Cell lines
BM41.322, 386, 390–391
BM41.440, 361–362, 364–370
Bombesin, 92
Bone marrow, 17, 19, 21, 23–24, 160–162, 165–
        169, 280–281, 284–285, 318, 324–326,
        334, 367–368, 370, 385, 387–389, 390–
        394, 495, 526, 559
Bootello, A., 43
Borgogone, A., 331, 602–603
Borowitz, M.J., 225
Bortin, M.M., 171, 280
Bovine serum albumin. *See* BSA
Boyse, E.A., 413
Bradner, W.T., 431
Bradykinin, 448

Brain, 30, 291–292, 303, 365, 505
Brennan, P.J., 378
Brenner, S.O., 59–60
Brieva, J.A., 43
5-Bromo-4-chlorandoxyl phosphate (BCIP), 210
Bromophenol blue, 114
Bronchial washing analysis, difficulty in establish-
        ing diagnosis from, 165–171
Brown, R., 575
BSA, 112, 128, 132–133, 175, 209, 227, 237, 466,
    480
Buetti, E., 187
Bulloch, K., 62
Burchell, J., 243
Burkitt lymphoma, 127–128, 187, 217–221, 225,
    549
Burns, 3, 597–598, 600, 602, 604–606
Burritt, M.F., 4
Bursectomy, 547

Cachexia, 23, 30, 321
Cadwallader, B.D., 484
Callahan, R., 187
Calle, R., 602, 604
Caloric
    intake, 5
    requirements, 3
Camerino, M., 59
cAMP, 445
Campanelli, A., 602
Campling, B.G., 91
Campos, A., 43
Cancer, 150, 409–411, 413, 432, 438, 440–441,
        464, 472, 590, 598, 600–603, 605
    aging research, relevance of to, 97–100
    of biliary passages, 151
    bladder, 98, 149, 154–155, 284
    bone marrow, 152
    brain, 149, 152
    breast, 121–122, 150, 154–155, 214, 235–239,
        242, 284, 330, 502, 601
    postmenopausal, 285
    premenopausal, 279, 282
    cervical, 153, 189, 191–203, 373–375
    colorectal, 145, 150, 155, 178–180, 207–214,
        243, 249–261, 284, 424, 441, 559,
        571–575
    esophageal, 155, 601–602
    family histories of, 121–124
    gastrointestinal, 154, 284, 330, 559, 601–602
    genital, 153, 601
    of head and neck, 330, 463–473
    kidney, 151–152, 402
    of lip, 149–152
    liver, 151–152
    lung, 98, 150, 152, 155, 291–295, 375,
        429–431
    malnutrition induced by, 3

nasopharyngeal, 98, 217–221, 549
of oral cavity, 463–473
ovarian, 121, 155, 241–245
pancreatic, 155
pancreatic correlative studies on antigenicity of
    blood group types and, 145–148
of penis, 153
of perineum, 149, 151, 153
prostate, 150, 285, 450
rectal, 150–151, 153, 155
screening for, 231–234
skin, 149–152, 154–155
of spleen, 152
stomach, 121–124, 155, 333
in transplant patients given immunosuppressive
    therapy, 153–154
of uterine body, rarity of, 153
of uterine cervix, 99, 149–150, 152, 284, 330
of vulva, 149, 151, 153
see also different neoplasm and tumor types
Candiani, P., 602, 606
Candida, 45, 378, 458
Candidin, 375
Canon, C., 281
Cantrell, J., 412
Carbohydrates, 213, 242–243
    cell surface, 82, 128
    epitope structures of, 132
Carbonic anhydrase, 227
Carboxylmethylcellulose. *See* Poly-ICLC
Carboxypeptidase B, 445
Carcinogenesis, 87, 301, 307, 431, 447
Carcinogens, 97–100; *see also specific agents*
Carcinoids, 267
Carcinoma
    adenosquamous, 293
    basal cell, 151
    bronchioalveolar, 293
    C146, 251–252
    C168, 251–252
    C170, 251–253, 256, 258–259
    large cell, 293
    Lewis lung, 66, 361–362, 366, 370, 477–484
    LS174T, 252–253, 259, 261
    neuroendocrine skin, 263, 267–268
    small cell, 3
    squamous cell, 24, 149, 151, 154, 264, 266,
        463
    thymic, 549
Carcinomatosa, 338
Cardi, F., 602, 604
Carrageenan, 21, 432, 435
Catabolism, increased, 5
Catane, R., 448
Catania, G., 602, 604
Catecholamines, 58, 62
cDNA, 226

Cell lines
    729-HF-2, 212
    A549, 293–294, 296
    ABLS-8.1, 361, 367–368
    BL-2, 17
    B lymphoma, 207–208
    Bowes melanoma, 270
    Burkitt lymphoma, 127–128
    CD4, 619–625
    CD8, 619–625
    CEM, 132,504
    EBV immortalized tumor, 504
    EFM19, 237–238
    ESb, 74–78
    ESb-M, 73–78
    G2, 66–70
    H9, 494, 496–498, 504–505
    HB-100, 238
    HeLa, 174–178, 180
    HEp-2, 190–193
    HISL19, 265
    histiocytic, 127–131, 133–134
    HL60, 127, 132, 364
    HMFG-2, 245
    HMy-2, 212
    Hodgkin disease-derived, 127–134
    HSB-2, 272–274
    HTLV-III producer, 511
    HTLV-IT, 162
    Hut-78, 504–505
    hybridoma, 271
    K562, 51–54, 103–109, 270, 272, 274, 276,
        364, 572, 591
    KM3, 225, 227–228
    L428, 127, 132
    L540, 127, 132
    L591, 127, 134
    L662, 132
    L1210, 111, 361, 365, 367–368
    L5178Y, 111–119
    LCL660, 132
    LCL725, 132
    Leu7, 103–109, 377, 379
    Leu11, 103–108
    Lewis lung, 176–177
    lymphoblastoid, 127, 269–276, 549
    lymphoma, 128–131, 133–134
    MBL-2, 318, 320, 326
    MCF-7, 237–238, 245
    Mel 4, 352
    Molt-4, 272–273, 364
    MVE-2, 16, 20–24
    NCI-H125, 293–294, 296
    NCI-H460, 293–294, 296
    NCI-H969, 293–294
    Null, 502
    OKT4, 162–163

OKT8, 163
p24, 553–556
P815, 361, 367–368
P815Y, 111–119
P815-X2, 117
promyelocytic, 127–134
Raji, 132, 502
SK-BR-3, 237–238
Sternberg Reed, 127, 132–133, 559
T47D, 245
T lymphoblastoid, in AIDS, 498
U937, 127, 132
XG3AG, 270
YAC, 319, 361, 367–368
YAC-1, 184–186, 303, 386, 439
ZR75-1, 245
see also Antibodies, Antigens; B cells; Cells;
    T cell
Cell-mediated immunity, 1, 2, 4, 8–11, 53,
    409–410
Cells
    allogeneic, 137
    allokiller, 437–438
    autoreactive, 285
    basal, 81
    bone marrow, 17, 23, 318, 325–326, 385,
        387–388, 390–394, 526–530
    C, 266
    dark populations, 81
    decidual, 41
    dyskaryotic, 197
    effector, 23, 94, 385, 388–389
    epithelial, TPA-induced maturation of, 81–88
    eukaryotic, 311
    fetal suppressor, 41
    growth and differentiation of normal, 52
    hematopoietic, 517
    Hodgkin, 127–128, 132–134
    inflammatory, 203
    K, 17
    LOX, 293
    lymphokine-activated killer, 401, 403
    maternal suppressor, 41
    Merkel, 152, 263–267
    metaplastic, 196–197
    mononuclear, 5, 40, 53, 185, 458, 465, 544
    myeloid progenitor, 386
    NK, 2, 5, 8, 10, 16, 19–22, 24, 40, 51–54, 58,
        60, 62, 103, 108–109, 164, 286, 302,
        304–307, 317–326, 370, 379, 385–386,
        388–390, 394, 401, 426–427, 439, 445,
        448–450, 463–473, 515–516, 518–520,
        522, 552–554, 571–575, 578, 580, 589,
        591, 594, 597–600, 606, 616
    Null, 32, 34, 36, 152
    peripheral blood, 526–527, 529–531, 572,
        619–625

    polymorphonuclear, 605
    reticulum, 577–578, 580–582
    sorting of, 93
    surface markers, 225–229, 270, 591
    syncytial giant, 505
    target, 53
    see also Antigens; Antibodies; B cell; Cell
        lines; T cell
Cellular effector cells. *See* Cells, NK;
    Macrophages
Central nervous system (CNS), 160, 419
    HTLV-III/LAV and, 509–510
    lymphoma and, 549–550, 560, 562, 564
Cerebrospinal fluid, 378
    AIDS and, 509–510, 512–513
Ceruloplasmin, 433, 435
cGMP, 446
CGP, 478–479, 482–483
Chamaret, S., 615
Champagne, E., 615
Chastang, C., 282
Cheigson-Pau, R., 99
Chelation, 252
Chemoimmunotherapy, 282
Chemotaxis, 62, 446
Chemotherapy, 16, 23, 153, 166–168, 207, 282,
    291–295, 313, 316–317, 329, 335, 337–
    338, 340, 342, 345–346, 385, 387, 564,
    590, 598, 602
    adjuvant, 154, 280, 285, 323–324
    BACOD, 562
    CHOP, 562
    MOPP-ABVD, 562
    neoplastic consequences of, 149–156
    toxicity of, 3
    see also specific drugs
Chen, J.J., 219
Chen, S.S., 414
Chen, W.F., 418
Cheng, R., 91
Chiavaro, I., 602
Chimpanzees
    AIDS and, 509–511
    HIV and, 506
Chiodine, A., 603, 605
Chi-squared test, 122
Chlorambucil, 154, 377–382
Chloramine-T method, 480
Chlornaphazine, 155
N,N-bis (2-Chloroethyl)N-nitrosourea (BCNU),
    312–313, 316
4-Chloro-1-naphthol, 236–237, 264, 510
1-(p-Chlorophenyl)-3,3-dimethyltriazine (DM-Cl),
    311–312, 314–316
Chmielewska, D., 330–331
Cholangitis, 504
Choline, 8–9

Choriogonadotropin, human (hCG), 173–175, 177–178, 180, 477–484
Chou, J.Y., 180
Chromatin, 450
Chromatography, high-performance liquid, 312–314, 591
Chymotrypsin, 446, 450
Ciamexon. *See* BM 41.332
Cianci, A., 478
Cianci, S., 478
Cimetidine, 4, 413
Circulating immune complexes, 353–356
Cirrhosis, of liver, 5
Cirulli, G., 331, 602
Clamon, G. H., 3
Cloning, 211
Clostripain, 446
CNS. *See* Central nervous system
Cocaine, 535–537
Colcemid, 92
Cold agglutin disease, chronic, 153
Cold target inhibition studies, 111–112
Cole, S.P.C., 91
Collagenase, 250, 257
Collagen-vascular diseases, 153
Colloidal gold, 213
Colony-stimulating activity, 531
Colony-stimulating factor, 385–395, 423, 433–436
Colton life table statistics, 480
Comis, R.L., 142
Concanavalin A, 9, 33–34, 44, 75–76, 132–133, 412, 415, 417–418, 450, 546, 619, 621, 623, 625
Condyloma acuminatum, 149, 153
Coomassie blue, 133
Copper, 7
Corbino, N., 478
Cort, S.P., 615
Corticosteroids, 58, 61, 154, 159, 168, 378
Corynebacterium, 400
Corynebacterium parvum, 423, 432, 464, 472
Cote, R.J., 214
Couve, E., 287
Creatinine, 3, 23, 584
Creosote, 568
Crohn's disease, 5
Cryptosporidia, 502, 504
Cunningham-Rundles, S., 2
Cupissol, D., 450
2-Cyanaziridine, 390–391
Cyclooxygenation, 62
Cyclophosphamide, 16, 20, 150, 154–155, 166–168, 221, 325–326, 378, 385–386, 390–391, 400–401
    see also Cytoxan
Cyclosporine, 150, 165–166, 171
    A, 159–160, 162–164

Cytochalasin B, 92
Cytokines, 326, 399–404, 440
Cytolysis
    antibody-mediated, 65
    of immune competent cells, 94
Cytomegalovirus, 160, 162, 169–170, 330, 501–502, 583, 604, 620
    pneumonia, 165
Cytoplasts, 92–95
Cytosine arabinoside, 166, 168, 251
Cytosol, 212–213, 450
Cytotoxicity, antibody-dependent, cell-mediated, 445, 448, 450
Cytoxan, 317–318, 324–325, 385–387, 389–391, 394–395

Dalgleish, A.G., 99
Daniels, W.P., 295
Datura stramonium, 132
Daunomycin, 166–168, 249, 254, 258–261
Davidsohn, I., 146
Degradation, of extracellular matrix, 269
Deisseroth, A.B., 171
Del Buono, S., 602
Delogu, C., 602
Dermatomyositis, 153
De Simone, M., 602
Devillechabrolle, A., 605
DeVinci, C., 221
Dexamethasone, 166
N,N-Diallyltartardiamide, 191, 201, 203
Dialysis, 571
3-3'-Diaminobenzidine tetrahydrochloride, 132, 264–266, 554
Diaminobenzine, 209
Dibenzofurans, 568–569
2,4-Dichlorophenoxyacetic acid (2, 4-D), 567
Dicke, K., 171
Dietary history, 3
Diethyl dithiocarbamate, 409, 413–415, 419
Diethylstilbestrol (DES), 98
Digestion, proteolytic, 132
Diggelmann, H., 187
N,N-Dimethylamino-2-propanol, 329
7-12-Dimethylbenz(α)anthracene, 99
Dimethylguanosine, 589, 591–594
Dimethyl sulfoxide, 479
Dinarello, C., 418
Dioxins, AIDS and, 567–569
DiPaola, M., 330
DiPersio, L., 295
Diphtheria, 378, 458
    toxoid, 477–484
Diploidy, 549
Disease
    differential diagnosis of, 219
    early detection of, 219
    heterogeneity, 217

neoplastic, 21–22
parasitic, 21
prevention, 219
susceptibility, 218
DiSimone, C., 330
Dissection, radical, neck, 465
Dixon, D., 282
DMEM, 274, 362–365, 368
DMSO, 292
DNA, 98, 175, 192, 209, 484, 494
    AIDS proviral, 495–498
    metabolism, 450
    methylation, 311–316
    recombinant, 402–403
    recombinant MMTV proviral, 183
    retroviral sequences, 187
    synthesis, 44
Docosahexaenoic acid, 62
Donati, L., 607
Douglas cul-de-sac, 338
Dowell, B.L., 225
Downing, R.G., 99
Drexler, H.G., 272
Drohan, W., 187
Drug
    abuse, 554, 557–558, 584–585
    immune status of addicts, 535–540
    targeting, 249–261
    in vitro screening, 292, 293, 294, 295, 296
    in vivo testing, 295
Drugs, anticancer, 423–441
Drugs, thymomimetic. *See specific drugs*
DTPA-conjugated antibody, 252
Dunnet's test, 480
Dupont, D., 234
Durand, M., 282
Dye, E.S., 119
Dye fronts. *See specific dyes*
Dysplasia, 189, 192, 194–197, 200, 202–203

Eczema, 446
Edema, 59, 167, 169
Edgar, L.C., 47, 543, 547
Edsmyr, F., 285, 450
EDTA, 66, 227
Edwards, B.K., 63
Eghbali, H., 282
Eichler-Reiss, F., 281
Eicopentaenoic acid, 62
Eicosapentaenoic acid, 61
Eilber, F.R., 283
Elastase, 450
Electrolytes, 3
ELISA, 45–46, 162, 208–212, 526, 535–536,
        546–547, 579
    AIDS and, 505, 510–511, 513
Ellrodt, A., 498
Embryogenesis, 269

Emergence-associated tumor immunogen, 117–119
Encephalitis
    granulomatous, 504–505
    retroviral, 501
Encephalopathy, AIDS, 513
Endocarboxypeptidase, 446
Endorphins, 62
Endotoxins, 386, 409, 412, 414, 418–419
Eneroth, P., 59–60
Engleman, E.G., 521
Enkephalins, 62
Enolase, neuron specific, 263–267
Environmental contamination, by PBBs, 29–36
Enzymes
    Bg, 496
    Bgl II, 494–497
    E, 496
    Eco R1, 495–497
    Hind III, 494–495, 496, 498
    restriction, 493–494
    Sac I, 494, 496, 498
Eosin, 294, 297–298, 303
Eosinophils, 62, 413
Epidemiology, of AIDS, 487–489, 495
Epiillumination, 270
Epinephrine, 4
Epistaxis, recurrent, 166
Erythema, 59, 352, 354–356
Erythrina cristagalli, 132
Erythrocytes, 113, 209, 211, 237, 363, 369, 446,
        526, 622
Erythromycin, 171
Erythrosin B, 185
Esophagitis, 562
Esposti, P.L., 450
Essential fatty acid deficiency (EFAD), 62
Esterase, 318, 387
Estrogen therapy, 234
Ethanol, 237
Ethanolamine, 92, 210
Ethylene diamine tetraacetic acid. *See* EDTA
Etiology, 329–331
    of AIDS, 493
Euploidy, 549
Europe, AIDS and, 487–489
Evans, W.K., 3

Fab, 112–113, 115, 184
    anti-, 116, 118
Facial herpes. *See* Virus type, herpes simplex I
Factor substitution, B cell response in hemophil-
        iacs and, 43–47
Failly, E., 234
Fast red, 266
Fatty acids, as immune function mediators, 61–62;
        see also specific acids
Fauci, A.S., 47, 543, 547
Femur, 325, 388–391

Fenton, J., 602
Fenwick, M., 203
Fetal
    bovine serum (FBS), 16, 92–93, 386
    calf serum (FCS), 52, 74, 191, 208, 226, 271,
        362–363, 365, 367, 458, 465, 479, 572,
        622
Fibrinogen, 270, 273
Fibrinolysis, 269–276
Fibroblasts
    3T3, 173–180, 365, 369
    L929S, 365, 369
Fibrosarcoma, 427–428, 430, 438
    Meth A, 362–363, 365–369
    UV2237, 323–324
Fichelscher, M.T., 229
Ficoll-Hypaque gradient centrifugation, 185
Fidalgo, B.V., 446
Fishelevich, R., 203
Fisher, R., 282
Fisher exact test, 536
Fistula
    drainage, 3
    thoracic duct, 150
Flad, H., 450
Flow
    cytofluorometric analysis, 173–180
    cytometry, 93, 103–109, 255, 257, 515–522,
        611–617
Fluorescein isothiocyanate (FITC), 68, 74, 94,
        104–105, 128, 175, 255, 257, 270, 516,
        558, 612
Fluorescence, 69, 612
    -activated cell sorter, 418
    mean linear, 250
    punctuated, 70
5-Fluorouracil (5-FU), 334, 336
Focan, C., 284
Focan-Henrard, D., 284
Fogh, J. M., 295
Folate, 1, 8
Folic acid, 8
Foon, K.A., 283
Ford, W.L., 575
Formalin, 82, 146, 209, 211–212, 264, 293, 611
Formol-acetone, 209
Franke, W.W., 267
Franks, L.M., 99
Frere, M.H., 284
Fridman, H., 602, 604
Froldi, M., 602
Functional analysis, 103–107, 109
Fungi, 168–169, 404, 423
Furans, 569

Gaedicke, G., 272
Galactose, 74
β-Galactosidase, 195

Gale, R.P., 171, 284
Gallo, R., 498, 513
Gamma
    camera images, 252–254
    counting, 105
Gammaglobulin, 161, 221, 446
Gastrocnemius, 174
Gauher disease, 446
Gel electrophoresis, SDS-PAGE, 66, 75, 77–78,
        114, 118, 128, 133–134, 191, 193–195, 210,
        212–213, 227–228, 435, 497, 510
Gene
    env, 494–495, 498, 509, 513
    gag, 509, 513
    H-2D/K products, 112, 119
    Ig, 520
    MMTV, 183
    mutations, 121; *see also specific mutations or*
        syndromes
    nuclear, 95
    ontogeny, 98
    pol, 495, 509, 512
    T-cell, 518–520
Genomic variability, in AIDS, 493–497
Gerontology, 97–98
Gentamycin, 16, 174, 318, 591
Geodia cydonium, 128, 132
Giemsa technique, 92, 318, 387, 527
Gillis, S., 414
Gingivitis, necrotizing, 501
Ginseng, red, effect of on NK cell activity,
    301–307
Giovineto, A., 602
Girard, P., 378
Glioblastomas, 365
Glioma, 284
Globulin
    antilymphocyte, 150, 159, 160–161, 163, 378
    antithymocyte, 150
Glomerulonephritis, 153
Glover, J.S., 480
β-1,3-Glucan, 333
Glucans, 423
Gluckman, E., 171, 330, 498
β-1,3-Glucopyranoside, 333
β-1,6-Glucopyranoside, 333
H-Glucosamine, 114, 116, 118–119
Glucose, 23
Glutamic acid, 446
Glutamine, 74, 128, 303
L-Glutamine, 16, 92, 318, 386, 465, 527–528,
    622
Glutaraldehyde, 209–210
Glycerol, 139, 210, 362
Glycine, 128, 209, 264
    HCl, 66
Glycolipids, 87, 132

membrane, 128
see also specific compounds
Glycoproteins, 127–132, 134
    Dalton, 249
    isolation of lectin-binding, 74
    membrane, 183–187
    transblotted, 133
    viral, 615
    see also Lectins, plant
Glycosylation, 229
Goldstein, A., 418
Goldstein, G., 414
Goldstein, S., 98
Good, R.A., 414
Gottlieb, M.S., 543
Gould, V.E., 267
Gouzien, C., 414
Graft vs host reaction, 279–280, 284
Graft vs leukemia reaction, 279–280
Granulocyte-monocyte
    colony-forming units (GM-CFU-C), 53, 317–
        318, 324–325, 385
    colony-stimulating factor (GM-CSF), 386–391,
        393–394
Granulocytes, 21, 62, 165, 167, 171, 412, 518
Granulocytopenia, 385
Greaves, M.F., 225
Greenwood, F.C., 480
Griffonia simplicifolia, 132
Grimm, E.A., 403
Gross, R.L., 1
Growth inhibitors. *See specific compounds*
Guanine, 446
Gui, D., 331, 602, 604
Guillaumin, J.M., 414
Gupta, P.K., 203
Gynecomasty, 234

H-2 receptor blockers. *See specific blockers*
Hadden, J.W., 414
Haiti, AIDS and, 494–495, 497
Hajema, E., 506
Hakomori, S.I., 128
Halen, M., 285
Hall, E., 59–60
Hamid, J., 575
Haptoglobin, 433, 435
Harris, J.E., 285
Hartz, A.J., 171
Head injury, increased catabolism and, 5
Heart, 293–294, 303, 429
Heinsohn, H., 229
Heisel, J.S., 60
Helix pomanita, 132
Hematoma, 30
Hematapoiesis, 385

Hematoxylin, 209, 264, 266, 293, 296–297, 303,
    578, 581
Hemoglobin, 173
Hemopexin, 433, 435
Hemophilia, 536, 571, 584
    A, 43–45
    AIDS and, 538–539, 543
    B-cell response in, 43–47
Hemorrhage-inducing factor, 433, 435
Henle-Koch postulates, 217
Heparin, 622
Hepatisone, 414
Hepatitis, 153, 293, 536–537
    alcoholic, 5
Hepatocytes, 369, 433
Hepatoma, 429–430, 451, 478
Hepatomegaly, 167
Hepatosplenomegaly, 166
Herpes genitalis. *See* Virus type
Heteroantiserum225, 227, 228
Heterogeneity, genetic, in AIDS, 493, 495
Heterotransplantation, 133
1-Hexadecylmercapto-2-methoxymethyl-rac-
    glycero-3-phosphocholine. *See* BM 41.440
Hexamita, 501
Hirata, M., 446
Hische, E.A.H., 513
Histiocytes133, 505
Histocompatibility, major, 419
Hjelm, R., 59–60
Hochmann, J., 78
Hodgkin disease, 122, 137–138, 140–142, 152,
    155, 446, 554, 558
Hoerni, B., 282
Hoerni-Simon, G., 282
Holland, J.F., 283
Hollinshead, A.C., 284
Holmes, E.C., 283
Hoof growth, abnormal, 30
Hormones
    endocrine, 410, 419
    peptide, 263
    thymic, 409–411, 413–414, 418–419
    trophoblastic; *see specific hormones*
Host, syngeneic lymphoma-bearing, 111–113
Houghton, A.N., 214
Hsu,S-M., 133
Human T-cell lymphoma-leukemia virus. *See*
    Retrovirus
Humoral immunity, 1–2, 4
Humphrey, J.H., 59
Hunter, W.M., 480
Hyaline membrane formation, 169
Hybridization, 236–237
Hybridoma
    antiphosphorylcholine, 184
    escape of from cellular defense mechanisms,
        91–95

human-human, 207–214
  production of, 190
  supernatants, 235–239, 242, 271
  technique, 83
Hydrocortisone, 166, 168
4-Hydroperoxycyclophosphamide, 401
N-Hydroxysuccinimide, 255
Hypercarbia, 165
Hypergammaglobulinemia, 29
  polyclonal, 34
Hyperglobulinemia, 410
Hyperleukocytosis, 166
Hyperlipoproteinemia, 11
Hyperplasia
  follicular, 106, 503, 559
  intrahepatic bile duct, 30
  paracortical, 106
  sinus, 106
Hypersensitivity, delayed-type, 4–7, 11, 375, 377–
    378, 380, 382, 425, 427, 438–439, 445,
    448, 450, 457, 459–452, 545, 601
Hypoergy, 331
Hypogammaglobulinemia, 122
Hypomethylation, 311, 316
Hyposplenia, 446
Hypoxanthine, 270, 409
Hypoxia, 165
Hysterectomy, 373
  radical, 374

Ide, L., 378
Idiopathic thrombocythemia, 153
IgA, 2, 32–34, 58, 111, 116, 118, 218–219, 221,
    446, 545, 560
IgD, 558, 560
IgE, 2
IgG, 6, 8, 32–34, 44, 46–47, 66, 68, 111, 116,
    118, 175, 184–186, 208–212, 227–228,
    236–237, 242, 250–252, 258, 260, 271–
    272, 357, 378, 445–446, 544–547, 558,
    560, 585, 612–613
  response to AIDS virus, 509–513
Iglesia, G., 532
IgM, 6–7, 32–33, 43–44, 47, 111, 113, 116, 118,
    184, 186, 209–213, 236–237, 242, 271–
    272, 445, 544–547, 558, 560
Ikeda, S., 450
Ikehara, S., 414
Immune
  cells, 98
  dysfunction
    family clustering of, 36
    Michigan residents and, 29–36
  escape, 91–95
  response, 385–387, 390–395
  surveillance, 51–52
  system, 97–100
Immunity

activated cellular, 535, 536
  natural, 395
  natural antitumor reduced by protein defi-
    ciency, 15–23
  stress-related modulation of, 57–63
Immunization, 235–237, 242
Immunoadsorption procedure, 226
Immunobiology, tumor, 111
Immunoblot technique, 83, 207, 210, 213
Immunocompetence, 120
  in pregnancy, 39–41
Immunodeficiency, subclinical, 121–124
Immunodepression, 149–150, 153–156, 312, 450
  of diverse etiology, 329, 331
Immunodetection, 249–261
Immunodiagnosis, 231, 232, 233, 234
Immunofluorescence, 83, 160–161, 270–277, 545
  with anti-Tac antibody, 138–139
Immunoglobulin, 83, 152, 159, 208–209, 238,
    378, 518, 558, 572, 545
  concentrations unaffected by stress, 58
  gene ontogeny, 98
  heterogeneity, 160
  see also specific immunoglobulins
Immunology, of cancer, 189–203
Immunomodifiers, 286
Immunomodulation, 111–120, 301–307, 326, 333–
    334, 399–404, 425–441, 457–462
Immunoperoxidase technique, 264–265, 470
Immunopharmacology, 279–280, 283–286
Immunophenotyping, 515–522
Immunoprecipitation, 112, 118–119, 193–194, 226
  with monoclonal antibodies, 74–75
Immunoprophylaxis, of cancer, 477–484
Immunostimulation, 280, 329, 423
  stress and, 57, 60
Immunosuppression, 159–160, 163, 301–302, 323,
    377–382, 459, 464, 467, 563, 571
  neurotransmitters and, 62
  in nontransplant patients, 153–154
  stress and, 57
Immunotherapy, 285–286
  active, 279–283
  adjuvant, 282, 351–358, 373–375
  adoptive, 279–283
  local, 284
  passive, 279
  pulse, 457–462
  see also specific immunotherapies
Immunotoxicology, 29–36
Imreg, 411
Imunovir, 329, 331
Inada, K., 446
Indomethacine, 619–620, 624–625
Infection
  bacterial, 2, 502
  host defense against stress and, 60

opportunistic, 526, 528, 535, 557, 562, 584
parasitic, 330
respiratory, 446, 604
urinary, 604
viral, 330, 413, 419
Inflammatory
bowel disease, 7
cells, 62
functions, 61
responses, 153
Inosine, 329, 414
dimethylaminoisopropanol, 457
pranobex BAN. *See* Imunovir
Insulomas, 267
Intercourse, anal, 585
Interferon, 261, 401–402, 404, 468, 472, 597, 606
α, 402, 469, 473
β, 326, 402
γ, 40, 54, 164, 319, 402, 412, 473
production of related to stress, 58
Interleukin, 164
1, 326, 409, 411, 419, 423, 433–437, 473,
598, 606
2, 39–41, 54, 137–142, 164, 326, 358, 401–
403, 409–411, 413–415, 417–419, 437–
440, 473, 503, 525–527, 529–532, 584,
606, 619–625
3, 423, 433–435
Iodine, 270, 479–480
I-Iodo-deoxyuridine, 258
IPNX. *See* Isoprinosine
IRMA technique, 232
Iron, 7–8
Irradiation, beta, 99
Irving, M.H., 575
Ishihara, K., 450
Isoprinosine (IPNX), 377–382, 409, 411–415,
457–459, 461–462, 597–607, 611–617
Isotherapy, 457, 459–462

Jablon, S., 99
Jacobson, L., 221
Jaffe, E., 133
Johnson, A., 63
Jones, N.H., 225
Jones, S.E., 282
Jurst, M.W., 60

Kahler, C., 473
Kaplan-Meier method, 335, 601
Kaposi sarcoma, 99, 149–150, 153–155, 402, 410,
457–459, 461, 487–488, 526, 528, 545,
558, 561–564, 586, 589, 597, 612, 620
Agent orange and, 567–569
hair dyes and, 567–569
incidence of in African rain forest151
pesticide exposure and, 567–569
Kato, H., 99

Kausel, H., 284
Kay, H.E.M., 171
Kellen, J.A., 478
Keller, S.E., 59
Kennedy, M.S., 616
Keratins, cellular, 82
Keratitis, herpetic, 9
Keratoses, premalignant, 151
Kidneys, 293–294, 303, 334, 338
Kiloh, L.G., 59
Kinlen, L. J., 121
Klatzmann, D., 616
Klebs, M., 46–47
Klebsiella, 44, 544
Klein, H., 4
KLH test, 375
Klinger, M., 602, 606
Knojia, M., 171
Kolb, H.J., 171
Kolb, R., 575
Kolin, A., 478
Konopinska, D., 450
Koverech, A., 603, 605
Koyama, Y., 334
Kramer, B.S., 63
Krans, L., 60
Krensky, A.M., 521
Kripke, M.L., 21
Krutzke, J.F., 378
Kurdziel, S., 36
Kyriazis, A.P., 295

Lactalbumin, 8
Lactate, 23
Lactic dehydrogenase, 160
Lactoperoxidase procedure, 74–75, 114
Lactopropionic orcein, 92
Lagarde, C., 282
Lands pathway, 361–362
Lane, H.C., 47, 543, 547
Lange, M., 498
Lanier, L.L., 521
Lawrence, H.S., 373
Lazarus, L., 59
Lazzarin, A., 602, 606
Lectins, plant, 73–78
binding pattern of Hodgkin disease-derived cell
lines, 127–134
Lee, I., 267
Lehung, S., 284
Leloir, C., 234
Lens culinaris, 132–133
Lentinan, 333–348,
antitumor and metastasis inhibitory activities
of, 423–441
Lentiviruses, 498, 503, 505
Leptomeningitis, 560
Leucine aminopeptidase, 446, 450

Leukemia, 98, 100, 121–124, 151, 154–155, 187, 234, 271, 274–277, 280, 331
    ascitic, 312
    atomic bomb survivors, increased risk of in, 99
    childhood, 165–171
    DBA/2, 111–113
    lymphoblastic, 7, 154, 165–167, 225–229, 284
    lymphocytic, 154, 270
    lymphoid, 279–280, 282
    MBL-2, 318
    myelocytic, 225
    myeloid, 154–155, 269, 280, 283, 450
    see also specific leukemias
Leukocytes, 1, 62, 138, 373–374
    cell surface structures of, 515–517
    dialyzable extract of, 373–375
    polymorphonuclear, 449, 605
Leukonin, 446
Leukokininase, 446
Leukopenia, 377, 382
Leukotrienes, 62
Levamisole, 282–284, 409, 411–415, 419
Levi, L., 59–60
Levine, P.H., 221
Levy, R., 280
Lewis, R.T., 4
Li, W.J., 219
Li, Z.Q., 219
Lineage, myelohistiocytic, 127, 134
Lininger, G.284
Linoleic acid, 10, 61–62
Lipids, 11; *see also* Fatty acids, as immune function mediators
Lipopolysaccharide, 319–320, 412, 419, 423, 432
Lipotropes, 2, 11
Lipoxygenation, 62
Listeria monocytogenes, 8
Liver, 30–31, 160–162, 291–293, 296–297, 303, 323, 334, 338, 414, 419, 429
Locke, S.E., 60
Locniskar, M., 11
Locomotor activity, 448
Log rank test, 379
Lotus, 132–134
Lozzi, A., 602
Luckhurst, E., 59
Luczak, M., 450
Lumsden, C.E., 378
Luna, M., 171
Lung, 160–161, 291–293, 296–297, 303, 323, 338, 366, 477, 479–484
    biopsies, difficulty in establishing diagnoses from, 165–171
    tumor colonies, 321–322, 325–326
Lupus erythematosus, 153–154
Luteinizing hormone, 180

Luz de la Sen, M., 43
Lymphadenitis, 554
Lymphadenomegaly, 589–590, 592–594
Lymphadenopathy, 166, 354–356, 494–495, 502–503, 525–532, 553, 555–559, 561, 577–582, 612
    persistent generalized, 543–547, 549–552, 597–598
    risk groups for, 554
Lymphadenopathy-associated virus. *See* Retrovirus types LAV and HTLV-III/LAV
Lymph nodes, 111, 160, 292–293, 374, 410, 428–429, 504, 553–555, 558, 560–561, 564, 577–581, 592
    mesenteric, 207
    regional, 296–297, 463–473
    SIV and, 505
Lymphoblastogenesis, 613
Lymphocytes, 4, 6, 9–10, 62, 207–214, 280, 302, 374, 412, 545
    CD3, 516
    CD4, 515–516
    CD8, 515
    CD16, 516
    EBV-induced stimulation of, 221
    enucleated, 91–95
    impaired plaque formation of, stress and, 58, 60
    intraepithelial, 3
    large granular, 24, 464, 473, 519
    peripheral blood, 107–108, 142, 186, 457, 503–504, 612–613, 615
    tonsillar, 186
    in vitro response of, 619–625
Lymphocytopenia, 4, 10
Lymphoid
    tissues, innervation of, 62
Lymphokines, 10, 401, 403, 410, 412, 584; *see also specific agents*
Lymphoma, 78, 121–124, 149–150, 152–156, 159, 163–164, 266–267, 280, 311–316, 331, 428, 440, 448, 450–451, 593
    AIDS-associated, 557–564
    Burkitt, 127–128, 187, 549, 560
    CNS, 549–550, 560, 562, 564
    diffuse, 106
    follicular, 106
    histiocytic, 122, 127
    Hodgkin, 557, 559, 561–564
    large, noncleaved cell, 106
    LS178Y, 74
    macaque, 502
    Moloney virus-induced, 184, 303
    non-Hodgkin, 103–108, 150, 152–154, 282, 550, 557–559, 561–564
    small cleaved cell, 106
Lymphopenia, 162, 532

Lymphotoxin, 607
Lysine, 446
Lysophosphocholine, 361–362, 369–370
Lysozymes, 435

Macaca
    cyclopis, 501
    mulatta, 502, 504
Maclura pomifera, 132
Macrophage-activating factor, 439
Macrophages, 133, 286, 317, 319–321, 323, 326,
        361–363, 365, 367–370, 385–395, 401–
        403, 410–413, 432–434, 436, 439–440,
        445–446, 448, 450, 473, 505
Mador, N., 78
Magnesium oxide, 29–30
Makuch, R., 3
Malkin, J.A., 478
Malnutrition, 3–4
    childhood diarrheas and, 2
    in cancer patients, 23
    markers for, 6
Malnutrition-associated immune disfunction
        (MAIDS), 61
Mangebeys, sooty, 505
Mannick, J.A., 4
Mann-Whitney u-test, 599
Marbrook, J.T., 418
Marescot, M., 605
Markers, immunohistochemical, 263–267
Markow procedure, 122
Martin, P.J., 272
Martinez, J., 449
Mastocytomas, 111–112, 428
Masur, H., 47, 546–547
Mathe, G., 281, 283
Maturation, 81–88, 408
Matysiak, M., 330–331
Maver, C., 284
Mawle, A., 615
May, F.E.B., 187
Mazumder, A., 403
McAlpine, D., J.S., 615
McDaniel, S.M., 59
McGarry, R., 91
McIrvine, A.J., 4
McKneally, M., 284
Meade, T.W., 378
Measles, 2
Melanoma, 264–265, 267, 269–270, 282–283,
        291–292, 294–296, 317, 321, 323, 326,
        358, 361, 369, 375, 402, 448, 450,
        457–462
Melanotropin, 450
Meli, D., 330, 602
Melphalan, 294, 298
Membranes, human milk fat globule, 243
Meningiomas, 365

Menon, M., 273
2-Mercaptoethanol, 24, 92, 362
6-Mercaptopurine, 166
Meroni, P., 602
Mesotheliomas, 590
Metastasis, 73–78, 151–152, 208, 292–298, 326,
        364, 366, 423, 428–430, 441, 448, 463,
        465, 467
    potential for, 133, 180
Methionine, 9
L-Methionine, 191
S-Methionine, 191–193, 226–227
Methotrexate, 154, 166–168, 171, 221, 249, 254–
        255, 257–261, 279, 562
1-Methyladenosine, 589, 591, 593–594
Methylation, 311–316
Methyl-CCNU154
Methylcholanthrene, 427–429, 432–433, 448
5-Methylcytosine, 312–316
1-Methylinosine, 591, 593–594
Metropathia hemorrhagica, 99
Metzger, R.S., 225
Michael, G.T., 295
Micksche, M., 575
Microbacillus tuberculosis, 170
Microsomal lipoprotein fraction, 113
Midarm muscle circumference, 3
Midini, G., 330, 602
Miller, R.A., 280
Minowada, J., 272
Mirski, S., 91
Mitogens. *See specific mitogens*
Mitomycin C, 117, 334, 336
Miyawaki, T., 43, 47
Moll, I., 267
Moll, R., 267
Moller, P., 133
Monkeys
    African green, 488, 505
    macaques, 502–503, 506
Monocyte/macrophages, 16–17, 19–22, 24, 370
Monocytes, 280, 385, 395, 402, 410–411, 436,
        446, 473, 518, 606, 622
Mononucleosis, infectious, 60, 549
Monophosphoryl lipid A, 412, 418
Montagnier, L., 498, 513
Morin, A., 602, 604
Moroni, M., 602, 606
Morrissey, D.M., 214
Morse, H.C., 44
Morton, D.L., 283
Mosier, D.E., 44
Mougdil, G.C., 575
Moulias, I., 605
mRNA, 225–229
Mullen, J.L., 4
Multiple sclerosis, 154, 377–382

Mumps, 45
Muscle, 293–294
Myalgia, 166
Mycobacteriosis, 562
Mycobacterium avium, 410, 501
Mycoplasma, contamination by, 292
Mycosis fungoides, 152, 521
Myeloma, 122, 124, 127, 152, 155, 164, 184, 402
Myelopoiesis, 326, 385–395
Myoglobin, 133
Myosin, 133, 227

Nagaoki, T., 43, 47
Najjar, V.A., 446
Nakamura, H., 450
Nanni, G., 602, 605
Naslund, I., 450
Natural killer cells. See Cells, NK
Nauss, K.M., 11
Naxolone, 448
Neequaye, D., 221
Nemeto, N., 446
Neo-aminomel, 24
Neopterin, 535–540, 583–586
Nephelometric technique, 612
Neuraminidase, 76, 127–131, 133–134, 237, 283
Neuropeptides, 57–63
Neurotransmitters. *See specific transmitters*
Neutropenia, 60, 63, 446
Neutrophils, 6, 10, 59, 62, 169, 446
    phagocytosis of, stress and, 58
Newberne, P.M., 1, 11
Newman, R.A., 225
Newton, J., 506
Ni, L.Y., 146
Nicholson, J.K.A., 615
Nishijima, A., 446
p-Nitroaniline, 271
Nitro blue tetrazolium, 210
Nitrocellulose, 236–237
Nitrosoguanidine, 311
Niven, J.S.F., 59
Nkrumah, F.K., 221
Nocardiosis, 562
Nonkeratinocytes, 267
Norbury, K.C., 21
North, R.J., 119, 401
Nowinski, R.C., 279
Nucleosides, modified, 589–595
Nutrition
    imbalances, tumor-related, 24
    immunological requirements and, 1–10
    parenteral, 601

Obesity, 2
Ochai, T., 284
Ochoka, M., 330–331
Oenothera oil, 10

Oettgen, H.F., 214
Oka, T., 284
Okamura, K., 284
Oncogenes, 97–100, 285
    B-lym, 164
    c-myc, 164
Oncogenesis, 128
    prevention, 423–441
Oncology, viral, 221
Opiates, 537
Oral herpes. *See* Virus type, herpes simplex I
Orfeo, T., 295
Orr, T.W., 219
Ortho-phenylenediamine-dihydrochloride, 44, 544
Ortho-phenylenediamine (OPD), 209
Osteosarcoma, 283
Ota, K., 283, 450
Othmane, O., 414
Otsuka, K., 272
Ovalbumin, 133, 227
Ovaries, 303, 338

Pahwa, R., 414
Palmieri, G., 602
Palmieri, R., 602
Palumbo, G., 478
Pancreas, 292, 296–297, 303
    exocrine, 145
Pancreatitis
    adenovirus, 501
    necrotizing, 504
Panet, A., 78
Panning, 103–109
Paolozzi, F.P., 142
Papain, 446, 450
Paraffin, 82–83, 105, 146, 209, 211–212, 293
Paragangliomas, 267
Paraplasts, 264
Paraproteinemia, 410
Parasites, gastrointestinal infection and, 2; *see also specific parasites*
Pardo, A., 43
Parker, R., 412
Pascal, M., 414
PBB. *See* Biphenyls, polybrominated
PCB. *See* Biphenyls, polychlorinated
Peanut agglutinin (PNA), 75–76, 133–134, 415, 417–418
Pearson, G.R., 219
Pellet, H., 378
Penicillin, 128, 208, 363, 466, 572
Penny, R., 59
Pentachlorophenol, 568–569
Pentapeptides, 446
Pepoli, R., 603, 605
Pepsin, 446, 450
Peptides

synthetic hCG conjugate, 477
thymic286
Pereira, L., 203
Peritonitis, 153, 338
Peroxidase, 209, 264, 467, 510
   antiperoxidase technique, 558
   avidin-conjugated horseradish, 128
   immunocytochemistry, 183
Pertechnetate, 254
Pesando, J.-M., 280
Pesce, A.-J., 296
Petrini, B., 59, 60
Pettersson, I.-L., 59, 60
Peyer patches, 410
Phagocytosis, 6, 412, 440, 446, 448, 605, 606
Phase contrast microscopy, 83–84
Phaseolus vulgaris, 132
Phenobarbitol, 364
Phenotypic analysis, 103–107, 109
P-Phenylene-diamine, 83, 138
Phenylmethylsulfonylfluoride, 114, 128, 191, 210
Pheochromocytomas, 267
Phlebotomy, 154
Phorbol esters, 81, 132
Phosphate-buffered saline (PBS), 66, 74, 83, 112–
      113, 128, 139, 184–185, 192–193, 209–210,
      236–237, 272, 325, 363, 388, 390–394,
      480, 612
Phospholipids, 361, 368, 370
Phosphorylase-b, 133, 227
Phosphorylation, 128
Phycoerythrin, 516, 612
Phytohemagglutinin, 33–34, 36, 39, 60, 137–142,
      330, 374, 378–380, 457, 460, 503–504,
      527–530, 584, 604, 612–613, 619, 621–625
Picari, M., 602, 605
Picibanil (OK432), 317–327, 390, 394–395
Piette, A., 605
Pisum sativum, 133
Pittiruti, M., 331, 602, 604
Pizza, G., 221
Pizzo, P.A., 63, 171
Plant toxins. *See specific toxins*
Plasma cell lymphomas. *See* Myeloma
Plasmin, 269–270, 273
Plasminogen, activators, 269–274
Pleomorphism, 504
Pneumocystis carinii, 410, 488, 501, 562, 590,
      620
Pneumonia, 501, 620
   adenoviral, 504
   fungal, 165
   interstitial, 545
Pneumonitis, 170
Pneumothorax, 170
Poiesz, B.J., 142
Pokeweed mitogen (PWM), 33–34, 36, 44, 46–
      47, 208, 212

PolyA-polyU, 284, 414
Polycythemia rubra, 154
Polyethylene glycol (PEG), 66, 264, 270
Poly-ICLC, 24, 318–320, 385–387, 390–392, 394
Poly-L-lysine, 24, 208
Polymorphism, 280, 498
   restriction fragment, 495
Polymyxin B, 418
Polynosinic-polycytidylic acid poly-L-lysine. *See*
      Poly-ICLC
Polypeptides
   acidic keratin, 86
   glycosylated, 225
   keratin, 82
Polysaccharides, 333
Polysomes, 229
Polyriboinosinic-polycytidylic acid. *See* Poly-L-
      lysine
Polyunsaturated fatty acids, 10–11
Polyurea, 18
Ponceau, S., 128
Popovic, M., 615
Prealbumin, 5, 18–19, 23
Prednisone, 150, 159, 166–168
Pregnancy, immunocompetence and, 39–41
Preimmunization, 477
Primary amyloidosis, 153–154
Probands, 122–124
Prolactin, 58
Pronase, 435, 446
β-Propiolactone, 92
Prostaglandins, 11, 62
   E, 386
   E2, 472
Protease, 272
   inhibition, 450
Protein, 3, 6, 11
   A, 184–185, 191, 194, 463
   acute phase transport, 433
   calorie malnutrition, 1–5
   deficiency, 61
   deficiency and reduction of natural antitumor
      immunity, 15–23
   deficiency caused in mice by poor feed, 17–19,
      24
   HSVII, 189–192
   P24 HTLVIII, 553–556
   profiles, 75
   retinol-binding, 3–4
   S-100, 580–581
Proteus, 378, 458
Prothymocytes, 414
Protozoans, 168; *see also specific microorganisms*
Proust, M.R., 605
Pseudouridine, 589, 591, 593–594
Psoriasis, 153
Psychoimmunology, 58

Pteridine, 584
Purpura
    idiopathic thrombocytopenic, 446
    mucocutaneous, 166
Pyran copolymer, 21
2-Pyridone-5-carboxamide-N'-ribofuranoside
        (PCNR), 591, 593–594
Pyridoxine. *See* Vitamin B6
Pyronine G, 210
Pyruvate kinase deficiency, 571

Radiotherapy, 23, 166–167, 219, 282, 329–330,
        385, 598, 601–602
    for colorectal cancer, 207
    for Kaposi sarcoma, 153
    upper cervical spine, 168
Raman, S., 285
Receptors
    CRII, 520
    CR3, 521
    IL2, 526
    muscle cell, 450
    purine, 414
    Tac, 624
    transferrin, 625
Reed, F.C., 431
Reeves, W.G., 142
Reizenstein, P., 281–282
Renoux, G., 414
Renoux, M., 414
Resection, 429–431
Retinyl acetate, 9
Retransplantation, autologous, 279
Retrovirus
    ARV, 493–494, 498
    D, 502, 506
    HTLV, 164
    HTLV-I, 160, 504
    HTLV-II, 504
    HTLV-III, 410, 497–498, 545, 550, 553, 555,
        557, 615
    HTLV-III/LAV, 43, 99, 160, 162, 457–459,
        461, 487–489, 494, 498, 509, 511–513,
        535–540, 543, 547, 556, 585–586, 590,
        598, 607, 620–621
    LAV, genetic comparison of related isolates,
        493–497
    SAIDS D type 1, 503
Rheumatoid arthritis, 62, 153–154
RIA technique, 232
Ribi, E., 412, 418
Riboflavin. *See* Vitamin B2
Ribonucleotide reductase, 203
Ricca, D., 330
Richin, 261
Ricinus communis, 132
Riggs, C.W., 283
Rimm, A.A., 171

Ritz, J., 279
RNA, 411, 484
rRNA, 98
Robichaud, K.J., 63, 171
Robinson, E., 284
Rochefort, H., 187
Roder, J.C., 91
Roizman, B., 203
Ronconi, P., 331, 602, 604
Rook, A.H., 47, 543, 547
Rose, W.C., 431
Rosenberg, S.A., 403
Rosettes
    E, 601–602, 604
    EA, 601–602, 604
    E-active, 330
Roxas, M.A., 602
Rozenbaum, W., 498
Rubinstein, P., 498

Sagebiel, R., 283
Saito, T., 334
Sallan, S.E., 279
Salmon, S. E., 282
Salmonella, 44, 544
    typhimurium, 8–9, 17, 318, 386
Salovaara, H., 59–60
Salovaara, L., 59–60
Sandor, I.E., 473
Sanhadji, K., 414
Saphora japonica. 132
Sarcoma, 424, 426, 428
    immunoblastic, 106
    Meth A, 361
    mouse virus system, 221
    osteogenic, 375
    Ridgeway osteogenic, 482
    soft tissue, 155
    Yoshida, 478
Sarin, P., 461
Schaison, G., 330
Scheid, M.P., 414
Schliefer, S.J., 59
Schlom, J., 187
Schumaker, C., 63
Schwartzman, S., 412
Schyns-Mosen, J., 284
Scintigraphy, 208
Scollay, R., 417–418
Scott, A.L., 221
Seki, H., 43, 47
Se-Selenomethionine, 255
Selye-Levi concept, 59
Sepharose, 184, 191, 194
    lectin, 75
Sepsis, 3–5, 11, 604, 606
Sequi, J., 43
Serine, 243

Seroconversion, 60
Serrou, B., 450
Serum. *See specific sera*
Severe-combined immunodeficiency disease
        (SCID), 411
Sharkey, F.E., 295
Sheikh, K., 378
Shortman, K., 378
Shmookler-Reir, R.J., 98
Sialic acid, 76, 133
Sickle cell anemia, 571
SIgA, 2–3
Signorini, M., 602, 605
Sign test, 622
Silica, 21, 432
Siminoff, P., 431
Skin, 338, 293
        carcinogenesis in mice, 21
        hypersensitivity of, 59
Skinner, M., 418
SK-SD, 45
Sligh, J.M., 615
Smaley, R.V., 283
Smith, D.S., 378
Smith, R.G., 59
Sodium dodecylsulfate, 114, 210
Solomons, N.W., 3
Sonnet, J., 498
Souillet, J.F., 330
Southern blotting analysis, 498
Souyri, M., 498
Sparks, F. C., 283
Sperm, 585
Spinal cord, 152
Spitler, L.E., 283
Spleen, 8–10, 111, 119, 160–161, 169, 292–293,
        303–305, 319–321, 324, 363–367, 370, 439
        SIV and, 505
Splenectomy, 150, 446
Splenomegaly, 503, 560
Squalene, 478–479
Squames, in TPA-treated cultures, 84
Stains. *See specific agents*
Staphylococcus, 464
        aureus, 43–44, 114, 543
        cowan 1, 611–614, 616
Stein, M., 59
Stejskal, R., 146
Steroids, 41, 160
Stewart, T.H.M., 284
Stinnett, J.D., 295
Strander, H., 283
Streptococcus, 29, 44, 60, 378, 458, 544
        α, 168
        pyogenes, 317, 465
Streptomyces olivoreticuli, 445, 450
Streptomycin, 128, 208, 303, 363, 458, 465

Stress
        academic examinations and, 57
        bereavement and, 58–59, 61–62
        depression and, 57–58
        divorce and, 61–62
        everyday events and, 58
        grief and, 57, 61
        host defense against infection and, 60
        hypnosis and, 58
        loneliness and, 61
        -related immunodeficiency, 57–63
        sleep deprivation and, 57–58
        social-stress, lifelong chronic, 100
        space flight and, 57–58
        unemployment and, 58–60
Student's t-test, 17, 259, 325, 379–380, 388, 429,
        480, 573, 613
Substance P, 62
Subtilisin, 446
Suda, H., 450
Suemasu, K., 428
Summerhayes, I.C., 99
Supernatants, 271, 275, 436, 502, 546, 612
        thymic epithelial, 418–419
        see also Hybridomas
Surface markers. *See* Cells, Null
Sutherland, A., 225
Syndrome
        Duncan, 550
        human toxic PBB, 36
        infectious lymphoproliferative, 160–161,
                163–164
        lymphadenopathy, 525–532, 543–547, 553,
                555–559, 561, 577–582, 612
        MEN, 121
        respiratory distress, 169–171
        nephrotic, 153
        Sezary, 269, 274–275, 279
        short bowel, 7

T cell
        function, 3–5, 8–10, 20–21, 23, 29, 32–34,
                36, 39–41, 43–44, 46–47, 54, 59, 92,
                99, 105–106, 111, 119, 127, 137, 150,
                152, 163–164, 225, 269–273, 275–276,
                280, 317–318, 324, 358, 377–380, 382,
                385, 401, 403, 409–419, 423–424, 433,
                438, 445, 448, 450, 457–462, 465,
                504, 515, 517–519, 525–527, 529, 531–
                532, 558, 560, 571–575, 583–586,
                597–598, 600, 607, 611–619
        see also T lymphocytes
T lymphocytes, 5, 16, 32–34, 36, 39–40, 51, 59,
        74, 137, 160, 164, 286, 323, 326, 333,
        374, 401, 409, 426–427, 434, 437, 458–
        459, 461, 464, 473, 487–488, 493, 498,
        501, 539, 543, 551, 556, 591, 594, 598,
        600, 604, 607, 612, 614, 622

Taga, K., 43, 47
Takayama, K., 412
Takita, T., 450
Tam, M.R., 279
Taniguchi, N., 43, 47
Taylor-Papadimitriou, J., 243
Tedder, R.S., 99
Tegafur, 333–334, 336–337, 339, 341–342
Tempelis, L., 280
Teniposide, 168
Teodorczyk-Injeyan, J.A., 478
Tetanus toxoid, 378, 458
2,3,7,8-Tetrachlorodibenzo-p-dioxin (TCDD), 567–568
12-O-Tetradecanoylphorbol-13-acetate, 81–88
Tetrapeptides, 445–446
Tetraploidy, 211
Thalassemia, 571
Theorell, T., 59–60
Thiabendazole, 413
Thiamine. *See* Vitamin Bone1
6-Thioguanine, 30, 208
Thoracoscopy, 170
Thornton, J.C., 59
Threonine, 243
Thrombocytopenia, 377
Thrombopenia, 382
Thromboxanes, 62
^{3}H Thymidine, 43–44, 270, 362–365, 367, 380, 415, 458, 544, 622–623
Thymocytes, 412, 415, 417–418, 436–438
Thymopoietin, 411–413, 418
Thymosin, 410–411, 413–414, 418
Thymostimulin, 411
Thymulin, 410–411, 413, 418
Thymus, 30, 303, 433
  zinc deficiency and, 10
Thyroid, 266
Tilly, R., 243
Tiso, J., 296
Tomar, R.H., 142
Tonsillectomy, 185
Touraine, L.L., 414
Toxoplasma gondii, 8
TPA, epithelial cell maturation induced by, 81–88
Tranquilizers, intake increased during stress periods, 61
Transfer factor, 373–375, 411, 413–414
Transferrin, 3–23, 625
Transfusion
  AIDS and, 535, 583–584
  granulocyte, 165
  perioperative blood, 571–575
Transplantation
  bone marrow, 149–150, 495
  heart, 150
  heart/lung, 150
    kidney, 150, 153, 159, 161, 563
    of Lewis lung cell carcinoma, 477, 479–484
    liver, 150
    neoplastic consequences of, 149–156
    pancreatic, 150, 159, 161
    thymic, 419
Travade, P., 282
Triazene, 311–312
2,4,5-Trichlorophenoxyacetic acid, 567
Trichosantes kinlowii, 132
Trimethoprim-sulfamethoxazole, 171, 330
Tripeptides, 446
Tritium, 436
tRNA, 589–590
Tronick, S., 187
Trophoblasts, 478
Trychopyton, 378, 458
Trypan blue
  assessment, 175, 321, 480
  exclusion, 363, 364, 466
Trypanosoma lewisi, 8
Trypsin, 174, 428, 446, 450, 479, 484
  -EDTA, 293
Trypsinogen, 114, 118
Tuberculin, 59, 378, 458
Tuberculosis, 167
  miliary, 165
Tuftsin, 286, 445–446, 448–450, 451
Tumor
  biopsies, 217–221
  burden, 16, 24, 324, 472
  cell markers, 173–180
  immunity, 51, 111–120
  immunology, 231–234
  induction, racial differences in susceptibility, 98–99
  influence of host age on induction, 98–99
  latent period of development, 21
  markers, 145, 189–203, 207–214, 231
  necrosis factor, 401–402, 404
  see also specific neoplasms

Uchida, A., 575
Ulcerative colitis, 153
Ultraimmunohistochemistry, 577–582
Umezawa, H., 450
United States, AIDS and, 487–489, 497–498
Urea, 3
Uremia, 10
Urethan, 301–302, 304–307
Uricemia, 160
Uridine, 312, 314–315
Urikinase, 270
Urokinase, 269–270, 272, 275

Vaccines
  hCG, 478, 484
  HIV, 509–513

melanoma, 351–358
    tumor cell, 324
Vaccinia melanoma oncolysates (VMO), 351–358
H,D-Valyl-L-leucyl-L-lysine-p-nitroanilide dihy-
    drochloride, 270
Vancomycin, 169
Van der Helm, H.J., 513
Varidase, 375
Vellekoop, L., 171
Vibrio cholerae, 128, 237
Vicia
    faba, 132
    villosa, 75, 132
Vietnam, Agent orange exposure in, 568
Vincristine, 166–168
Vindesine, 249
Virchow's node, 338
Virus type
    adenovirus, 160, 502
    AIDS-related (ARV), 493–494
    Bittner mammary tumor, 478, 484
    Charlotte Friend, 283
    cytomegalovirus, 47, 160, 162, 330, 410, 501–
        502, 583, 604, 620
        pneumonia, 165
    Ectromelia, 292
    Epstein-Barr, 47, 162, 211, 272, 410, 549–552,
        583
    antigens, 217–221
    immunological markers for, 217–221
    infections, 159–160, 163–164
    herpes simplex, 9–10, 47, 51–54, 160, 162,
        189–197, 200–201, 330–331, 410
        I, 52–54, 192, 203
        II, 149, 153, 604
    herpes zoster, 160, 604
    HIV, 503–506, 577, 580
    HTV-III/LAV, 510
    influenza, 160, 607
    lactic dehydrogenase, 292
    LAV, 410, 568, 614
    lymphocytic choriomeningitis, 292
    Mason-Pfizer monkey, 502
    murine mammary tumor, 78, 183–187
    myeloproliferative sarcoma, 531
    parainfluenza, 160
    paramyxovirus, 502
    reovirus type 3, 292
    Rous sarcoma, 448
    SIV, 501, 503–506
    SV40, 365, 502
    varicella zoster, 330–331, 604
    see also Retrovirus; Lentiviruses
Viscum album, 132
Vitamin
    A, 1, 2, 7
        deficiency, 9–10

B complex, 374
    B1, 1
    B2, 1
        deficiency, 1, 61
    B6, 1, 10
        intrauterine deficiency of, 2
    B12, 8–9
Viza, D., 221
Vose, B.M., 575
Vriz, N., 286

Wada, S., 446
Wain-Hobson, S., 498
Wallace, J., 599
Ward, B., 244
Ward, C., 575
Wasik, M.R., 280
Wasserman, J., 59–60
Watanabe, H., 428
Webster, A.D.B., 121
Wegener granulomatosis, 154
Weight
    development and protein-deficient feed, 17–18
    loss, 3, 23, 321, 504, 545, 590
Weiner, R.S., 171
Weiss, L., 449
Weiss, R.A., 99
Western blotting analysis, 213, 266, 505, 526,
    535–536
Westley, B.R., 187
Whalen, G., 47, 543, 547
Wheat germ agglutinin (WGA), 132–133
Whole cell fusion, 91–95
Wilcoxon's rank sum test, 44, 335, 341, 441, 537,
    546, 622
Williams, R. M., 60
Winternitz, F., 450
Wistaria floribunda, 132
Wlekuk, M., 450
Wolff, M.H., 203
Wright, D.G., 171

Xenogenization, chemical, 311–316
Xenografts
    colorectal carcinoma, 251–261
    human tumor, 291–292, 294–295
Xenotransplantation
    of hybrid cells, 93
Xylol, 466
d-Xylose, 7

Yang, K., 133
Yetter, R.A., 44

Zabay, J.M., 43
Zamkoff, K.W., 142

Zander, A., 171
Zanjani, S., 36
Zanussi, C., 602
Zatz, M., 418
Zhang, H.Z., 403

Ziegler, J.L., 564
Zinc, 4, 7–8, 285
    deficiency,1–2, 10
Zyogma, 168